Management of Impotence and Infertility

Management of Impotence and Infertility

Edited by

E. Douglas Whitehead, M.D.
Associate Clinical Professor of Urology
Mount Sinai School of Medicine
Associate Attending Urologist
Department of Urology
Beth Israel Medical Center
New York, New York

Harris M. Nagler, M.D.
Professor of Urology
Mount Sinai School of Medicine
Chairman, Department of Urology
Beth Israel Medical Center
New York, New York

With 41 additional contributors

J. B. Lippincott Company
Philadelphia

Acquisitions Editor: Mary K. Smith
Production Manager: Janet Greenwood
Assistant Editor: Anne Geyer
Indexer: Robert Zolnerzak
Production: TechEdit Production Services
Compositor: Techset Composition, Ltd.
Printer/Binder: R.R. Donnelley & Sons, Inc.

1 3 5 6 4 2

Library of Congress Cataloging-in-Publication Data

Management of impotentce and infertility / edited by E. Douglas Whitehead, Harris M. Nagler; with 41 additional contributors.
p. cm.
Includes bibliographical references and index.
ISBN 0-397-51153-1
1. Impotence. 2. Infertility, Male. I. Whitehead, E. Douglas. II. Nagler, Harris M., 1949–
[DNLM: 1. Impotence—therapy. 2. Infertility, Male—therapy. WJ 709 M2659 1994]
RC889.M349 1994
616.6'92—dc20
DNLM/DLC
for Library of Congress 94-15543
CIP

This book is printed on acid-free paper.

The authors and publisher have exerted every effort to ensure that drug selection and dosage set forth in this text are in accord with current recommendations and practice at the time of publication. However, in view of ongoing research, changes in government regulations, and the constant flow of information relating to drug therapy and drug reactions, the reader is urged to check the package insert for each drug for any change in indications and dosage and for added warnings and precautions. This is particularly important when the recommended agent is a new or infrequently employed drug.

Contributors

Arnold M. Belker, M.D. Clinical Professor of Urology, University of Louisville School of Medicine; Jewish Hospital, Louisville, Kentucky

Richard E. Berger, M.D. Professor of Urology, University of Washington School of Medicine; Director of Male Reproductive and Sexual Medicine, University of Washington Medical Center, Seattle, Washington

Joseph N. Biase, M.D. Chief Resident in Urology, Department of Urology, Beth Israel Medical Center, New York, New York

Richard Bronson, M.D. Associate Professor of Urology, State University of New York at Stony Brook, School of Medicine; Director, Division of Reproductive Endocrinology, SUNY Health Sciences Center, Stony Brook, New York

Michael D. Carter, M.D., F.R.C.S.(C). Clinical Lecturer, Department of Surgery, Division of Urology, University of Calgary Faculty of Medicine; Calgary General Hospital, Calgary, Alberta, Canada

Michael Condra, Ph.D. Assistant Professor, Department of Psychology, Director of Student Counseling Service, Queen's University Faculty of Medicine, Kingston, Ontario, Canada

Charles J. Devine, Jr., M.D. Professor of Urology, Eastern Virginia Medical School; Director, The Devine Center for Genitourinary Reconstructive Surgery, Sentara Norfolk General Hospital, Norfolk, Virginia

Craig F. Donatucci, M.D. Associate Professor of Clinical Surgery, Division of Urology, Department of Surgery, University of Chicago Pritzker School of Medicine; University of Chicago Medical Center, Chicago, Illinois

Irwin Goldstein, M.D. Professor of Urology, Boston University School of Medicine; University Hospital–Boston University Medical Center, Boston, Massachusetts

Dimitrios G. Hatzichristou, M.D. Lecturer, Department of Urology, School of Medicine, Aristotelian University of Thessaloniki, Thessaloniki, Greece

Jeremy P.W. Heaton, F.R.C.S.C., F.A.C.S. Associate Professor, Department of Urology, Queen's University Faculty of Medicine; Kingston General Hospital, Kingston, Ontario, Canada

Mitchell B. Hollander, M.D. Clinical Instructor, Department of Urology-Gynecology, St. John's Medical Center, Detroit, Michigan

Jonathan P. Jarow, M.D. Associate Professor of Urology, Bowman Gray School of Medicine; Wake Forest University Medical Center, Winston-Salem, North Carolina

Gerald H. Jordan, M.D. Professor of Urology, Eastern Virginia Medical School; Director, Adult Reconstruction, The Devine Center for Genitourinary Reconstruction, Sentara Norfolk General Hospital, Sentara Leigh Memorial Hospital, Children's Hospital of the King's Daughter's, Norfolk, Virginia

John N. Kabalin, M.D. Assistant Professor of Urology, Stanford University School of Medicine; Chief of Urology, Palo Alto VA Medical Center, Palo Alto, California

Nabet G. Kasabian, M.D. Physician in charge of Neuro-Urology and Female Urology, Beth Israel Medical Center; Assistant Professor of Urology, Mount Sinai School of Medicine, New York, New York

Barry J. Klyde, M.D. Assistant Professor of Clinical Medicine, Division of Endocrinology, Cornell University Medical College; Assistant Attending Physician, The New York Hospital, New York, New York

Ronald W. Lewis, M.D. Professor of Urology, Mayo School of Medicine and Mayo Clinic, Rochester, Minnesota

Larry I. Lipshultz, M.D. Professor of Urology, Scott Department of Urology, Baylor College of Medicine, Houston, Texas

Tom F. Lue, M.D. Professor of Urology, University of California, San Francisco School of Medicine; Attending Physician, UCSF Hospital, San Francisco, California

Eric I. Mitchnick, M.D. Clinical Assistant Professor, SUNY Health Science Center at Stony Brook, Stony Brook, New York; Attending Urologist, John T. Mather Memorial Hospital, St. Charles Hospital, Port Jefferson, New York

Alvaro Morales, M.D., F.R.C.S.(C)., F.A.C.S. Professor and Chairman, Department of Urology, Queen's University Faculty of Medicine; Urologist and Chief, Kingston General Hospital, Hotel Dieu Hospital, Kingston, Ontario, Canada

Perry W. Nadig, M.D. Clinical Professor of Urologic Surgery, University of Texas Health Science Center in San Antonio; Staff Urologist, Santa Rosa Medical Center, San Antonio, Texas

Harris M. Nagler, M.D. Professor of Urology, Mount Sinai Medical School; Chairman, Department of Urology, Beth Israel Medical Center, New York, New York

Daniel Navot, M.D. Professor of Obstetrics and Gynecology, New York Medical College, Valhalla, New York; Director, Division of Reproductive Endocrinology, West Chester County Medical Center; Director of Reproductive Endocrinology, Pascack Valley Hospital, Westwood, New Jersey

Robert D. Oates, M.D. Assistant Professor of Urology, Boston University School of Medicine; University Hospital, Boston, Massachusetts

Dana A. Ohl, M.D. Assistant Professor, Department of Surgery, Section of Urology, University of Michigan Medical School, Ann Arbor, Michigan

Terry Payton, R.N., B.S. Urological Nurse Clinician, Boston University School of Medicine, Boston, Massachusetts

Inder Perkash, M.D., F.R.C.S., F.A.C.S. Professor of Urology, Stanford University School of Medicine; Chief, Spinal Cord Injury Service, Palo Alto VA Medical Center, Palo Alto, California

Pedro Puech-Leão, M.D., Ph.D. Instituto H. Ellis, São Paulo, Brazil

Ivan Rothman, R.N., M.N. Research Nurse-Clinician, Department of Urology, University of Washington School of Medicine; Health Care Specialist, University of Washington Medical Center, Seattle, Washington

Paul Salkin, M.D. Assistant Clinical Professor, New York Medical College; Attending Physician, Department of Medicine, Lenox Hill Hospital, Beth Israel North, New York, New York

Steven M. Schlossberg, M.D. Associate Professor of Urology and Anatomy, Department of Urology, Eastern Virginia Medical School; Associate Director, Adult Reconstruction, The Devine Center for Genitourinary Reconstruction, Sentara Norfolk General Hospital, Norfolk, Virginia

Richard T. Scott, M.D. Chief, Reproductive Endocrinology, Clinical Director, Federal Fellowship in Reproductive Endocrinology, Uniformed Services University, University Hospital System, Bethesda, Maryland

Mark Sigman, M.D. Assistant Professor of Urology, Brown University Program in Medicine; Staff Urologist, Department of Urology, Rhode Island Hospital, Providence, Rhode Island

Rebecca Sokol, M.D. Associate Professor of Medicine, UCLA School of Medicine, Los Angeles, California; Department of Medicine, Harbor–UCLA Medical Center, Torrance, California

Ronald S. Swerdloff, M.D. Professor of Medicine, UCLA School of Medicine, Los Angeles, California; Chief, Division of Endocrinology, Harbor–UCLA Medical Center, Torrance, California

Anthony J. Thomas, Jr., M.D. Head, Section of Male Infertility, Department of Urology, Cleveland Clinic Foundation, Cleveland, Ohio

Christina Wang, M.D. Professor of Medicine, UCLA School of Medicine, Los Angeles, California; Director of Clinical Studies Center, Harbor–UCLA Medical Center, Torrance, California

Robert I. White, Jr., M.D. Professor and Chairman, Department of Diagnostic Radiology, Yale University School of Medicine; Director, Diagnostic Imaging, Yale–New Haven Hospital, New Haven, Connecticut

E. Douglas Whitehead, M.D. Associate Clinical Professor of Urology, Mount Sinai School of Medicine; Associate Attending Urologist, Department of Urology, Beth Israel Medical Center, New York, New York

Adrian W. Zorgniotti, M.D. Professor, Department of Urology, New York University School of Medicine, New York, New York

Shirley Zussman, Ed.D. Private Practice, New York, New York

Preface

Sexuality and sexual functioning are regarded as important for most men, and erectile dysfunction is recognized as a major disease and an important public health problem. Unfortunately, physicians and other health professionals infrequently discuss sexuality during evaluation of men with medical and psychological problems, and therefore erectile dysfunction is underdiagnosed and undertreated.

Because there are multiple determinants of sexual functioning, it is necessary to understand indications and management principles for the evolving use of new tools of putative value. Furthermore, because sexual dysfunction and particularly erectile dysfunction frequently are multifactorial, with coexisting psychogenic and organic etiologies, very often a multidisciplinary approach to diagnosis and treatment is advisable, particularly because multiple treatment options are available and highly effective. It is important that the patient and, where possible, his partner actively participate in this approach by defining goals and selecting an appropriate treatment.

This book reviews the fundamental advances in our understanding of the pathophysiology of male sexual dysfunction, particularly erectile dysfunction, and emphasizes that we have come to recognize the predominance of organic and mixed etiologies, and the importance of understanding the infrastructure and dynamics of a couple's relationship and other psychologic determinants.

The section on male sexual dysfunction reviews the rapid advances in the expanding field of sexual medicine and effective treatment options and allows us to formulate appropriate paradigms and algorithms for diagnosis and treatment, using a multidisciplinary approach that, when necessary, frequently optimally serves the patient and his sexual partner.

Of equal importance in this book is the assembly in one place of the experience, thoughts, and visions of some of the leading authorities treating men with sexual *and* reproductive abnormalities.

The section on infertility provides the practitioner with the information necessary to appropriately and effectively treat the infertile man in the nineties. Although the advent of assisted reproductive techniques such as in vitro fertilization have had an immense impact on the treatment of the infertile couple, the urologic community has embraced these techniques as adjuncts to treatment. In the last several months, and since the preparation of this book, great strides have been made in the field of in vitro fertilization and micromanipulation. The preliminary reports from doctors Palermo et al. indicate that intracytoplasmic injection of sperm (ICSI) may achieve exceedingly high fertilization rates utilizing specimens that hitherto would not have been sufficient for any micromanipulation technique. Nevertheless, the necessity to evaluate and treat causes of male infertility continues.

Infertility may be the presentation of significant medical disease. Furthermore, as outlined herein, infertility may be treated effectively without the great emotional and financial cost of assisted reproductive technologies. It is imperative that the practicing andrologist/urologist attempts to identify and correct causes of infertility to restore normal reproductive function. The use of assisted reproductive techniques, although useful and at times mandatory, is merely a strategy and should not be looked upon as a cure. The approach and techniques that have been established in the prior decade are chronicled and updated, emphasizing recent advances. Many refinements in approaches have been made in the treatment of previously recognized conditions, and new conditions have been recognized. Previously recognized but untreatable conditions now can be treated with a multidisciplinary approach. The approaches presented in this book will both enable the physician to benefit from the experience of others and allow him or her to share in the joy of enabling an infertile couple to become parents.

E. Douglas Whitehead, M.D.
Harris M. Nagler, M.D.

Contents

Part I Impotence

Part I
Impotence

1

Noninvasive Pharmacotherapy of Impotence: An Update

Alvaro Morales
Jeremy P. W. Heaton
Michael Condra

Other chapters in this volume refer to the large amount of progress achieved over the last decade in the diagnosis and treatment of erectile failure. Surgical techniques have proven effective in dealing with some vascular problems, while the intracavernosal administration of vasoactive drugs has been shown to be capable of producing erections of sufficient quality for intercourse in many cases. However, there is still a large group of patients who may not be, or choose not to be, candidates for these invasive forms of treatment or, as in the case of vasoactive medication, reject further use because of pain, fibrosis, or merely dissatisfaction with the results.

Unquestionably, oral medication effective in restoring or improving the quality of erections would be a most welcome addition to the urological armamentarium. Although many attempts have been made at finding systemic agents with activity in impotent men, conclusive results have been elusive. Nevertheless, our improved understanding of the physiology of penile tumescence (and detumescence) augurs well for the finding of effective compounds. This optimism is somewhat tempered by the complexity of clearly identified, as well as putative neurohormonal pathways involved in erectile function.[1] It appears entirely reasonable, therefore, to anticipate that a combination of agents could provide the best results. At this early stage in the search for an effective, easily administered pharmacological cure, however, it is mandatory to investigate the individual merits of various drugs and later on to determine their synergistic activity (see Table 1-1).

Hormonal Therapy

A serum testosterone determination or a complete hormonal screen is commonly part of the assessment of an impotent man.[2] Endocrine abnormalities are relatively rare, which is unfortunate, since they are, in general, amenable to effective treatment. Current methods allow the

Management of Impotence and Infertility, edited by Douglas Whitehead and Harris Nagler,

Table 1-1 Systemic Therapy for Impotence

1. Neuropharmacotherapy
   a. Dopaminergic agonists
      - L-dopa
      - Amphetamine
      - Deprenyl
      - Apomorphine
      - Pergolide
      - Quinelorane
      - Methylenedioxypropyl-noraporphine
      - Fenfluramine
   b. Adrenergic antagonists
      - Yohimbine
      - Phentolamine
   c. Serotonergic agonists
      - Trazodone
      - Methysergide
   d. Opiate antagonists
      - Naltrexone
      - Naloxone
   e. Oxytonergic agonists
      - Oxytocin
2. Hormonal
   a. Hypogonadism
      - Testosterone
   b. Hyperprolactinemia
      - Bromocryptine
3. Vascular
   - Nitric oxide derivatives
   - Pentoxyfillene
   - Minoxidil

clinician to pinpoint defects in the hypothalamic–pituitary–gonadal axis with a high degree of accuracy and to institute specific therapy for the abnormality present.

The following abnormalities are most commonly associated with erectile disturbances.

Hyperprolactinemia

This is an exceedingly uncommon cause of impotence, with an estimated incidence of less than 5%. In most cases the elevation in serum prolactin levels is the result of medication known to induce an excessive production of prolactin, most commonly estrogens or α-methyldopa. The initial treatment, of course, includes the appropriate changes in medication. A small number of individuals with hyperprolactinema are found to harbor pituitary tumors (prolactinomas). Most of these patients have microadenomas that respond to the judicious use of bromocryptine. It is commonly agreed that only those with large tumors that do not respond adequately to the administration of the drug require hypophysectomy. Bromocryptine is normally started at small doses because it frequently induces gastric intolerance; the dose is progressively increased until a total daily dose of 5 to 7.5 mg is reached. These patients require periodic determinations of serum prolactin, radiological evaluation of the sella turcica, and visual-field examinations. Normalization of serum prolactin may not be sufficient to bring back normal erections. Some of these patients require supplemental androgens and, as in most cases of organic impotence, variable degrees of counseling are necessary before satisfactory restoration of function is achieved.

Hypogonadism

Both hyper- or hypogonadotropic hypogonadism require the administration of exogenous androgens. For androgen replacement, preference should be given to the injectable preparations: testosterone enanthate 300 mg intramuscularly every 3 to 4 weeks. The amount and frequency of administration vary and may require adjustments with chronic use. The sublingual and oral administration of testosterone is simpler and more readily acceptable to the patient; unfortunately drug absorption by these routes is somewhat unpredictable. Newer preparations may provide a more stable absorption of the hormone by the gut. Recent investigations suggest that the transcutaneous administration of testosterone may be a simpler viable alternative.[3] The transscrotal route has been used with promising results.

Nonhormonal Therapy

Patients with organic impotence rarely are candidates for hormonal manipulation, and, as a general rule, such an approach should be limited to those in whom hormonal deficiencies are thoroughly documented. There is, therefore, a large population of men with erectile dysfunction in whom other organic factors (vascular, neurological) are the underlying cause for their problem and who could benefit from nonhormonal pharmacological treatment. Furthermore, a significant group of impotent men with a predominantly psychogenic etiology could also derive significant benefit from pharmacological therapy. A number of studies have been carried out in an effort to elucidate the value of drugs thought to be effective, and active research is being conducted to find new compounds that may one day be useful in the treatment of one or more causes of erectile failure. A few drugs have been investigated in small phase I or II clinical trials, in some cases with encouraging results. Among the preparations tested were glyceryl trinitrate,[4] zinc,[5] oxytocin,[6] and luteinizing hormone-releasing hormone.[7] None of these, however, has found a place in the armamentarium. On the other hand, the introduction of intracavernosal therapy fundamentally changed our approach to the treatment of impotence; the injection of single or multiple agents is currently the first therapeutic choice for many patients. Slower and much less dramatic progress is being made in developing noninvasive, preferably oral, alternatives. However, basic research is providing an increasing understanding of the physiology of libido and erection, which is about to translate into significant therapeutic developments.

For instance, detailed studies have resulted in the identification of zones in the medial preoptic area (MPOA) of the diencephalon that are strongly associated with erectile function and sexual behavior. Other studies have brought up the recognition of a peripheral neural network controlling sexual reflex responses. Equally important has been the determination of the fundamental role of adrenergic, dopaminergic, and serotonergic activities in the regulation of erections in men. These developments are beginning to provide a basis for the development of an effective pharmacological therapy in erectile failure. There is, for instance, convincing evidence that alterations in catecholamine metabolism result in alteration of sexual behavior, thus suggesting an important participation of both adrenergic and dopaminergic receptors in sex drive.

Central Mechanisms

Adrenergic Receptor Antagonists

A large number of compounds are included in this group. The most commonly used have been phentolamine and yohimbine. Phentolamine is employed either alone or in combination with papaverine by intracorporeal administration (this route is discussed in the following chapter). Very preliminary evidence indicates that oral phentolamine exhibits erectogenic activity[8]; additional studies should provide a better understanding of its effectiveness.

Yohimbine, on the other hand, has received much attention as an oral treatment for impotence. It is an indole alkaloid with well-defined properties as an α_2-adrenoceptor antagonist, with profound central and peripheral effects in animals and humans.[9] It has been widely touted as an aphrodisiac for over a century, but it has not been properly investigated until relatively recently. The early reports on the effectiveness of yohimbine, which were quite remarkable,[10] were later supported by Wolpowitz and Barnard.[11] Despite its early promise in these and other trials, the drug produced no significant clinical impact. Several reasons account for the waning of interest in the role of yohimbine in the treatment of impotence. Most important, early uses of the drug were entirely empirical and its pharmacology poorly understood. Further damage to its reputation was caused by combining it with other drugs (testosterone, caffeine, strychnine, vitamin E), thus making it impossible to determine its individual effectiveness. Finally, the procedures used to establish the etiological diagnosis of impotence were inappropriate even for those days and certainly unacceptable for today's standards. There was, however, sufficient evidence in the literature to justify a careful and objective look at the effects of yohimbine in sexual function.

A pilot investigation on the treatment of impotence with yohimbine was published in 1982.[12] The study found a positive response in 43% of the sample of impotent men with a predominantly organic etiology. Of these, 26% became able to achieve full, sustained erections. Although the findings were significantly lower than those reported in earlier studies, there was enough activity attributable to the drug to justify further trials. A controlled randomized study in patients with organic impotence receiving 6 mg of yohimbine orally three times a day for 10 weeks versus placebo demonstrated a response similar to the one noted in the pilot study: 42% of the patients experienced a positive response that, in half of them, was a complete recovery of erectile function. Thirteen percent of the patients receiving placebo also experienced a positive response; although the trend was in favor of the active compound, the differences between yohimbine and placebo did not reach statistical significance.[1] A more definite response to yohimbine was found in a controlled study of patients with a diagnosis of psychogenic impotence: the positive response in the yohimbine cohort was 62%, while in the control group it was only 16%; this difference was statistically highly significant.[13] Further controlled studies have indicated that yohimbine favorably affects erectile function in impotent patients and have also rekindled interest in the development of new α_2-adrenoceptor antagonists with improved selectivity.[14] They are still at the investigational level, and it may be several years before their activity is known. It is evident from available studies that, under the best circumstances, yohimbine is of limited effectiveness. The drug, however, is well tolerated, and it can be recommended as the first line of treatment. It is possible that larger amounts (i.e., 30 mg daily in divided doses) may be more effective. Recently, an empirical combination of yohimbine and the serotonergic agonist trazodone (to be discussed under serotonergic receptors) has been reported to be more effective than yohimbine alone. Very early experience with this approach at our center tends to support this concept, but a larger study is needed to determine the synergistic value of these two drugs.

Although the mechanism of action of yohimbine on sexual functioning has not been established, recent evidence indicates that its effects are primarily central. Clark[15] conducted a series of revealing experiments in rats in which complete inhibition of sexual performance (mounting, intromission, and ejaculation) was achieved by administration of clonidine into the MPOA. Total restoration of sexual functioning was accomplished by administration of yohimbine either systemically or directly into the MPOA. He concluded from these studies that α_2-adrenoceptors are important in the control of male sexual behavior and that alterations of adrenergic mechanisms in the MPOA may underlie sexual dysfunctions from multiple etiologies. It is conceivable that in this particular portion of the diencephalon there is an integration of a number of neurotransmitter interactions that is important in the regulation of penile erections.

Dopamine Receptor Agonists

As mentioned previously, numerous studies have documented some of the details of the central neurotransmitter systems contributing to the control of sexual behavior. In addition to norepinephrine, interest has focused on the role of dopamine, which is also widely distributed in brain tissues.[16] Dopamine has long been recognized to be a facilitator of male copulatory performance in animals, while the administration of dopamine-blocking agents inhibits their copulatory behavior. The administration of the dopamine agonist apomorphine has been shown to induce bouts of yawning and penile erections both in animals and humans. This effect has permitted the development of important animal models for the investigation of potency.[17] Clinical studies have indicated that apomorphine may have a role to play in the treatment of erectile dysfunction in men. Lal et al.[18] have shown that apomorphine induces erections in both normal subjects and impotent men when administered subcutaneously. Trials are currently in progress to determine the effectiveness of apomorphine and other dopaminergic agonists (i.e., bromocryptine) in the treatment of impotence from various causes. Table 1-1 provides additional examples of the many dopaminergic agonists that have been investigated as possible erectogenic compounds.

Serotonergic Receptors

A further system with a recognized major involvement in the erectile process includes serotonin-related compounds. Serotonergic compounds appear more complex to study than either adrenergic or dopaminergic compounds since they seem to have an inhibitory effect on sex drive centrally but an erectogenic effect peripherally. The enhancement of serotonergic activity has been implicated as the mechanism of action of trazodone in normal and impotent patients. More recently, however, Saenz de Tejada et al.[19] have suggested that an alternative possible mechanism would be related to the α-adrenergic blocking properties of trazodone by interference with the sympathetic control of penile detumescence. It is evident that much more needs to be understood about serotonergic receptors and the drugs affecting them. At this particular juncture they appear to play an important role in the erectile process, and their pharmacological manipulation may translate into a significant avenue of treatment in disturbance of sexual function.

Other receptors are believed to be involved in the human penile response. For example, opiate antagonists such as naloxone can enhance sexual performance and induce erections. It has been suggested[20] that the additive effect of a psychopharmacological agent such as yohimbine and a neuropharmacological agent such as naloxone may be a more fruitful approach. Although this hypothesis is attractive, the categorization of drugs as neuro- or psychopharmacological agents is artificial, probably inappropriate, and certainly confusing. Regardless of nomenclature, reliable information about synergistic effect of class compounds is, unfortunately, lacking, but it is a crucial consideration to be discussed later. In any case the use of two agents may be necessary since evidence has been presented indicating that for an appropriate response to a neuropharmacological agent, an adequate hormonal environment is mandatory.[21]

Peripheral Mechanisms

Oral and transcutaneous drugs may have profound effects in the penis. There is undisputable and not surprising evidence that nitric oxide (NO) mediates the relaxation of cavernosal smooth muscle as it does in other vascular beds. Organic nitrates and nitrites are well recognized vasodilators through their relaxant effect on vascular smooth muscle.[22] Among the best known of these compounds is nitroglycerine, which is absorbed readily after topical administration. Several years ago we felt that nitroglycerine deserved to be investigated in patients with impotence. Initially a pilot study was conducted under laboratory conditions,[23] and this was followed by a further assessment also performed in the laboratory.[24] In the latter, the effect of 2% nitroglycerin paste applied to the penile shaft of impotent subjects was evaluated in a placebo-controlled double-blind study. After application of nitroglycerin paste or a placebo ointment base, penile tumescence was recorded while subjects viewed an erotic video presentation. Relative to the placebo paste, the number of patients demonstrating an increase in penile circumference after nitroglycerin was significantly larger than all other outcome possibilities. In an additional study it has been shown that the topical administration of nitroglycerin to the penile shaft is rapidly followed by a significant dilatation of the cavernosal arteries with a concomitant increase in blood flow.[25] Although other investigators have confirmed these observations,[26] nitroglycerin and related compounds have not yet been truly investigated outside laboratory conditions. Their effect in the treatment of impotence remains speculative. It would be anticipated, however, that their main role would be in those patients with an underlying vascular etiology. Nevertheless, the newly discovered role of NO or endothelium-derived relaxing factor (EDRF) as a powerful vasodilator with a putative role in cavernosal physiology[27] has opened new avenues for therapeutic research. Recent work suggests that EDRF and nitric oxide[28] are identical. Thus, the trickle down from mainstream vascular physiology and pharmacology may open new possibilities in manipulating the humble penile vascular bed with NO-derived or other simple nitrogen-based compounds. In a recent report, Cavallini[29] presented the intriguing results of a study in which the topical application of minoxidil (best known for its capacity to reverse alopecia androgenetica) was found to be more effective than nitroglycerine in enhancing penile tumescence in impotent men. Confirmation of such findings further supports the value of local vasodilation. Needless to say, an erection requires more than simple vasodilatation. The point is that if a deficiency in blood supply is the main or a significant contributor to the problem, it could be treated with a relatively simple local measure, thus circumventing the potential side effects of systemic therapy.

Conclusion

It is evident that any effective pharmacological agent would require, at least, some preservation of the erectile mechanisms in the penis. It would be absurd to anticipate, for instance, any response from a penis with severely occluded cavernosal arteries. On the other hand, we suspect that, until recently, undue emphasis has been given to the pharmacological events at the level of the target organ (penis) leading to a considerable neglect of mechanisms at higher centers. This imbalance is understandable given the relative accessibility of the former for a variety of animal and clinical investigations. It is our contention, however, that a more comprehensive and integrated approach is mandatory in the search for successful strategies in male sexual dysfunction.

We seem to have come in a complete circle to the therapies advocated in the 1960s when multiple ingredients were combined in a single tablet for the generic treatment of impotence with reportedly good results. The level of understanding of the mechanisms of sexual functioning has increased considerably in three decades, and the sophistication of the diagnostic process is also a whole new game. But let us not be smug about it. The multipronged approach to the treatment of impotence should be considered carefully again. A sample of drugs with recognized erectogenic properties is listed in Table 1-1.

The discovery of a noninvasive pharmacological cure for erectile failure has proven to be a difficult one. Part of the problem may be the enormous complexity of mechanisms involved in the development of an erection. As examples, one can think of the recent finding of regularization of substantia nigra dopamine cell firing by adrenergic neurotransmitters[30] or the effect of adrenergic antagonists on the hydroxytryptamine receptor-mediated inhibition in the same area of the brain of experimental animals.[31] Findings such as these suggest a scenario in which all neurotransmitters influencing sexual behavior work in a very close and interdependent fashion. Certainly, there is a multiplicity of central and peripheral neurotransmitter systems involved in the sexual human response; therefore, it is likely that a combination of agents, or a highly specific diagnostic process with a specifically defined therapeutic target, will be needed for successful treatment.[1] A combined treatment approach may be most appropriate until the individual contributions of each of the various central and peripheral systems are further understood.

REFERENCES

1. Morales A, Condra MS, Owen JE, Fenemore, J, and Surridge DH: Oral and transcutaneous pharmacological agents in the treatment of impotence. Urol Clin NA 1988; 15:87–93.
2. Leonard M, Nickel JC, Morales A: Hyperprolactinemia and impotence: Why, when and how to investigate. J Urol 1989; 142:992–994.
3. Carey PO, Howards SS, Vance ML: Transdermal testosterone treatment of hypogonadal men. J Urol 1988; 140:76–79.
4. Muddi JW: Impotence response to glyceryl trinitrate. Am J Psychol 1977; 134:922–926.
5. Antonio L, Shalbhoub R, Sudhkar T: Reversal of uremic impotence by zinc. Lancet 1977; 2:895–896.

6. Lidberg L, Sternthal V: A new approach to the hormonal treatment of impotentia erections. Pharmaco-psychiat 1977; 10:21–24.
7. Levit N, Vinik A, Sive A. Synthetic LHRH in impotent male diabetics: A double blind cross-over trial. S Afr Med J 1981; 59:10–14.
8. Gwinup G: Oral phentolamine in non-specific erectile insufficiency. Ann Intern Med 1988; 108:162–163.
9. Grunhaus L, Tiongco D, Zelnik T: Intravenous yohimbine. Selective enhancer of norepinephrine and cortisol secretion and systolic blood pressure in humans. Clin Neuropharmacol 1989; 12:106–114.
10. Margolis A, Prieto P, Stein L: Statistical summary of 10,000 male cases using Afrodex in the treatment of impotence. Curr Ther Res 1971; 13:616–620.
11. Wolpowitz A, Barnard CN: Impotence in heart transplantation. S Afr Med J 1978; 53:693.
12. Morales A, Surridge DH, Marshall PG, Fenemore J: 1982; Non-hormonal pharmacological treatment of organic impotence. J Urol 1982; 128:45–47.
13. Reid K, Surridge DH, Morales A, Condra M, Harris C, Owen J, Fenemore J: Double-blind trial of yohimbine in treatment of psychogenic impotence. Lancet 1987; 2:421–423.
14. Susset JG, Tesier CD, Wincze J, Bansal S, Malhotra C, Schwacha MG: Effect of yohimbine hydrochloride on erectile impotence: A double-blind study. J Urol 1989; 141:1360–1363.
15. Clark JG: Suppression of copulatory behavior in male rats following central administration of clonidine. Neuropharmacology 1991; 30:373–382.
16. Crowley WR, Zelman FP: The neurochemical control of mating behavior. In: Adler NT, ed. Neuroendocrinology of reproduction, physiology and behavior. New York: Plenum, 1981: 451.
17. Heaton JPW, Varrin S: The validation of an innovative bio-assay for potency in an animal model. J Urol (in press).
18. Lal S, Larya E, Thavunadyil JX, Vasavan NNP, Negrete J, Ackman D, Blundell P, Gardiner RJ: Apomorphine-induced penile tumescence in impotent patients—preliminary findings. Progr Neuropsychopharmacol Biol Psychol 1987; 11:235–242.
19. Saenz de Tejada I, Ware JC, Blanco R, Pittard JT, Nadig PW, Adzazoi KM, Krane RJ, Goldstein I: Pathophysiology of prolonged penile erection associated wtih trazodone use. J Urol 1991; 145:60–64.
20. Foreman MN, Wenicke JF: Approaches for the development of oral drug therapies for erectile dysfunction. Sem Urol 1990; 8:107–112.
21. Heaton JPW, Varrin SJ, Gee SP, Morales A: Manipulation of the hormonal milieu and penile tumescence: Effects of castration, diethylstilbestrol, flutamide and cyproterone acetate. Urology (subm).
22. Needleman P, Corr PB, Johnson EM Jr: Drugs used for the treatment of angina: Organic nitrates, calcium channel blockers and β-adrenergic antagonists. In: Gilman AG, Goodman LS, Rall TW, Murad F eds: The pharmacological basis of therapeutics. New York: Macmillan, 1985: 806.
23. Morales A: Clinical use of systemic erectile agents. J Urol 1986; 135:31A.
24. Owen JA, Saunders F, Harris C, Fenemore J, Reid K, Surridge D, Condra M, Morales A: Topical nitroglycerin: A potential treatment for impotence. J Urol 1989; 141:546–548.
25. Heaton JPW, Morales A, Owen J, Saunders FW, Fenemore J: Topical glyceryltrinitrate causes measurable penile arterial dilatation in impotent men. J Urol 1990; 143:729–731.
26. Claes H, Baert L: Transcutaneous nitroglycerin therapy in the treatment of impotence. Urol Int 1989; 44:309–312.
27. Vanhoutte PM: The end of the quest. Nature (London) 1987; 327:459–460.
28. Palmer RMJ, Ferridge AG, Moncada S: Nitric oxide accounts for the biological activity of endothelium-derived relaxing factor. Nature (London) 1987; 327:524–552.
29. Cavallini G: Minoxidil versus nitroglycerine: A prospective double blind controlled trial in

transcutaneous erection facilitation for organic impotence. J Urol 1991; 146:50–53.
30. Grenhoff J, Svensson TH: Clonidine regularizes substantia nigra dopamine cell firing. Life Sci 1988; 42:2003–2009.
31. Schoeffter P, Hoyer D: 5-Hydroxytriptamine 5-HT1B and 5-HT1D receptors mediating inhibition of adenylate cyclase activity. Pharmacological comparison with special reference to the effects of yohimbine, rauwolscine, and some beta adrenoceptor antagonists. Nauyn Schmiedebergs Arch Pharmacol 1989; 340:285–292.

ANNOTATED BIBLIOGRAPHY

de Groat WC, Steers WD: Nueroanatomy and neurophysiology of penile erection. In: Tanagho EA, Lue TF, McClure RD, eds. Contemporary Management of Impotence and Infertility. Williams & Wilkins, Baltimore, 1988: 1–27.

This chapter and other publications on the same subject by Drs. de Groat and Steers are mandatory reading for all persons interested in understanding the fundamentals of the erectile process. In a very clear and concise form they explain the very complex mechanisms involved in producing the final events of penile tumescence and rigidity.

Wein AJ, Van Arsdalen KN: Drug-induced male sexual dysfunction. Urol Clin NA 1988; 15:23–31.

In our search for a pharmacological therapy for impotence we may tend to forget that a number of sexual dysfunctions are drug-induced. Physicians treating erectile dysfunction should have good knowledge of drugs that have been implicated as "erectolytic." This review provides an excellent overview of the subject.

2 Intracavernous Injection Therapy for Impotence

Dimitrios G. Hatzichristou
Terry Payton
Irwin Goldstein

The most important advance in the diagnosis and treatment of impotence over the past decade has been the intracavernosal administration of vasoactive agents.

Historically, such agents were first introduced in the diagnosis and treatment of erectile dysfunction in the early 1980s. In 1982, Virag reported the ability of intracavernous injection of papaverine to induce an erection. In 1983, Brindley described that injection of phenoxybenzamine, an α-adrenergic receptor blocking agent, could induce and sustain an erection. In 1985 Zorgniotti introduced the combination of papaverine with phentolamine, and in 1986, Ishii documented the results of intracavernous PGE_1 injections.[1]

Numerous studies have been published with different drug combinations in therapeutic pharmacologic erection programs (PEP).[1] Widespread popularity has developed as this therapy has been found to offer patients the opportunity to achieve safe, predictable, reversible, functional erections without the need for surgery or any external mechanical devices.

It is the goal of this chapter to review the clinically applicable vasoactive agents, to develop a hypothesis explaining the difference between the physiologic and the pharmacologic erection, to describe the indications and technical principles of intracavernosal self-injection therapy, and to review the literature concerning the results and complications of patients utilizing this therapy.

Vasoactive Agents

Papaverine Hydrochloride

Papaverine hydrochloride (6,7-dimethoxy-1-veratryl-isoquinolone hydrochloride) is a benzylisoquinoline alkaloid obtained from the opium papaver somniferum; however, there are no known associated narcotic properties. Papaverine, which is metabolized in the liver, has a plasma half-life of 1–2 hours.[1,2]

Papaverine's major action is to relax smooth muscle, which it achieves through multiple

Management of Impotence and Infertility, edited by Douglas Whitehead and Harris Nagler,

mechanisms. Papaverine increases intracellular cAMP by reducing both transmembrane calcium transport and cyclic nucleotide phosphodiesterase activity.[2] Papaverine also induces low intracellular concentration of calcium by inhibiting both extracellular influx and the storage of intracellular Ca^{2+}. In vascular smooth muscle, papaverine depletes intracellular calcium stores by inhibiting calcium-activated chloride and potassium currents.[2]

Papaverine (Papaverine HCL, Lilly) induces an erection when injected as a single agent. In the corpora cavernosa, papaverine relaxes the smooth muscle cells of the lacunar trabeculae and the helicine arteries.[3]

Side effects from papaverine include hypotension, nausea, vomiting, weakness, flushing, dizziness, and sinus tachycardia. These occurrences are rare, presenting most commonly in patients with severe venoocclusive dysfunction, who use large volumes of drugs. Fibrosis in the corpora cavernosa has been reported as long-term side effect of papaverine.[1] The pH of the papaverine is between 3 and 4 and may be, in part, responsible for the intracorporeal scarring.[2] Elevations in liver transaminases have been rarely reported with the use of papaverine.[1]

Phentolamine Mesylate

Phentolamine mesylate (4,5-dihydro-2-[*N*-(*m*-hydroxyphenyl)-*N*-(*p*-methylphenyl)aminomethyl]-1*H*-imidazole 1:1-methanesulfonate) is an α-adrenergic antagonist with a plasma half-life of 30 minutes. It can also block receptors for 5-hydroxytryptamine, release histamine from mast cells, and may have a direct, nonspecific relaxant effect on vessels.[1,2]

It is well documented that phentolamine blocks sympathetic vasoconstrictive activity by blocking both α_1- and α_2-adrenergic receptors. In the penis, phentolamine appears to relax preferentially the smooth muscle of the helicine and cavernosal arteries over the corporal smooth muscle of the lacunar trabeculae.[3]

Phentolamine does not produce a rigid erection by itself as its action does not involve direct corporal smooth muscle relaxation. In combination with papaverine, phentolamine (Regitine, CIBA) reduces the volume of vasoactive drug administered and increases the successful response rate of the pharmacologically induced erection in impotent men. Studies on the physicochemical stability of papaverine–phentolamine mixture have been performed in room temperature or at −4°C. They have shown that over a period of 6 months, there was no change in pH over time, no alteration in color, and no precipitation or formation of new moieties.

Phentolamine may be responsible for hypotension, tachycardia, cardiac arrhythmias, weakness, dizziness, nasal stuffiness, nausea, and vomiting.

Prostaglandin E_1 (PGE_1)

Prostaglandin E_1 (PGE_1) or (11α,13*E*,15*S*)-11,15-dihydroxy-9-oxoprost-13 en-1-oik acid is one of the endogenically produced eicosanoids with smooth muscle relaxant properties. In clinical use, PGE_1 (Prostin VR, Upjohn) is mixed in dehydrated alcohol solution.

Intravenously, PGE_1 has been found to produce vasodilatation, significantly increase the cardiac output, inhibit platelet aggregation, and decrease LDL influx into the arterial wall. Its action may be on blocking α_2-adrenoreceptors.[2]

In the corpora cavernosa, PGE_1 has resulted in a pharmacologically induced erection.[1] PGE_1 relaxes smooth muscle in the corpora as well as in the helicine arteries.[2] It has also a synergistic action with papaverine alone and with papaverine and phentolamine in combination, thereby reducing the dosage required for pharmacologic erection and increasing the effectiveness of either therapy.[4]

Side effects noted have been penile discomfort and pain, redness, and burning sensation of the penile skin. Systemic side effects with intracavernosal use have not been reported, probably as the drug metabolizes in the penis.

Other Drugs

Agents producing penile erections include the smooth muscle relaxant nitroglycerine,[2] the α- adrenoceptor blockers phenoxybenzamine[1] and thymoxamine (moxisylyte),[5] the K^+ channel opener minoxidil,[2] the antidepressant trazodone,[2] and the peptides vasointestinal (VIP) and calcitonin gene-related peptide (CGRP).[2] Recently, linsidomine (SIN-1), an active metabolite of the antianginal drug molsidomine, which acts by liberating nitric oxide, has been reported to produce erection.[2]

Vasoconstrictive Agents for Priapism

Pharmacologically-induced prolonged erections are successfully being treated with α-adrenergic agonists, such as phenylephrine, metaraminol, epinephrine, norepinephrine, adrenaline, and dopamine.[1,2] Complications such as acute hypertension, bradycardia, cardiac arrythmias, and even death have been reported.

Terbutaline, β_1-agonist, has been reported to successfully treat priapism when administered orally or intravenously.[6] When administered intracavernously, however, it produces tumescence. Its mechanism of action in inducing detumescence is unknown.

Cascade Hypothesis of Pharmacologic Erections

There has been recent extensive research on the physiology of penile erection. On the other hand, there are few studies investigating the mechanism of pharmacologically induced erection.

The mechanisms that regulate the process of penile erection will be summarized in detail. Such information will then be utilized to develop a hypothesis of pharmacologic erection.

Neurophysiology of Erection

Erection is a neurovascular phenomenon.[7] Cavernosal nerve stimulation causes relaxation of the vascular smooth muscle that surrounds the helicine arteries. The helicine arteries, which open directly into the lacunar spaces, act as resistance arteries controlling blood flow to these spaces. Relaxation of the helicine artery smooth muscle increases blood inflow to the lacunar spaces, from approximately 3–5 to approximately 25 ml/minute in the flaccid state.

Cavernosal nerve stimulation simultaneously induces relaxation of the trabeculae surrounding the lacunar spaces. Such relaxation enables dilation of the lacunar spaces.[7] The systemic blood pressure, now transmitted through the dilated helicine arteries, expands the relaxed trabecular walls against the tunica albuginea. This reduces cavernosal venous outflow by compression of the subtunical venules against the tunica albuginea, a mechanism known as corporal venoocclusion. This mechanism seems to be passive as erection can be pharmacologically induced by the intracavernosal injection of smooth muscle relaxants (i.e., papaverine, prostaglandin E_1).[8] These drugs not only relax the smooth muscle of arteries, trabeculae, and veins, but also interfere with the ability of the smooth muscle to contract in response to adrenergic agonists or adrenergic nerve stimulation. Such data suggests that active constriction of veins is not necessary for the restriction of outflow from the corpora cavernosa. Venous outflow is regulated by the tone of the trabecular smooth muscle. When the smooth muscle is contracted there is low resistance to outflow. This allows for the easy detumescence of the corporal bodies and may contribute to the maintenance of penile flaccidity. On the other hand, when smooth muscle is relaxed the resistance to venous outflow is high.

Vascular endothelium influences the surrounding corporal smooth muscle tone in addition to that produced by neurogenic stimulation.[9] This is achieved through the release of endothelium-derived relaxing factor (EDRF), endothelium-derived hyperpolarizing factor, endothelium-derived eicosanoids, and endothelin[7–11] (Figure 2-1).

Locally, corporal smooth muscle relaxation is mediated by a parasympathetic nonadrenergic–noncholinergic neutrotransmitter (NANC) as well as by the endothelium–derived relaxing factor (EDRF).[7] Recent studies have found both NANC and EDRF in corpus cavernosum to be nitric oxide.[9] Nitric oxide, from either neurologic or endothelial sources, diffuses into the smooth muscle. This stimulates soluble guanylate cyclase resulting in accumulation of cyclic guanosine monophosphate (cGMP), leading to smooth muscle relaxation.

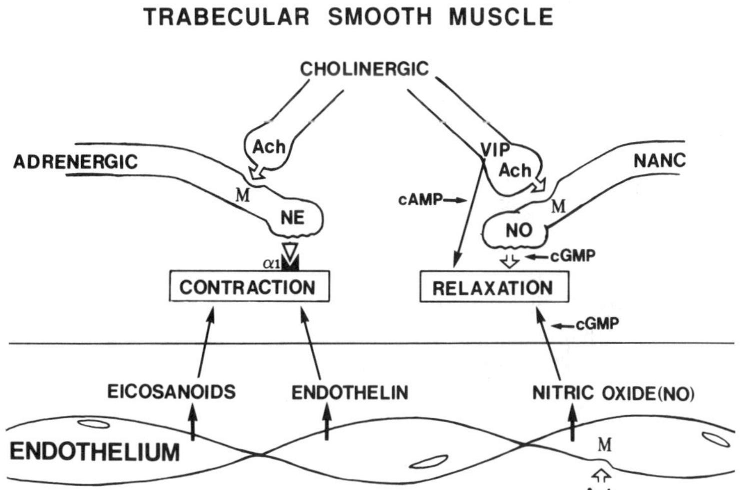

Figure 2-1 Mechanisms controlling trabecular smooth muscle tone. Neurogenic mediation involves (1) adrenergic contraction via the neurotransmitter norepinephrine, (2) cholinergic prejunctional neuroinhibition of adrenergic nerves and prejunctional ncurocxcitation of nonadrenergic, noncholinergic nerves, and (3) nonadrenergic, noncholinergic nerve relaxation via the neurotransmitter nitric oxide. Endothelial mediation involves (1) vasoconstriction factors such as endothelin and eicosanoids and (2) vasoactive agents such as nitric oxide and other eicosanoids such as prostaglandin E_2.

The physiologic regulation of the release of endothelium-derived nitric oxide may also be related, as proposed in blood vessels, to shear stress.[11] This occurs most likely as mechanical tangential frictional forces at the endothelial surface associated with neurologically mediated arterial flow-induced increases.

Activation of sympathetic constrictor nerves is mediated by norepinephrine acting on α_1-adrenoceptors.[12] The excitatory action of norepinephrine is due to an increase of calcium influx from the extracellular space, release of calcium from intracellular stores, and suppression of calcium extrusion or sequestration in smooth muscle. Such biochemical activities cause an increase in the tone of the smooth muscle of the helicine arteries and the trabeculae, resulting in detumescence. This results in a reduction of arterial inflow and collapse of the lacunar spaces with decompression of subtunical venules and increased lacunar space venous outflow returning the penis to the flaccid state.[12] Recently endothelin-1, one of the most potent vasoconstrictors yet described, has been shown to synthesize by human corpus cavernosum endothelium and elicits strong, sustained contractions of corpus cavernosum smooth muscle.[10] This has led to the speculation that endothelin may contribute to the maintenance of penile flaccidity by providing sustained tone to the trabecular smooth muscle.

The "Cascade" Hypothesis

Application of the above mechanisms involved in penile erection may be utilized to formulate a hypothesis concerning the mechanism of pharmacologic-induced erection. A hypothesis is presented based on clinical observations to explain the mechanism of intracavernosal vasoactive drug-induced erections.

The endogeneous physiological mechanisms that relax penile smooth muscle and elicit a normal sexually stimulated erection can be mimicked by the intracavernosal administration of vasoactive drugs. These agents either directly relax the corporal smooth muscle or block adrenergically induced smooth muscle tone.[1,2]

Vasoactive drugs do not appear to diffuse from the injection site throughout the entire corpora inducing smooth muscle relaxation equally. This is most obvious in a neurogenically impotent patient with a spinal cord injury who develops an erection within minutes following a volume of 0.1 ml (3 mg) injection of papaverine. The small 0.1 ml volume could not diffuse to the opposite crus and induce travecular smooth muscle relaxation. The erection response in such an individual suggests that a "cascade" phenomenon is established by the intracavernosal injection.

It is hypothesized that a concentration profile of vasoactive agents occurs around the injection site. Smooth muscle relaxation, which is concentration dependent, occurs in the region of the appropriate vasoactive drug concentration. In the region of concentration-dependent smooth muscle relaxation, there occurs (1) local increases in blood inflow, (2) activation of endothelium-mediated relaxing factors, (3) enlarged zone of regional smooth muscle relaxation, and (4) the "cascade" initiation of relaxation–inflow-relaxing factor, relaxation–inflow-relaxing factor, relaxation–inflow-relaxing factor, etc.

Therefore, the pharmacologic erection is initiated by a local injection. Spread or dissemination of factors that result in an erection is based on increased blood flow mediating release of endothelium-derived nitric oxide. Further support for the hypothesis that endothelium-derived relaxing factors are the "transmitter" for pharmacologic erection is based on the observation that high doses of agents are required for erection in impotent patients with endothelial cell dysfunction such as diabetes and hypercholesterolemia. In addition, incracavernosal methylene blue, a guanylate cyclase blocker preventing nitric oxide-induced smooth muscle relaxation, was found to significantly inhibit the erectile response to intracavernosal injection of vasoactive substances.

Indications

In general, intracavernosal pharmacotherapy is offered to most patients with impotence. The therapeutic goal is to achieve an erection satisfactory for sexual intercourse.

The quality of the erectile response to the pharmacologic erection is based on the arterial inflow perfusion pressure and the function of the corporal venoocclusion mechanism. Patients with neurogenic or psychogenic impotence and normal hemodynamic parameters, therefore, are expected to achieve the best erectile response.[13,14] Such patients are also most at risk for the development of prolonged erection or priapism.

Patients with arterial insufficiency also respond by virtue of the long-acting nature of the smooth muscle relaxation provided by the vasoactive agents.[1,7] Patients with significant corporal venoocclusive dysfunction, however, would be the least likely to respond to this form of therapy.

There are few outright contraindications for this therapy in impotence. Patients with significant psychiatric disease or potential for mistreatment or abuse of this therapy should be excluded from treatment. Patients with poor manual ability, morbid obesity, and visual inadequacy, or those in whom even a passing hypotensive epidose may have an adverse effect should be carefully considered prior to being offered this therapeutic option. Patients who are concomitantly taking aspirin or coumadin have successfully been treated without obvious deleterious effect.[6]

Patients with psychogenic impotence have also been treated with intracavernosal pharmacotherapy alone or in conjunction with sex therapy.[14] These patients, however, must fully understand the undesired side effects of this therapy especially the potential for the formation of fibrotic nodules within the corpora.

Pharmacological Erection Program (PEP)

Patients who enter a nurse–physician pharmacologic erection program should be first asked to complete an informed consent concerning complications such as priapism and intracavernosal masses. A handout with a diagram of the injection technique along with a detailed explanation of the program is useful. The objective of the program is to train impotent patients to safely self-administer the lowest dose required for achieving an appropriate erectile response for satisfactory sexual performance.

The Training Program

The training program consists of several phases, including the dose determination phase, and the self-injection phase, and the inhome self-injection phase. Suitable training can usually be achieved with three visits.

Visit #1

Patients with neurogenic impotence should receive an extremely low dose. Patients with vascular disease will usually begin the dosage determination phase with a higher dose and subsequently require higher increments in dose.

The initial injection consists of low volume and concentration of vasoactive agents designed to achieve only a slight penile swelling of poor quality and short duration. No masturbatory practices or intercourse should be attempted. The patient is simply instructed to observe the techniques involved in self-injection. This includes attention to compression of the site of injection for 3 minutes. The patient then assesses his erection over the ensuing 1–2 hours, generally not in the office. Such a failed dose is helpful to allay patient anxiety. Should a prolonged erection occur despite these precautions, appropriate instructions are provided.

Visit #2

The results of the first injection are reviewed in terms of erection duration and quality. If a weak erection of short duration was achieved with the first dose, the second dose of vasoactive agents is increased. The patient is again encouraged to observe the self-injection techniques including careful compression of the injection site. The patient is then instructed to stimulate himself within 1 hour of the second injection. No pressure is put on the patient to perform intercourse.

Visit #3

If a 50–60% erection response occurs with the second injection that becomes more rigid with stimulation, then several prefilled syringes are provided to the patient for home use, on a trial basis. Instructions are described regarding precise sites of injection and side effects (Figure 2-2). A rubber model of a penis can be used to practice injection techniques. The patient is instructed in sterile injection techniques. Reinforcement is provided to compress the site of injection for 3 minutes. In cases where there continues to be inadequate erectile responses, further testing with increasing doses of vasoactive agents is indicated. In cases where the erection response is overly prolonged, the dose of agents is lowered.

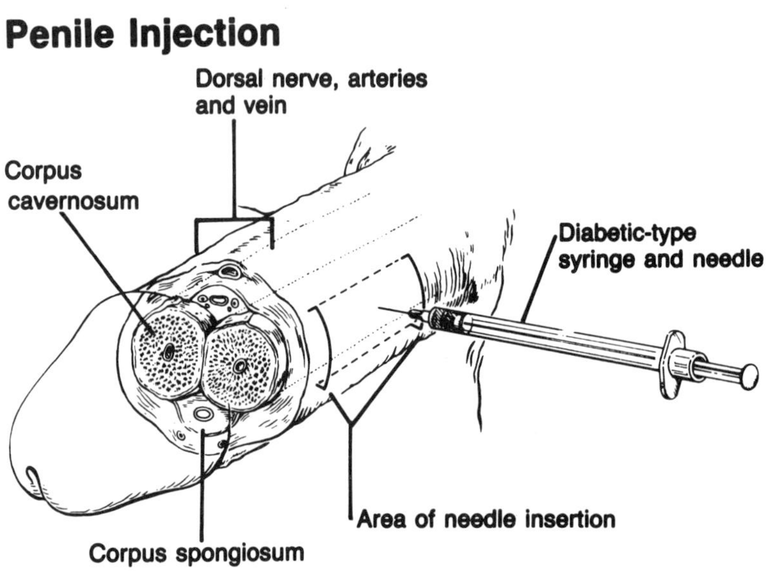

Figure 2-2 Technique of penile self-injection showing location of needle insertion to be lateral to the ventral corpus spongiosum and the midline dorsal neurovascular bundle.

At Home Use

The patient is instructed to inject the last known dose should this prove satisfactory. Patients are told not to inject more frequently than once per day. Doses may be tailored to individual needs as it is very common that dosages determined in the office will be decreased by the patient at home.

The Pharmacologic Erection Program[15]

Once the patient has successfully utilized his prefilled syringes, he is then eligible to join the self-injection program. Syringes and medication are provided as needed. Nurse–physician follow-up should occur at regular intervals. Patients should keep all medication vials in a refrigerator at home. All syringes must be stored in a secure place. Following use, disposal of used syringes must be accomplished in appropriate containers. Patients must be cautioned to call their physician if an erection persists for 4 hours or longer, although there is no general agreement on the time limits at which treatment of prolonged erection is necessary. Irreversible histologic changes of the erectile tissue have been identified after 12 hours of priapism. The majority of pharmacologically induced prolonged erections will detumesce on their own; however, some will require an intracavernosal injection of an α-agonist to produce detumescence. α-Agonists that have been used for this purpose include epinephrine, phenylephrine, adrenaline, noradrenaline, ethylephrine, and metaraminol.[8,16,17] At present, we use an initial intracavernosal injection of 200 μg of phenylephrine. This may be repeated as necessary until detumescence. It is important to mention that α-adrenergic agents lose their efficacy in sustained "blood statis" and low pH.[1,17] In such cases, irrigation of the corpora with an adrenergic agonist solution has been an effective alternative to intracavernosal injections of adrenergic agonists. Following the dosage determination phase the complication of prolonged erection is quite rare and is seen in less than 1% of injections.

Principles of Self-Injection

There are three basic principles for safe intracavernosal pharmacotherapy as a treatment option for impotence. The first principle is to use low drug volumes. The volume should not exceed 1 ml and should be adjusted if possible to 0.5 ml or less. This will maximally reduce the potential systemic complications. Also, minimizing drug volume can make this therapy cost effective for the patients.

The second principle is to use polypharmacotherapy with agents such as papaverine, phentolamine, and prostaglandin E_1 (Table 2-1). Multiple vasoactive agents have a synergistic action on the erectile tissue.[4] This principle is based on the "cascade" hypothesis of the mechanism of pharmacologically induced penile erection. These agents possess different

Table 2-1 Vasoactive Drug Combinations

Vasoactive Agents Combinations	Papaverine	Phentolamine	PGE_1
Bimix	300 mg (10 ml)	15 mg (3 ml)	
Trimix	300 mg (10 ml)	10 mg (2 ml)	100 mg (0.2 ml)
Super trimix	300 mg (10 ml)	20 mg (4 ml)	200 mg (0.4 ml)

mechanisms of action inducing relaxation of the trabecular smooth muscle. Such use of multiple vasoactive agents has the best possibility of achieving the largest zone of smooth muscle relaxation around the injection site. In our facility, the three agents papaverine, phentolamine, and prostaglandin E_1 have been utilized as a "trimix" in the following doses: papaverine 300 mg (10 ml), phentolamine 10 mg (2 ml, reconstituted by the papaverine), and prostaglandin E_1 100 μg (0.2 ml). The total volume in the ampule is 10.2 ml. Each milliliter solution has approximately 29 mg papaverine, 1 mg phentolamine, and 10 mg PGE_1.

The third principle is to maximally compress the specific site of the injection. This is best achieved either using two fingers, one at the needle puncture site and the other positioned at the opposite side of the penile shaft or by using the clenched fist. Compression should be maintained for a full 3 minutes after each intracavernosal injection. One has to assume that each intracavernosal injection has induced some intracavernosal bleeding. This will maximally reduce the potential local complication of scarring or fibrosis.

Failures of Therapy

Using the "cascade" hypothesis, treatment failures with intracavernosal administration of vasoactive agents would theoretically occur because of (1) inadequate drug concentration around the injection site to cause concentration-dependent smooth muscle relaxation, (2) inadequate increases in blood inflow in the region of concentration-dependent smooth muscle relaxation, and (3) inadequate activation of endothelium-mediated relaxing factors in the region of concentration-dependent smooth muscle relaxation and blood inflow increases. However, the effect of sympathetic trunk stimulation seems to antagonize the relaxing action of papaverine on the cavernous smooth muscles and the cavernous arterioles.[3] High sympathetic tone may explain the poor response to intracavernous injection of vasoactive agents.

Treatment failures with intracavernosal self-injection occur most often in patients with severe corporal venoocclusive dysfunction or severe arterial insufficiency. One possible explanation may be that these patients have the most pathology involving the corporal lacunar endothelium, especially with vascular risk factors such as hypercholesterolemia, cigarette smoking, diabetes mellitus, and hypertension. Therefore, in these patients the "cascade" is unable to be activated easily.

Based on the "cascade" hypothesis, the following strategies should be considered for treatment failures to intracavernosal self-injection: (1) increase the vasoactive drug concentration and (2) use pharmacologic agents with different sites of action (smooth muscle cell, endothelial cell, to cause release of endothelium-mediated relaxing factors). Such a strategy aims at achieving around the injection site a sufficient high concentration of vasoactive agents, inducing local smooth muscle relaxation, increasing blood inflow to the region, activating endothelium-mediated relaxing factors, widening the zone of relaxation, and activating a cascade effect of maximum arterial inflow and corporal venoocclusion throughout the corpora.

In patients who have failed to achieve an adequate erectile response using the standard three mixture polypharmacotherapy solution, we have had some success increasing the dose of phentolamine to 20 mg and PGE_1 to 200 μg, keeping the amount of papaverine the same (300 mg). In this "super trimixture" solution, the total volume of the mixture is 10.4 ml with approximate doses of papaverine 29 mg, phentolamine 2 mg, and prostaglandin E_1 19 μg in each milliliter of the solution. This mixture is also best maintained in a refrigerator.

Intracavernosal discomfort is most frequently associated with the pharmacologic agent prostaglandin E_1. Elimination of the prostaglandin E_1 from the "trimix" solution might be successful. The use of solution 300 mg papaverine and 15 mg phentolamine is suggested. This "bimix" solution has a total volume of 10 ml and each milliliter contains 30 mg papaverine and 1.5 mg phentolamine.

There are several patients who have failed all of the above mixtures. Such patients may choose an alternate treatment between vacuum constriction devices and penile prosthetic implants.

Results and Complications: Literature Experience

Response Rate

The response rate of pharmacologic erection therapy is described in terms of achieving an erection sufficient for intercourse. Different series have reported varied response rates. Erectile responses have been reported as high as 97%.[1] In specific groups, such as the elderly, aged 60–84 years, the response has been as low as 19%.[19]

In a recent review, a total of 482 patients were identified who underwent intracorporal injections with several vasoactive agents.[20] A full erection was achieved with papaverine as monosubstance in 36% of the patients, with a combination of papaverine and phentolamine in 68% and with PGE_1 alone in 76%. McMahon reported an improved erectile response with the combination of the three drugs, papaverine, phentolamine, and PGE_1, compared to any one of the previously reported combinations.[21]

Patient Satisfaction

The lack of prospective, double-blind studies in the literature makes it difficult to reach valid unbiased conclusions concerning patient satisfaction. Often patient satisfaction has been assessed by simplistic criteria such as the presence of an adequate erectile response. Assessments of patient satisfaction are typically based on patient responses to questionnaires or to interviews.

Sidi et al. reported that 78% of 239 patients were satisfied with self-injection therapy.[22] Virag, reporting 8 years of experience with 615 patients with follow-up ranging from 12 to 96 months (mean 24 months), observed 90% full sexual activity and 80% patient satisfaction.[23] Althof et al. reported that when pretreatment and postinjection sexual functioning were contrasted, statistically significant improvements in quality of erection with foreplay and intercourse, sexual satisfaction, and frequency of intercourse were seen.[24] In another study the same authors evaluated partner satisfaction with self-injection therapy.[25] They found significant increases in sexual satisfaction, sexual arousal, frequency of coital orgasm, and frequency of intercourse. The women reported feeling more at ease in their relationships and characterized sex as more leisurely, relaxed, and assured. Negative responses focused on the lack of spontaneity and hesitation about initiating sex.

Early Local Complications

Prolonged erection or priapism has been reported in 0–19% of cases.[1,5,13–15,20–25] Most authors accept an erection lasting more than 4 hours as consistent with priapism. Junemann and Alken reviewed the literature experience prior to 1989 and identified 2134 patients treated with the pharmacological agents papaverine, 2914 with the combination of papaverine and phentolamine, and 1284 with PGE_1 as monosubstance.[1] Prolonged erections were noted in 10, 5, and 2%, respectively. These data are derived from intracavernosal agents utilized for diagnosis and not for treatment.

In a survey of several controlled studies where 428 patients were tested with papaverine, papaverine and phentolamine, and PGE_1, the incidence of prolonged erection was 3, 3, 6, and 1%, respectively.[20] Other more recent studies have shown that the prevalence of priapism is less than 1% of the total number of injections, but it occurs in 3–19% of patients during diagnostic work-up.[5] Virag reported that 10% of 615 patients experienced 114 episodes of prolonged erections or 0.3% of the total number of injections.[23] In a randomized cross-over study of 228 impotent men, McMahon compared the combination of papaverine and phentolamine to PGE_1 and to the combination of the three drugs.[21] He found that the combination of the three drugs was superior. The "trimix" combination had the best success rate in patients with vasculogenic impotence and was associated with a lower incidence of priapism (0.9%) compared to PGE_1 (1.3%) or to the combination of papaverine and phentolamine (7%).

Postinjection pain and discomfort have been reported in 17% of 1284 patients treated with PGE_1 and appeared to be dose dependent.[1] In another review, pain was noted in 23% of 428 patients who injected various intracavernosal vasoactive agents. The only agent that was associated with penile pain in these patients was PGE_1.[20] McMahon[21] reported burning pain at the time of injection to be less of a problem when prostaglandin E_1 was mixed with other agents.

Hematomas and ecchymosis were noted in 2–10% of patients undergoing self-injection therapy and usually resolved within a few days without any permanent sequelae. Cavernositis or infections have rarely been observed.[1]

Late Local Complications

The most frequent late side effect of intracavernosal pharmacologic therapy is self-injection therapy-associated penile fibrosis. This may include either the formation of painless intracavernosal masses or painless tunica albuginea plaques or both. The incidence of fibrotic changes has been related to the frequency of injection use as well as to the duration of the self-injection treatment.[1] Current hypotheses on the pathogenesis of fibrotic reactions include the reaction to the low pH of papaverine, the result of faulty injection with hematoma formation, the consequence of repeated needle trauma, and the resultant hypertrophy of corporal smooth muscle fibers.[1] Such fibrotic reactions have been reported to vary between 0 and 57% of cases.[1,19–26] In the review of the literature, Junemann and Alken reported fibrotic lesions in 5.4% of 1573 patients reviewed.[1] Such lesions may be reversible after discontinuation of the treatment.[23] PGE_1 has been associated with lower percentage of fibrotic changes in the corpora.[20] Recently, thymoxamine hydrochloride (moxisylyte), an α-adrenergic blocking agent, has been found to have a moderate success rate, producing rigid erection in 68% of 72 patients studied, but only 1.3% of the patients developed fibrotic lesions.[5]

There have been several cases of diffuse fibrosis of the corpora following intracorporal injections almost invariably associated with markedly prolonged erections.

Systemic Side Effects

Systemic side effects of self-injection treatment have included vasovagal episodes and syncope, probably related to hypotension. These side effects remain infrequent and are usually seen during the dosage determination phase.[1] It would be expected that patients with significant corporal venoocclusive dysfunction will require larger volumes of agents. Such patients may exhibit an increase in systemic absorption of intracavernosal agents and therefore be more susceptible to postinjection hypotension.

Intracavernosal pharmacotherapy with papaverine has been rarely associated with hepatotoxicity. During a mean follow-up of 26 months, three cases of abnormal liver function tests in the first 201 patients (1.5%) were reported.[15]

α-Adrenergic agents used to treat priapism may cause peripheral vasoconstriction and hypertension. Several fatalities due to myocardial infarction or rupture of arterial aneurysms have been reported following intracavernosal administration of adrenergic agonists.[16]

The Drop-out Rate

Those patients who initiate management with the therapy but terminate because of dissatisfaction with the therapy are considered drop outs from the program. The drop-out rate for the self-injection therapy has been reported to vary between 29 and 66%. Most studies acknowledged that the highest percentage of the drop-out occurs early in the therapy.[1,25] In one study, 29% of 76 patients discontinued self-injection during the initial PEP training, while later in the therapy the drop-out rate had increased to 66% of the original population.[26] Of the remaining patients who continued in the study, 88% were satisfied with the rigidity of their erection and 40% reported improvement in orgasm satisfaction. Finally, 90% of the remaining patients and 70% of their partners answered "yes" when considering if they would have started the therapy again. Althof et al. reported a drop-out rate of 3% of 131 patients after the first month of therapy, and 5, 18, and 3% drop-out at 3, 6, and 12 months, respectively, after therapy.[27] Several reasons were identified for patient drop out prior to test dosing. These included the idea of injecting self (40%), possible side effects (37%), artificiality (31%), disagreement with treatment (25%), and fear of a new procedure (19%). The reasons for dropping out during the test dosing were dissatisfaction with treatment (40%), ineffectiveness (35%), scheduling conflicts (25%), pain (20%), injecting self (20%), and lack of spontaneity (20%). The reasons for late drop out included ineffectiveness (50%), dissatisfaction with treatment (33%), financial (25%), lack of spontaneity (17%), follow-up appointments (17%), pain (8%), injecting self (8%), and partner resistance (8%). Kursh suggested that close cooperation with a psychologist or psychiatrist who is knowledgeable and interested in impotence is important, since two-thirds of the drop outs occur early in the therapy.[13] He believes that such cooperation among disciplines would be beneficial to the patient to provide a more accurate assessment of an individual's problem, permitting a more intelligent approach to self-injection.

Conclusions

Cavernosal injection of vasoactive agents has been one of the most important contributions to the urologist's armamentarium in treating the patient with erectile dysfunction. The relative lack of side effects and the ease of delivery have made this therapy well accepted worldwide. Furthermore self-injection has the advantage of being a reversible treatment, contrary to prosthesis implantation.

Recent studies in our department on the 5 to 7 year long-term follow-up of self-injection patients have found them to have (1) excellent satisfaction with the therapy, (2) absence of systemic complications and (3) local complications consisted mainly of intracavernosal masses, which are related to the number of injections, but do not interfere with overall patient satisfaction. Such long-term follow-up information is needed to establish the safety and efficacy of this therapeutic option and therefore determine the direction the therapy takes over the ensuing decade.

Anticipated approval by the Federal Drug Administration will enable wide dissemination of information concerning the therapy. It should be expected in the future that continued development of basic and clinical research in this field will result in further advances in the pharmaceutical agents for medical management of impotence.

REFERENCES

1. Junemann KP, Alken P: Pharmacotherapy of erectile dysfunction: A review. Int J Impotence Res 1989; 1:71–93.
2. Andersson KE, Holmquist F, Wagner G: Pharmacology of drugs used for treatment of erectile dysfunction and priapism. Int J Impotence Res 1991; 3:155–172.
3. Juenemann KP, Lue TF, Fournier GR, Tanagho EA: Hemodynamics of papaverine and phentolamine-induced penile erection. J Urol 1986; 136:158–161.
4. Goldstein I, Borges FD, Fitch WP, Kaufman J, Moreno J, Payton T, Yingst J, Krane RJ: Rescuing the failed papaverine phentolamine erection: A proposed synergistic action of papaverine, phenotolamine and prostaglandin E1. Int J Impotence Res 1990; 2, Suppl. 2:277.
5. Buvat J, Buvat-Herbaud M, Lemaire A, Marcolin G: Reduced rate of fibrotic nodules in the cavernous bodies following auto-intracavernous injections of moxisylyte compared to papaverine. Int J Impotence Res 1991; 3:123–128.
6. Shantha TR, Finnerty DP, Rodriquez AP: Treatment of persistent penile erection and priapism using terbutaline. J Urol 1989; 141:1427–1429.
7. Krane RJ, Goldstein I, Saenz de Tejada I: Impotence. N Engl J Med 1989; 321:1648.
8. Lue TF, Tanagho EA: Physiology of Erection and Pharmacological Management of Impotence. J Urol 1987; 137:829.
9. Kim N, Azadzoi KM, Goldstein I, Saenz de Tejada I. A nitric oxide-like factor mediates nonadrenergic noncholinergic neurogenic relaxation of penile corpus cavernosum smooth muscle. J Clin Invest 1991; 88:112–118.
10. Saenz de Tejada I, Carson MP, de las Morenas A, Goldstein I, Traish, AM: Endothelin: Localization, synthesis, activity and receptor types in the human penile corpus cavernosum. Am J Physiol 1991; 260 (Heart Circ Physiol 29): H1078–H1085.
11. Rubanyi GM, Romero JC, Vanhoutte PM: Flow-induced release of endothelium-derived relaxing factor. Am J Physiol 1986; 250:H1145–1149.
12. Andersson KE, Holmquist F: Mechanisms for contraction and relaxation of human penile smooth muscle. Int J Impotence Res 1990; 2:209–225.
13. Kursh ED, Bodner DR, Resnick MI, Althof SE, Turner L, Risen C, Levine SB: Injection therapy

for impotence. Urol Clin North Am 1988; 15:625–629.
14. Weiss JN, Ravalli R, Badlani GH: Intracavernous pharmacotherapy in psychogenic impotence. Urology 1991; 37:441–443.
15. Padma-Nathan H, Goldstein I, Payton T, Krane RJ: Ultracavernosal pharmacotherapy: the pharmacologic erection program. World J Urol 1987; 5:160–165.
16. Watters GR, Keogh EJ, Carati CJ et al.: Prolonged erections following injections of medications to overcome impotence. Br J Urol 1988; 62:173–175.
17. Lue TF, Hellstrom WJG, McAninch JW, Tanagho EA: Priapism: A refined approach to diagnosis and treatment. J Urol 1986; 136:104–108.
19. Richter S, Gross R, Nissenkorn: Cavernous injection therapy for the treatment of erectile dysfunction in elderly. Int J Impotence Res 1990; 2:43–47.
20. Junemann KP, Schmitt P, Persson-Junenmann Ch, Tschada R, Alken P: Review of therapy: pharmacology, surgery. Methods Clin Urodynam 1991; Spec Vol: 24–27.
21. McMahon CG: A comparison of the response to the intracavernosal injection of a combination of papaverine and phentolamine, prostaglandin PGE1 and a combination of all three agents in the management of impotence. Int J Impotence Res 1991; 3:113–121.
22. Sidi AA, Reddy PK, Chen KK: Patient acceptance of and satisfaction with vasoactive intracavernous pharmacotherapy for impotence. J Urol 1988; 140:293–294.
23. Virag R, Shoukry K, Floresco J, Nollet F, Greco E: Intracavernous self-injection of vasoactive drugs in the treatment of impotence: 8-year experience with 615 cases. J Urol 1991; 147:287–293.
24. Althof SE, Turner LA, Levine SB, Risen CB, Bodner D, Kursh ED, Resnick MI: Sexual, psychological and marital impact of self-injection of papaverine and phentolamine: a long-term prospective study. J Sex Marit Ther 1991; 17:101–112.
25. Levine SB, Althof SE, Turner LA, Risen CB, Bodner DR, Kursh ED, Resnick MI: Side effects of self-administration of intracavernous papaverine and phentolamine for the treatment of impotence. J Urol 1989; 141:54–57.
26. van Driel MF, Mooibroek JJ, van de Wiel HBM, Mensink HJA: Intracavernous pharmacotherapy: Psychological, sexological and medical aspects. Int J Impotence Res 1991; 3:95–104.
27. Althof SE, Turner LA, Levine SB, Risen C, Kurssh E, Bodner D, Resnick M: Why do so many people drop out from injection therapy for impotence? J Sex Marital Ther 1989; 15:121–129.

ANNOTATED BIBLIOGRAPHY

Andersson KE, Holmquist F, Wagner G: Pharmacology of drugs used for treatment of erectile dysfunction and priapism. Int J Impotence Res 1991; 3:155–172.

A review of the literature on the pharmacology of drugs and drug combinations used orally, transcutaneous, intravenously, and intracavernosally for treatment of impotence and priapism. Possible mechanisms of action and the literature experience on different doses and combinations in humans and in animals are discussed.

Junemann KP, Alken P: Pharmacotherapy of erectile dysfunction: A review. Int J Impotence Res 1989; 1:71–93.

The authors summarized the literature experience on 7 years of intracorporeal drug administration with papaverine monosubstance, 4 to 5 years with the combination papaverine and phentolamine, and 2–3 years with prostaglandin E_1 as a diagnostic and treatment modality for impotence. The authors concluded that (1) prostaglandin E_1 has at least the same response rate as the combination of papaverine and phentolamine and higher than papaverine alone, (2) pharmacologically induced prolonged erection, the most severe early complication, occurs mostly during the diagnostic work-up and the pharmacological test period, (3) PGE_1 has the lowest incidence of priapistic episodes, but is associated with post-injection intracavernosal pain in a significant percentage of cases, (4) the most significant long-term side effect of this treatment is the development of fibrotic lesions or nodules in the corporal bodies, and (5) in general pharmacotherapy of erectile dysfunction should be considered as a well-established and safe treatment modality.

Kim N, Azadzoi KM, Goldstein I, Saenz de Tejada I: A nitric oxide-like factor mediates nonadrenergic noncholinergic neurogenic relaxation of penile corpus cavernosum smooth muscle. J Clin Invest 1991; 88:112–118.

The vascular endothelium, when stimulated with chemical or physical stimuli, releases an endothelium-derived relaxing factor (EDRF) that diffuses to the underlying smooth muscle, causing its relaxation. The principal neurotransmitter mediating trabecular smooth muscle relaxation has been characterized as a nonadrenergic noncholinergic neutrotransmitter (NANC). The authors reported experimental results that show that in corpus cavernosum tissue, the endothelium-derived relaxing factor (EDRF) released by acetycholine has the chemical properties of nitric oxide. Furthermore, the authors observed that in the presence of muscarinic and adrenergic blockade, transmural electrical stimulation of corpus cavernosum tissue in which the endothelium has been mechanically or chemically disrupted elicits NANC neurogenic relaxation. This response is significantly attenuated or blocked by substances that interfere with the synthesis or the effects of nitric oxide. These experiments strongly support the fact that nitric oxide mediates NANC relaxation in trabecular smooth muscle. Therefore, nitric oxide released by the endothelium and the dilator nerves is a key mediator in the relaxation of the trabecular smooth muscle.

McMahon CG: A comparison of the response to the intracavernosal injection of a combination of papaverine and phentolamine, prostaglandin PGE1 and a combination of all three agents in the management of impotence. Int J Impotence Res 1991; 3:113–121.

In a randomized cross-over study of 228 impotent men, McMahon compared the combination of papaverine and phentolamine to PGE_1 and to the combination of the three drugs. He found that the combination of the three drugs is superior, as it has the higher response rate in patients with vasculogenic impotence and is associated with lower incidence of priapism.

Virag R, Shoukry K, Floresco J, Nollet F, Greco E: Intracavernous self-injection of vasoactive drugs in the treatment of impotence: 8-year experience with 615 cases. J Urol 1991; 147:287–293.

This is a study on the mid- and long-term follow-up of 533 patients during an average period of 24 months (range 12 to 96 months). Sexual acitivity index (SAI) was determined on a scale from 0 to 10, taking into account the number of sexual acts, the possibility and quality of penetration, and the control of ejaculation. In addition, the authors asked each patient to grade from 0 to 10 the satisfaction of his sex life (satisfaction index = SI). The sexual activity index and the satisfaction index were higher than 6 in 90 and 80%, respectively. Fifty-one patients (10%) experienced prolonged erections, and palpable subcutaneous nodules in contact with albuginea were reported in 14% of the cases, but 11% were temporary.

3 Implantation of Penile Prostheses

E. Douglas Whitehead

The first use of paired rigid polyethylene intracorporal penile prosthesis implanted in the United States, referred to as the "first modern intracorporal penile prosthesis,"[1] was reported in 1973 (Figure 3-1).[2] In the same year the first paired silicone intracorporal multicomponent inflatable penile prosthesis was reported.[3] In 1975 the first semirigid paired silicone intracorporal prosthesis was reported.[4] This prosthesis quickly became popular for the next 10 years.[5] The early multicomponent inflatable penile prosthesis, popularized by Scott, were plagued by malfunctions and an unacceptably high rate of mechanical failure, ranging up to 50% over many years.[6] Due to constant improvement in engineering, materials, and surgical techniques, the later models have had a significantly lower malfunction rate.[7,8] In the United States in recent years between 20,000 and 30,000 prostheses are inserted each year. Today the patient and his partner have a wide variety of reliable devices to choose from with advantages and disadvantages accruing to each.

Selection of Patients for Implantation of Penile Prostheses

Patients being considered for penile prostheses should be emotionally stable, have a strong libido, ideally a desiring sexual partner and reasonable health. They should be appropriately evaluated for the cause or causes of their impotence. Frequently a multispecialty approach is advisable.[9,10] After evaluation, penile implantation is indicated for the treatment of organic impotence in patients with various etiologies (Table 3-1) who are (1) not candidates for or do not wish treatment by nonsurgical means such as pharmacologic erection programs (PEP) or vacuum erection assistance device programs (VEADP), (2) dropouts from PEP and VEADP programs, (3) not candidates or not desirous of, or have not been successfully treated with, revascularization or venous ligation surgery, or (4) unsuccessful with psychotherapy or have refused to consider or to continue psychotherapy. Patients referred by psychologists, sex therapists, or psychiatrists for

Management of Impotence and Infertility, edited by Douglas Whitehead and Harris Nagler,

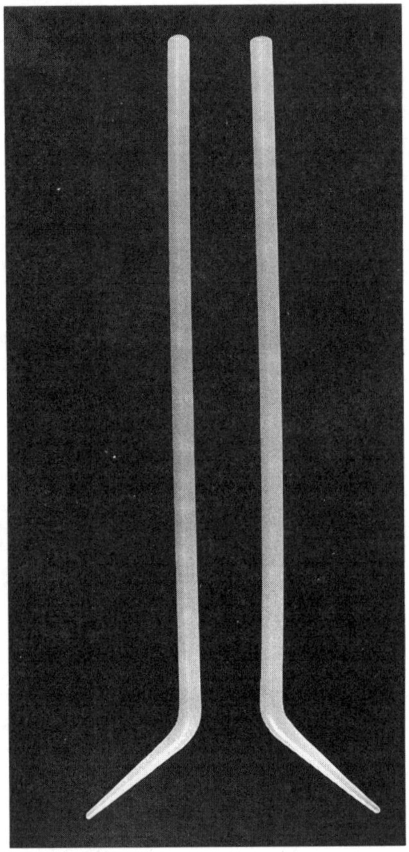

Figure 3-1 Polyethylene intracorporal penile prosthesis.

Table 3-1 Etiologies Of Impotence Amenable To Penile Prostheses

Arteriogenic impotence
Venogenic impotence
Mixed arteriogenic-venogenic impotence
Neurogenic impotence
Mixed arteriogenic-venogenic and neurogenic impotence
Psychogenic impotence

implantation are frequently suitable candidates. In younger men penile implantation is more cost effective over the long-term than PEP.[11] Approximately two-thirds of patients implanted are between the ages of 50 and 69 and 10% are over the age of 70.

Preoperative Counselling and Informed Consent

The patient and his partner should have realistic expectations from the planned surgery[12] and know that while the functional success rate (mechanical capability for coitus and vaginal penetration) of implantation is approximately 95%,[13] with any of the currently available prostheses a satisfaction rate, in terms of sexual intercourse and cosmetic appearance, of between 80 and 90% may be expected.

Sometimes it is beneficial for the patient to speak with a patient who has had a similar implant and for his sexual partner to speak to the sexual partner of a man who has had the same implant.[14] Patients who have had an excellent result are asked to sign a consent form allowing their name to be given to a prospective patient. In my practice, in addition to the above, I occasionally introduce two patients in the office, one who has had the same implant a prospective patient is considering. The former patient may demonstrate in the office to the prospective patient the action and cosmetic appearance of the implant.

Because implantation of a penile prosthesis may expose the urologist to a relatively high risk of malpractice suit, the implanting urologist must thoroughly understand the design limitations and functional limitations of each prosthesis and must document the patient's informed consent. The patient should be given printed material on the subject of penile prostheses and be aware of possible alternative methods of surgical and nonsurgical management. He should understand that the decision to undergo penile implantation is a major and irreversible decision that should be seriously considered only after careful discussion and consideration of alternative treatment modalities. He and if possible his sexual partner should have realistic expectations of what a penile prosthesis can provide and understand the possible problems and complications from this surgery. This author uses a "Preimplantation Certification" document to be certain informed consent is obtained.

A representative sample device from each major category should be demonstrated. In my practice I offer the patient a choice from the three major categories of prosthesis: noninflatable, unitary inflatable, and multicomponent inflatable (two-piece and three-piece). The patient and his partner should be aware of the advantages and disadvantages of each of these types of prostheses and that the ideal penile prosthesis does not presently exist, but some of the characteristics it would embody are shared by several of the available penile prostheses[15] (Table 3-2).

Table 3-2 Characteristics of the Ideal Penile Prosthesis

Technically easy surgical implantation
Short operative procedure
Complication-free surgical implantation and postoperative course
Low cost
Freedom from mechanical complications
Little patient education and manual dexterity required
Partner unawareness of the device
Easy concealability
Restoration of preimpotence penile girth, length, rigidity, and flaccidity

Generally, the older patient selects a noninflatable or two-piece inflatable prosthesis. Some men with incomplete arteriogenic impotence and many men with psychogenic impotence are able to obtain some natural tumescence around the prosthesis after implantation, particularly after insertion of an inflatable prosthesis. Prior to implantation the patient and his sexual partner should understand that after implantation of any type of prosthesis the erection will not be "normal" and that irreversible damage to a variable degree occurs to the erectile tissue. Furthermore, they should know that (1) the prosthesis does not create tumescence of the glans or corpus spongiosum; (2) the penis may not be as long or have as much girth as a previously normal erection; (3) the prosthesis will not harm the partner; (4) prostheses rarely solve interpersonal difficulties and do not ensure sexual gratification; (5) prostheses do not affect the ability to have orgasm and ejaculation. If the patient was able to ejaculate and have orgasm before implantation he should continue to do so after the surgery. Many men after implantation are able to resume a satisfactory sex life and feelings of inadequacy caused by their impotence resolve. Some men find that after implantation their erections are better than prior natural erections, due to their ability to engage in sexual intercourse for a longer time and to develop an erection on demand. Should significant interpersonal problems be noted prior to implantation, a referral to a mental health professional, either a sex therapist, psychologist or pscychiatrist[16] is indicated.

PRE-IMPLANTATION CERTIFICATION

ALL OF THE FOLLOWING HAS BEEN DONE PRIOR TO SURGERY:

(1) The function of all major categories of penile prostheses (implants) and selected specific types; nonsurgical alternatives (vacuum constriction devices, injection of vasoactive agents and medications, and vascular surgery—arterial and venous) has been discussed.

(2) Printed material on the subject of impotence, including various available implants has been made available.

(3) That the erection produced after implantation might be slightly shorter and narrower than the normal erection prior to the development of impotence and that it is not a natural or "normal" erection has been discussed.

(4) The possible surgical, medical, and device-related risks and complications, including but not limited to the following have been discussed: infection, erosion of the implant through the skin or urethra (possibly requiring removal of the implant and later inability to reimplant), malposition or suboptimal position of the implant, occasional severe pain in the surgical area, loss of penile sensation, mechanical failure of the implant (particularly with the inflatable implant resulting in removal of the implant), loss of remaining spontaneous erectile capabilities, and other risks of a general nature inherent in any type of surgical procedure such as: a bad reaction to anesthesia, contracting pneumonia, phlebitis, or dangers arising from existing heart problems.

(5) That this is an "irreversible" procedure that might require further surgery if complications or dissatisfaction should occur has been discussed.

(6) The patient's motivation and expectation as well as those of his partner, when appropriate, have been discussed and are believed to be realistic.

(7) That if scar tissue is present as a result of priapism, or other causes, then a suboptimal cosmetic result might follow injection of vasactive agents, has been discussed.

(8) That with respect to silicone, to date the benefits of these prostheses seem to outweigh by far any unforeseen long-term problems, has been discussed.

(9) That three-component inflatable implants with an abdominal reservoir and tubes in the abdomen can be injured during subsequent abdominal surgery has been discussed.

(10) The fact that the durability and long-term biocompatibility of materials of any implant is not completely known has been stressed.

(11) That antibiotic prophylaxis should be considered in the future prior to any type of surgery has been discussed.

I CERTIFY THAT I HAVE READ AND FULLY UNDERSTAND THE ABOVE AND HAVE RECEIVED A COPY OF THIS DOCUMENT.

Date	Witness to Signature
Signature of Patient	Name of witness (printed or typed)
Name of patient (printed or typed)	Signature of physician

Multicomponent Inflatable Penile Prostheses

Multicomponent inflatable penile prostheses are appropriate for patients who desire the most natural appearing erection and flaccidity, patients who do not wish to have constant corporal hardness, and some patients who require multiple endoscopic procedures. Inappropriate patients are those who lack manual dexterity needed to operate the device, are unwilling or unable to learn how to operate the device, and have severe pelvic scarring or abnormalities of the abdomen that preclude implantation of a reservoir into the paravesical space although it may be placed into the flank. A three-piece inflatable penile prosthesis might be contraindicated in patients with adhesions of the pelvic organs resulting in bowel fixation that may result in reservoir migration into the bladder or bowel.[17] Some paraplegic patients are good candidates for multicomponent or unitary inflatable penile prostheses. However, quadraplegic patients due to absence of manual dexterity are rarely candidates for inflatable prostheses unless they have a sexual partner to activate the device.

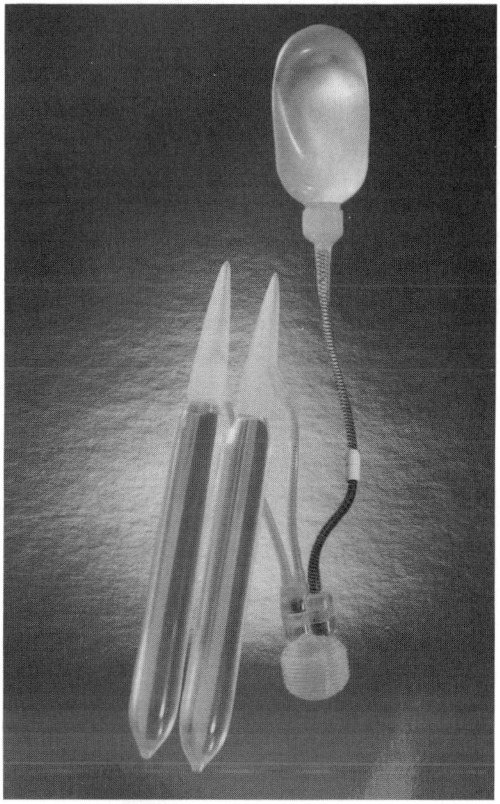

Figure 3-2 Alpha I inflatable penile prosthesis. (Courtesy of Mentor Corporation, Goleta, California.)

Mentor Penile Prostheses

Alpha I Inflatable Penile Prosthesis

The Mentor Alpha I three-piece multicomponent inflatable prosthesis, introduced in May 1989, was the first three-piece device that required only one connector between the pump and reservoir (Figure 3-2). The cylinders are preattached to the pump. This device consists of two cylinders constructed of Bioflex, a polyurethane elastomer, that are fully inflatable to the tip. They have significantly higher tensile strength than silicone and are extremely erosion resistant that minimizes mechanical failure due to aneurysm or cylinder abrasion. It has a separate abdominal reservoir and an intrascrotal pump. Maximal girth expansion of each cylinder is 22 mm. It has a lifetime replacement policy. The list price is $3,775.00.

Mark II Inflatable Penile Prosthesis

This multicomponent single two-piece inflatable penile prosthesis, introduced in 1988, uses a fully preassembled and connectorless system (Figure 3-3). The Bioflex cylinders are connected to an intrascrotal inflate/deflate Resipump (a single unit reservoir and pump) with a fluid injection port. The cylinder lengths range from 12 to 22 cm and produce excellent girth, rigidity, and flaccidity. Two different volume Resipumps are available, a 20 ml capacity for shorter length cylinders and a 25 ml capacity for longer length cylinders. Normal saline is injected into the Resipump through a penetrable injection port on the inferior aspect. Surgical implantation is relatively simple and considerably easier than implantation of a three-piece prosthesis that requires placement of a reservoir into the abdomen. Technical ease of implantation results in less potential for operative injury to the cylinders. The ability for transcrotal injection of fluid into the Resipump permits postoperative fluid adjustment. These devices are ideal for most patients, particularly patients with an average or slightly smaller than normal penis where an excessive amount of fluid need not be transferred. However, for the patient with a long and wide penis requiring more fluid than can be accommodated in the Mark II prosthesis, a three-piece inflatable prosthesis might be desirable. It is not advisable to implant the Mark II prosthesis in a patient with a long and wide penis who has had a failed three-piece prosthesis due to possible unsatisfaction with the rigidity obtained from the limited amount of fluid in the Resipump. It has a lifetime replacement policy. The list price is $3,750.00. Patient satisfaction with this device exceeds 90%.

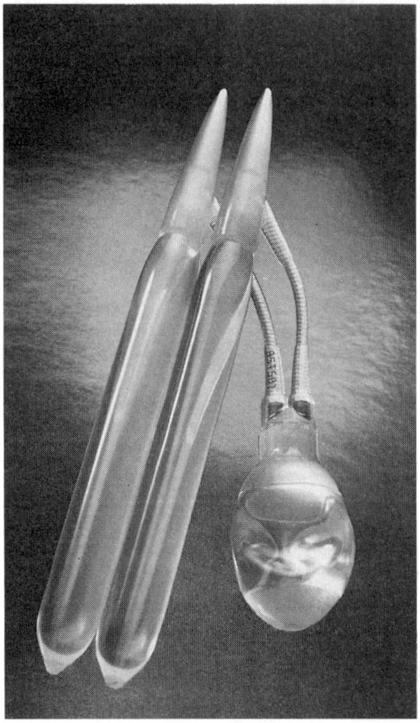

Figure 3-3 Mark II inflatable penile prosthesis. (Courtesy of Mentor Corporation, Goleta, California.)

Acu-Form Penile Prosthesis

This malleable prosthesis is easily positioned and almost eliminates spring-back (Figure 3-4). This prosthesis requires trimming at indicated lengths and capping with a tail cap. The distal end is blunt and soft. There have been no reported mechanical failures. It has a lifetime replacement policy. The list price is $1,695.00.

Mentor Malleable

This malleable prosthesis is similar to the Acu-Form (Figure 3-5). It has a lifetime replacement policy. The list price is $1,450.00.

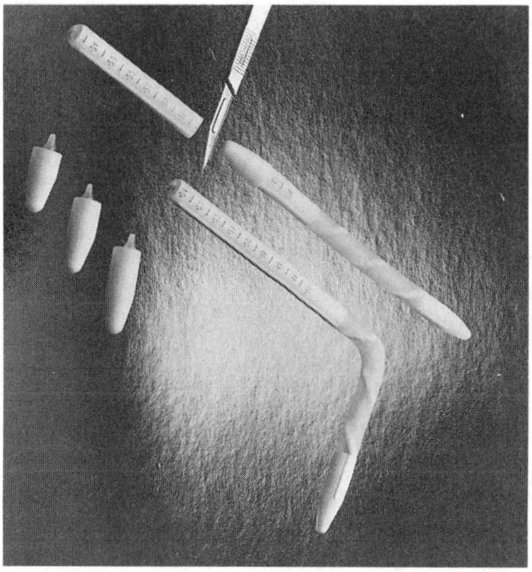

Figure 3-4 Acu-Form malleable penile prosthesis. (Courtesy of Mentor Corporation, Goleta, California.)

Dacomed Penile Prostheses

Dura-II Prosthesis

This second-generation prosthesis, introduced in 1992, may be the premiere malleable implant because no other malleable device provides the degree of positionability and concealment that the Duraphase Prosthesis has in the past (Figure 3-6).[18] This device consists of a cylinder body of 10 or 12 mm diameter and proximal and distal tips. It may be implanted by a subcoronal or penoscrotal approach. Surgical technique is simple. With this prosthesis an excellent cosmetic result may be expected and no spring-back is noted. Its axial rigidity is excellent and it can be positioned in the upright or dependant state with one hand. Patient and partner satisfaction is superior. This prosthesis is ideal for patients who (1) do not wish an inflatable prosthesis, (2) wish a less expensive device, (3) lack the manual dexterity

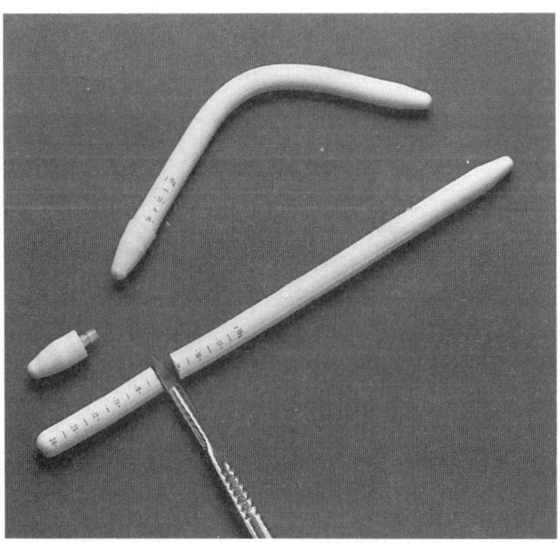

Figure 3-5 Mentor malleable. (Courtesy of Mentor Corporation, Goleta, California.)

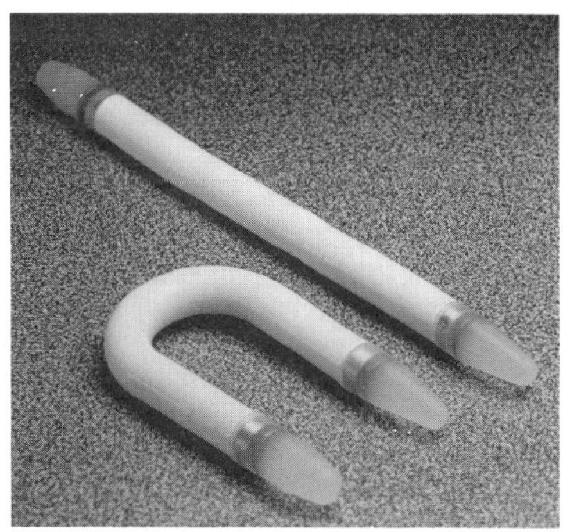

Figure 3-6 Dura-II prosthesis. (Courtesy of Dacomed Corporation, Minneapolis, Minnesota.)

or intellectual capability to utilize a more complex device, or (4) have spinal cord injury and require a prosthesis for erectile dysfunction or condom catheter use. It has a limited lifetime warranty. The list price is $2,295.00.

American Medical Systems Penile Prostheses

AMS 700 Series

The AMS 700 Series include the 700 CX, 700 CXM, 700 Ultrex, and 700 Ultrex Plus. These multicomponent inflatable penile prostheses are silicone-elastomer prostheses. Each device consists of the following components: a scrotally located inflate/deflate pump, a spherical seamless reservoir, and a pair of controlled expansion cylinders. These prostheses have a limited warranty policy.

700 CX and 700 CXM

The 700 CX prosthesis is a three-piece inflatable prosthesis (Figure 3-7). The cylinders are 3-ply—an inner silicone surface, a middle woven fabric surface, and an outer silicone surface. They are available in various lengths and have rear-tip extenders. The cylinders have controlled girth expansion from 12 to 18 mm. Due to the three-ply construction the risk of cylinder buckling and aneurysmal dilatation is minimized making them ideal for implantation in patients with a weakened tunica albuginea. The reservoir is placed in the paravesical space. These cylinders provide excellent rigidity and girth. The 700 CXM prosthesis is used for patients who have a short and narrow penis. The complete device price is $3,595.00.

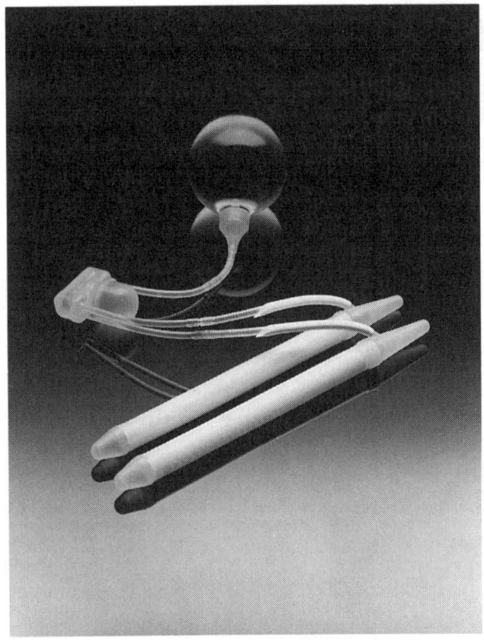

Figure 3-7 AMS inflatable 700CX™ penile prosthesis. (Courtesy of American Medical Systems, Inc., Minnetonka, Minnesota. Medical Illustrations by Michael Schenk.)

700 Ultrex

The 700 Ultrex prosthesis is similar to the 700 CX but after maximal girth expansion of the cylinders they lengthen by up to 20%. This tissue expander effect is limited only by tissue elasticity and the patient's ability to fully inflate the device. This feature is particularly valuable because after a period of time increased corporal pliability frequently occurs sometimes resulting in a suboptimal erection. The ability of fluid to extend into the expandable tip obviates this problem and if the corpora are slightly undersized during insertion of the cylinders, the expandable cylinder tip will fill the fractional distances within the corpora. This feature is not available with other prostheses. However, due to this phenomena, the Ultrex prosthesis should not be used for reconstructive surgery such as Peyronie's Disease but rather the AMS 700 CX or a Mentor multicomponent prosthesis should be used. The complete device price is $3,595.00.

700 Ultrex Plus

This prosthesis differs from the 700 Ultrex in that the 700 Ultrex Plus comes with the inflate/deflate pump and cylinders already prepared and preconnected, and the reservoir is prepared with normal saline so that fluid only needs to be removed before inserting the reservoir into the paravesical space (Figure 3-8). Only one connector is utilized between the pump and reservoir. The complete device price is $3,895.00.

Cylinders that are preassembled, prepared, and preconnected without connectors or with only one connector decrease the chance for damage to the device during preparation in the operating room or subsequent connector problems such as leakage, and decrease operative time that may also decrease the incidence of infection.

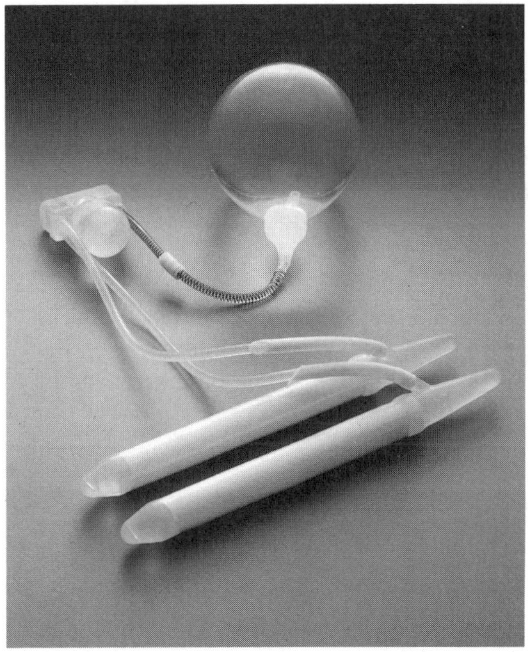

Figure 3-8 AMS inflatable 700 Ultrex Plus penile prosthesis. (Courtesy of American Medical Systems, Inc., Minnetonka, Minnesota. Medical Illustrations by Michael Schenk.)

Dynaflex

This unitary self-contained inflatable penile prosthesis, introduced in 1990, consists of two cylinders (Figure 3-9). It is available in two diameters with the reservoir and pump integral to the cylinders. It presents several desirable features: (1) ease of surgical insertion, (2) absence of extra penile parts, (3) easy inflation due to the long pump inflation control surface at the distal end, and (4) a time-delay release valve that virtually eliminates inadvertent deflation. Inflation is accomplished by pressing the inflation area under the glans several times and deflation by flexing the prosthesis for 10 seconds. These prostheses are prefilled to a fluid volume appropriate to each cylinder size. Therefore, no fluid adjustment is necessary. Rear-tip extenders are available. Erections attained with this device may not be as full or as firm as with the multicomponent devices. It has a limited warranty policy. The price of this device is $3,570.00.

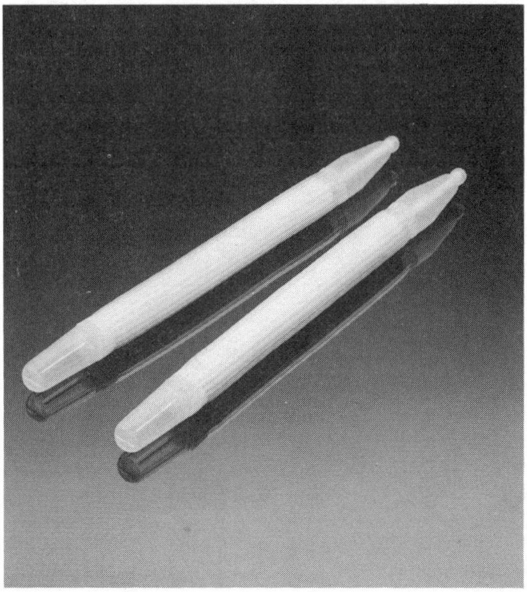

Figure 3-9 AMS Dynaflex penile prosthesis. (Courtesy of American Medical Systems, Inc., Minnetonka, Minnesota. Medical Illustrations by Michael Schenk.)

Malleable 600 and Malleable 600 M

The Malleable 600 prosthesis, introduced in 1983, provides various diameters and lengths by removal of the silicone jacket and rear-tip extenders (Figure 3-10). Each rod has a stainless steel core wrapped with synthetic fibers and covered with silicone. While this prosthesis is permanently firm, the malleability allows the patient to bend it to a comfortable position while the enhanced rigidity allows positioning without buckling during intercourse. However, with larger diameter and longer prostheses concealment may be a problem. The Malleable 600 M prosthesis is identical to the 600 but is for patients with narrower corpora. It has a limited warranty policy. The price of this device is $1,425.00.

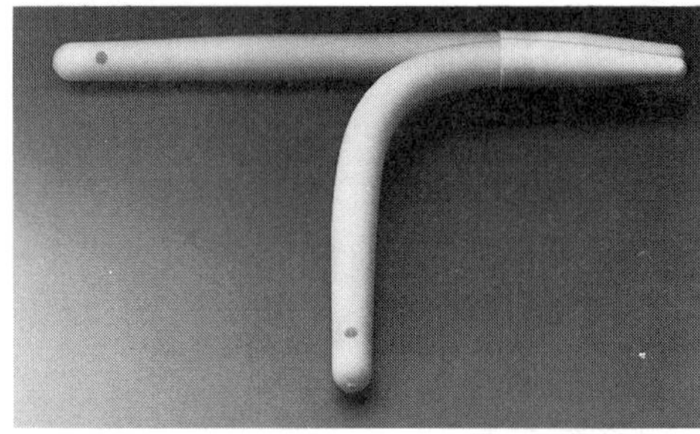

Figure 3-10 AMS malleable 600^{TM} penile prosthesis. (Courtesy of American Medical Systems, Inc., Minnetonka, Minnesota. Medical Illustrations by Michael Schenk.)

Local and Regional Anesthesia

While most patients prefer general anesthesia, local penile anesthesia may be accomplished with or without instillation of anesthetic agent into the corpora cavernosa. Intravenous injection should be avoided and total dosage must be closely monitored. It may be combined with a pudendal nerve block. A tourniquet may be placed around the base of the penis or perineal pressure may be applied and the corpora infiltrated with 0.25% Lidocaine solution using a 23-G scalp vein needle. Ideally an anesthesiologist should be on standby.

The author favors a 1:1 mixture of 0.5% Bupavicaine and 1% of Lidocaine without epinephrine because Lidocaine provides a rapid onset of anesthesia and bupavicaine obviates the need for narcotic analgesic for the first 6 hours after surgery. Intracorporal infiltration of anesthesia is not used. When using Bupavicaine care should be taken to aspirate prior to injection to ensure that it is not injected into the systemic circulation, i.e., the corpora cavernosa. If the patient has large venous leakage Bupavicaine should not be used. The author's technique of local penile anesthesia and pudendal nerve block is illustrated in Operative Report Number I. After adequate anesthesia an infrapubic, penoscrotal or penile shaft incision may be made. If a Foley catheter is used 2% Lidocaine jelly may be inserted into the urethra. Local anesthesia may not be appropriate in patients who are anxious, have cardiovascular problems, lung disease, or other significant medical problems.

Table 3-3 Preoperative Orders for Penile Prosthesis Implantation

Betadine shower HS and AM before OR
Ancef or Kefzol 1 g iv, 1 hour before OR
Tobramycin 80 mg iv, 1 hour before surgery
(If patient is allergic to penicillin, RX vancomycin 500 mg, iv piggy-back, Q6H instead of Ancef or Kefzol)
Fleets enema AM before OR, before AM Betadine shower
Shave and prep pubis, perineum, abdomen in OR
NPO after midnight day before OR
Urine culture on admission

Outpatient Implantation of Penile Prostheses

All types of prostheses can be implanted in an outpatient setting using an infrapubic or penoscrotal incision, including the three-piece multicomponent inflatable prosthesis with a reduction in costs compared to inpatient surgery.[19] Outpatient implantation is safe and may reduce the incidence of infection. The anesthesia may be general, spinal, regional, or local. Many urologists, however, prefer to admit the patient to the hospital to observe him for 24 to 48 hours postoperatively and to give 48 hours of prophylactic intravenous antibiotics. The author's preoperative and postoperative orders are noted in Tables 3-3 and 3-4. Sexual intercourse is prohibited for 4 to 6 weeks after implantation.

Intraoperative Considerations for All Penile Prostheses

Surgical Technique

While implant techniques are essentially standardized, familiarity with specialized instruments and the ability to adapt technique to anatomical variations and intraoperative problems is essential to attain a high success rate.

Technical considerations necessary for successful results include (1) accurate selection of appropriate length and diameter prosthesis, (2) adequate dilation of the entire corpora and separation of distal corporal septations when present, (3) avoiding intraoperative complications, (4) use of long-term absorbable suture, and (5) correct location of corporotomy sites. Distal dilatation should always be at least 1 cm greater than the width of the prosthesis. Proximal dilatation generally need not exceed 9 Hagar. In order to prevent perforations, dilators smaller than 9 mm should not be used.

Incisions

While the subcoronal, dorsal penile and perineal incisions are used, most implanting urologists prefer either the penoscrotal or infrapubic incision depending on the type of prosthesis implanted. The penoscrotal approach is ideal for implantation of noninflatable prostheses, unitary inflatable prostheses,

Table 3-4 Postoperative Orders for Implantation of Penile Prosthesis

Recovery room VS, then Q 8 hours	
Resume preoperative diet when fully awake after nausea	
Ivs: D/5% 1/3 NS to run 100 ml/hour	
Insert heparin lock	
D/C iv when diet well tolerated	
Ice packs to scrotum × 48 hours	
TED stockings × 3 days	
OOB and ambulate in AM	
Medications:	Demerol 50–75 mg im, Q 3–4 hours, PRN pain
	Phenergan 25 mg im, Q 4–6 hours PRN, N or V
	Tylenol #3, 1 TAB PO Q3 hours, PRN pain
	Dalmane 30 mg, PO, H.S. PRN sleep
	Laxative of choice, PRN constipation
	Tobramycin 80 mg, iv or im, Q8 hours × 48 hours[a]
	(If patient allergic to penicillin, RX Vancomycin 500 mg, iv piggy-back, Q 6 hours instead of Ancef or Kefzol)[a]
	May shower 5th postoperative day
	No tub baths or soaks
	No scrotal supports if scrotal device present
	No bandages or ointments to wound
	Daily BUN and creatinine
	If not void by ________ call House Physician/Resident to insert Foley—leave in
Discharge Medication:	1. Keflex or Velosef or Ceclor 500 mg PO QID × 14 D
	2. If allergic to penicillin: RX Vibramycin 100 mg PO Q 12 H × 14 D
Renal transplant pt.—antibiotics	
Cefobid 1 g iv Q 12 hours × 48 hours	
Vancomycin 500 mg iv Q 6–Q 12 hours × 48 hours	

[a] If patient not afebrile for 48 hours, continue iv antibiotics.

and many believe for multicomponent inflatable penile prostheses, and in patients in whom one expects difficult cavernosal dilatation. With this incision a more proximal corporotomy may be made with the option to extend it as far proximally and distally as necessary. Indeed, virtually the entire corpora can be exposed through this incision. It may also be the approach of choice in the obese patient and when extensive corporal reconstruction is necessary. The Scott Ring Retractor with elastic stays and hooks is very useful. When the three-piece multicomponent inflatable penile prosthesis is placed through a penoscrotal approach the Scott Reservoir Insertor or a long nasal speculum may be used to insert the reservoir through the inguinal canal into the paravesical space. Occasionally herniation of the reservoir may occur. With the infrapubic incision no pressure dressing is used due to the increased chance of significant penile or scrotal edema.

Infection Control

In order to reduce the possibility of intraoperative infection the following is important: immediate skin shave and preparation should take place in the operating room, operating room traffic should be limited, and the prosthesis should be soaked in an antibiotic solution. The surgeon and assistant apply a light layer of Betadine to their hands prior to gloving. No drains are used. An intraoperative antibiotic solution is used to irrigate the corpora and exposed tissues that consists of a solution of 1 g of Kanamycin and 50,000 units of Bacitracin in 1 liter of saline.

Dilamezinsert

The rounded or pointed tip dilamezinsert instrument reduces operating time and is particularly useful for intracorporal measurement and for uniform dilatation to approximately 13 Hagar in patients with a wide penis. This prosthesis utilizes a plastic stretching blade that with one pass eliminates multiple passages that may occur with multiple passes of the Hagar, Pratt or Mentor dilators. This instrument may also be used for passage of the Keith needle attached to the cylinder tip suture. However, many implanting urologists prefer to use the Furlow Insertor for this maneuver due to complete control of the needle tip.

Special Considerations for Implantation of Multicomponent Inflatable Penile Prostheses

Frog-Leg Position of Armboard for Feet Extension at Foot of Table

When using a multicomponent inflatable penile prosthesis with a scrotal pump or reservoir/pump and the infrapubic approach, a frog-leg position of the lower extremities or placement of armboards at the foot of the table for the patient's feet facilitates access to the scrotum. Alternatively, the frog-leg position, utilizing a sandbag placed on the lateral aspect at the break of the knees with the heels together or by placing several rolled sheets transversely under the knees, permits easy access to the scrotum.

Infrapubic Incision

The infrapubic incision is preferred for implantation of multicomponent inflatable penile prosthesis due to the following: (1) there is virtually no possibility of urethral injury, (2) the tubing can be concealed under the subpubic fat, (3) inflation and deflation of the device can take place soon due to the absence of a scrotal incision, (4) skin and subcutaneous elastic stays with hooks are not necessary, lessening the possibility of cylinder damage, and (5) stirrups are not required, decreasing the O.R. setup time.

In the author's opinion this approach is ideal for the insertion of two-piece and three-piece multicomponent inflatable penile prosthesis, allowing placement of the reservoir into the paravesical space under direct vision and easy placement of the pump or reservoir/pump into the scrotum.

Corporotomy Placement

When implanting a multicomponent inflatable penile prosthesis, the corporotomy incision should be as far proximal as technically feasible to conceal the input tubing and input tubing junction beneath the subpubic fat (infrapubic approach) or beneath the pubis (penoscrotal approach) and to conceal the cylinder crease sometimes noted with the Bioflex cylinder in patients with a thin penis. The input tubing should exit the tunica albuginea directly at the most proximal aspect of the corporotomy to avoid cylinder and tubing abrasion.

Air Evacuation

Virtually all the air should be removed from the system prior to implantation. With the cylinder input tubing junction toward the ceiling evacuation of air bubbles is easily accomplished. The pump or reservoir/pump should also be tilted so that the air bubble is toward the ceiling and easily evacuated.

Cylinder Fluid Volume

Particularly with two-piece multicomponent inflatable penile prostheses, it is essential that the maximum amount of fluid that is consistent with an ideal cosmetic result both in the erect and flaccid state to permit maximum rigidity and optimum flaccidity be selected. Reference to the fluid fill instruction guidelines of the manufacturer is advisable.

Rear Tip Extenders

The longest cylinders possible should be implanted to prevent the input tubing and rigid part of the prosthesis from being palpable on the penile shaft and possibly interferring with patient utilization and cosmetic result. Rear-tip extenders should be used only as necessary. As a result, more of the collapsable inflatable cylinder is positioned in the pendulous penis resulting in maximal dependency and an optimal cosmetic result in the deflated flaccid state.

Difficult Cylinder Insertion

If insertion of the second cylinder to midglans level is difficult, deflation of both cylinders and placement of a rubber shod clamp over the tubing of the *in vivo* cylinder will allow space for the second cylinder, which may then be inserted by simply inserting the inflated cylinder into the contralateral corpus using standard technique. Removal of the rubber-shod clamp and inflation of both cylinders will usually result in optimal distension of both corpora. If it is difficult to insert the proximal part of the cylinder, a Kelly clamp with its tip grasping and pointing to the tip of the prosthesis may allow easy insertion. Alternatively, if rear-tip extenders are used, placement of the largest rear-tip extender in the proximal corpus first, after which the rigid proximal part of the cylinder can easily be slipped into the rear-tip extender.[20]

Scott Reservoir Insertor

The Scott Reservoir Inserter, used during the penoscrotal approach, is designed to carry the reservoir of a three-piece multicomponent inflatable penile prosthesis safely through the inguinal canal into the paravesical space with minimal trauma.

Operative Report Number I

Insertion of DuraPhase Penile Prosthesis

The patient was prepped in the low lithotomy position after which a penile block and pudendal block were obtained utilizing 1% Lidocaine and 0.5% Marcaine in equal volumes. The penile block was accomplished using a 25-G 1.5-in. needle by injecting infrapubically 5 ml under Buck's faschia on the left and 5 ml on the right, after which each spermatic cord was infiltrated with 5 ml of the solution. Following this a pudendal block was accomplished after inserting a finger into the rectum and palpating the ischial tuberosities. After making a skin wheel using a 15-cm 25-G needle, 10 ml of the solution was injected medial and anterior to the ischial tuberosity on each side and then toward the scrotum in a fan-like fashion anesthetizing the pudendal nerve and its branches. Adequate anesthesia was then noted.

The patient was reprepped and draped. A Scott Ring Retractor was placed over the genitalia. Following instillation of 5 ml of Betadine ointment into the urethra, a 12 French 5 ml

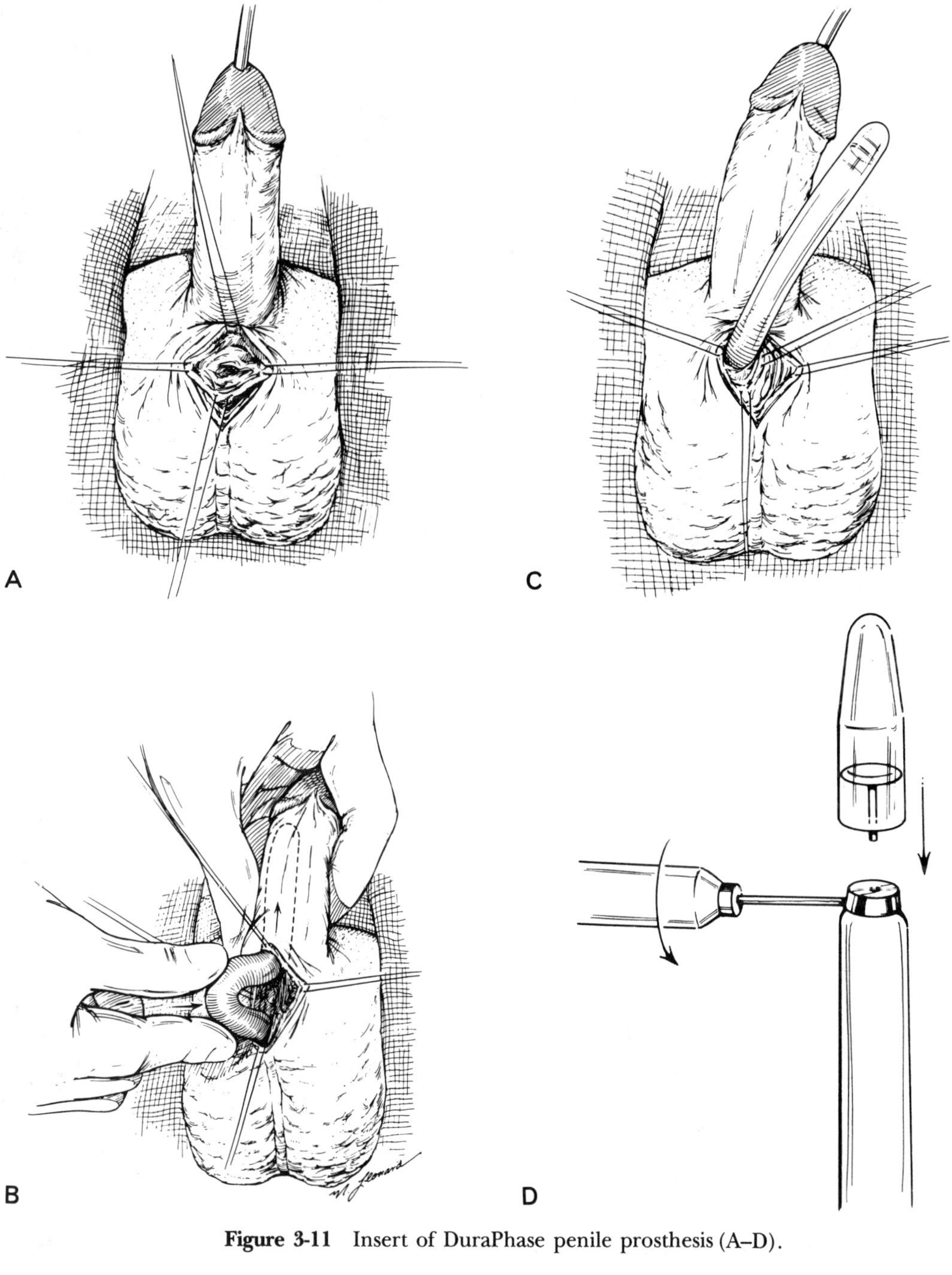

Figure 3-11 Insert of DuraPhase penile prosthesis (A–D).

Foley catheter with 10 ml in the balloon was passed into the bladder. Four milliliters of the anesthetic solution was then used to anesthetize the scrotal raphe at the penoscrotal junction. Anesthesia was complete.

The pubis to midglans measurement was 10 cm. A 3-cm midline raphe incision was made. Using sharp and blunt dissection the corpora on each side were identified and Buck's fascia was incised and tunica albuginea was clearly visualized. The urethra was visualized and the Foley catheter palpated. A stay suture of 0-Prolene was placed on the left side approximately 1 cm lateral to the urethra and another stay suture was placed 1 cm lateral to the first. An identical procedure was performed on the contralateral side. Using a 15 blade scalpel and a Pott's scissors a generous corporotomy measuring approximately 7 cm was made on each side. No intracorporal anesthesia was necessary.

Using the Dialamezinsert instrument a distal measurement of 7 cm was noted and the dilation was performed in one pass. The proximal measurement was 10 cm and was also performed in one pass with slightly less dilatation. An identical procedure was performed on the contralateral side with the same measurements obtained. The Scott Ring Retractor stay hooks were utilized throughout the procedure for exposure and were particularly valuable at the most proximal aspect of the corporotomy by holding it up and open for insertion of the prosthesis.

Reference to the company provided sizing chart indicated that a 2 cm tip was necessary proximally and a 2 cm tip was necessary distally. The tips were attached to a 12-mm-diameter body using a Hex wrench in the standard fashion. Copious corporal and wound irrigation were performed throughout the procedure. The prosthesis was soaked in antibiotic solution. Two large straight sounds (36 French) were simultaneously inserted distally. Dorsal to ventral palpation between the sounds revealed a satisfactory space between them. The prostheses were then inserted without difficulty.

Confirmation of the correct location was made by palpation proximally outside the corpora toward the crus and also outside the corpora distally as well as careful palpation of the midglans, noting that the tips were identically located, bilaterally equal, and symmetrical. Upward axial rigidity was excellent and no bowing was present on the downward phase. It appeared that an ideal cosmetic result was obtained. The corpora were closed with interrupted sutures of 3-0 PDS. Subcutaneous tissue was closed with a 3-0 plain gut and the skin was closed with a subcuticulous stitch of 4-0 Vicryl. Steri-strips and a Telfa dressing was applied.

Operative Report II

Insertion of Mentor Mark II Inflatable Penile Prosthesis

The patient was placed on the operating room table in the supine position with the lower extremities in a frog-leg position. Following induction of general anesthesia the lower abdomen and genitoperineal area were shaved and prepped with Betadine and draped in the usual sterile fashion. After this a 5-cm infrapubic transverse incision was made using a 15 scalpel blade two finger breadths above the base of the penis. The incision was carried through subcutaneous tissue and Scarpa's fascia. Hemastasis was achieved with electrocartery.

Sharp and blunt dissection was used to expose the tunica albuginea of the corpus cavernosum of each side of the midline after identifying the suspensory ligament and midline neurovascular structures. Care was taken not to disturb the neurovascular structures. Using sharp dissection Buck's fascia was incised for approximately 4 cm. The tunica albuginea was then dissected as far proximally as technically feasible. Following exposure of each corpus cavernosum, a Allis clamp was placed on the tunica albuginea 2 cm lateral to the midline structures. Two 0-Prolene stay sutures, 1 cm apart, replaced each Allis clamp. An identical procedure was performed on the contralateral side. The left corpus cavernosum was then incised between the stay sutures with a 15 scalpel blade. The corporotomy was extended proximally using Pott's scissors. Proximally number 9 Hagar dilators and then 10 Hagar dilators were used. Each corpus was then serially dilated distally to midglanular level with 10 Hagar then 11 Hagar dilators. However, some distal tightness was noted under the glans. Therefore, a long, blunt Mayo scissor was inserted obliquely, to avoid injury to the urethra, to spread the fibrous tissue within the glanular area. The Mayo scissor tips were placed slightly distal to the area of restriction, opened, and then locked with a finger at the fulcrum while retracting the scissors. Following this maneuver it was easy to place the 12 Hagar dilators to midglanular level. An identical procedure was performed on the contralateral side. Measurement of the distal left corpus cavernosum from the proximal aspect of the corporotomy to midglanular level was 14 cm. The intracorporal measurement from the proximal aspect of the corporotomy to the crus was 7 cm. Total intracorporal length was 21 cm. The identical measurement was obtained on the right side. Following this, using the company provided sizing chart, a 18-cm prosthesis and a 3-cm rear-tip extender was selected. These were placed in antibacterial solution. The corpora were then copiously irrigated with antibacterial solution.

All air was evacuated from the cylinder and Resipump in the standard fashion using the Quick Fill guidelines provided by the manufacturer. Following these instructions 56 ml of normal saline was injected into the Resipump injection port and cylinders. The entire prosthesis was then cycled several times to ensure good operation. Cylinder tip sutures were inserted through the left and right side of the glans with the Keith needles and the Furlow insertion tool was used in the standard fashion before the cylinders were drawn through into the distal corpora in the deflated state then inflated to hydraulically dilate the corpora. Both cylinders were then deflated. The rear-tip extenders were inserted first into the proximal corpora. These maneuvers aided in insertion of the proximal ends into the proximal corpora. After placement of both prostheses an additional 3 ml of fluid was added to the Resipump in order to create what appeared to be optimal rigidity and flaccidity of the penis. The tips of the cylinders were then palpated at midglanular level. The tubing exited at a right angle from the most proximal aspect of the corporotomy. Both corporotomies were closed with the cylinders in the flaccid position with interrupted 3-0 PDS sutures that had been preplaced. After closure of the corpora inspection of the function of the device revealed that inflation produced bilateral good rigidity and deflation satisfactory flaccidity. The cylinders were inflated. The wound was again copiously irrigated with antibacterial solution.

The Resipump was placed in the midaspect of the right hemiscrotum in the most dependant position after blunt digital scrotal dissection creating a subdartos scrotal pocket. The scrotal compartment was copiously irrigated with antibacterial solution. After placement of the Resi-

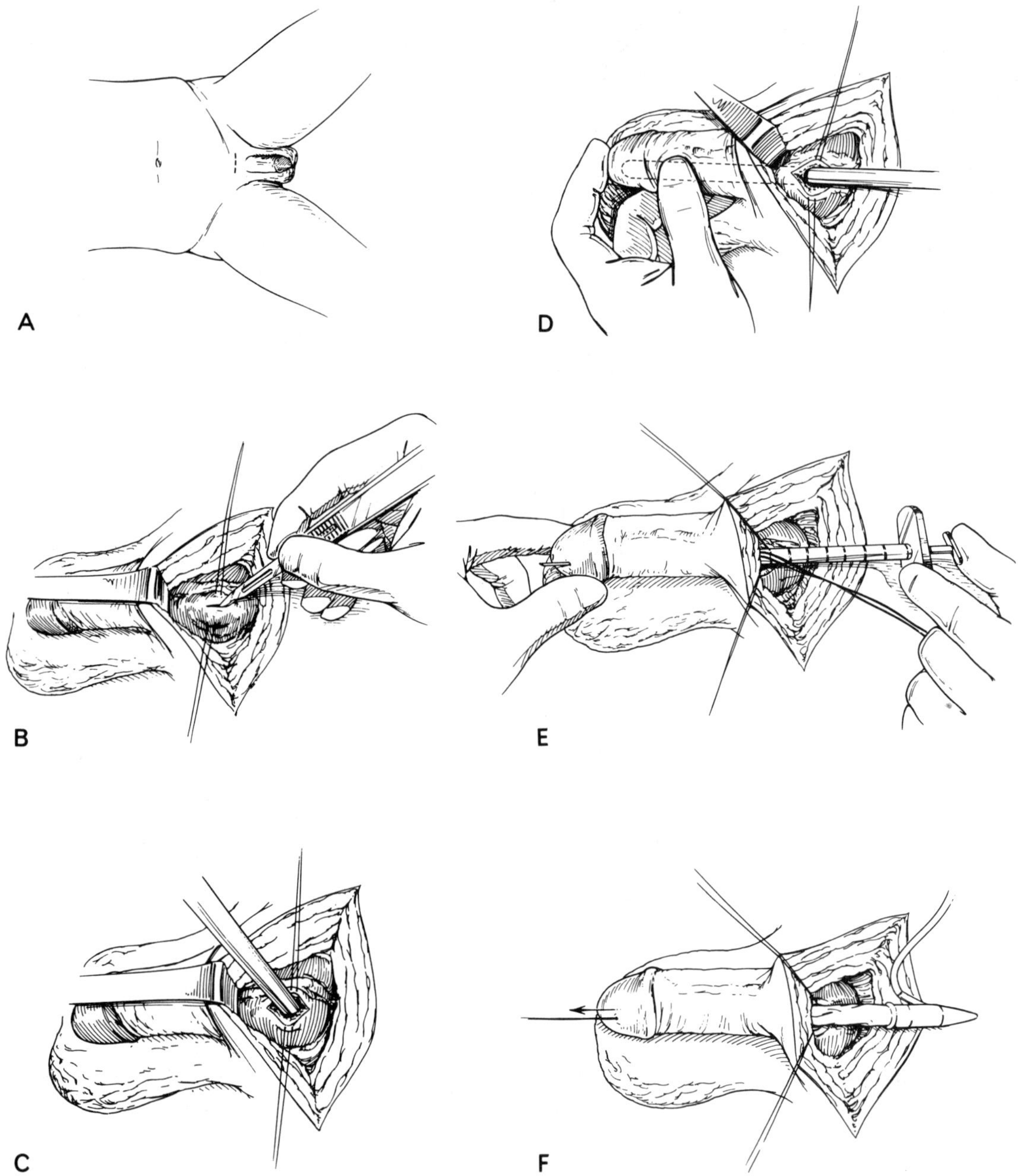

Figure 3-12 Insert of Mark II prosthesis (A–I).

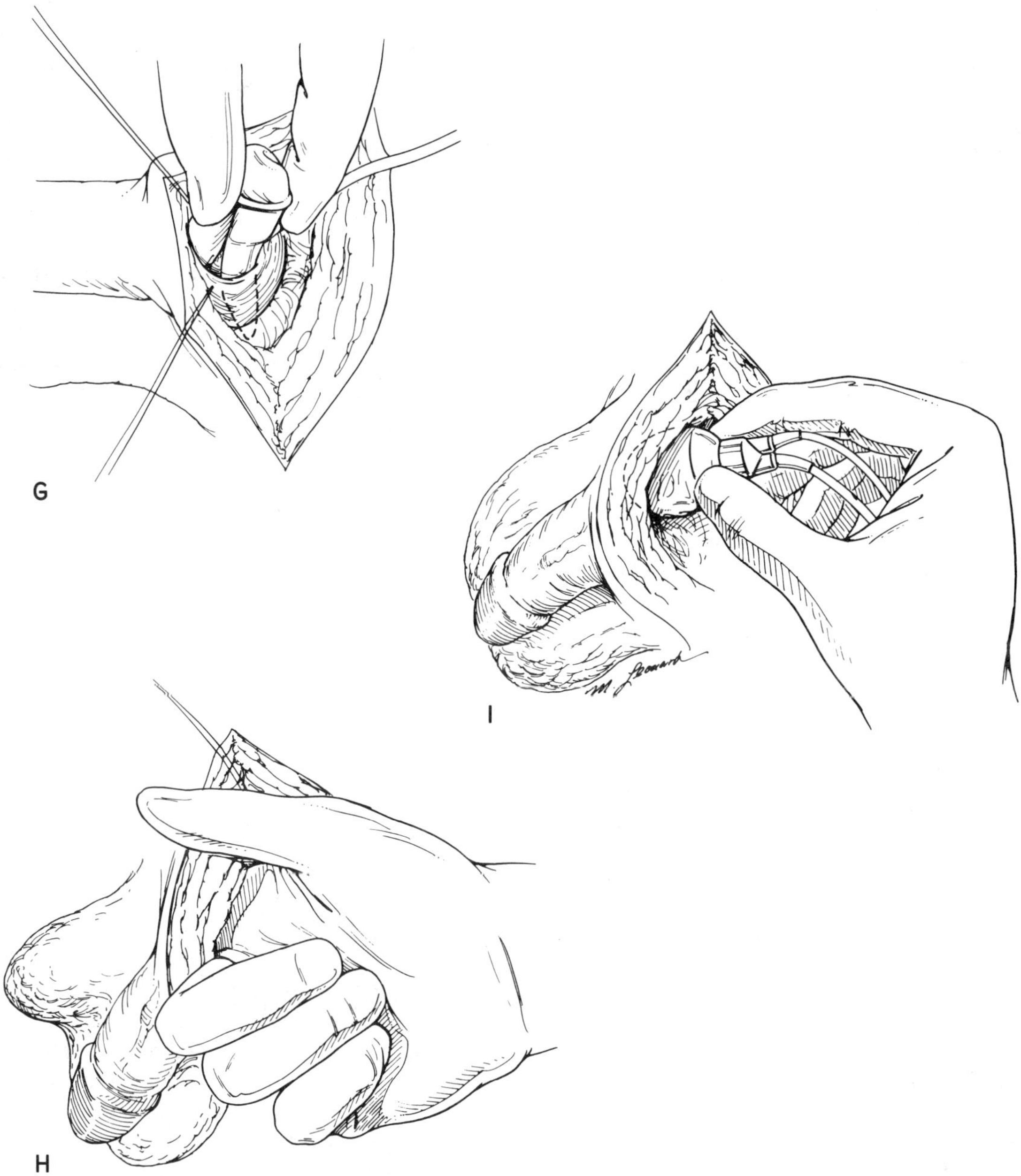

Figure 3-12 (continued)

pump the tubing was noted to lie smoothly without kinks. Several sutures of 3-0 plain gut were utilized to maintain the Resipump in the most dependant part of the hemiscrotum. The subcutaneous tissue was approximated in several layers with interrupted 3-0 plain gut sutures. The skin was closed with a running subcuticular 4-0 Vicryl suture. The cylinder tip sutures were cut and the device was left in the semiinflated state for hemostasis. Steri-strips were placed after which several layers of collodian were placed and finally a small Telfa dressing was applied to seal the incision.

Postoperative Management

Some urologists use Jackson-Pratt drains for 18 hours and the Trendelenberg position in patients that have a scrotal pump mechanism to prevent postoperative edema and hematoma. Postoperative discomfort is variable. Most patients require only mild anelgesics and many require none. Sexual intercourse and all strenuous activity that might result in contact with the prosthesis, incision, or components, must be avoided for 4 to 6 weeks after surgery.

Ideally the inflatable penile prosthesis should be cycled for the first month every second day by the patient and once a week by the urologist. The two-piece inflatable prosthesis should be left in the inflated state for approximately 30 minutes per day to allow for the fibrous pseudocapsule to form around the distended cylinders rather than the deflated cylinders. The device should be fully deflated at all other times so that a constricting pseudocapsule does not form around the reservoir/pump of the two-piece inflatable prosthesis. The unitary inflatable prosthesis should be left inflated for 4 to 6 weeks and taped to the abdomen to prevent constricting bands from developing in the corpora precluding optimal distension of the prosthesis. With the three-piece multicomponent inflatable prosthesis, the abdominal reservoir must be full for as much time as possible to allow for the fibrous pseudocapsule to form around the filled reservoir so that fluid restriction does not occur which would compromise cylinder deflation.

It is essential that followup visits be requested to determine the patient's ability to manipulate the device and to determine if he is utilizing the prosthesis correctly. If necessary, additional literature and instructions are given. Sometimes at a remote date further instruction is necessary due to patient reluctance, anxiety, fear, or marital problems precluding successful initial use of the device.

Postoperative Counselling

Sex Therapy

When first attempting intercourse after implantation some patients and their partners find use of the device unnatural and mechanical. However, most adjust without difficulty. Some patients notice a decrease in sexual desire and a difficulty with orgasm, usually due to not being fully aroused and failing to engage in foreplay prior to vaginal penetration, or as a result of psychological concerns. The sexual partner may note vaginal dryness due to anxiety or due to a lack of or too short a period of foreplay. Sometimes after implantation sexual techniques may need to be varied and new techniques learned. Gynecologic consultation may be indicated.

Complications

Due to relatively standardized surgical techniques, special instruments, antibiotic guidelines, and current generations of penile prostheses, a low incidence of complications has been attained.

Infection

The most serious complication resulting from implantation of a penile prosthesis is infection, which can occur in the immediate postoperative period or up to several years after implantation in spite of meticulous attention to surgical technique and prophylactic preoperative, intraoperative, and postoperative antibiotic coverage. Infection usually manifests as fixation of the skin to the prosthetic component or swelling of erythema prior to a purulent discharge. Extrusion and erosion of the prosthesis or component may follow. The incidence of prosthetic infection ranges between 2%[21] and 8%.[22]

Preoperative and Postoperative Antibiotic Regimens

Most prosthetic infections are due to staphylococcus epidermidis, acquired from the operating room environment or personnel. A smaller number are due to Gram-negative enteric species, noted in association with urinary tract infections, neurogenic bladder or an ileal conduit. Therefore, most prophylactic antibiotic regimens include an aminoglycoside to cover Gram-negative rods and a cephalosporin to cover Gram-positive cocci, or an aminoglycoside and vancomycin. Vancomycin may be substituted for cephalosporin in penicillin-allergic patients or in patients who might have a cephalosporin-resistant staphylococcus, and perhaps in diabetic patients due to their increased susceptability to *S. epidermidis.* Most prophylactic antibiotic regimens continue postoperatively with oral antibiotics for up to 1 or 2 weeks.[23]

Risk Factors

Risk factors predisposing to infection include (1) reoperation such as implant revision or reimplantation, (2) implantation in patients at risk of chronic urinary tract infections such as spinal cord injury patients or infection of the genitalia or intertrigenous areas such as in diabetic patients, (3) inadequate antibiotic coverage, (4) break in sterile technique, (5) protracted length of surgery, and (6) simultaneous placement of an artificial urinary sphincter.[22]

Infections in Spinal Cord Injury Patients

Patients with spinal cord injury have a significantly higher risk for prosthetic infections of about 15%[21] and have a higher incidence of erosion than the general population irrespective of the type of prosthesis used due to development of urinary tract infections and decubitus ulcers and because of lack of sensation of early signs of infection.[24] Some patients benefit from a prosthesis to facilitate intermittent catheterization or for condom management. In these cases a noninflatable prosthesis might be appropriate recognizing the erosion rate of up to 25%.[25] It does not appear that intermittent self-catheterization results in increased risk of infection.[26]

Infection in Diabetic Patients

Diabetic patients are at no greater risk of infection following penile implantation than nondiabetic patients if they are under optimal diabetic control.[27] The glycosalated hemoglobin value is useful to evaluate long-term glucose control prior to implantation. A level greater than 11% indicates poor control and a 10% risk of infection, whereas only 5% of patients develop infections if the diabetes is adequately controlled.[28]

Infection in Immunosuppressed Patients

Immunosuppressed renal transplant recipients who are impotent are suitable candidates for penile prosthesis implantation because there does not appear to be an increased incidence of infection or erosion of the prosthesis.[29] Necessary precautions include extended postoperative intravenous antibiotic therapy and increased steroid coverage, in addition to the routine preoperative, intraoperative, and postoperative antibiotic management.

Device Malfunction or Device-Related

Silicone prostheses may shed silicone particles that can be found in the fibrous capsule and draining lymph nodes. However, it appears that the benefits of these prostheses outweigh any long-term problems.[30]

Inflatable Penile Prostheses

Prior to 1981 the failure rate of the American Medical Systems multicomponent inflatable prosthesis had as high as a 61% overall 5-year complication rate of which 38% were due to fluid leak.[31] With the latest generations of inflatable prostheses, cylinder and reservoir fluid leaks, and cylinder aneurysm and pump failure are exceedingly rare.

With earlier models reoperation rates due to device failure varied between 14 and 44%.[32,33] Today it is estimated that the mechanical failure rates of multicomponent inflatable prostheses is less than 5% for the first 5 years after implantation.

Noninflatable Penile Prostheses

The major device-related problems with the noninflatable prostheses are due to their rigidity. Erosion and extrusion of the prosthesis through the penis, glans, or urethra, particularly in spinal cord-injured patients due to their lack of sensation and increased incidence of pressure necrosis may occur, particularly if the prosthesis is oversized. Mechanical malfunction such as fracture or internal derangement has also been noted with noninflatable prostheses.[34] As with inflatable prostheses, recent design modifications and introduction of superior prostheses have reduced the incidence of device failure and increased the percentage of patients satisfied with these types of prostheses. The failure rate of noninflatable prostheses is estimated at less than 5% over 5 years.

Furthermore, it may be expected that in the next 10 to 20 years, 10 to 25% of patients having a current generation inflatable or noninflatable device implanted will require reoperation due to device failure.

Technical

Oversizing

Oversizing of the prosthesis or incorrect prosthesis placement, particularly of noninflatable prostheses, may produce pain, bowing of the penis, and erosion of the prosthesis into the urethra, tunica albuginea, glans, or crura. Inflatable prostheses have a lower erosion rate than noninflatable prostheses.

Undersizing

Undersizing of the prosthesis or proximal corporal perforation and prosthesis migration can result in a flexion deformity known as the SST deformity. It may be corrected by placement of the correct size prosthesis or plication of the tunica albuginea and glans.

Cavernosal Septum Crossover

Cavernosal septum disruption and prosthesis crossover proximally or distally and prosthesis disruption of the corporotomy incision may also occur. Cavernosal septal crossover usually occurs distally and only requires repositioning. If this situation is not recognized during placement of an inflatable prosthesis, a Keith needle may injure the first implanted cylinder during insertion of the second cylinder.

Crural or Proximal Tunical Albugineal Perforations

Perforation or erosion of the crus, or the proximal or distal tunica albuginea may be due to (1) intrinsically weak tunica albuginea, (2) overvigorous dilatation, (3) oversizing, (4) clinical or subclinical infection, and (5) fibrotic corpora. Usually proximal crural perforations may be suspected when total intracorporal length measurement reveals an asymmetry or when a "give" is felt during proximal dilatation. However, it may not be noted until postoperatively when proximal migration is detected. The prosthesis may be palpated in the perineum. If suspected and confirmed intraoperatively stabilization may be accomplished by (1) repositioning the prosthesis and bypassing the perforation, (2) intraoperative or postoperative repair with a Gore-tex (R) vascular graft fashioned into a cup or a single velour woven Dacron (R) graft fashioned into a sleeve sutured to normal tunica albuginea, (3) attaching a rear-tip extender to the albuginea with nonabsorbable sutures and inserting the proximal tip into the rear-tip extender, or (4) immediate perineal exploration and repair of the crura with prosthesis repositioning. Sexual intercourse should be postponed for 6 to 8 weeks after surgery.

Distal Urethral or Distal Albugineal Perforation or Erosion

Perforation into the urethra may be suspected with blood at the meatus and may be confirmed by cystoscopy. If this occurs implantation only on the other side should be performed. A Foley catheter should be used for urinary diversion or a trocar cystotomy tube. Reimplantation should be delayed for at least three to six months.

If the perforation of the distal tunica albuginea is noted at the time of surgery it can sometimes be corrected by suturing the defect and placement of a shorter prosthesis or preferably repositioning the prosthesis in a different track. Occasionally, perforation of the distal tunica albuginea is noted postoperatively. If the prosthesis is correctly positioned and the patient has no discomfort nothing else need be done.

Glanular Perforation

If glanular perforation occurs, a vascular graft cup or sleeve using Gore-tex (R) or Dacron (R) may be attached to the distal end of the prosthesis and sutured to normal tunica albuginea. However, explantation or corporoplasty without reimplantation may be necessary.

Treatment of Infected Penile Prostheses

Because a prosthetic infection usually occurs between the prosthesis and the pseudocapsule, infection with or without extrusion may mandate removal of the entire device. Various management strategies have been employed.

Immediate Prosthesis Removal and Delayed Reimplantation

Many urologists believe that infection of the prosthesis mandates immediate removal combined with irrigation and drainage of the corpora. With two-piece and three-piece multicomponent prostheses, the scrotum and possibly the paravesical space should be irrigated and drained. If the entire prosthesis is immediately removed reimplantation may be performed either after 6 to 8 weeks obviating the formation of dense fibrotic scarring precluding reimplantation at a later date, or in 3 to 6 months. At the latter date reimplantation may be exceedingly difficult and may require a full-length corporotomy with excision of fibrous tissue and Dacron (R) or Gore-tex (R) patch grafting.[35] If two prostheses cannot be inserted due to fibrosis, a satisfactory result may be obtained using only one prosthesis. Occasionally it is not possible to implant a prosthesis on either side.

The results obtained with delayed reimplantation are frequently inferior to those obtained from the original procedure due to loss of tissue pliability, penile length and cavernosal deformity. A functional implant and a satisfaction rate of approximately 60% may be expected.[36]

Immediate Prosthesis Removal and Early Reimplantation

An alternative approach is to remove the entire prosthesis, irrigate the infected area using DABS solution (500 mg of Neomycin, 80 mg of Gentamicin, and 100 mg of polymyxin in 1000 ml of normal saline), and Jackson-Pratt drains every 8 hours for approximately 3 to 7 days, and reimplant the prosthesis prior to discharge during the same hospitalization.[37]

Salvage Procedure

The salvage procedure for infected or eroded prostheses has been advocated if the infection is low grade and appears focal. In this procedure only the involved components are explanted, repositioned or replaced. The other components are left *in situ*. However, the entire prothesis may be removed if a newer generation device is available. Postoperative antibiotic irrigation utilizes DABS solution, Jackson-Pratt drains, and irrigation usually for 3 to 5 days. The wound is closed primarily around the drains. A success rate of 73% for pump erosion and a success rate of 100% for reservoir infection is reported.[38] The Mulcahy salvage procedure utilizes a sequence of solutions (Table 3.6) and red rubber 18 French catheters for precise and complete irrigation of all tissue spaces in contact with the device. Solution 4 uses an

Table 3-6 Sequence of Solutions Used in Penile Implant Salvage

1. Kanamycin 1 Gram and Bacitracin 50,000 units per litre
2. 1/2 Strength Hydrogen Peroxide
3. 1/2 Strength Betadine
4. Pressure Irrigation (Simpulse)
   5 liter bag containing Vancomycin 1 gram - Gentamicin 80 mg.
5. 1/2 Strength Betadine
6. 1/2 Strength Hydrogen Peroxide
7. Kanamycin 1 Gram and Bacitracin 50,000 units per litre

orthopedic pressure system. After the irrigation, Solution 3, then Solution 2, and finally Solution 1 are again utilized. No drains are placed.

A salvage or exchange procedure may be appropriate in non-diabetic patients with device infection and: (a) absence of bacteria, (b) Gram positive Cocci, (c) absence of frank pus or significant tissue induration, because approximately 80% of patients treated in this fashion will retain their prosthesis for 18 months or longer. Drains are placed in the infected area but the incision is closed primarily without drainage.

Rescue Procedure

The rescue procedure has been advocated for patients with early detected infection. In this technique a new prosthesis is immediately implanted after removal of all components of the infected prosthesis. Copious irrigation of all component sites with antibiotic solution is performed. However, in patients with purulence and a fulminating infection the entire prosthesis is removed and only the wound is drained. A success rate of approximately 82% is reported.[39]

Penile Prostheses and Peyronie's Disease

For patients with Peyronie's disease, inflatable or noninflatable penile prostheses may be indicated if they have (1) severe Peyronie's disease with failed attempt at conservative management and are unable to engage in intercourse due to pain or angulation of the penis; (2) significantly impaired or absent rigidity; (3) preserved erectile function with pain and angulation precluding intromission; and (4) failed placque incision, excision, or grafting. The success rate of penile prosthesis in patients with or without placque incision or excision approximates 90%.[40]

In patients with mild deformities in whom a prosthesis is indicated, the AMS 700 CX or the Mentor Alpha I or Mark II prostheses will frequently result in penile straightening and optimal rigidity without corporoplasty. In patients in whom complete straightening does not occur with prosthesis insertion, incision of the placque over the prosthesis will result in penile straightening. Aneurysmal dilatation does not occur due to the girth limiting expansion of these cylinders. If the defect is significant, grafting with autologous material such as dermis or tunica vaginalis or synthetic material such as Dacron (R) or Gore-tex (R) is appropriate. Placque excision is rarely necessary when a penile prosthesis is used. If complete straightening after the above does not occur, plication or excision of a diamond-wedged piece of tunica albuginea from the opposite side at the point of maximal angulation will usually result in penile straightening.

Penile Prostheses and Cavernosal Reconstruction

Cavernosal infection, Peyronie's disease, priapism, prosthesis removal, long-term PEP, particularly with high dosage of Papaverine, and untreated penile fracture[41] may result in dense fibrotic scarring of the cavernosal tissue. If such scarring is present extensive surgery may be required to expose the entire length of the corpora and to adequately dilate it to accommodate placement of a noninflatable or inflatable prosthesis. Such an extended unilateral or bilateral corporotomy may be accomplished through a generous penoscrotal incision or by degloving the penis using a circumferential circumcision type incision. The latter is not advisable in diabetic patients due to the possibility of ischemia. A combined incision may be necessary. Sometimes no prosthesis or only one suboptimal sized prosthesis can be implanted, but at a later date a larger prosthesis may be considered.

Conclusion

At the present time, due to their high success rate, penile prostheses remain an important management alternative and are considered by some the gold standard to which other treatments should be compared for many patients with organic erectile dysfunction and some patients with psychogenic dysfunction. Realistic expectations and patient and partner satisfaction are related to full knowledge of the capabilities of the various types of prostheses, necessitating presentation to the patient of at least one type from each of the three major categories.

REFERENCES

1. Small MP: Surgical treatment of erectile impotence. Contem Surg 1980; 16:64.
2. Morales PA, Suarez JB, Delgado J, Whitehead ED: Penile implant for erectile impotence. J Urol 1973; 109:641.
3. Scott FB, Bradley WD, Timm GW: Management of erectile impotence: Use of implantable inflatable prosthesis. Urology 1973; 2:80.
4. Small MP, Carrion HM, Gordon JA: Small-carrion penile prosthesis: New implant for management of impotence. Urology 1975; 5:479.
5. Small MP: Semi-rigid penile prostheses. In: Whitehead ED, Leiter E, eds. Current operative urology, Second ed. Philadelphia: Lippincott, 1984.
6. Joseph DB, Bruskewitz RC, Benson RC Jr: Long-term evaluation of the inflatable penile prostheses. J Urol 1984; 131:1670.
7. Furlow WL: Inflatable penile prostheses: Mayo Clinic experiences with 175 patients. Urology 1979; 13:166.
8. Malloy TR, Wein AJ, Carpiniello VL: Improved mechanical survival with revised model inflatable prosthesis using rear-tip extenders. J Urol 1982; 128:489.
9. Whitehead ED: Cooperative professional relationships needed in diagnosing and treating male sexual dysfunction. A.U.A. Today 1992; 5:4.
10. Whitehead ED, Klyde BJ, Zussman S, Wayne M, Shinbach K, Davis DM: Male sexual dysfunction and diabetes mellitus: Multidisciplinary approach to diagnosis and management alternatives. NY State J Med 1983; 83:1174.

11. Buch JP, Zorn BH, Taylor RJ: Cost-benefit analysis of pharmacologic erection program (PEP) versus penile prostheses. Urology 1991; 37:116.
12. Whitehead ED, Leiter E: New frontiers in alloplastic genitourinary prostheses II. The surgical management of erectile impotence. NY State J Med 1982; 82:1806.
13. Zorgniotti AW, Lizza EF: Diagnosis and management of impotence. Philadelphia: B.C. Decker, 1991.
14. Whitehead ED: Impotence. Diabetes Forecast 1982; 37:35.
15. Whitehead ED: Commentary: Malleable penile prostheses. In: Whitehead ED ed. Current operative urology 1989. Philadelphia: Lippincott, 1989.
16. Whitehead ED: Erectile impotence in the diabetic: Evaluation and treatment. In: Serrano-Rios M, Lefebvre PJ, eds. Diabetes 1985. New York: Elsevier Science Publishing, 1986.
17. Singh I, Godec CJ: Asynchronous erosion of inflatable prosthesis into small and large bowel. J Urol 1992; 147:709.
18. Whitehead ED, Klyde BJ, Zussman S, Salkin P: Treatment alternatives for impotence. Postgrad Med 1990; 88:139.
19. Lubensky JD: Outpatient three-piece inflatable penile prosthesis. J Urol 1991; 145:1176.
20. Whitehead ED: Ten "pearls" from my practice of penile prosthesis implantation. Urology 1981; 38:550.
21. Kabalin JN, Kessler R: Infectious complications of penile prosthesis surgery. J Urol 1988; 139:953.
22. Thomalla JV, Thompson ST, Rowland RG, Mulcahy JJ: Infectious complications of penile prosthetic implants. J Urol 1987; 138:65.
23. Blum MD: Effective control of genitourinary prosthesis infection. Cont Urol 1990; 2(2):51.
24. Collins KP, Hackler RH: Complications of penile prostheses in the spinal cord injury population. J Urol 1988; 140:984.
25. Van Arsdalen JN, Klein FA, Hackler RH, Brady SM: Penile implants in spinal cord injury patients for maintaining external appliances. J Urol 1981; 126:331.
26. Diokno AC, Sonda LP: Compatability of genitourinary prostheses and intermittent self-catheterization. J Urol 1981; 125:659.
27. Montague DR: Periprosthetic infections. J Urol 1987; 138:68.
28. Bishop JR, Moul JW, Sihelnik SA, Peppas DS, Gormley TS, McLeod DG: Use of glycosylated hemoglobin to identify diabetics at high risk for penile periprosthetic infections. J Urol 1992; 147:386.
29. Sidi AA, Peng W, Sanseau C, Lange PH: Penile prosthesis in the treatment of impotence in the immunosuppressed man. J Urol 1987; 137:L681.
30. Barrett DM, O'Sullivan DC, Malizia AA, Reiman HM, Abell-Aleff PC: Particle shedding and migration from silicone genitourinary devices. J Urol 1991; 146:319.
31. Kabalin JN, Kessler R: Five-year followup of the Scott inflatable penile prosthesis and comparison with semirigid penile prosthesis. J Urol 1988; 140:1428.
32. Kaufman, JJ, Lindner A, Raz S: Complications of penile prosthesis surgery for impotence. J Urol 1982; 128:1192.
33. Kessler R: Surgical experience with the inflatable penile prosthesis. J Urol 1980; 124:611.
34. Levinson K, Whitehead ED: OmniPhase penile prosthesis: Delayed bilateral central cable breakage. J Urol 1989; 141:618.
35. O'Donnell PD: Operative approach for secondary placement of penile prosthesis. Urology 1986; 28:108.
36. Gasser TC, Larsen EH, Bruskewitz RG: Penile prosthesis reimplantation. J Urol 1987; 137:46.
37. Petrou SP, Barrett DM: The use of penile prostheses in erectile dysfunction. Sem Urol 1990; 8:138.
38. Furlow WL, Goldwasser B: Salvage of the eroded inflatable penile prosthesis: A new concept. J Urol 1987; 138:312.
39. Fishman I: Perforation and erosion of penile prostheses. Cont Urol 1991; 3 (8):51.
40. Eigner EB, Kabalin JN, Kessler R: Penile implants in the treatment of Peyronie's disease. J Urol 1991; 145:69.

41. Biase JN, Whitehead ED, Miller F, Hoffman S: Unilateral Dynaflex penile prosthesis to correct impaired tumscence and severe penile deformity resulting from traumatic rupture of one corpus cavinosum. J Urol (submitted for publication).

ANNOTATED BIBLIOGRAPHY

Barrett DM, O'Sullivan DC, Malizia AA, Reiman HM, Abell-Aleff PC: Particle shedding and migration from silicone genitourinary prosthetic devices. J Urol 1991; 146:319.

This study comprised 30 patients undergoing penile prostheses and 10 patients undergoing artificial urinary sphincters. In 18 of the 25 periprosthetic specimens and in all four lymph nodes examined silicone was found. Foreign body granulomas were noted in 14 of these 29 specimens. Most devices prior to implantation or after explantation demonstrated free particles of silicone or silicates on the surface. It was concluded that genitourinary prostheses shed silicone particles that can be found in the fibrous capsule and draining lymph nodes. However, the authors concluded that the clinical implication of the shedding, migration, and tissue response remains unclear. Furthermore, they state that to date the benefits of the prostheses seem to outweigh by far any unforeseen long-term problems.

Buck JP, Zorn BH, Taylor RJ: Cost-benefit analysis of pharmacologic erection program (PEP) versus penile prostheses. Urology 1991; 37:116.

The authors noted that in the elderly who require only a limited time span of impotence therapy PEP is more cost-effective than penile prosthesis implantation. Furthermore, when cost modifiers were considered PEP became even more cost-effective. However, they noted that in younger men penile prosthesis implantation is more cost-effective as therapy for long-term (greater than 5 years) treatment.

Lubensky JD: Outpatient three-piece inflatable penile prosthesis. J Urol 1991; 145:1176.

With an aim to reduce costs of penile prosthesis implantation the author implanted 74 consecutive organic impotent patients in an outpatient setting. All patients received the AMS 700 three-piece inflatable penile prosthesis. The author concluded that the outpatient setting is an effective, safe, and efficient milieu for implantation of the inflatable penile prosthesis.

Thomalla JF, Thompson ST, Rowland RG, Mulcahy JJ: Infectious complications of penile prosthetic implants. J Urol 1987; 138:65.

In this review article more than 300 penile prostheses implanted between 1979 and 1984 were studied. An overall infectious complication rate of 8.3% was noted. The authors make the following recommendations to reduce the incidence of infectious complications: perioperative administration of antibiotics (aminoglycoside plus vancomycin or a similar combination), vigorous perineal and genital cleansing preoperatively, intraoperative use of antibiotic irrigating solutions, technical perfection with primary placement, circumcision at implantation in uncircumcised recipients, and avoidance of simultaneous placement of an artificial urinary sphincter. They noted that no group of patients or type of prosthesis was more susceptible to the development of a postoperative infection.

4 Microvascular Arterial Bypass Surgery for Arteriogenic Impotence

Dimitrios C. Hatzichristou
Irwin Goldstein

The inspiration for microvascular arterial bypass surgery in the treatment of organically impotent patients with arterial insufficiency is the desire of the patient to return to normal erectile function. Such patients wish to have their own sexually stimulated spontaneous rigid erection, without mechanical devices (external or internal) or pharmacologic assistance.[1] The aim of any microvascular arterial bypass surgery for impotence, either by arteriovenous, or by artery-to-artery anastomoses, is to increase blood flow and arterial perfusion pressure to the erectile tissue bypassing hypogastric–cavernous arterial inflow obstruction.[1,2]

Microvascular arterial bypass procedures were first introduced for the treatment of erectile dysfunction in the mid-1970s.[3] Almost two decades later, penile microvascular arterial bypass procedures have expanded to utilize the inferior epigastric artery, the dorsal penile artery, and a saphenous vein graft as neoarterial inflow sources. Recipient vessels have included the dorsal artery, an isolated segment of the deep dorsal vein, or the cavernosal artery, depending on the location of the hypogastric–cavernous arterial occlusions.[1,2]

Published reports on surgical success have varied widely between 20 and 80%.[1–11] The reason for this variability may be dependent on diagnostic criteria, patient selection, and type of procedure. In our own institution, patient follow-up data has been accumulated in over 300 patients over a 10-year period. As indicators of clinical outcome, data are available concerning patient questionnaire responses, as well as preoperative and postoperative cavernosometric, cavernosographic, and arteriographic findings. In a 1 year follow-up study, improvement in erectile function was realized in 72% of cases.[11]

This chapter will review epidemiologic pathophysiologic data of arteriogenic impotence. More detailed information will be provided concerning indications and surgical principles involved in microvascular arterial bypass proce-

Management of Impotence and Infertility, edited by Douglas Whitehead and Harris Nagler,

dures for the treatment of arteriogenic impotence. Furthermore, our evolving experience within this field will be updated.

Epidemiology of Impotence

There has been a lack of epidemiologic data concerning the prevalence of impotence in a normative population and the relationship of impotence to intervening physiological and psychological variables. The majority of the attempts to determine the causes of impotence have been conducted in patients with medical disorders and have not been performed in healthy normative populations.[12]

The most comprehensive population-based data on male sexual behavior have been the Kinsey survey, conducted over 40 years ago in a social and medical context vastly different from that of the present. In this study impotence was found to be an age-dependent disorder with an incidence of 1.9% at 40 years of age and 25% at 65 years of age.[12] Recently, a large random community-based sample of healthy, noninstitutionalized men was performed.[13] The prevalence of erectile dysfunction in this normative population of men was found to be approximately 50% between the ages of 40 and 70. This would imply that impotence in some degree is found in an estimated 30 million American men and may be considered a major health concern. Furthermore, impotence was found significantly related to heart disease, hypertension, diabetes, and low levels of HDL.

Pathophysiology of Arteriogenic Impotence

Impotence is considered to be the persistent inability to attain and maintain an erection adequate to permit satisfactory sexual performance. Potency, which assumes a functional state of penile erection, may exist even when there is some degree of erectile impairment in terms of diminished penile rigidity or decreased capability to sustain an erection.[14]

Alterations in the inflow and outflow of blood to and from the penis are thought to be the most frequent causes of organic impotence. Atherosclerotic or traumatic arterial occlusive disease of the hypogastric–cavernous arterial bed can decrease the perfusion pressure and arterial flow to the lacunar spaces, thus decreasing the rigidity of the erect penis and the time to maximum erection, respectively.[12]

Several studies in impotent men report that the proportion of abnormal penile vascular findings significantly increased as the number of vascular risk factors were identified in their histories. Virag investigated the vascular risk factors in 440 impotent men.[15] He found diabetes, heart disease, cigarette smoking, and hypercholesterolemia as major risk factors. He reported that in 80% of cases, the cause of impotence was organic in origin. Other investigators, using an exclusive diabetic population, have found a relationship between impotence and diabetes, with a prevalence of impotence in diabetics varying between 35 and 75%.[12]

Cigarette smoking has been found as a statistically significant independent risk factor in the development of angiographically proven arterial occlusive disease to the hypogastric–cavernous arterial bed.[16] Five, 10 and 20 pack-year histories of cigarette smoking exposure was associated with 15, 30, and 70% incidence of arterial occlusive disease within the common penile artery. Nicotine may adversely affect erectile function by blocking corporal smooth muscle relaxation and thus prevent normal corporal venoocclusive function.

Blunt pelvic and perineal trauma is another important risk factor associated with arterial insufficiency in the hypogastric–cavernous arterial bed. A recent series evaluated the arteriograms of impotent men following blunt pelvic and perineal trauma and found that the patterns of arteriographically demonstrated occlusive disease within the distal hypogastric–cavernous arterial bed were consistent with the site of the traumatic injury. Patients with persistent impotence immediately following blunt pelvic trauma were found to have different locations of distal occlusive disease than similar patients with blunt perineal trauma.[17] Those who sustained blunt pelvic trauma revealed arterial occlusive lesions mainly in the internal pudendal, common penile, cavernosal, and dorsal arteries, while those who sustained blunt perineal trauma demonstrated a more focal pattern of arterial occlusive pathology primarily in the cavernosal and dorsal arteries. The incidence of arterial lesions in the distal internal pudendal or common penile artery was significantly higher in patients with blunt pelvic trauma (92%) than in patients with blunt perineal trauma (35%). The incidence of a solitary arterial lesion in the cavernosal artery without proximal disease was significantly higher in patients with blunt perineal trauma (48%) than in patients with blunt pelvic trauma (8%). It was further hypothesized in the study that blunt trauma without immediate impotence was a potential risk factor for the later development of arterial vasculogenic impotence, and that unrecognized or seemgingly innocuous trauma was a factor in cases of "idiopathic" impotence. Patients without trauma and with the previously discussed vascular risk factors of hypertension, cigarette smoking, diabetes mellitus, and hyperlipidemia were found in the study to have a more diffuse pattern of arteriographically demonstrated arterial lesions compared to the patients with either blunt pelvic or perineal trauma.

How Should Candidates for Microvascular Arterial Bypass Surgery Be Evaluated?

The purpose of the diagnostic evaluation of the impotent patient is to reveal the etiology of the erectile dysfunction.

The evaluation begins with a sexual, psychosocial, and medical history, a physical examination, and routine laboratory tests. Typical history of patients with arteriogenic impotence is of constant diminished erectile rigidity, spontaneity, and duration of sustaining capability adversely influencing morning masturbation and coital erections. Morning erections are often slightly more rigid and may have a greater sustaining capability than the coital erections. Vascular risk factors, such as blunt perineal trauma, cigarette smoking, and hypercholesterolemia, are often identified in the history.[13,15]

Several studies exist to evaluate the integrity of the penile arteries in a patient with suspected anteriogenic impotence. Flaccid state evaluations, such as the penile-brachial index or penile plethysmography, cannot be depended on to detect cavernosal artery occlusions, nor can they provide data concerning flow, perfusion pressure, or changes in the cavernosal artery diameter during maximal dilation. Furthermore, abnormal arterial responses to such testing may be the result not only of cavernosal artery pathology but may occur secondary to excessive adrenergic constrictor tone in the cavernosal artery due to anxiety.[12]

Hemodynamic investigations in the dynamic state following intracavernosal vasoactive agent administration provide more information concerning arterial function. Adrenergic activity is diminished by administering repeat doses of intracavernosal vasoactive agents until consistent testing results are recorded.

An office screening test of vascular integrity is performed by observing the erectile response following administration of vasoactive agents with or without visual or mechanical stimulation. Normal venoocclusive vascular status is implied if a rigid erection results within 5–10 minutes and is sustained in rigidity for approximately 1 hour. Arterial integrity is unable to be assessed by identifying a rigid erectile response in this test. Arterial and venoocclusive hemodynamic impairment may be presumed if only a delayed, partial, short-lived, or absent erection results following several repeat doses of intracavernosal agents on different study sessions. However, excessive adrenergic activity cannot be ruled out and may induce inappropriate conclusions.

The integrity of the cavernosal artery and the corporal venoocclusive mechanism may be directly evaluated at the same time, under the same dynamic state during dynamic infusion cavernosometry and cavernosography (DICC).[18] This four-phase procedure has the ability to evaluate both vascular components of the erection following pharmacologically induced smooth muscle relaxation. In phase one of this study, the rise from baseline corporal body pressure is evaluated in response to the administration of intracavernosal pharmacologic agents. The normal intracavernosal pressure response to intracavernosal pharmacologic stimulation (equilibrium pressure) may be said to approximate the mean arterial blood pressure and the time to equilibrium intracavernosal pressure in normal patients is generally under 10 minutes. Those patients with predominantly arterial occlusive disease demonstrate an abnormally prolonged time to equilibrium, usually greater than 15 minutes, as well as reduced intracavernosal pressures compared to the mean arterial pressure. An axial loading force of 2 kg may be applied to the glans penis at this time to assess if the penis at equilibrium is able to resist buckling or deformation. This determination assesses the ability of the penis to develop rigidity. Rigidity is a function of intracavernosal pressure and penile volume and can be found in all patients at 70 mm Hg and in some patients, with smaller volume corpora, at pressures as low as 50 mm Hg.

Corporal venoocclusive function is evaluated in phase two by determining the flow of heparinized saline necessary to maintain selected intracavernosal pressures typically chosen as 30, 60, 90, 120, and 150 mm Hg. Venous outflow resistance is constant and is implied by a linear relationship between these flow-to-maintain values. A nonlinear relationship is indicating incomplete smooth muscle relaxation.[19] Redosing of intracavernosal agents and reassessing changes in flow-to-maintain values have been successful in converting responses to a linear, constant resistance relationship. A wide range of normal and abnormal parameters for venoocclusive testing exists in the literature. In our experience, the normal flow-to-maintain values for various intracavernosal pressures is 3 ml/minute or less, in contrast to values of 5–30 ml/minute previously proposed. Such discrepancy in the literature is most likely the result of testing in the presence of adrenergic constricting influences.

A second evaluation of venous outflow resistance is performed by assessing the decay in intracavernosal pressure following termination of the saline infusion. Once the intracavernosal pressure of 150 mm Hg is reached, the flow of heparinized saline is discontinued and the corporal body pressure fall over a 30-second period is determined. In patients with intact venoocclusive mechanism, the fall of corporal body pressure over a 30-second period from a suprasystolic pressure of 150 mm Hg is less than 45 mm Hg. If the decay is excessive, the study is repeated in the presence of perineal compression. If this maneuver normalizes the pressure fall over 30 seconds, it is likely that subsequent cavernosography will demonstrate abnormal venous drainage confined to the crural region.

Cavernosal artery hemodynamics are evaluated in phase three by determining both the right and left cavernosal artery systolic occlusion pressures, which are compared to the brachial artery systolic pressure. The Doppler ultrasound is placed at the mid-shaft overlying the left and right cavernosal arteries before, during, and after termination of intracavernosal infusion of heparinized saline. The intracavernosal pressure is determined where respective cavernosal artery pulsations return. This value is the effective cavernosal artery systolic pressure and implies the maximal right or left cavernosal arterial pressure that can be delivered to the corporal body during erection. The cavernosal artery systolic occlusion pressure should be within 35 mm Hg of the brachial artery systolic occlusion pressure.

The last phase of the DICC includes the radiologic examination of the corporal venous drainage system during erection (phase four). Normally, there is no visualization of any venous drainage during cavernosography. Patients with Peyronie's disease and corporal venoocclusive dysfunction show plaque-associated site-specific leak. Patients with diabetes or peripheral vascular disease typically show diffuse patterns of drainage involving visualization of the dorsal, cavernosal, or crural veins, the glans, and the corpus spongiosum.

In patients with suspected arterial occlusive disease, another evaluation of the integrity of the cavernosal arteries is focused, pulsed Doppler ultrasonography.[20] This study is performed in conjunction with intracavernosal vasoactive agent administration. The focused ultrasound has the unique capability to determine changes in the diameter of the cavernosal artery and in blood flow velocity in the cavernosal artery. Atherosclerotic cavernosal arteries will show only minimal dilation and a low blood flow velocity. Cavernosal arterial dilation may be normal, however, despite proximal arterial occlusive pathology. This may be seen especially in the patient felt to be the optimal revascularization candidate, that is, the young man with traumatic occlusive injury to the internal pudendal or common penile artery. Duplex ultrasound studies may be useful to provide an objective assessment of the postoperative follow-up of a patient undergoing a penile arterial bypass procedure.

Selective internal pudendal pharmacoarteriography is indicated only in those selected impotent patients who are interested in arterial bypass surgery for treatment of their arteriogenic impotence.[1,2,18] Such patients have a history consistent with arteriogenic impotence and have cavernosometric findings consistent with an abnormal response to intracavernosal pharmacologic agents, normal veno-occlusive function, and abnormal cavernosal artery systolic occlusion pressures. Patients who exhibit diffuse venoocclusive dysfunction are discouraged from undergoing selective arteriography since the success rate of reconstructive surgery with such a pattern of corporal venoocclusion is too low. The study is performed under local anesthesia and intravenous sedation. Intracavernosal and intraarterial vasoactive agents allow for optimal visualization of the penile arterial tree in the dynamic state. This study is utilized to define the anatomic pattern of arterial occlusive disease in the hypogastric–cavernous arterial bed. Such information enables the appropriate arterial bypass procedure to be selected.

Which Patients Are Candidates for Microvascular Arterial Bypass Surgery?

Patients with arterial occlusive disease secondary to atherosclerotic vascular risk factors, such as aging, hypertension, cigarette smoking, diabetes, and hypercholesterolemia, have been commonly found to have an associated corporal venoocclusive dysfunction. The basis for this hemodynamic impairment is most likely related to a pan-cavernosal, abnormal compliance of the erectile tissue, possibly secondary to an excess of cross-linked collagen or advanced glycosylated end-products. Such morphologic changes in the corporal tissue have been found in impotent patients with severe arterial obstructive disease. Such data strongly support the concept that atherosclerotic vascular disease affects the physiology of erection in many different levels: at the level of large inflow vessels, at the level of the penile microvasculature, at the level of the lacunar space endothelium, and at the level of the penile fibroelastic frame. In the presence of associated diffuse corporal venoocclusive dysfunction, such patients do not experience success with microvascular arterial bypass surgery.[1,2]

In our experience, this microvascular arterial bypass procedure is most successful in a highly selected group of young patients who have arteriogenic impotence following blunt pelvic or perineal trauma. Such patients with discrete lesions in the pudendal and/or common penile arteries secondary to pelvic or perineal trauma are most likely to have arteriogenic impotence without a corporal venoocclusive dysfunction. These patients arteriographically demonstrate occlusions within the distal hypogastric–cavernous arterial bed at the site of the traumatic injury. Moreover, young patients, being at the beginning of their sexual lives, are more likely to consider a lengthy surgical procedure designed to restore erectile function than average impotent elderly men.[1]

Microvascular Arterial Bypass Options

The goal of microvascular arterial bypass surgery is to increase the arterial perfusion pressure and blood inflow to the erectile tissue, thus enabling a more rigid, spontaneous penile erection. To achieve this, a variety of surgical techniques have been developed.[1–11]

The first described microvascular arterial bypass procedure included a direct anastomosis of the inferior epigastric artery to the tunica albuginea of the corpus cavernosum. This Michal I operation was largely abandoned due to the high incidence of immediate postoperative priapism as well as short-term anastomotic occlusion. A second procedure involved an end-to-side microvascular arterial anastomosis between the inferior epigastric artery and one dorsal penile artery (Michal II).[3] McDougal and Jeffery modified this latter procedure using bilateral inferior epigastric arteries end-to-side to both dorsal arteries.[7] Sharlip utilized the same vessels in an end-to-end anastomosis in the proximal aspect of the dorsal artery, thus allowing retrograde flow to the cavernosal artery.[2] Direct anastomosis of the inferior epigastric artery to the cavernous artery was reported by MacGregor and Konnak.[5] Crespo utilized a branched saphenous venous graft *in situ* to divert blood flow from the femoral or external iliac arteries to the dorsal or cavernosal arteries.[6]

Virag in the early 1980s introduced the use of the deep dorsal vein as recipient vessel.[4] The vein, used as graft, was either left unligated, isolated only proximally, or isolated proximally and distally. Several modifications of the original operation followed.[4,10] Hauri, using both dorsal artery and deep dorsal vein, described a side-to-side anastomosis between those two vessels, leaving a common arteriovenous lumen.[8] The inferior epigastric artery was then anastomosed end-to-side to this arteriovenous fistula. The goal was to achieve low peripheral vascular outflow resistance enabling improved arterial blood runoff distal to the anastomosis, thereby reducing the potential for postoperative thrombosis. However, none of these operations and their modifications received broad acceptance as the rationality of these procedures remains unclear and the long-term results are controversial.

Which Surgical Procedure?

Different arterial occlusive lesion combinations have been observed, depending on the pathogenesis of the lesions and the presence of coexisting vascular risk factors. What is the most appropriate surgical procedure for specific patterns of arterial occlusive disease?

Traditionally, each surgeon uses his or her favorite technique, independent of the hemodynamic status and the arteriographic data of each patient. Some surgeons have even advocated that the arteriogram is superfluous as their individual choice of vascular reconstruction is uninfluenced by this diagnostic study, especially if the surgical option is restricted to venous arterialization.

The goal of the microvascular arterial bypass surgery is to increase the arterial perfusion pressure and blood inflow to the erectile tissue. It is our experience that the best means to achieve this goal is by individualizing the new blood inflow pathways, based on the results of the arteriogram. In this fashion, the minimally invasive technique that allows maximal transmission of systemic blood pressure to the cavernous bodies through the most anatomically accesible available pathway can be realized.

Four types of arteriographic patterns are able to be described in patients with arteriogenic impotence. These patterns lead us to the "ideal" choice of the arterial bypass.[18] The application of the preoperative decision is, of course, dependent on modifying intraoperative factors such as the length of the inferior epigastric artery and the quality of the recipient vessels.

The first arteriographic pattern of arterial occlusive disease shows bilateral focal lesions proximal to the cavernosal artery in the internal pudendal or common penile artery (Figure 4-1). These patients may be treated with an anastomosis of the inferior epigastric artery to the proximal dorsal penile artery if a communication between the dorsal and cavernosal arteries is shown to exist distal to the occlusion. The rationale is to increase perfusion pressure and inflow to the cavernosal artery retrograde from the proximal dorsal artery with the presumption that there will be adequate arterial runoff in the unaffected cavernosal artery.

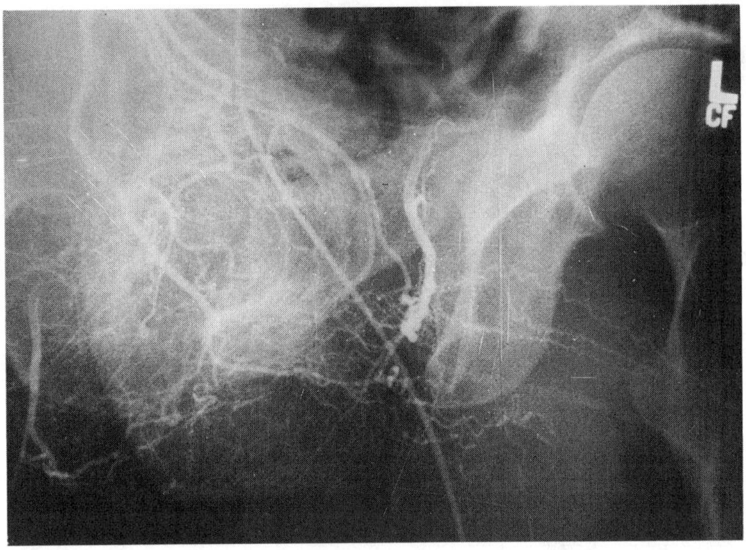

Figure 4-1 The selective internal pudendal arteriogram demonstrates complete obstruction of the common penile artery with reconstitution of the dorsal and cavernosal arteries through pelvic collaterals. This patient suffered blunt pelvic trauma. The arteriogram is representative of the pattern 1 type of arterial occlusive disease.

The second pattern consists of arterial occlusive disease within both cavernosal arteries (Figure 4-2). These patients have been treated successfully with an anastomosis of the inferior epigastric artery to an isolated deep dorsal vein segment. The rationale is to increase perfusion pressure and inflow to the lacunar spaces retrograde from the dorsal vein segment through the emissary and subtunical venules. The regulation of arterial blood inflow in the retrograde direction through the deep dorsal vein bypass is unknown. In the flaccid state, the normal high tone of trabecular smooth muscle may provide a high resistive vascular bed restricting retrograde flow, thus preventing high flow priapism. Arterial blood in the flaccid state may preferentially flow through low resistive circumferential veins or through veins in the corpus spongiosum away from the corpora. This would enable blood flow to remain high through the anastomosis between the inferior epigastric artery and the deep dorsal vein. During the initiation of the erection, however, the trabecular smooth muscle relaxes, and the retrograde pathway is converted to a low resistance pathway. An alternative surgical approach is by direct arterialization of the cavernous arteries in which successful results have been documented. This technique has, however, not gained wide popularity because of the possibility of iatrogenic injury to the surrounding erectile tissue.

A third pattern of arterial occlusive disease may consist of combinations of arterial lesions. This may include unilateral cavernosal artery occlusion with an ipsilateral occluded dorsal artery (similar to one side of pattern two) in conjunction with proximal contralateral proximal arterial occlusive disease and a communication between the contralateral dorsal penile artery and the contralateral proximal cavernosal artery (similar to one side of pattern one). These patients may be treated with a modification that involves two microvascular anastomoses. The first anastomosis would be to an isolated dorsal vein segment in a side-to-side fashion and the second would involve an end-to-end anastomosis to the proximal dorsal penile artery. The rationale is to increase perfusion pressure and inflow to the cavernosal tissue

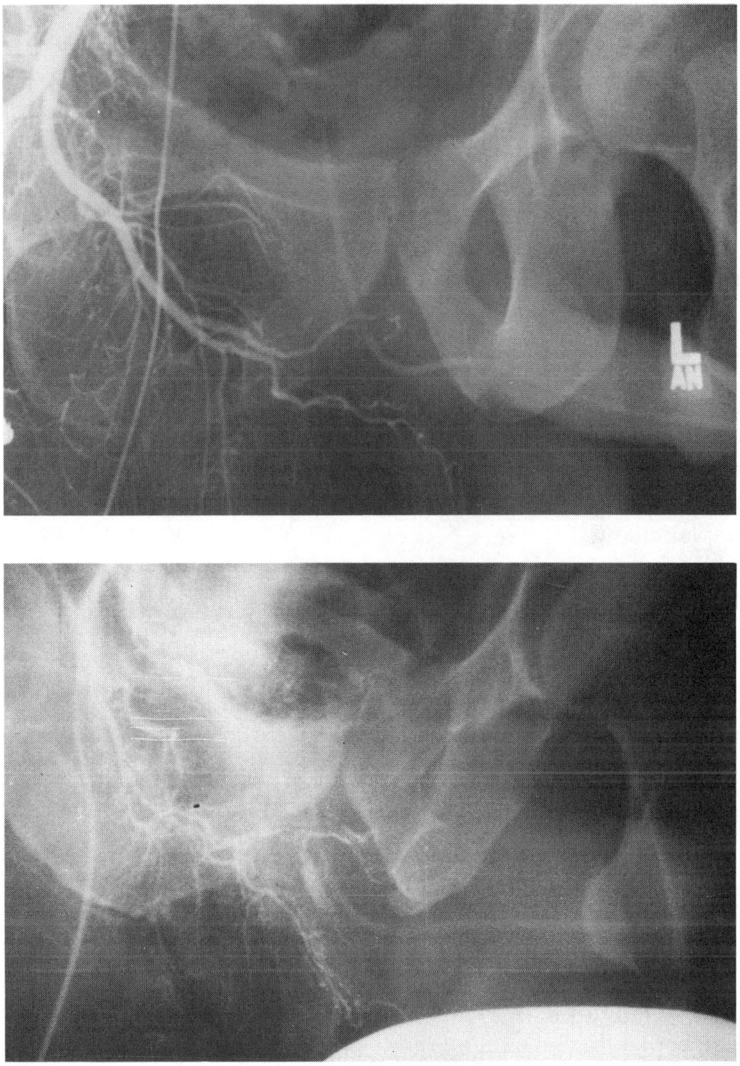

Figure 4-2 (A) This selective internal pudendal arteriogram demonstrates arterial occlusive disease within the distal common penile artery with obstruction of the dorsal and cavernosal arteries at their origins off the common penile artery. This patient experienced an episode of blunt perineal trauma. The anteriogram is representative of the pattern 2 type of arterial, occlusive disease. (B) This selective internal pudendal arteriogram demonstrates arterial occlusive disease within the distal internal pudendal, common penile, dorsal, and cavernosal arteries. This patient had a history of hylerlipidemia, cigarette smoking, and hypertension.

retrograde from the dorsal vein segment and proximally through the cavernosal artery through the proximal dorsal artery. The inferior epigastric artery flow should be high through deep venous low resistance runoff channels and thus should help maintain anastomosis patency.

The fourth pattern may involve a unilateral cavernosal artery occlusion with an ipsilateral normal dorsal artery. There may be diffuse arterial pathology in the contralateral system, with no communication between the dorsal and cavernosal artery. These patients may be treated with anastomosis of the normal dorstal artery to an isolated deep dorsal vein segment or to the ipsilateral cavernosal artery. Use of the dorsal artery as the neoarterial inflow source avoids an abdominal incision to harvest the usual inflow source, the inferior epigastric artery.

Other patterns of arterial occlusion within the hypogastric–cavernous bed exist, especially in patients with atherosclerotic vascular risk factors. Such patients often reveal multiple sites of arterial occlusion in the large vessels as well as in the distal vasculature within hypogastric–cavernous arterial bed. Atherosclerotic-associated pathology within the microvasculature and fibroelastic frame of the erectile tissue in these patients is expected. These patients are usually encouraged to seek alternative treatments, such as intracavernosal injections, vacuum erection devices, or penile prosthesis implantation.

In conclusion, it is emphasized that there is no "gold standard" procedure for all occlusive patterns in patients with arteriogenic impotence. It is our experience that each case be treated individually.

Microvascular Principles in Arterial Bypass Surgery for Impotence

Arterial reconstructive surgery for occlusive disease within the hypogastric–cavernous arterial bed is based on the same vascular and microvascular surgical principles utilized in arterial reconstructive procedures for occlusive disease within the coronary, cerebral, or peripheral vascular beds.

Venous bypass grafts have been utilized for years in the treatment of arterial occlusive disease in the coronary and peripheral arteries. These latter bypass procedures are some of the most common operative procedures performed in the United States with estimated use exceeding 220,000 cases per year. Veins are optimal conduits to bypass small vessel arterial occlusive disease because they possess intrinsic biologic properties that modulate the blood–graft interface and foster maintenance of vascular patency. In the last decade, use of the saphenous vein in peripheral artery occlusive disease as an *in situ* graft has become very popular with success rates reported in 90% of selected cases.[21]

In the penis, the deep dorsal vein may also be used as an *in situ* graft, with the purpose of bypassing arterial occlusive disease within the cavernosal artery. Alternative means of bypassing pathology within the cavernosal artery involve directly anastomosing a neoarterial inflow source directly to the cavernosal artery in its course within the corpus cavernosum.[9] Such procedures, however, may worsen erectile function by inducing iatrogenic injury to the surrounding erectile smooth muscle and developing focal corporal venoocclusive dysfunction.

Controversy exists in the literature as to the longevity of arterialized vein grafts.[22] Some believe that vein grafts have a short life span due to postoperative morphologic alterations that either lead to early occlusion by thrombosis and late stenosis by myointimal proliferative lesions. Although it is generally accepted that early occlusions are due to technical error, the pathogenesis of myointimal proliferation lesions is unknown. Some authors believe that the intimal lesion is the consequence of associated vein graft exposure to systemic blood pressure and arterial flows. Others suggest that the vein graft morphologic changes are the result of injury from prolonged ischemia, thermal or mechanical injury during surgical preparation, or during venous valve ablation. We have histologic evidence in a functioning deep dorsal vein graft, examined prior to and following "arterialization" for over 10 months, demonstrating that the endothelium of the vein is preserved. This would imply that myointimal proliferative lesions are the result of endothelial injury secondary to surgical preparation trauma rather than secondary to exposure of systemic blood pressure and flow.

Such observations make obvious the role of endothelium-preserving techniques not only of the deep dorsal vein, but of the donor and other potential recipient vessels such as the dorsal artery during this vascular procedure. Healthy vascular endothelium secretes factors such as endothelium-derived relaxing factors (EDRF). Such factors are not only potent vasodilators but they are also strong inhibitors of platelet adhesion and aggregation.[18]

At all times during this vascular surgery, maximal smooth muscle relaxation is desired to decrease the endothelial damage.[18] This is very critical as the room temperature of the operating room, the use of room temperature irrigating solution, and even the skin incision can induce vasoconstriction, spasm, and possible endothelial cell damage. Topical papaverine hydrochloride irrigation preserves endothelial and smooth muscle cell morphology during vein graft preparation and its frequent use is encouraged. For intraluminal irrigation, we utilize a dilute papaverine, heparin, and electrolytic solution. Heparin may inhibit the early development of vein graft myointimal proliferative lesions following endothelial injury.

Preparation of the *in situ* deep dorsal vein for such arterial bypass surgery requires limited dissection. Thus ischemic, mechanical, and thermal trauma to the vein wall should be minimized. Careful avoidance of mechanical twisting, stretching injury of the vessel, excessive dissection, or endothelial damage from high pressure vascular occluding clamps is of critical concern. Vascular hemostasis may be achieved with low pressure vascular occluding clips or by vessel loops under minimal tension for minimal operating time. Thermal injury is avoided by using low current microbipolar cautery set at the minimum level necessary for adequate coagulation.

The deep dorsal vein has several valves within the lumen, however, they are often variable and unpredictable in number and location. The most common pattern of valves includes one proximal valve at the junction of the suspensory and fundiform ligaments and one distal valve near the glans penis. If this pattern exists and the anastomosis to the neoarterial inflow source is placed between these two valves, then valve ablation maneuvers may not be necessary. If alternative valve configurations exist and valve ablation is required to ensure arterial runoff, then ablation should be achieved with extreme caution, usually with a 2-mm Leather valve cutter.

The adventitia should be preserved in all vessels by minimizing the surgical dissection to the vessel. It is well documented that when intraluminal blood flow is interrupted, the vasa vasorum provides a nutritional role to the vessel wall. The preservation of the adventitia is additionally important in terms of vessel innervation. It has been demonstrated that grafted vessels possess a supersensitivity to catecholamines, secondary to denervation during surgical preparation. This may account for the enhanced vascular reactivity observed in reversed saphenous vein bypass grafts. The only location where the adventitia must be carefully removed is at the site of the vascular anastomosis.

The integrity of the recipient vessels that provide outflow runoff is of paramount concern. Interference with arterial runoff to the deep dorsal vein and the dorsal artery may place any subsequent arterial anastomosis at risk for occlusion. Atherosclerotic occlusive disease in the dorsal artery has been observed clinically at the time of surgery as well as during subsequent histomorphologic evaluation. Atherosclerotic lesions in the deep dorsal vein are not usually clinically evident at the time of surgery, but subsequent histomorphologic evaluation has revealed structural changes within the veil wall (unpublished data).

We will describe the surgical technique performed in our hospital, which emphasizes the above vascular and microsurgical principles. As we have already described, we use the inferior epigastric artery as donor and both the dorsal artery and a segment of the deep dorsal vein as recipient vessels.[18]

The Operation

The success of any type of distal microvascular repair in restoring potency depends on several vascular and microsurgical principles including (1) endothelium-sparing vascular technique, (2) adequate flow and perfusion pressure in the neoarterial inflow source, (3) a technically sound anastomosis, and (4) sufficient arterial runoff into the distal penile vessels. If care is not taken to ensure that these principles are specifically attended to, failure may occur.

A curvilinear inguinal–scrotal incision, two fingerbreadths lateral to the shaft of the penis, commences at the public tubercle and continues to the median scrotal raphe. The advantage of this incision is that excellent proximal and distal exposure of the penile neurovascular bundle may be achieved, and, in particular, the proximal aspect of the deep dorsal vein may be easily exposed. In addition, no subsequent scars will exist on the penile shaft or at the base of the penis with this incision.

A basic surgical principle in this procedure is to preserve the two ligaments of the penis, the fundiform and the suspensory ligaments, during dissection of the penis (Figure 4-3). The fundiform contains cutaneous nerves important for sensation at the base of the penis. The integrity of the fundiform, along the with suspensory ligament, is important to the preservation of penile length.

Blunt finger dissection along the tunica albuginea is performed proximally to the ipsi-

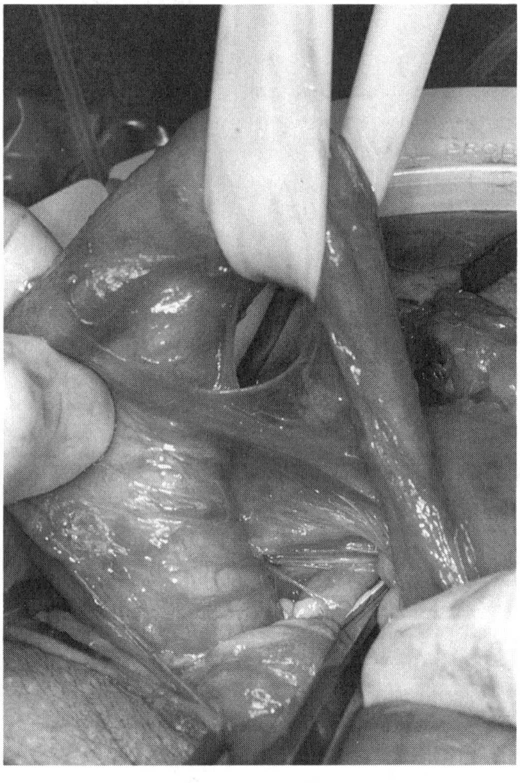

Figure 4-3 Intraoperative picture showing the fundiform ligament, the continuation of Scarpa's fascia onto Buck's fascia. Cutaneous sensation loss overlying the base of the penis and shortening of penile length may result with excision of this ligament.

lateral crus to the level of the ischiopubic ramus. Further dissection will fascilitate exposure of the suspensory and the fundiform ligament, the continuation of Scarpa's fascia onto Buck's fascia. At the junction of the fundiform and suspensory ligament, at the level of the pubic symphysis, a second defect is fashioned, which is secured with a penrose drain. The neoarterial inflow source, the inferior epigastric artery, will be introduced through this defect.

Exposure of the neurovascular bundle and, in particular, the deep dorsal vein is then performed. The vein is first approached at the distal end of the penis near the corona of the glans. Distal branches that appear to communicate directly to the glans penis are ligated to prevent postoperative glans hyperemia. Exposure of the proximal deep dorsal vein is ultimately gained within the suspensory ligament. The vessel is ligated under the pubic symphysis midway between the onset of the suspensory ligament and the urogenital diaphragm. To establish the capability of retrograde arterial flow from the deep dorsal vein to the corpora, one corpus may be cannulated with a 19-gauge butterfly needle and free flow of corporal blood established. Evans blue or diluted methylene blue solution is then injected into the isolated venous segment and the corporal effluent is observed (Figure 4-4). In approximately 60% of cases a retrograde communication exists through "valveless" emissary veins and the effluent reveals staining of Evans or methylene blue. Low venous outflow resistance implies that there are few obstructing venous valves in the emissary and circumferential veins.

A few vein valves are commonly found in the deep dorsal vein. In such cases valve ablation is mandatory, in a fashion that least injures the surrounding deep dorsal vein endothelium. At present, in our institution, we use a 2-mm Leather valve cutter, introducing it through a 2.5-mm venotomy.

The abdominal incision that provides excellent operative exposure of the inferior epigastric artery is a unilateral transverse abdominal incision. The starting point of the incision

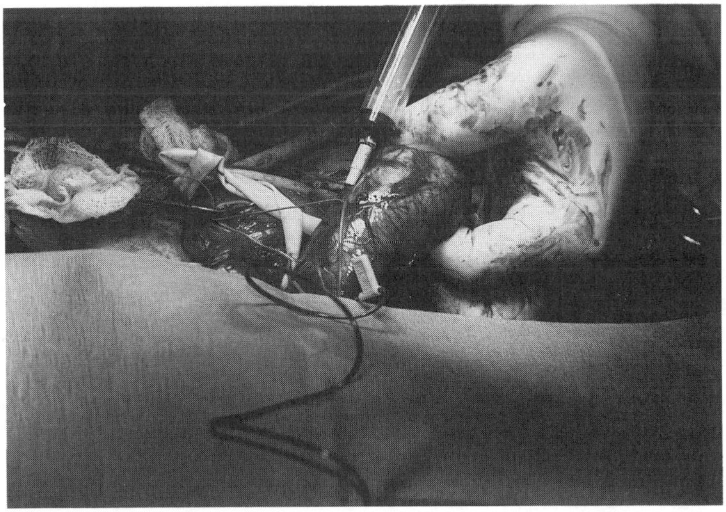

Figure 4-4 Methylene blue solution is injected into the isolated venous segment. Recovery of the methylene blue in the corporal bodies implies that there exists retrograde communication from the deep dorsal vein to the lacunar spaces not impeded by emissary vein valves.

transects a line connecting the umbilicus to the pubic bone at approximately mid-way to two-thirds. The incision is then extended laterally along the skin lines of Langer to the lateral abdominal wall. This incision heals with a more cosmetic scar compared to the scars observed after the previously utilized paramedian skin incision. Although the skin incision is transverse, the rectus fascia is transected horizontally. The rectus muscle is subsequently reflected medially to identify the inferior epigastric artery and its two accompanying veins.

It is critical to harvest an inferior epigastric artery of appropriate length so that there will be no tension on any microvascular anastomosis. The transfer route of the neoarterial inflow source is prepared prior to transecting the vessel distally. The internal ring is identified lateral to the origin of the inferior epigastric artery in the pelvis. The artery is passed between the fundiform and suspensory ligaments at the base of the penis. Following transfer, the bundle should remain vigorously pulsatile. The abdominal incision may be temporarily closed with staples.

Using a Scott retractor and its elastic hooks on the inguinal–scrotal incision, exposure of the 2-cm segment of deep dorsal vein graft is made in the mid-third of the penile shaft, within the lower aspect of the fundiform ligament. Factors involved in the decision of where to create the arteriovenous anastomosis include location of emissary branches in the dorsal vein segment, absence of tension in the inferior epigastric artery, and depth in the incision of the vein segment. The distal adventitia of the inferior epigastric artery and the anterior adventitia of the deep dorsal artery in the region of the anastomosis must be carefully removed.

Under miscroscopic control at ×10 magnification, a vertical venotomy is fashioned in the deep dorsal vein segment. A similar sized vertical arteriotomy is made in the inferior epigastric artery for a side to side anastomosis. Typically 8-0 sutures are used to fashion an inferior epigastric artery to deep dorsal vein anastomosis while 10-0 sutures are used for the inferior epigastric artery to dorsal artery anastomosis. Following release of the low pressure angled temporary occluding vascular clamp on the inferior epigastric artery, the deep dorsal vein segment should reveal arterial pulsations along its length.

A second anastomosis may be subsequently completed between the distal inferior epigastric artery and the dorsal artery in an end-to-end proximal fashion (Figure 4-5A). The inferior epigastric artery and the dorsal artery are approximated and the anastomosis is created using interrupted 10-0 nylon sutures under ×10 magnification. Long-term patency of an anastomosis is dependent on accurate microvascular technique.

Following completion of both microvascular anastomoses, cannulation of the distal deep dorsal vein may be performed to identify post-operative oxygen tension and deep dorsal vein pressures. In our experience, the pressure in the deep dorsal vein graft approaches the systemic brachial arterial blood pressure. After hemostasis has been achieved, closure of the abdominal and inguinal–scrotal incisions may begin in routine fashion. We occasionally place a Jackson-Pratt drain in the scrotum. A Foley catheter is left to straight drainage overnight.

Modifications of the above described procedure are utilized for patterns one, two, and four described above. In pattern one, no deep dorsal vein segment is used and the anastomosis is performed with the end of one proximal dorsal artery segment to the end of the inferior epigastric artery. If appropriate, an end-to-side anastomosis is made and if indicated both dorsal arter-

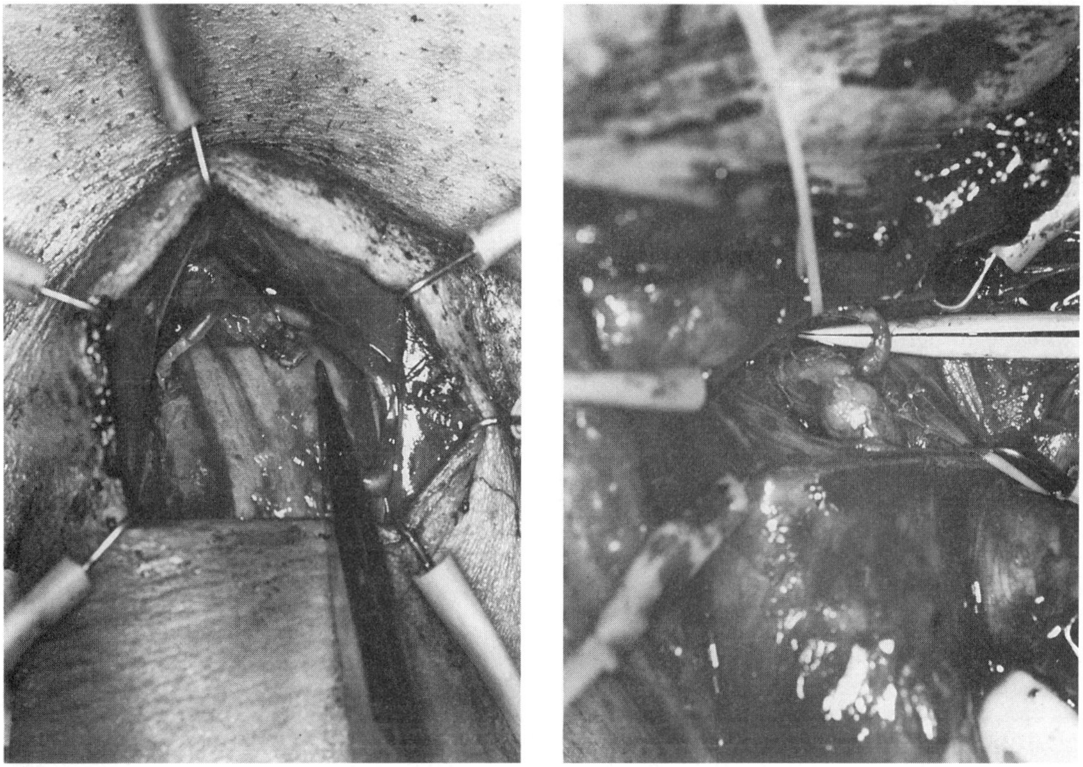

Figure 4-5 (A) Intraoperative photograph showing a microvascular arterial anastomosis of the inferior epigastric artery end-to-side to the deep dorsal vein bypass graft and end-to-end (the microvascular instrument points to the arterial–arterial anastomosis) to the proximal dorsal artery. (B) Intraoperative photograph showing an end-to-side microvascular arterial bypass of the inferior epigastric artery to the deep dorsal vein graft. Note that the fundiform ligament is well preserved in this view.

ies may be used to anastomose to two branches of the inferior epigastric artery end-to-end or one dorsal artery is anastomosed end-to-end while the other is anastomosed end-to-side to the inferior epigastric artery.

In pattern two, no dorsal artery anastomosis is used. Therefore the end of the inferior epigastric artery is anastomosed directly to the dorsal vein segment in an end-to-side fashion (Figure 4-5B). Finally, in pattern four, no abdominal incision is required and the dorsal artery is anastomosed, as in pattern two, end-to-side in an anterolateral position to the deep dorsal vein segment.

Postoperative Care

Most patients spend one evening in the hospital and are discharged the following day. Intercourse, humping, masturbation, or any trauma to the infrapubic area is considered potentially dangerous for a minimum of 6 weeks following surgery. Patients are evaluated at 7 days postoperatively to assess wound healing, remove skin sutures, and identify any problems. Patients are seen again at 6 weeks to test Doppler ultrasound recording of the anastomosis. If possible, patients undergo a follow-up duplex ultrasound for the evaluation of anastomoses patency and dynamic infusion cavernosometry and cavernosography for the evaluation of the hemodynamic status at 6 months. Preoperative and postoperative data are compared.

Conclusions

Some impotent patients will always expect that their abnormal erectile function will be able to be restored naturally without the use of mechanical or pharmacologic support. This concern is particularly important in young impotent patients, who are at the beginning of their personal lives, and have potentially many years of sexuality ahead of them.[1] In our experience, vascular reconstructive surgery for impotence has successfully restored erectile function in such a select group of young patients who have arteriogenic impotence following blunt pelvic or perineal trauma.

To help them achieve this goal, marked improvements in surgical technique have been made in the last decade in arterial reconstructive surgery for impotence. Such technical advances have been founded on sound vascular and microvascular principles. Concomitantly, the diagnostic evaluation for impotence has become more sophisticated, enabling more accurate decisions concerning hemodynamic integrity. It is anticipated that such advances will translate into improved long-term results of arterial reconstructive surgery for impotence.

REFERENCES

1. Hatzichristou DG, Goldstein I: Arterial bypass surgery for impotence. Current Opinion Urol 1992; 1:114–148.
2. Sharlip ID: The role of vascular surgery in arteriogenic and combined arteriogenic and venogenic impotence. Sem Urol 1990; 8:129–137.
3. Michal V, Kramar R, Pospichal J, Hejkal L: Arterial epigastricocavernous anastomosis for the treatment of sexual impotence. World J Surg 1977; 1:515–517.
4. Virag R, Zwang G, Dermange H, Legman M: Vasculogenic impotence: A review of 92 cases with 54 surgical operations. Vasc Surg 1981; 15:9–17.
5. MacGregor RJ, Konnack JW: Treatment of vasculogenic erectile dysfunction by direct anastomosis of the inferior epigastric artery to the central artery to the corpus cavernosum. J Urol 1982; 127:136–139.
6. Crespo E, Soltanik E, Bove D, et al.: Treatment of vasculogenic sexual impotence by revascularizing cavernous and/or dorsal arteries using microvascular techniques. Urology 1982; 20:271–275.
7. McDougal WS, Jeffery RF: Microscopic penile revascularization. J Urol 1983; 129:517–521.
8. Hauri D: A new operative technique in vasculogenic erectile impotence. World J Urol 1986; 4:237–249.
9. Konnak JW, Ohl DA: Microsurgical penile revascularization using central corporeal penile artery. J Urol 1989; 142:305–308.
10. Barada JH, Bennet A: Penile revascularization: Where do we stand? Int J Impotence Res 1990; 2:79–86.

11. Levine FJ, Goldstein I: Vascular reconstructive surgery in the management of erectile dysfunction. Int J Impotence Res 1990; 2:59–78.
12. Krane RJ, Goldstein I, Saenz de Tejada I: Impotence. N Engl J Med 1989; 321:1648–1659.
13. Feldman H, Goldstein I, Hatzichristou DG, Krane RJ, McKinley J: Impotence and its medical correlates: Results of the Massachussets Male Aging Study. In preparation.
14. Breza J, Aboseif SR, Lue TF, Tanagho EM: Cavernous vein arterialization for vasculogenic impotence. An animal model. Urology 1990; 35:513–518.
15. Virag R, Bouilly P, Frydaman D: Is impotence an arterial disorder? A study of arterial risk factors in 400 impotent men. Lancet 1985; 1:181–184.
16. Rosen MP, Greenfield AJ, Walker TG, et al.: Cigarette smoking: An independent risk factor for atherosclerosis in the hypogastric-cavernous bed of men with arteriogenic impotence. J Urol 1991; 145:759–763.
17. Levine FJ, Greenfield AJ, Goldstein I: Arteriographically determined occlusive disease within the hypogastric-cavernous bed in impotent patients following blunt perineal and pelvic trauma. J Urol 1990; 144:1147–1153.
18. Hatzichristou DG, Goldstein I: Penile microvascular arterial bypass surgery: Indications and surgical considerations. Surg Annu (in press).
19. Saenz de Tejada I, Moroukian P, Tessier J, Kim JJ, Goldstein I, Frohrib D: Trabecoular smooth muscle modulates the capacitor function of the penis. Studies on a rabbit model. Am J Physiol 1991; 363:H1590–H1595.
20. Lue TF, Hricak H, Marich KW, Tanagho EA: Vasculogenic impotence evaluated by high resolution ultrasonography and pulsed Doppler spectrum analysis. Radiology 1985; 155:777–781.
21. Bergamini TM, Towne JB, Bandyc DF, Seabrook GR, Shhmitt DD: Experience with in situ saphenous vein bypasses during 1981 to 1989: Determinant factors of long term patency. J Vasc Surg 1991; 13:137–149.
22. Clowes AW, Reidy MA: Prevention of stenosis after vascular reconstruction: Pharmacologic control of intimal hyperplasia—a review. J Vasc Surg 1991; 13:885–891.

ANNOTATED BIBLIOGRAPHY

Barada JH, Bennet A: Penile revascularization: Where do we stand? Int J Impotence Res 1990; 2:79–86.

A review of the different modifications the deep dorsal vein arterialization, including the authors'experience with these methods.

Clowes AW, Reidy MA: Prevention of stenosis after vascular reconstruction: Pharmacologic control of intimal hyperplasia—a review. J Vasc Surg 1991; 13:885–891.

An overview of the problem of intimal thickening of vein grafts with specific references to the role of iatrogenic arterial injury. Furthermore, the mechanisms of local control of vascular deriving factors and the results of various pharmacologic agents in order to prevent intimal hyperplasia are discussed.

Levine FJ, Greenfield AJ, Goldstein I: Arteriographically determined occlusive disease within the hypogastric-cavernous bed in impotent patients following blunt perineal and pelvic trauma. J Urol 1990; 144:1147–1153.

The authors identified characteristic angiographic patterns of arterial occlusion disease for impotent patients with a history of blunt pelvic and perineal trauma.

Saenz de Tejada I, Moroukian P, Tessier J, Kim JJ, Goldstein I, Frohrib D: Trabecoular smooth muscle modulates the capacitor function of the penis. Studies on a rabbit model. Am J Physiol 1991; 363:H1590–H1595.

At this study in an animal model, the authors documented that the corporal venoocclusive mechanism depends on smooth muscle relaxation. In the presence of corporal smooth muscle contraction, venous outflow resistance varies over the range of intracavernosal pressures from 30 to 150 mm Hg. Within this range of intracavernosal pressures, in the presence of complete corporal smooth muscle relaxation, a linear relationship was identified between flow-to-maintain values at different intracavernosal pressures. This observation implied that at complete smooth muscle relaxation conditions, venous outflow resistance was constant.

Sharlip ID: The role of vascular surgery in arteriogenic and combined arteriogenic and venogenic impotence. Sem Urol 1990; 8:129–137.

A review of the literature and the author's comments and experience on patient selection criteria and the different types of arterial bypass procedures for vasculogenic impotence.

5 Venous Ligation for Venogenic Impotence

Ronald W. Lewis

It is well recognized that venous occlusion is a necessary component for normal human erection. This venoocclusive mechanism depends on development of an intracorporeal pressure of 90–110 mm Hg. This increase in intracavernosal pressure depends on good arterial inflow into the cavernous tissue and a normal compliance and elasticity of the cavernous tissue, which is a manifestation of relaxation of the perisinus smooth muscle. For the most part, the veins that drain the corpora cavernosa are found to coalesce as venules in the subtunical space on the outer surface of the corpora cavernosal tissue. These vessels exit as emissary veins through the tunica albuginea into either circumflex veins or, less often, directly into the deep dorsal vein of the penis. The passage of the emissary veins through the thick wall of the tunica in an oblique fashion may also be involved in venous occlusion since, as the penis expands, in the presence of normal elasticity of the tunica albuginea, there is a further curtailment of venous efflux from the deep cavernous tissue.

The problem with venous surgery for the treatment of erectile dysfunction is readily apparent. Since venous occlusion depends to a large degree on compliance of the cavernous tissue and arterial inflow into that tissue, it is imperative that diagnosis of disease in the arterial or the sinus-smooth muscle compartment be extremely accurate. We have certainly witnessed evolving sophistication in arterial disease diagnosis. Now we await methods to diagnose smooth-muscle disease in the cavernous tissue, which might help us to better select those patients who might benefit from venoocclusive surgery.

A defect in the venoocclusive mechanism that is due to a congenital or secondary abnormal vein as a single cause of impotence is not that common. There are many patients with both arterial disease and disease in the smooth muscle of the cavernous tissue, so each or both cause a secondary defect in the venoocclusive mechanism. Since these disorders prevent good arterial inflow or development of good intracavernous pressure, simple venous dissec-

Management of Impotence and Infertility, edited by Douglas Whitehead and Harris Nagler,

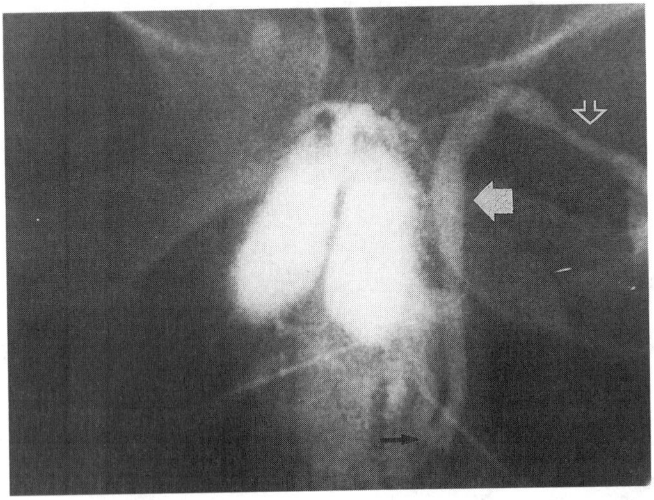

Figure 5-1 This is the cavernosography in a 30-year-old primary impotent male who was found to have a large abnormal sinus draining the corpora cavernosum through a defect in the tunica albuginea (small black arrow) that drain into a large superficial subcutaneous vein on the left side of the penis (large white arrow) and eventually into the external pudendal vein (open white arrow).

tion and ligation surgery may not aid these patients. There are a small number of individuals who have congenital venoocclusive disease, i.e., a large venous sinus that drains directly into aberrant cavernous venous drainage, such as the superficial system, which can be improved with simple ligation of these aberrant veins. Figure 5-1 represents a patient who had a large sinus coalition of vessels that drained aberrantly through the tunica albuginea of the corpus cavernosum on the left side of the penis into a large superficial penile vein. Through a simple circumcision incision, ligation of this vein and closure of the defect in the tunica albuginea led to normal erections for this primary impotent patient. However, it should be stressed that this type of patient is rare. Stief et al. have also described this abnormality.[1]

Similarly, there are iatrogenic causes for runoff from the sinuses of the corpora cavernosa, such as that originally described by Ebbehøj and Wagner.[2] Their description was in a patient who had a shunt between the glans and the distal corpora for the treatment of priapism. The patient persisted with impotence after treatment for the priapism and had sub-

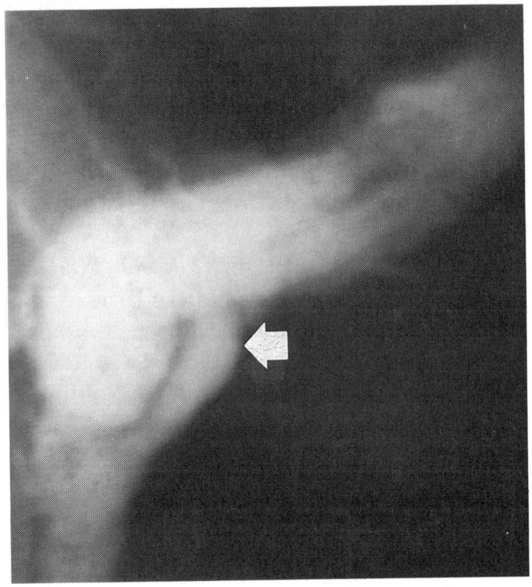

Figure 5-2 This is a young male who had a severe penile scrotal stricture that had been treated by optical internal urethrotomy, and there was a direct communication between the spongiosum and the cavernosum as a result of this surgery. See dense staining of the spongiosum (large white arrow) during filling of the corpora cavernosa with contrast at the time of infusion cavernosography.

sequent successful surgical closure of the corpora to glans shunt. In addition, a cutting of a stricture at the 12 o'clock position in patients with dense bulbar urethral strictures that focally involve the entire wall of the corpus spongiosum may lead to direct communication between the spongiosum and the cavernosum. Figure 5-2 illustrates a representative case in a young man who had a bulbar urethral stricture treated by optical internal urethrotomy with cutting into what was thought to be normal spongiosum. This patient was impotent for approximately 9 months, at which time scarring finally closed the direct fistula to the cavernosa; the patient then regained potency. Patients with Peyronie's disease, treatment of this disease with patch graft, or severe inflammatory disease due to strictures can also have abnormal venous drainage from the cavernous tissue due to effects of a focal defect in the elasticity of the tunica albuginea.[3]

I have prepared several recent review articles in this field.[4–7] Wespes has also recently reviewed penile venous surgery for cavernous impotence.[8] The reader is referred to these articles for more extensive bibliographies. Table 5-1 is a history of very early surgical approaches to the venoocclusive mechanism and significant references in the early modern history of the treatment of venoocclusive dysfunction.

Diagnosis of Venogenic Impotence

The diagnosis of venogenic impotence is based on history and some type of cavernosometry and cavernosography. Venoocclusive dysfunction can be found in cases of primary and secondary impotence. Patients may describe

Table 5-1 Early Surgical Reports of Venous Surgery for Impotence

Study/Year	Reference Number	Comment
Duncan/1895	9	Single case
Wooten/1902	10	Single case
Lydston/1908	11	Superficial results–"second series of 100 patients"–50% successful; 25% improved
Lowsley and Bray/1936	12	Multiple plication procedures, including plication of suspensory ligament to compress dorsal vein—61% successful
Lowsley and Reuda/1953	13	Later follow-up—same operation loosely followed series—37% successful in 273 patients—27% improved
Ebbehøj and Wagner/1979	2	Four cases repaired after infusion cavernosography diagnosis
Virag/1982	14	Mentions in a chapter on penile revascularization that he had treated six cases successfully with deep dorsal vein ligation
Lewis/1984	15	First deep dorsal vein dissection and ligation in October 1981, and 12 subsequent cases reported at the First World Meeting on Impotence in 1984
Wespes and Schulman/1985	16	Report of 20 patients with deep dorsal vein ligation

brief rigid erections with an inability to maintain adequate rigidity or complain of soft erections insufficient for penetration. Nocturnal penile tumescent (NPT) studies usually show REM-associated erections and normal tumescence (circumference changes). Rigidity of the erection is deficient in degree and/or duration. If the patient describes any use of tobacco, we insist on elimination of its use before consideration for venogenic surgery, since this can affect normal venoocclusive function. The patient with significant venoocclusive dysfunction does not get a rigid erection from intracavernosal smooth-muscle relaxant injections or gets a rapid rigid erection with early detumescence by 10–20 minutes.

As mentioned previously, venoocclusive dysfunction can be present secondary to arterial disease. Therefore, we feel that it is imperative to evaluate the arteries with sophisticated tests, such as a color duplex Doppler sonography.[17] If bilateral cavernosal arteries show a velocity of flow >30 cm/second and the diameter of the arteries increase to at least 0.7 mm or greater after the injection of smooth muscle relaxing agent, this is indicative of no significant arterial disease. These velocities of flow and diameter should be followed over a period of 20 minutes with measurement of the values every 5 minutes. We have also found that the end diastolic velocities of flow at 15–20 minutes are good screening indicators for venoocclusive dysfunction, if it is elevated above 3–5 cm/second.[18] In addition, we have found that velocity of flow measured in the deep dorsal vein is not diagnostic of venogenic impotence. Others have also reported this.[19]

We recommend either 10–20 μg of PGE_1 or preferably 0.25 ml of a mixture of papaverine (4.4 mg), phentolamine (0.15 mg), and PGE_1 (1.5 μg) as an injection agent for the color duplex Doppler test or for office testing. A patient who responds with a full rigid erection within 10–15 minutes and sustains it for at least 30 minutes or greater does not have venoocclusive dysfunction that will be improved by venous surgery. If this clinical response is obtained, then it can also be stated that there is no major vascular cause for the erectile dysfunction, and other nonvascular causes should be determined.

If the patient has normal arterial inflow and does not have a rigid erection from the smooth-muscle agent, this is not diagnostic of venoocclusive disorder but is suggestive. Patients who wish to pursue vascular surgery options to solve their erectile dysfunction instead of vacuum constriction devices, penile implants, or trials of other doses of pharmacological injection agents then should have further invasive studies. Invasive tests to diagnose venogenic impotence consist of three major variations of cavernosometry: pump infusion pharmacocavernosometry, gravity pharmacocavernosometry, or decay pressures over given times after steady-state plateau pressures are established by intracavernous saline infusion. In addition, most doctors will prefer pharmacocavernosography to delineate the pattern of venous leakage in the patient who is a candidate for venogenic surgery. We have discussed in a previous publication some of the early history of cavernosometry and cavernosography, and the reader is referred to that study.[4]

At this time, I prefer infusion pump pharmacocavernosometry and pharmacocavernosography (see Table 5-2 for a description of our current technique). We are continuing to look at infusion pump cavernosometry and pharmacocavernosometry along with gravity pharmacocavernosometry in attempts to determine the efficacy of the gravity test. We do believe that the maintenance flow rate on pharmacocavernosometry is the most important measurement that is indicative of venoocclusive dysfunction. Ten to fifteen minutes after the injection

Table 5-2 Technique of Cavernosometry/Cavernosography

Two 19-gauge needles placed into each corpus cavernosum (obliquely, toward patient's head), without anesthesia, laterally along shaft of penis under sterile conditions
One needle connected for pressure measurement via a transducer connected to a physiologic recorder or monitor
Other needle connected to an infusion roller pump for infusion of heparinized saline solution (1000 units/1000 ml)—prewarmed to body temperature
Record baseline pressure
Infuse fluid at 50 ml/minute increments until full erection occurs (90–100 mm Hg), then decrease flow to obtain flow rate needed to maintain erection (do not infuse above 300 ml/minute)
Inject through needle pharmacologic agent (usually 45 mg of papaverine and 2.5 mg of phentolamine)
Record baseline pressure 10 minutes later
Repeat flow study obtaining flow rate to maintain erection (do not infuse above 150 ml/minute)
Inject 30% diatrozoate or iothalomate meglumine (60 ml full strength or 120 ml 50% dilution with saline) at same rate as last maintenance flow rate and obtain cine, fluoroscopic images, or spot static X-ray images (AP and oblique) for cavernosography

of 45 mg of papaverine and 2.5 mg of phentolamine, we define any maintenance flow rate >50 ml/minute as a definite indication of venoocclusive dysfunction. If a flow rate of 30–50 ml/minute is necessary to obtain an intracavernous pressure of 100 mm Hg, this is considered borderline and suggestive of venoocclusive dysfunction. Finally, anything <30 ml/minute of flow is an indication of no active venoocclusive dysfunction (see Table 5-3 for other infusion cavernosometry data that have appeared in the literature).

After completing pharmacocavernosometry studies, we perform pharmacocavernosography with 60 ml of iothalomite meglumine or diatrozoate (30%) infused into the corpora at the same rate as the postinjection maintenance flow rate to produce an intracavernous pressure of at least 90–100 mm Hg. Non-sodium-containing water-soluble contrast medium is used to limit discomfort. Rapid runoff of contrast into dilated deep dorsal penile vein or veins, cavernosal veins, crural veins, or into the superficial system with eventual runoff into the external pudendal vein can be seen in patients with a venous leak[26,32] (see Figures 5-3–5-6).

In 1990, Puech-Leao and his associates introduced gravity cavernosometry.[33] Meuleman and his associates compared the diagnostic values of infusion pump and gravity cavernosometry in the evaluation of the cavernous venoocclusive mechanism.[34] In this study, two groups of patients were studied by various pharmacocavernosometry criteria, either infusion pump or gravity studies. Group 1 consisted of patients who obtained a positive response to the injection of 50 mg of papaverine intracavernously in the office with a rigid erection within 10 minutes after injection (performed on two separate occasions). Group 2 were patients who had a consistently negative test on both of the injections (see Table 5-4 for the results of comparison between the two tests found most significant for diagnosing venoocclusive dysfunction). It was the conclusion of these authors that maintenance flow rates obtained by infusion pump cavernosometry followed by steady-state intracavernous measurements obtained on gravity cavernosometry are the two most accurate parameters to separate patients with from patients without venoocclusive dysfunction. They did feel that there was a higher risk of dislocation of the intracavernous needles with pump cavernosometry compared to gravity cavernosometry.

Table 5-3 Cavernosometry and Pharmacocavernosometry Findings in Patients with Venoocclusive Dyfunction

Study (year)	Infusion Flow Rates (ml/minute) Initiation	Maintenance (Range)
Without Pharmacologic Agents		
Virag (1982)[14]	>200	>100
Puyau and Lewis (1983)[20]	>180	
Buvat et al. (1986)[21]		
Severe leak		120
Moderate leak		80–120
Wespes et al. (1986)[22]	202	111
Delcour et al. (1986)[23]	215.5	145
Porst et al. (1987)[24]	139.3 (53–230)	116.7 (35–230)
Stief and Wetterauer (1989)[25]		
Primary impotence		205 (173–350)
Secondary impotence		238 (136–326)
Lewis (1990)[26]		
Possible leak		75–100
Definite leak		>100
After Pharmacologic Agents		
Wespes et al. (1986)[22]	103	43.5
Delcour et al. (1986)[23]	124.1	73.4
Bennett and Garofalo (1989)[27]		> 60
Knoll et al. (1989)[28]		≥150
Lewis (1990)[26]		
Possible leak		30–50
Definite leak		> 50
Knoll et al. (1990)[29]		
Mild leak		24–45
Moderate leak		45–65
Severe leak		> 65
Kropman et al. (1990)[30]	> 35	> 20
Weiske (1990)[31]		
Possible leak		15–30
Definite leak		> 30

Other diagnostic tests that purport to diagnose venoocclusive dysfunction are Phase II of Goldstein's dynamic infusion cavernosometry and cavernosography (DICC).[35] This is performed following intracavernosal injection of 45 mg of papaverine and 2.5 mg of phentolamine. The pressure drop over 30 seconds from 150 ml steady state reached with infusion pump, which is turned off after the steady state is reached, should not be over 30–50 mm Hg in

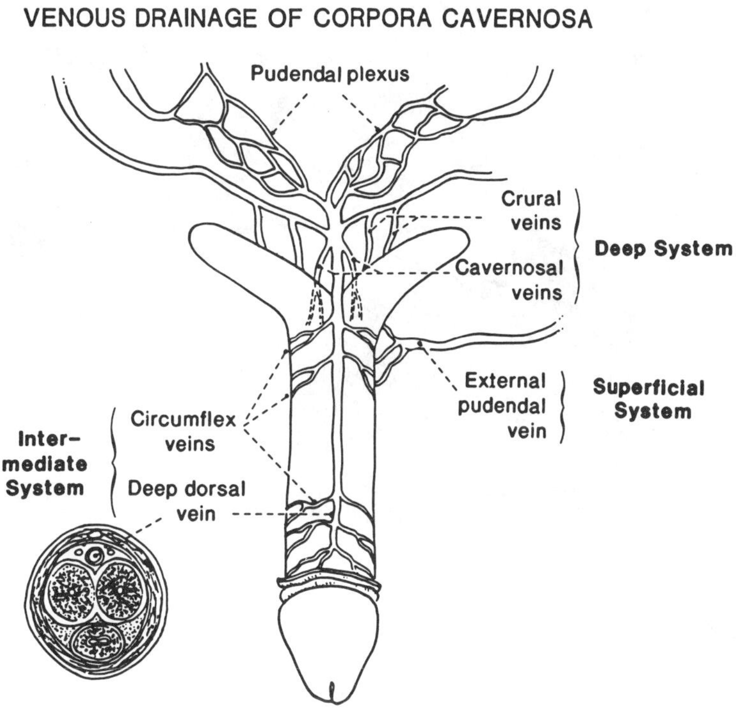

Figure 5-3 Diagrammatic representation of the different areas of venous leakage divided into the superficial, intermediate, and deep system of veins.

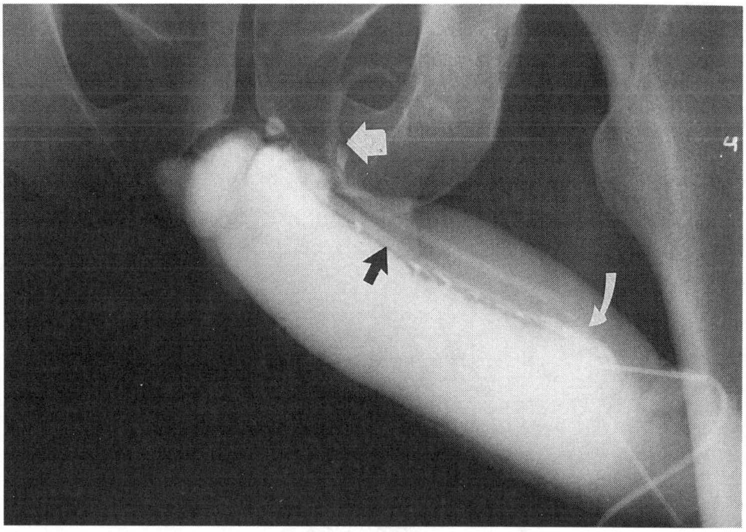

Figure 5-4 Excellent example of the deep dorsal vein filling on pharmacocavernosography (small black arrow). Note there is also communication between the deep dorsal vein and a more superficial vein (small curved white arrow); the superficial vein eventually empties into the external pudendal system (large white arrow).

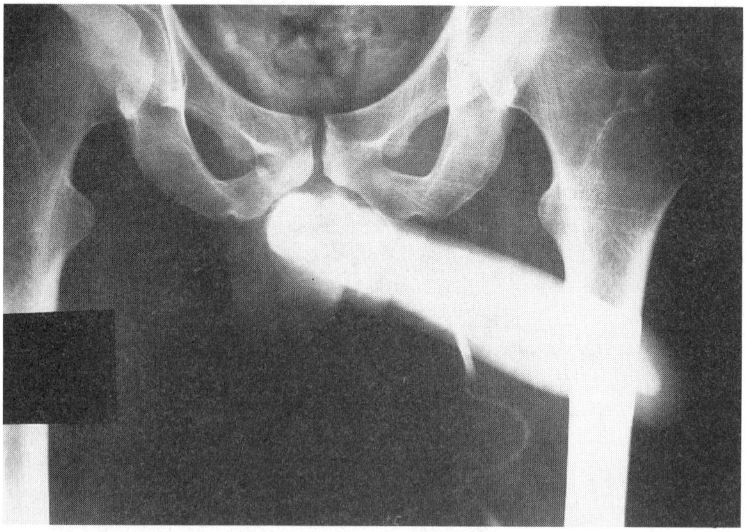

Figure 5-5 Normal rigid corpora cavernosa that shows no significant venous drainage at the time of pharmacocavernosography.

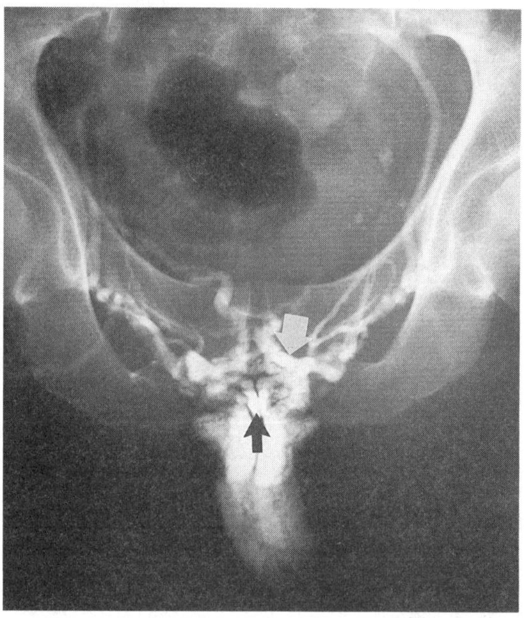

Figure 5-6 This shows drainage into a large retropubic venous complex (large white arrow) through two large cavernosal veins (small black arrow) at the base of the penis.

normal individuals. However, we have not found this to be an accurate test.[4]

Freidenberg and his associates calculated a venous outflow resistance measurement based on flow necessary to maintain corporeal pressure 20 mm Hg above the mean arterial pressure 20 minutes or so after the injection of 60 mg of papaverine into the corpora.[36] In 48 patients with significant leakage on cavernosography, venous outflow resistance was <14.2 mm Hg minute/ml. A later study using this criterion compared decay pressure measurement, maintenance flow rates, and venous outflow resistance in impotent and potent men.[37] The conclusion was that resistant values were probably the most sensitive method to diagnose venous leaks, based on the fact that it was normal, i.e., >5 mm Hg minute/ml, in 95% of their 20 potent controls and this value corresponded to <30 ml/minute to maintain an intracavernous pressure of 150 mm Hg in those impotent patients who are not thought to have venoocclusive dysfunction. It was felt that the

Table 5-4 Comparison of Pump and Gravity Pharmacocavernosometry[a]

Test	Patient Group	Number of Patients	Mean ± Standard Deviation	Median (range)	p Value (Comparison Groups 1 and 2)
Steady state intracavernous pressure (mm Hg)—parameter of gravity cavernosometry	1	22	97 ± 19	102 (35–120)	<0.001
	2	26	59 ± 35	66 (10–108)	
Maintenance flow ml/minute–parameter of infusion pump cavernosometry	1	46	14 ± 13	10 (0–60)	<0.001
	2	41	89 ± 82	50(5–200)	

[a] From Meuleman and associates.[34]

resistant values >5 mm Hg minute/ml were more likely to represent normal than values of ≤5.

In summary, the patients selected for venoocclusive surgery should have no evidence of concomitant arterial disease, should not smoke, and should demonstrate venoocclusive dysfunction by cavernosometry, pharmacocavernosometry, and pharmacocavernosography. We discuss other options of treatment with every patient. Particularly relevant here is the discussion of penile implants. Penile implants do have a high success rate, but are of a more permanent nature. Options after penile implant are few should there be a complication, such as infection requiring removal of the device. Vacuum constriction devices should be offered to every patient who has venoocclusive dysfunction as a first line of attack. Finally, pharmacological injection therapy, which may not work with a patient with moderate or severe venoocclusive dysfunction, might be effective in patients with minor venous leakage problems. Some patients who have venoocclusive dysfunction have preferred a combination of pharmacological injection therapy and the use of vacuum constriction devices. Patients should be clearly presented with the high failure rate of venoocclusive surgery, ranging from 30 to 40%. These patients are encouraged to carefully study the other options. We wholeheartedly agree with the concept that Dr. Tom Lue has described of patient goal-directed therapy.[38]

Surgical Technique

Some of the early surgical approaches to venoocclusive dysfunction were directed at simple ligation of the deep dorsal vein alone. We have always advocated complete penile vein dissection and ligation of any of the vessels that have been demonstrated on pharmacocavernosography. We believe in complete deep dorsal vein dissection with ligation of all direct emissary veins that are feeding into this deep dorsal vein in the midline, as well as ligation of the circumflex veins feeding into the deep dorsal vein. This dissection is taken to approximately 1 cm from the glans. It is at this level that the multiple tributaries that drain from the glans into the deep dorsal vein coalesce to form a single or double trunk. In addition, we carefully inspect the junction of the corpora cavernosa to the spongiosum and ligate any communicators between the circumflex veins and the spongiosum or veins draining the spongiosum (see Figure 5-7 for a detailed description for the operation).

We prefer the anterior scrotal incision as described by Doctor Lue.[39] We also recommend complete taking down of the suspensory ligament to reach the infrapubic area. It should be mentioned that great care should be given to staying in the midline if cavernosal veins are ligated. These vessels can be identified as veins by using an intraoperative Doppler probe.

Figure 5-7 Steps in penile vein dissection and ligation. (A) The standard anterior scrotal peripenile incision. Penile edema is less likely to occur with this incision. (B, C) The inversion of the penile shaft into the perpenile incision. The entire penile shaft can be approached by this inversion, and the infrapubic region can easily be reached through it. (D) As the penile skin is stripped away from the penile shaft, there is often a connection between the deep penile veins and the superficial penile veins. The junction between these two systems can be identified and ligated at this step. (E) Two important steps are shown. A 19-gauge needle is placed into one of the corpora, usually on the side of the incision. After the injection of a pharmacological agent, indigo carmine can be injected to demonstrate effluxing veins. In addition, as shown in the last portion of this figure, this same line can be used for controlled infusion cavernosometry. The fixation of the butterfly wing by the chromic suture allows for less chance of dislodgement during the procedure. This step also shows a sharp dissection of the infrapubic suspensory ligament. Please note that care should be taken in this area because often superficial draining veins from the pubis can join the more superficial of the penile veins. This step shows a deeper incision of the suspensory ligament. The less defined superficial fundiform ligaments have already been cut. The suspensory ligament will be reapproximated with silk ligature at the end of the procedure. (F) This shows placement of a large silk suture around the deep dorsal vein in the infrapubic region. This particular diagram shows the vein fully exposed with the artery to its left margin. Buck's fascia has been removed for the sake of the illustration to show the orientation of the arteries and vein. Sometimes, the deep dorsal vein consists of more than one trunk along the shaft of the penis, but usually in the infrapubic region, these coalesce to form one large draining vein. This vein also has to be eliminated to approach the deeper cavernosal veins, which sometimes join directly to this vein as a common trunk in the infrapubic region or sometimes drain directly into the pudendal plexus or the internal pudendal veins. (G) This shows a careful dissection of the deep dorsal vein along the shaft of the penis until the region of the glans where several trunks can be seen to coalesce to begin the deep dorsal vein. Circumflex and direct emissary veins that drain into this deep dorsal vein are identified as this vein is dissected, divided between clamps or divided between ligatures, as the deep dorsal vein is dissected. It is extremely important to stay in the midline because of the dorsal arteries and penile nerve bundles that lie in close proximity just lateral to this vein on either side. The dissection is taken to approximately 1–2 cm from the glans edge since the nerves tend to fan out over the veins in this area. Any ligatures used on the penile shaft are absorbable. (H) This demonstrates the controlled cavernosometry that is performed after penile vein dissection and ligation to compare with preoperative cavernosometry data. This is accomplished after another 30 mg of papaverine has been injected into the corpora. Ten minutes later this controlled cavernosometry is obtained. If adequate venous dissection has been performed, maintanance flow rate is usually well below 5–10 ml/minute. (From Lewis RW: Diagnosis and management of corporal venoocclusive dysfunction. Semin Urol 1990; 8:119. Reproduced with permission of Mayo Foundation.)

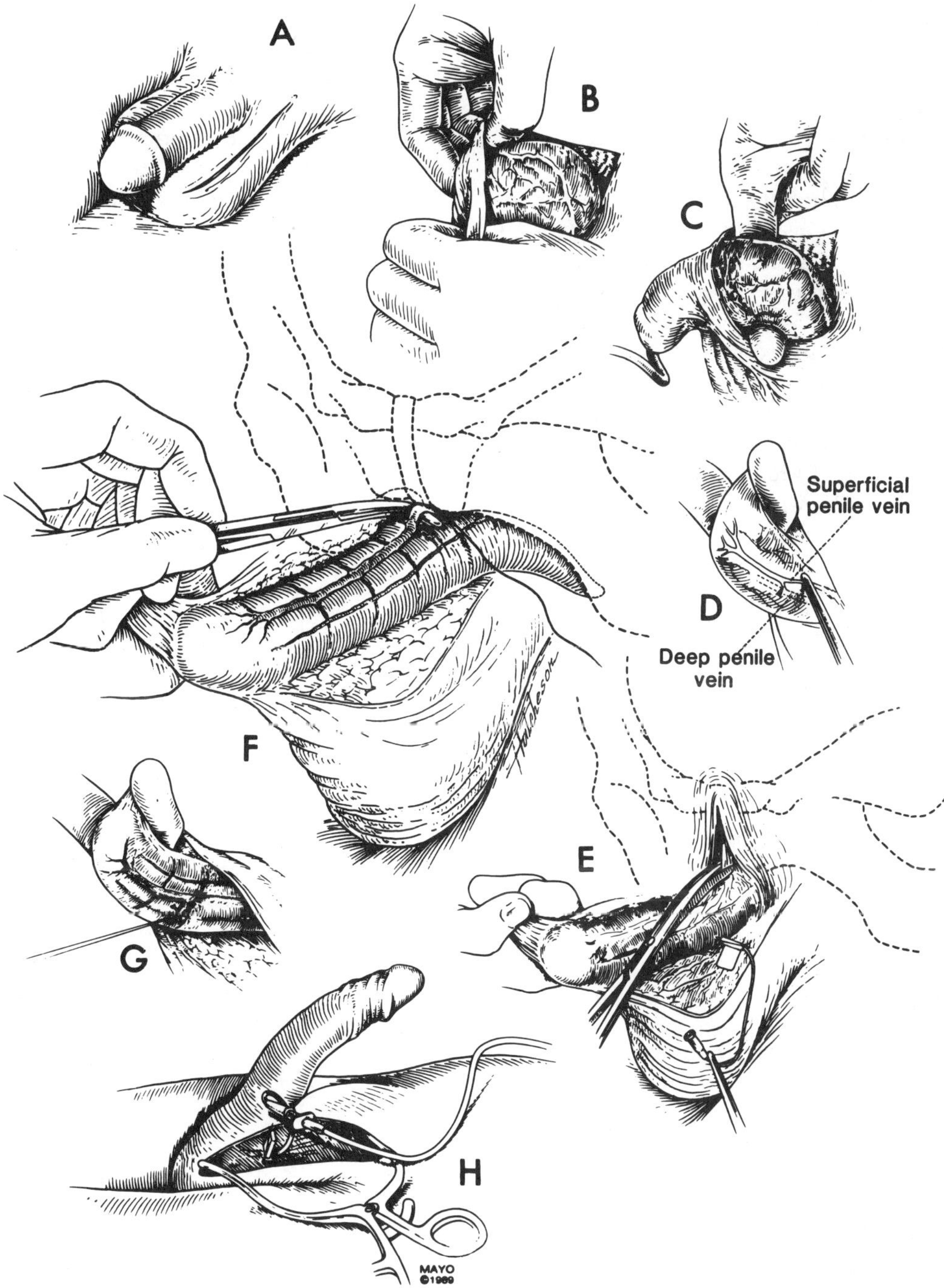
A
B
C
Superficial penile vein
D
Deep penile vein
F
E
G
H
MAYO
©1989

There has been a case in the United States where deep vein dissection led to complete ligation of the urethra, mistaking this for a large cavernosal vein.

We originally performed deep vein dissection and ligation through a circumcision-type incision, but found that it was inadequate to get to the deeper veins. We have found that it is still useful in patients who have a large sinus draining vein into the superficial system, such as shown in Figure 5-1. We have also tried vertical or horizontal infrapubic incisions, but do not feel that they are as adequate in approaching the complete infrapubic region as the anterior scrotal incision. In addition, they are more apt to be associated with significant penile edema postoperatively. A perineal incision is used only if we feel that the leakage is through major crural veins, and we plan crural banding or occlusion. We have used these techniques only as a secondary procedure.

We usually prefer placing a small round fenestrated suction-type drain in the infrapubic region exited out of a separate stab wound lateral to the infrapubic scrotal incision. The penis is wrapped gently with a self-adherent elastic dressing, and we usually leave a urethral catheter in place overnight after surgery.

Results of Surgery

There have been many reports of the results of surgery for venoocclusive disease. The review articles that I have written have tabulated this as information has become available. Table 5-5 shows the results of the surgery for venoocclusive surgery for sexual dysfunction from what I think are the better documented series: those series with large number of patients and with adequate follow-up. The surgery used by the different authors in these series has varied immensely. I will speak in detail to the results of surgery from the Mayo Clinic since I am more familiar with the long-term results of these patients and have followed them closely.

There are two groups of patients that are reported by me and listed in Table 5-5: the Tulane series performed at that institution from 1981 to 1987 and the Mayo series operated on from 1987 to 1989. In Table 5-5, the "excellent" category is return to full erectile capacity without any need for supplementation and the ability of the patient then to have full sexual intercourse to his and his partner's satisfaction. Most of the 1987 and 1988 Mayo series patients had vein dissection in the infrapubic region after complete division of the suspensory ligament, and all of the patients in the Mayo 1988–1989 series had this approach. There has been some minor improvement in the excellent and improved groups in the Mayo later series than the earlier series. We feel that one of the main reasons for this is an improvement in the diagnosis of arterial disease with the color duplex Doppler test.

In an analysis of the systolic artery velocity of flow when successes (excellent or improved) were compared to failures (immediate success/later failure or failures), it was found that 52% of the failures had either both or one-sided velocities of 25–29 cm/second compared to 23% of the successes. The mean cavernous artery systolic velocity of flow in the failure group was 35.5 cm/second compared to the success group with a mean velocity of flow was 43 cm/second. We originally used a normal value of systolic velocity of flow equal to or greater than 25 cm/second, but have modified our criteria and now consider normal flow in patients who have a velocity of flow >30 cm/second. We feel those who have a systolic vel-

Table 5-5 Results of Surgery for Venoocclusive Sexual Dysfunction

Study (Year of Study)	Number of Patients	Excellent	Improved	Immediate Success/Later Failure	Failures	Average Follow-up (Months)
Lewis—Tulane Series (1981–1987)[40]	49	12 (24%)	12 (24%)	8 (16%)	17 (35%)	15
Wespes et al. (1982–1986)[41]	67[a]	31 (46%)	16 (24%)		20 (30%)	24
Austoni et al. (1987)[42]	234	129 (55%)		21 (9%)	84 (36%)	9
Lue (1986–1988)[43]	68[b]	36 (53%)	17 (25%)	4 (6%)	11 (16%)	Unknown
Bondil et al. (1981–1988)[44]	60	25 (42%)[c]			35 (58%)	22
Lunglmayr et al. (1984–1986)[45]	29	9 (31%)[c]		10 (34.5%)	10 (34.5%)	to 24
Weidner et al. (1984–1988)[46]	51	28 (55%)		8 (16%)[d]	15 (29%)[d]	20
Treiber and Gilbert (1985–1987)[47]	115	28 (24%)	39 (34%)		48 (42%)	12.9
Lewis—Mayo Series						
(1987–1988)	28	7 (25%)	4 (14%)	8 (29%)	9 (32%)	36
(1988–1989)	32	9 (28%)	13 (41%)	5 (15.5%)	5 (15.5%)	18
Knoll et al. (1987–1989)[29]	41	22 (54%)	Unknown	Unknown	19 (46%)	18
Kropman et al. (1987–1989)[30]	20	6 (30%)	4 (20%)	8 (40%)	2 (10%)	15
Rossman et al. (1985–1988)[48]	16	2 (12.5%)	2 (12.5%)	10 (62.5%)	2 (12.5%)	Unknown
Claes and Baert (1987–1989)[49]	72	30 (41.7%)	23 (31.9%)		19 (26.4%)	>12

[a] Sixty-seven patient questionnaire responses to 105 letters sent.
[b] Four not reported because too soon after surgery or no follow-up.
[c] Series reported as excellent or improved as a group not in each individual category.
[d] Fourteen of 23 are now able to get pharmacologic agent injection erection.

ocity of flow 25–30 cm/second fall into the borderline area where arterial disease may exist and more invasive arterial evaluations, such as pudendal arteriography, would be performed before attempting venous surgery in these patients. Also, in patients where there is a discrepancy between the changes in arterial diameter compared to velocities of flow or if suspicion for arterial disease is high because of history of trauma, we would also tend in these cases to perform pudendal arteriography before attempting venous dissection and ligation surgery.

We believe that the improved category of patients, which represents approximately 20–25% of our patients, is a valid group in which to consider venous surgery helpful. These patients for the most part require pharmacologic erection therapy to supplement their erections. But in multiple trials with injection therapy prior to venoocclusive surgery, these patients have not been able to obtain a rigid erection for vaginal penetrance. Some authors have criticized considering this group of patients successes, but I disagree since these patients were not able to use one of the types of treatment (pharmacologic erection therapy) until after the surgery. The patients with immediate success and later failure certainly suggest the development of collateral vein circulation. Any series that reports results only before 12 months should be viewed with some skepticism since early results can dissipate as collaterals develop over the first year postoperatively. Importantly, as we study the results of Table 5-5, the failure rate of venous surgery is still 30–50%. This failure rate is certainly what should be stressed to the patient who is a candidate for venoocclusive surgery prior to selection of the therapy by the patient.

Three of the 60 patients in the Mayo series have had prior venous surgery elsewhere, and these patients subsequently have had improvement from their venoocclusive surgery at our institution. Five of our patients have had other subsequent surgery directed at venoocclusive dysfunction, two with a retropubic approach, two with an approach to veins other than a deep venous system, such as crural veins or veins between the corpus cavernosa and the spongiosum (spongiosolysis), and one who has had crural compression by banding. Four of these five patients with subsequent surgery have had improvement after the second surgery. We have found the approach to the crural vessels, spongiosolysis or crural banding, necessary only as a secondary procedure, and similar results have been reported by Treiber and Gilbert.[47]

Four of the 60 patients at Mayo Clinic have had simultaneous Peyronie's excision with a patch graft repair along with a deep vein dissection and ligation, and only one of these patients has had success from this type of surgery. As mentioned, we do not presently recommend venous occlusion surgery in patients with Peyronie's plaque.

When we compare successes and failures in the Mayo series, there was no difference in the mean ages of the patients, NPT findings, cavernosometry or pharmacocavernosometry maintenance flow rates, or baseline pressures after intracorporeal injection of vasoactive agents. Rossman et al. report similar findings of no correlation of the visible site of the leak, age of the patient, duration of disease, and rate of initial maintenance infusion between those who have had success and those who have had failures.[48] On the other hand, a very recent report by Claes and Baert suggests that there may be a greater improvement in subsets of patients according to maintenance flow rates.[49]

Complications

Short-term minor complications with vein ligation surgery occur quite commonly and consist of mild to moderate penile edema and superficial scrotal and penile shaft bruising of the skin. This usually resolves completely within 5–10 days after surgery. I found penile edema to occur less often with the anterior scrotal incision of Lue than with vertical or horizontal infrapubic incisions.

There are two major complications that are seen frequently with penile venogenic surgery. The first is numbness or anesthetic areas in the penis, particularly in the glans area. This is usually not total anesthesia. Sixteen of our 60 patients have had focal numbness or anesthesia of a portion of the glans of the penis. Almost all of the patients who have had a full return of sensation have noted early hyperesthesias, and we have found this sign to be a very excellent prognostic indicator for return of full sensation. I have found that patients usually regain feeling quite late after surgery, but the majority, in approximately 80–90% of the cases, develop complete return of sensation 7 to 9 months after surgery.

Another major complication described by the patient is a complaint of postoperative penile shortening. We have taken care to reapproximate the penis to the pubic periosteum and infrapubic region with a permanent suture and attempt to approximate all layers, but we have had a complaint of penile shortening in approximately 20% of our patients. There has been significant decrease in penile length requiring a revision with freeing of scar tissue and release of penile contracture in approximately 12% of our patients (7 of 60).

Seven patients have complained of prolonged discomfort up to 2 months after surgery, but this has gradually resolved. Ten of the patients have complained of decreased ability for orgasm, probably related to decreased sensations, since this complaint was present in almost all of these patients. Actual worsening of erectile function in patients who are able to have some partial erection prior to surgery is extremely rare and has been associated with only a few patients who have had Peyronie's plaque excision and a patch graft repair along with venous dissection surgery. In fact, our results with venous occlusion surgery in association with Peyronie's plaque excision and patch graft repair has been so dismal that we do not recommend venous surgery in this type of patient; instead we recommend placement of a penile prosthesis in the presence of Peyronie's disease of a severe nature in the impotent patient with venoocclusive disease. In our early series, we had to evacuate hematomas in one or two patients. Leaving a fenestrated suction type surgical drain in place after venous surgery has decreased the rate of postoperative wound hematomas measurably. We leave the drain in until the drainage has significantly decreased, sometimes from 48 to 72 hours. We have not performed operation for a hematoma since placing drains immediately postoperative.

Reasons for Failure of Venoocclusive Surgery

The surgery for venoocclusive disease, in my opinion, can be explained by four possible mechanisms. The first, and I think a major area of failure in some of the earlier series, was the inability to diagnose concomitant arterial disease. Newer techniques for arterial evaluation, such as a color duplex Doppler and a high index of suspicion in patients with history of vascular disease or other vascular risk factors, have allowed us to appreciate some improvement in the eradication of this particular factor. Another reason for some of the earlier failures is that surgery was not directed at completely removing all of the veins that are found to be responsible for the defective venoocclusive mechanism. The newer complete surgery, which has been outlined in this chapter, helped eliminate this as a major factor of failure. A third important mechanism for failure in venoocclusive surgery is development of collateral circulation. This probably accounts for the majority of patients who have had immediate success with later failure. Other papers have addressed the persistence of veins that were missed at surgery or the development of collateral veins, such as runoff into the spongiosum.[50,51] From this last category of patients, it is imperative that follow-up beyond 12 months be given before final results from individual groups surgical experience with venoocclusive surgery be given.

It is appropriate to end this chapter with a reiteration of what has been truly a major problem from venous surgery. This is for the most part that we are not treating a pathological venous abnormality but are trying only to eliminate venous runoff, which aids a defect in one of the components of erection that appears to be passive, and that is venoocclusion. This passive phase of the erectile cycle depends on two active components of erection, arterial inflow and the compliance of the corporeal space accomplished by relaxation of the sinus-smooth muscles. We have certainly improved the diagnosis of arterial disease, but yet we do not have a practical test for diagnosing sinus-smooth muscle disease that may be so severe that eliminating some of the channels that carry blood away from the corporeal tissue may not be able to produce enough aid in venoocclusion to benefit the patients from surgery. The veins that we dissect and ligate on the outer surface of the tunica albuginea are, in fact, usually not pathological veins, but are ultimate draining sites of the emissary veins that do not shut down in these patients with venoocclusive disorder. There are a significant number of patients who have had penile vein dissection and ligation who obtain a long-term benefit from this surgery, but the failure rates of 30–50% are still an area of concern.

It is my opinion that there are fewer patients who are candidates for venoocclusive surgery, and the choice of surgery for these patients has to be a highly selective process. In addition, it is imperative that the patients be informed of these failure rates and also be informed of the alternative treatments available to them so that they may goal-direct their therapy.

REFERENCES

1. Stief CG, Gall H, Scherb W, Bähren U: Erectile dysfunction due to ectopic penile vein. Urology 1988; 31:300.
2. Ebbehøj J, Wagner G: Insufficient penile erections due to abnormal drainage of cavernous bodies. Urology 1979; 13:507.
3. Dalkin BL, Carter MF: Venogenic impotence following dermal graft repair for Peyronie's disease. J Urol 1991; 146:849.
4. Lewis RW: Venous ligation surgery for venous leakage. Int J Impotence Res 1990; 2:1.
5. Lewis RW: Results of surgery for venoocclusive disease. J Sex Mar Ther 1991; 17:129.
6. Lewis RW, Fallen MJ: Diagnosis and management of venogenic impotence. AUA Update Series, Lesson 31 1991; 10:242.
7. Lewis RW: Venogenic impotence: Diagnosis, management, and results. In: Lewis RW, Barrett DM, eds. Problems in urology: The impotent man. Philadelphia: Lippincott, 1991; 5:567.
8. Wespes E: Penile venous surgery for cavernous impotence. World J Urol 1990; 8:97.
9. Duncan JA: Old age—a myth. Toledo Med Surg Reporter 1895; 3:163.
10. Wooten JA: Ligation of the dorsal vein of the penis as a cure for atonic impotence. Texas Med J 1902–3; 18:325.
11. Lydston GF: The surgical treatment of impotency. Am J Clin Med 1908; 15:1571.
12. Lowsley OS, Bray JL: The surgical relief of impotence: Further experiences with a new operative procedure. JAMA 1936; 107:2029.
13. Lowsley OS, Rueda EA: Further experience with an operation for the cure of certain types of impotence. J Int Coll Surg 1953; 19:69.
14. Virag R: Revascularization of the penis. In: Ben-

net AH, ed. Management of male impotence. Baltimore: Williams & Wilkins, 1982: 219.
15. Lewis RW, Puyau FA, Kerstein MD, Kaack MG: Corpora cavernosa outflow as defined by dynamic cavernosography—implications in the evaluation and treatment of impotence. In: Virag R, Virag-Lappas H. eds. Proceedings of the First World Meeting on Impotence. Paris: les Editions des CERI, 1984: 172.
16. Wespes E, Schulman CC: Venous leakage: Surgical treatment of a curable cause of impotence. J Urol 1985; 133:796.
17. Quam JP, King BK, James EM, et al.: Duplex color Doppler sonographic evaluation of vasculogenic impotence. JAR 1989; 153:1141.
18. Hattery RR, King BF, Lewis RW, James EM, McKusick MA: Vasculogenic impotence: Duplex and color Doppler imaging. Radiol Clinics NA 1991; 29:629.
19. Vickers MA, Benson CB, Richie JP: High resolution ultrasonography and pulsed wave Doppler for detection of corporovenous incompetence in erectile dysfunction. J Urol 1990; 143:1125.
20. Puyau FA, Lewis RW: Corpus cavernosography-pressure flow and radiography. Invest Rad 1983; 18:517.
21. Buvat J, LeMaire A, DeHaene JL, Buvat-Herbaut M, Guieu JD: Venous incompetence: Critical study of the organic basis of high maintenance flow rates during artificial erection test. J Urol 1986; 135:926.
22. Wespes E, Delcour C, Stryven J, Schulman CC: Pharmacocavernometry—cavernography in impotence. Br J Urol 1986; 48:429.
23. Delcour C, Wespes E, Vandenbosch G, Schulmann CC, Struyven J: Impotence: evaluation with cavernosography. Radiology 1986; 161:80.
24. Porst H, van Ahlen H, Vahlensieck W: Relevance of dynamic cavernosography to the diagnosis of venous incompetence in erectile dysfunction. J Urol 1987; 137:1163.
25. Stief CG, Wetterauer U: Quantitative and qualitative analysis of dynamic cavernosographies in erectile dysfunction due to venous leakage. Urology 1989; 34:252.
26. Lewis RW, Parulkar BGF, Johnson CM: Radiology of impotence. In: Lytton B, Catalona WJ, Lipshultz LI, McGuire EJ, eds. Advances in urology, Vol. 3. Chicago: Year Book Medical Publishers, 1990: 132.
27. Bennett AH, Garofalo FA: Enhanced cavernometry: Procedure for the diagnosis of venogenic impotence. Br J Urol 1989; 64:420.
28. Knoll LD, Furlow WL, Benson RL: Infusion cavernosometry and cavernosography: our experience as an office procedure. Int J Impotence Res 1989; 1:131.
29. Knoll LD, Furlow WL, Benson RC: Penile venous surgery for the management of cavernosal venous leakage. Int J Impotence Res 1990; 2:21.
30. Kropman RF, Nijeholt AABL, Giespers AGM, Swarten IJK: Results of deep penile vein resection in impotence caused by venous leakage. Int J Impotence Res 1990; 2:29.
31. Weiske WH: Pharmacocavernosometry and pharmacocavernosography in erectile dysfunction. Urologe 1990; 29:126.
32. Shabsigh R, Fishman IJ, Toombs BD, Skolkin M: Venous leaks: Anatomical and physiological observations. J Urol 1991; 146:1260.
33. Puech-Leao P, Chao S, Glina S, Reichelt AC: Gravity cavernosometry: A simple diagnostic test for cavernosal incompetence. Br J Urol 1990; 65:391.
34. Meuleman EJH, Wijkstra H, Douesburg WIMH, Debruyne FMJ: Comparison of the diagnostic value of pump and gravity and cavernosometry in the evaluation of the cavernous veno-occlusive mechanism. J Urol 1991; 146:1266.
35. Goldstein I: Vasculogenic impotence—its diagnosis and treatment. In: DeVere White R, ed. Sexual dysfunction problems in urology. Philadelphia: Lippincott, 1987: 547.
36. Freidenberg DH, Berger RE, Chew DE, Ireton R, Ansell JS, Schwartz AN: Quantitation of corporeal venous outflow resistance in man by corporeal pressure flow evaluation. J Urol 1987; 138:533.
37. Lowe MA, Schwartz AN, Berger RE: Controlled trial of infusion cavernosometry in impotent and potent men. J Urol 1991; 146:783.

38. Lue TF: Impotence: A patient's goal-directed approach to treatment. World J Urol 1990; 8:67.
39. Lue TF: Treatment of venogenic impotence. In: Tanagho EA, Lue TF, McClure RD, eds. Contemporary management of impotence and infertility. Baltimore: Williams & Wilkins, 1988: 175.
40. Lewis RW: Venous surgery for impotence. Urol Clin North Am 1988; 15:115.
41. Wespes E, Delcour L, Prejzerowiczl Struyven J, Schulman CC: Long-term follow-up of operated for venous leakage. In: Proceedings of Sixth Biennial International Symposium for Corpora Cavernosum Revascularization and Third Biennial World Meeting on Impotence. Boston: International Society of Impotence Research (ISIR), 1988.
42. Austoni E, Belloroforte C, Mantovani F: Improved results with intracavernous vasoactive drug infusion following new surgical techniques for vasculogenic impotence. World J Urol 1987; 5:182.
43. Lue TF: Penile venous surgery. Urol Clin NA 1989; 16:607.
44. Bondil P, Schauvliege T, Nguyen Qui JL: Venocavernous leakage: considerations in 60 operated cases. In: Proceedings of Sixth Biennial Corpora Cavernosum Revascularization and Third Biennial World Meeting on Impotence. Boston, International Society of Impotence Research (ISIR), 1988.
45. Lunglmayr G, Nachtigall M, Gindl K: Long-term results of deep dorsal penile vein transaction in venous impotence. Eur Urol 1988; 15:209.
46. Weidner W, Weiske WH, Rudnick J: Deep dorsal vein dissection for treatment of venous leakage review of the results after a four-year period. Urologe A 1989; 28:217.
47. Treiber V, Gilbert P: Venous surgery in erectile dysfunction: A critical report of 116 patients. Urology 1989; 34:22.
48. Rossman B, Mieza M, Melman A: Penile vein ligation for corporeal incompetence: an evaluation of short-term and long-term results. J Urol 1990; 144:679.
49. Claes H, Baert L: Cavernosometry and penile vein resection in corporeal incompetence: an evaluation of short-term and long-term results. J Impotence Res 1991; 3:129.
50. Kropman RF, Lycklama á Nijeholt AAB, Jansen FH, Kruyt RH: Results of repeated cavernography in 10 patients without good clinical late results after partial resection of the deep dorsal penile vein. World J Urol 1990; 8:101.
51. Rajfer J, Mehringer M: Cavernosography following clinical failure of penile vein ligation for erectile dysfunction. J Urol 1990; 143:514.

ANNOTATED BIBLIOGRAPHY

Hattery RR, King BF, Lewis RW, James EM, McKusick MA: Vasculogenic impotence: duplex and color Doppler imaging. Radiol Clinics NA 1991; 29:629.

Duplex ultrasonography and color Doppler imaging of the penis has become an integral part of the workup with a patient with male erectile dysfunction at the Mayo Clinic. This is a noninvasive means of assessing patients with suspected vasculogenic impotence. The addition of color Doppler enhances the examiners ability to detect small vessels, to define vascular anatomy, to demonstrate dynamic changes in blood flow, and to measure velocity more accurately. Accurate assessment of the Doppler angle is easier and more accurate beacause the color display of flow and vessel orientation is seen throughout the image field. Visualization of the vascular field in color allows for a more accurate acquisition of data in the study of penile vascular anatomy and hemodynamics.

This presentation is divided into four major sections. The vascular anatomy of the penis is first discussed in some detail to orient the reader to the anatomical data that are necessary for proper orientation and interpretation of color Doppler ultrasonography data. The second section is a discussion of the technique used at the Mayo Clinic for evaluation of the cavernosal artery with discussion of the intracavernosal agents used, the spectral wave form analysis, and the role of evaluation of the cavernosal artery diameter. The next two sections discuss the use of the data to diagnose venogenic competence or incompetence and arteriogenic competence or incompetence. End diastolic velocity measurements at the 15–20 minute postinjection phase of the evaluation has become a major diagnostic tool for determining venous competence in the erection reaction. Peak systolic velocities <30 cm/second when found in both cavernosal arteries are indicative of normal arterial inflow. Using these data, there is a brief discussion of the therapy that may be used in the management of impotence and how therapeutic decisions may be made with the knowledge obtained for color duplex Doppler ultrasonography. The authors point out that color Doppler imaging parallels earlier data generated by using standard sonography. However, by using color, there is an enhancement in the ability to obtain data, and the data appear to be more accurate and efficiently obtained.

Lue TF: Impotence: A patient's goal-directed approach to treatment. World J Urol 1990; 8:67.

With the rapid introductions of new tools for the evaluation of impotence and the multiple treatment approaches to male erectile dysfunction, the average clinician is often confronted with two questions: "What constitutes an adequate work-up?" and "What is the treatment of choice of the patient with male erectile dysfunction?" In this article, Tom Lue introduces the concept of a patient goal-directed approach for both the diagnosis and treatment of impotence. After the initial history, physical examination, and basic laboratory tests, the patients are given a pamphlet discussing all treatment options available at present. If patients are interested only in noninvasive treatment, then no further diagnostic work-up is performed. If patients wish to undergo further studies to identify causes of impotence or if they are interested in more invasive therapy, additional tests are carried out according to the desired treatment. Patients with probable psychogenic impotence are advised to have a nocturnal penile tumescence (NPT) test by a method in which both tumescence and rigidity can be obtained. Patients with abnormal testosterone may then have evaluation of the pituitary hormones. Neurological consultation is sought for patients with a history of neurological defect. What is particularly relevant for inclusion of this article in this annotated bibliography is Doctor Lue's discussion of the tests needed for vascular evaluation. It is his opinion that the combined intracavernous injection and stimulation test (CIS) is a crucial step in the evaluation of a patient who is thought to have a vascular cause for his impotency. In his article, he then discussed, after the results of this CIS test indicate a high probability of a vascular problem, the use of Doppler ultrasound scanning, cavernous arterial occlusion pressure, pharmacologic arteriography, and/or cavernosometry/cavernosography. According to the patients goals, he then describes the modern treatment options available for the patient with male erectile dysfunction in the face of correlation with the diagnostic data. This type of approach is a must for the modern practitioner dealing with male erectile dysfunction.

Meuleman EJH, Wijkstra H, Doesburg WM, Debruyne FMJ: Comparison of the diagnostic value of pump and gravity cavernosometry in the evaluation of the cavernous veno-occlusive mechanism. J Urol 1991; 146:1266.

This article is one of the few articles to compare various techniques of evaluation of the patient expected to have venoocclusive disorder. Two different techniques of evaluation of venoocclusion, pump cavernosometry, using a roler pump as the inflow source, and gravity cavernosometry, using an infusion set as the inflow source, are compared in two sets of impotent patients.

The first group who were considered not to have a venoocclusive disorder had at least one positive erection on injection of 50 mg of papaverine intracavernously on two occasions. The group that was suspected to have a venoocclusive disorder was those 44 patients who did not have an erectile response to the injection of 50 mg of papaverine on two occasions. Various criteria obtained by either pump or gravity cavernosometry data were compared between each of the groups, and a detailed statistical analysis of the data was used to determine which tests are more likely to be accurate to predict venoocclusive disorder. In pump cavernosometry, maintenance flow rate was the most accurate parameter of veno-occlusive function. The steady-state pressure obtained on gravity cavernosometry (although not quite as accurate as the maintenance flow rate) appeared to have an advantage because of its simplicity, cost-effectiveness and a lower complication rate. The authors concluded that the diagnostic value of both techniques were comparable. Every reader who is interested in understanding the finer diagnostic tests for evaluation of the venoocclusive mechanism must have an understanding of this article.

Treiber V, Gilbert P: Venous surgery in erectile dysfunction: a critical report of 116 patients. Urology 1989; 34:22.

Although this article was written in 1989, it is one of the best followed and presented results of a single series for the treatment of venoocclusive disorders. These are results of venous surgery in 116 patients operated on from June 1985 to December 1987 in which there is a long-term follow-up for over 1 year. This group of patients was divided into a group whose problem consisted of venous leakage exclusively, a second group consisting of patients with venous leakage and concomitant causes of impotence. Of course, as expected, the first group had a higher success rate (62.9%) compared to the group with concomitant disease (54.1%). The authors also presented a series of patients who had spongiosolysis, which for the most part was a secondary procedure in this group of patients. The authors pointed out that what has been seen by other authors is that there is an initial group of patients who have success in the first 6 months but who in long-term follow-up develop recurrent venoocclusive disorders. This one particular article with the results of venous surgery for venoocclusive disorder is selected because of the excellent analysis of the results.

6 Crural Ligation in the Treatment of Impotence

Pedro Puech-Leão

Surgical correction of venoocclusive dysfunction of the corpora cavernosa has been the most controversial aspect of the treatment of male sexual impotence in the last decade. The debate arises from the difficulties in characterization of the so-called venoocclusive dysfunction or venous leakage. To better understand the role of each surgical procedure in the treatment of these conditions, some considerations about the concept of venous leakage are needed.

Erection is a hemodynamic phenomenon that consists of entrapment of blood in the corpora cavernosa. Both an increase in arterial inflow and a decrease in the venous outflow are required to create a rigid erection. The role of venoocclusion has been the object of disagreement for decades, but today it is clear that it is an important part in the erectile process. The fact that the corpora cavernosa cannot be collapsed by squeezing during erection is the most simple and clear evidence of the existence of a venoocclusive mechanism.

Venous leakage and venoocclusive dysfunction are different concepts. Venous leakage may be defined as a condition in which the high pressure in the erect corpora is lost by drainage of blood through the venous system. Blood drainage from the sinusoids is a physiologic phenomenon; it occurs in every healthy man every time detumescence occurs after intercourse. Venoocclusive dysfunction is a condition in which venoocclusion cannot be reached, or is reversed before ejaculation and orgasm, causing an inopportune venous leakage.

Evidences have been collected by experimental research showing that corporal venoocclusion depends on the distention of the trabeculae of the sinusoidal tissue.[1] These trabeculae contain smooth muscle cells and connective tissue fibers, and both become distended to promote venoocclusion. Relaxation of the smooth muscle cells depends on the regulation of the autonomic nervous system, while elasticity of the connective tissue is related to local physical parameters that can be impaired by a number of conditions causing damage to the

Management of Impotence and Infertility, edited by Douglas Whitehead and Harris Nagler,

sinusoidal wall. These findings led us to classify venoocclusive dysfunction (VOD) in two different categories: functional VOD and organic VOD. The former is caused by either lack of relaxation or inopportune contraction of the corporal smooth muscle, which promotes reversion of the venoocclusive mechanism, and is related to psychological conditions such as performance anxiety. The latter is caused by structural damage to the trabeculae in diseases such as atherosclerosis[2] and Peyronie's disease.[3]

The differential diagnosis of the two kinds of VOD is of upmost importance when we treat impotent patients; functional VOD may be treated by sex counseling, while organic VOD requires surgical treatment.

Diagnosis of Venoocclusive Dysfunction

The two diagnostic tests for VOD are a pharmacoerection test and cavernosometry. Cavernosography is useful only for anatomic study of the venous pathways, if venous ligation is to be performed.

A rigid erection obtained with intracorporeal injection of smooth muscle relaxant rules out VOD. A negative response to injection does not always mean organic VOD, however, since adrenergic discharges may decrease the effect of drugs such as papaverine or prostaglandin E_1.

Obviously, the degree of confidence associated with the results of pharmacoerection as a diagnostic test depends on the reliance that smooth muscle cells were relaxed, to the maximum, by the vasoactive drug. Unfortunately, data from the literature and from personal experience of several investigators showed that the action of these drugs under laboratory conditions is inconstant and strongly influenced by adrenergic discharges, due to stress, during the test.

The most frequently used vasoactive drug has been papaverine HCl. Its ability to relax the corporal smooth muscle fibers is controversial. Virag et al.[4] reported in 1984 that 6 potent volunteers and 10 patients with normal NPT tests all had rigid erections with papaverine injections. In 1986 Buvat et al.[5] showed that in his series, 40% of patients with normal NPT did not respond to papaverine. Our experience with patients whose impotence subsequently was shown to be psychogenic was very similar to that of Buvat et al. Bennet and Garofalo[6] found a decrease in the incidence of VOD from 81 to 45% by simply adding phentolamine to the papaverine test, and Gerstemberg et al.[7] showed that 34 of 95 patients with negative papaverine tests became positive after vibration.

The experience with programs of self-injection performed at home showed that many patients have good responses when sexually stimulated, regardless of poor responses in laboratory conditions. In 1988, Glina and associates[8] showed that if the patient smokes a cigarette in the waiting room before the papaverine test, this may be enough to give us a false positive.

Thus, papaverine is not completely effective in conjunction with adrenergic discharges. Other drugs and combinations are under trial, but the accumulated experience so far is not enough to establish their effectiveness.

The Rationale for Crural Ligation

Since the description of the venoocclusive mechanism by Fourier et al.[1] in 1987, it has become clear that venous leakage is caused by impairment of corpora cavernosa expansibility, and not by an excess of veins or by anomalous veins draining the corpora. Because surgery cannot restore physical characteristics such as compliance or elasticity of the cavernous tissue, attention is more commonly turned toward correcting the leakage. Creation of venous stasis attempts to compensate for the loss of pressure caused by venous leakage, and thus to make drainage more difficult or corporeal filling easier. Crural ligation is one of the techniques proposed to achieve this goal.

The idea of ligation of the crura penis was based on data from anatomy, physiology, and diagnostic procedures:

1. Although blood drainage of the copora cavernosa in the flaccid state is done mainly by the deep dorsal vein, there are several veins arising from the infrapubic segment, and also from the medial side of the corporeal roots, which assume the most important role during erection.[9]
2. Compression of the crura penis during cavernosometry causes an immediate decrease in the flow needed to maintain erection, as well as an increase in intracavernous pressure in every patient; however, while in most cases the internal pressure tends to fall to previous levels despite continuous crural compression, in others it is kept at higher levels, as long as the compression is maintained.[10]
3. A number of veins leave the crura penis proximal to the point of entrance of the cavernous artery. Thus, exclusion of the first 2 cm of the crura may decrease blood drainage without impairing the arterial inflow to the remaining corpora.[11]

In 1986 we proposed crural ligation as a surgical technique for the correction of impotence caused by venoocclusive dysfunction. The rationale for the proposal was (1) to decrease venous drainage with a simple operation, and (2) to exclude part of the corpora from the distribution of flow, thus decreasing the area to be filled and making the venoocclusive mechanism easier to be triggered.

Technique of Crural Ligation

The operation can be performed by either a perineal midline or an infrapubic approach. The latter requires detachment of the suspensory ligament and is justified only when venous ligations are to be performed at the same time. We prefer the perineal incision, since the approach of the crura by its perineal side carries less risk of damage to the penile artery.

After incision of the skin and subcutaneous tissue, the bulbocavernous muscle is identified and divided midway from the bulb to the crura. Retraction of the bulbocavernous muscle allows visualization of the albuginea, with its characteristic white aspect.

The medial surface of the corpora is carefully dissected, exposing the albuginea up to 1 cm below the point of junction of the two crura. The dissection must be close to the tunica, so that all the tissue that lies between the two crura is retracted medially, because the arteries are located in that tissue. After dissection around the medial aspect of the crura, the periostium of the ischium may be seen, as well as the attachment of the corpora to the bone. Positioning the tip of a large needle at that point (Figure 1-1), a number 2 silk suture is passed below the crura from the medial to the lateral border, allowing the needle tip to be recovered at any point lateral to the crura. If the tunica is completely visualized at its medial border, one can be sure that the only structure

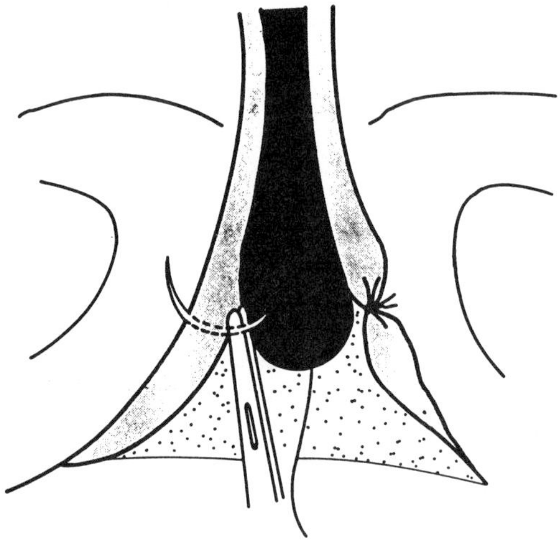

Figure 6-1 Crural ligation: positioning the tip of the needle.

ligated is the corpora, and the nerves and arteries that lie between the two crura are spared. The same procedure is repeated on the other side.

Results of Crural Ligation

In a review of 23 patients submitted to crural ligation, 1 month after the operation, we found 15 claiming to have erections that were more rigid and lasted longer than before. The other 8 patients had no improvement.[10] Reviewing the same group after a longer period (mean 18.9 months) we found 3 patients who considered themselves cured, 8 claiming to be better than before but not cured, and the 12 remaining having the same degree of erectile dysfunction than before the procedure. There were only mild complications: one incisional hematoma that required drainage under local anesthesia, and severe perineal pain in one case, which spontaneously disappeared 10 days after the operation.

Effectiveness of Crural Ligation

Our experience showed that crural ligation is effective on a short-term basis in a high percentage of cases. However, long-term follow-up data were not encouraging.[12] Since it does not approach the cause of the dysfunction, collateral outflow pathways tend to develop in a few months.

In our series, the procedure was effective in only 11 of 23 cases after a 1-year follow-up. We did not consider it ethical to perform invasive tests such as cavernosometry on patients who have a normal sexual life. Therefore, the question of how effective the operation has been in reversing psychological secondary blockage caused by performance anxiety in patients by increasing the intracavernous pressure is still unanswered.

Current Indications

In recent years, our indications for crural ligation have been restricted to a few selected cases. The selection of candidates is based on the following:

1. Absence of arterial insufficiency, demonstrated by cavernous artery occlusion pressure above 90 mm Hg and by Duplex-scanning.
2. Absence of peripheral neuropathy, demonstrated by normal bulbocavernous reflex latency and somatosensory genitocerebral-evoked potentials.

3. Lack of response to pharmacoinjection in any circumstance, including self-injection at home with 20 μg of PGE_1. When the patient has no erection in a laboratory injection test, but has rigid erections with self-injections at home, the problem is considered to be with the laboratory and not with the patient.
4. Good elasticity and compliance of the cavernous tissue. Intracavernous pressures above 110 cm H_2O in gravity cavernosometry perfusion are considered an indication that rigidity can be obtained if the inflow/outflow rate is adequate.[13]
5. Substantial increase in rigidity during gravity cavernosometry when the crura are compressed during a time not shorter than 1 minute.
6. Because corporal tissue damage increases with aging, patients older than 65 years are not considered candidates.

When a patient is selected as a candidate for crural ligation, he receives a detailed explanation of the possibilities and results of the procedure, as well as of the advantages and disadvantages of other treatment modalities, such as penile implants or venous ligation. Only those willing to accept the low possibility of long-term positive results are chosen.

The meaning of the term "potent" is not the same to every person. To some men, being potent means to be able to have a rigid erection and to penetrate; to others, it means achieving an erection, starting from the flaccid state. In the first case, an implant would achieve the expectation of the patient in a high percentage of cases. But in the last case, especially in primary impotence, when the patient never had the experience of achieving an erection by his own means, short-term recovery of physiologic erections may be an important step before an implant is performed.

The Future of Crural Ligation

The place of this treatment modality in the future, as well as that of all surgical techniques to correct venoocclusive dysfunction, will depend on increases in the accuracy of our diagnostic tests. The study of the electrical activity of the corpora cavernosa appears to offer a promising tool to avoid false diagnosis of organic impotence by monitoring the smooth muscle relaxation after pharmacoerection. Better selection of patients and better understanding of the pathology related to VOD may lead us to revisit venous and crural ligation.

REFERENCES

1. Fournier GR, Juenemann KP, Lue TF, Tanagho EA: Mechanism of venous occlusion during canine penile erection: An anatomic demonstration. J Urol 1987; 137:163–166.
2. Gasior B, Levine F, Goldstein I, Payton TR, Beyer S, Krane RJ: Cavernosometric and cavernosographic findings in patients with idiopathic Peyronie's disease: Plaque-associated corporal venoocclusive dysfunction. Int J Impotence Res 1990; 2(suppl. 2):111–112.
3. Azadzoi K, Saenz de Tejada I, Goldstein I, Krane RJ: Atherosclerosis and high cholesterol diet induce corporal venoocclusive dysfunction. Proceedings of the III World Meeting on Impotence, Boston, 1988: 17.
4. Virag R, Frydman D, Legman M, Virag H: Intracavernous injection of papaverine as a diagnostic and therapeutic method in erectile failure. Angiology 1984; 35:79–87.
5. Buvat J, Lemaire A, Marcolin G, Dehaene JL, Buvat-Herbaut M: Injections intra-caverneuses de drogues vaso-actives—evaluation de leur interet diagnostique et therapeutique dans 65 cas d'impuissance erectile. J Urol (Paris) 1986; 92(2):111–116.

6. Bennet AH, Garofalo FA: Enhanced cavernometry: Procedure for the diagnosis of venogenic impotence. Br J Urol 1989; 64:420–422.
7. Gerstemberg TC, Nordling J, Hald T, Wagner G: Standardized evaluation of erectile dysfunction in 95 consecutive patients. J Urol 1989; 141:857–862.
8. Glina S, Reichelt AC, Puech-Leao P, Reis JMSM: Impact of cigarette smoking on papaverine-induced erection. J Urol 1988; 139:1–2.
9. Newman HF, Puech-Leao P, Chao S: Relative role of the deep dorsal, crural and superficial veins on corporeal drainage. Proceedings of the III World Meeting on Impotence, Boston, 1988: 14.
10. Puech-Leao P, Reis JMSM, Glina S, Reichelt AC: Leakage through the crural edge of corpus cavernosum—diagnosis and treatment. Eur Urol 1987; 13:163–165.
11. Puech-Leao P, Chao S: Venous drainage of the crura—an anatomic study. Int J Impotence Res 1990; 1:105–110.
12. Glina S, Puech-Leao P, Reis JMSM, Reichelt AC, Chao S: Surgical exclusion of the crural ending of the corpora cavernosa: Late results. Eur Urol 1990; 18:42–44.
13. Puech-Leao P, Chao S, Glina S, Reichelt AO: Gravity cavernosometry—a simple diagnostic test for cavernosal incompetence. Br J Urol 1990; 65:391–394.

ANNOTATED BIBLIOGRAPHY

Buvat J, Marcolin G, Lemaire A, Dehaene JL, Buvat-Herbaut M: Impuissance par fuite veneuse. A la recherche de criteres diagnostiques fiables. J Urol 1989; 95:396–401.

In this study, results of the Artificial Erection Test (AET) performed in 9 controls and in 81 impotent patients were analyzed. Among very interesting data obtained, it is remarkable that 1 of 9 normal controls needed a flow of 160 ml/min to maintain erection. Also, among 68 patients who required more than 75 ml/min to maintain erection on AET, 16 were cured or significantly improved by sex therapy. The results of AET were different at a second test in 12 of 24 patients, showing that the test is not always reproducible. The article calls attention to the limits of cavernosometry as a diagnostic test for venoocclusive incompetence. After reviewing these data, one cannot avoid considering how many patients with psychogenic impotence underwent venous ligations, all around the world, based on false-positive AETs.

Desai KM, Gingell JC: Saline-induced artificial erection without papaverine—a potential source of error in diagnosing cavernosal venous leakage. Br J Urol 1982; 62:176–178.

The authors report two cases in which cavernosometry, performed without any previous injection of vasoactive drugs showed absence of erection with flows as high as 240 ml/min. In both cases, after intracavernous administration of papaverine, erection could be obtained with perfusion at a rate of 20 and 5 ml/min, and maintained with 5 to 10 ml/min. Nocturnal penile tumescence tests were normal in both cases and one of them was successfully treated with self-injections. The authors emphasize the need to be careful in interpreting results of cavernosometry when performed without efficient relaxation of the cavernous smooth muscle.

Puech-Leao P, Chao S: Venous drainage of the crura—an anatomic study. Int J Impotence Res 1990; 2:105–110.

The anatomy of the veins draining the crura penis was studied by casting the venous system with subsequent acid corrosion. The crura is drained by two to four trunks, which receive branches from the dorsomedial face of the corpora from all extensions from the subpubic segment to the crural tip. The number of small branches arising from the corpora and contributing to these trunks is such that ligation of the trunks in one site may be easily bypassed by collateral circulation. The anatomic findings also make clear that a complete venous ligation, if possible, can be performed only after complete detachment of the suspensory ligament.

7

External Devices for Erectile Dysfunction

Perry W. Nadig

The hope that some external device could cause or maintain an erection is as old as the problem of impotence. A 1908 catalog offered several "penis congesters" consisting of a cylindrical vacuum chamber with attached pump, but no provision for constriction.[1] Then, in 1917, a Doctor Otto Lederer, who described himself as a "subject of the Emperor of Austria," was granted a U.S. patent (number 1,225,341, May 8, 1917) for a "surgical device," prototype of all vacuum constriction devices (VCD's) currently available. "By creating a vacuum," Dr. Lederer claimed, "the blood is compelled to enter the cavernosum, whereby an erection is produced. By means of the ring remaining on the root of the penis, the erection is maintained for a considerable time after the sleeve has been removed, since owing to the existing compression, the blood can only flow back gradually."

But the medical profession either ignored or remained ignorant of the VCD until the first scientific report of its use was published in 1986.[2] Since that time the VCD has gained popularity among physicians and patients and is now the most widely prescribed treatment for impotence.

External devices currently in use are of three types: vacuum devices to cause penile rigidity, constriction devices to maintain rigidity, and a combination of the two, the VCD. A variant, the vacuum entrapment (VE) device, does not rely on constriction to keep the penis hard, but instead maintains the vacuum in a plastic sheath worn during intercourse.[3]

Physiology

When the penis is placed in a vacuum of greater than 100 mm Hg it becomes tumescent and rigid enough for vaginal penetration. This tumescence and rigidity can be maintained by a constricting device placed about the base of the penis either before or during the application of the vacuum. Constriction can safely be maintained for at least 30 minutes.[2] No serious injury from the proper use of a VCD has ever been reported.

Since the first report of the physiological effects of the VCD appeared, several investigators have increased our understanding of how the vacuum causes penile tumescence and

Management of Impotence and Infertility, edited by Douglas Whitehead and Harris Nagler,

rigidity and how the constricting band effects the penis.[4–7] We now know that the mechanism of action by which negative pressure induces penile rigidity is unlike that of a normal erection. In studies of the simian penis, Diederichs and his associates[5] showed that the increase in cross-sectional area of the corpora cavernosa that resulted from subatmospheric pressures was only 50% of that induced by intracavernous papaverine. These investigators concluded that contracted smooth muscle limited the expansion of the corpora cavernosa, and found no evidence that the suction induced any active mechanism for erection. They also demonstrated that intracavernous pressure can increase after suction to the same level as seen after intracavernous papaverine injection. They found the cross-sectional area of the simian penis to be almost the same during use of the VCD as after papaverine (0.61 vs. 0.60 cm^2), but the cross-sectional area of the three corpora significantly less (0.28 vs. 0.35 cm^2). In man, the VCD induces a penile diameter greater than that attained during a normal erection. Blood trapped in the extracorporal tissues accounts for these differences.

Beyond the constricting bands venous stasis and decreased arterial blood flow result in cyanosis and distention of the superficial veins and a lowering of the skin temperature of the penis. Because the penis is rigid only distal to the constricting bands, it pivots at its base. Constriction of the urethra traps all or most of the ejaculate until the constriction is relieved.

The VCD creates penile rigidity sufficient for vaginal penetration in up to 98% of impotent men.[8] Patients with scarring or deformity of the penis due to Peyronie's disease or from an infected penile prosthesis are those most likely to be unable to attain adequate rigidity, but a few men fail without apparent cause. Some patients, fewer than 2% of those who try the VCD, experience intolerable pain from a vacuum of little more than 100 mm Hg or from the pressure of the constricting band at the base of the penis, but the majority have little or at least tolerable discomfort.

The Vacuum Constriction Device

Equipment and Technique

The VCD consists of a vacuum chamber, a vacuum pump, and a constriction band, ring, or disk (Figure 7-1). The vacuum chamber should be transparent and of a length and

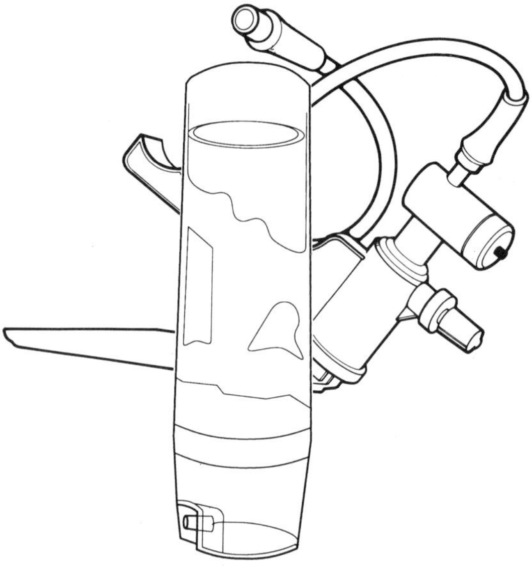

Figure 7-1 Equipment for a VCD includes a vacuum pump with a safety valve, a vacuum chamber, and constricting bands or disks (not shown).

(From Nadig PW: Vacuum erection devices. World J Urol 1991; 8:114–117, with permission.)

diameter that will accommodate penises of various sizes and configurations. It is open at one end. The diameter of the opening must allow the tumescent penis to fill it exactly. Inside diameters of 4.14, 4.45, and 4.76 cm are those most commonly required. The vacuum pressures must exceed 90 mm Hg. As the negative pressure increases, the incidence of ecchymosis and hematoma formation rises. A hand pump is adequate, but electric pumps are available. To maintain rigidity a band, ring, or disk of plastic or latex rubber is used to constrict the base of the penis. This band must be tight enough to maintain penile rigidity, but not so tight that it injures the penis.

The constricting band may be placed about the base of the penis before the vacuum is applied, but most available devices are designed to allow the user to apply the band after the penis is tumescent and rigid. To do this, the cylinder is prepared by stretching the band around the chamber near its open end. Lubricating jelly is then applied generously to the base of the penis to form an air-tight seal. The penis is placed in the chamber and the vacuum is applied for 6 minutes or until the penis becomes rigid (Figure 7-2). The constriction band is then pushed off the end of the chamber (Figure 7-3) to grip the base of the penis, the vacuum is released, and the chamber is removed.

Instead of applying the vacuum continuously, improved penile rigidity results if the vacuum is relieved momentarily after 1 to 2 minutes, then reapplied for another 3 to 4 minutes.[9]

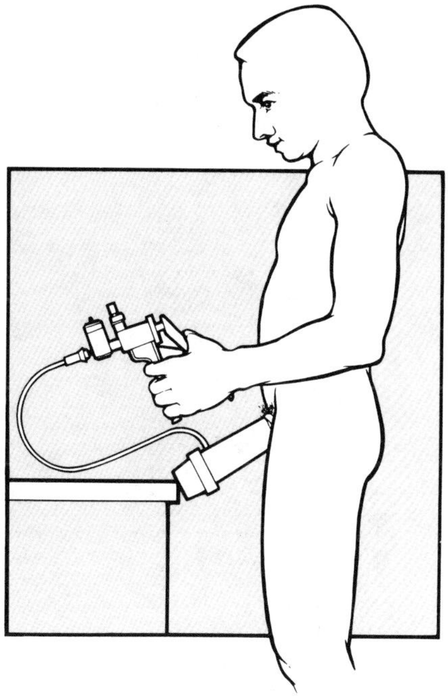

Figure 7-2 Applying the vacuum to the penis. It takes 3 to 6 minutes for the penis to become rigid. The man should be sitting or standing.

(From Nadig PW: Vacuum erection devices. World J Urol 1991; 8:114–117, with permission.)

Complications

The majority of complications from the use of the VCD have been minor and have required no treatment. No serious injury has been reported. Petechiae often develop on the skin of the penis after use of the VCD, presumably as a result of capillary rupture. These are painless and disappear within 48 hours. Ecchymoses can occur, particulary in men taking aspirin or other anticoagulant drugs, but have not caused problems. Men whose foreskin is tight risk developing paraphimosis when the penis becomes tumescent and should be circumcised before trying the VCD.

Men with spinal cord injuries and other neurological problems that impair sensation in the penis should use the VCD with caution. Skin necrosis has occurred in a paraplegic man

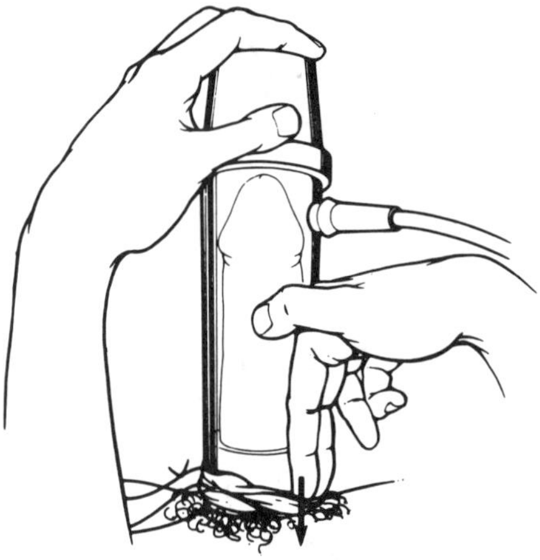

Figure 7-3 When the penis has become rigid, the constricting band is transferred from the chamber to the base of the penis.

(From Nadig PW: Vacuum erection devices. World J Urol 1991; 8:114–117, with permission.)

who used his VCD three times daily for three successive days.[10]

Men vary widely and unpredictably in their sensitivity to vacuum pressures. Some men have little or no discomfort with vacuums of as much as 600 mm Hg.[2] These latter, along with spinal cord injury patients, may repeatedly develop hematomas and ecchymoses of the penis.[11] Because negative pressure beyond 100 mm Hg is unnecessary and unrestricted vacuums could harm some patients, a safety valve should be used to limit the maximum degree of vacuum. A VCD lacking a safety valve should not be used.

Patient Acceptance and Satisfaction

The VCD will cause penile rigidity sufficient for vaginal penetration for most men, regardless of the cause of impotence, and including even those men with a malfunctioning penile prosthesis in place. Only men with extensive scarring and deformity of the penis such as that caused by an infected penile prosthesis can be predicted to fail to obtain rigidity with the VCD.

Successful use of a VCD requires careful instruction. Patients who rely only on the manufacturer's printed or video taped instructions are less likely to master the use of the VCD than those given a demonstration by a physician or experienced medical assistant. In our practice, every man interested in trying the VCD is shown how to use it on himself. Of those men who try the VCD, 89% chose to obtain one for continued use. Of these 70% report continued regular use after an average of 29 months (unpublished observations). Those who discontinue regular use usually do so within the first 3 months.

The great majority of men who continue to use the VCD report satisfaction with the rigidity, length and circumference, frequency of intercourse, and partner satisfaction. They also report improvement in their self-esteem and sense of well being.

The most frequent complaint by men using VCD is the unnatural interruption of the act of love-making to use the VCD. Some men complain of discomfort on ejaculation, but most do not describe this as objectionable. Other complaints include numbness of the penis, coldness of the penis, and difficulty in achieving orgasm.

Use of the VCD in Conjunction with Injections and Prostheses

The VCD can augment the effect of intracavernous injections in patients for whom the injections alone fail to induce penile rigidity adequate for vaginal penetration.[12] Fifteen minutes should be allowed to pass from the time of injection before the vacuum is applied.

Patients who have had a penile prosthesis explanted can use the VCD successfully.[9,13] Some men have observed that use of the VCD compared favorably with the prosthesis. Even if a malfunctioning prosthesis is still in place the VCD can be used to obtain rigidity or increase the girth of the penis.

The Vacuum Entrapment Device

The VE device uses a vacuum to draw blood into the penis, but the vacuum is maintained during use and constriction is unnecessary. The penis is placed in an individually fitted semi-rigid silicone sheath that conforms to the shape of the tumescent penis. When the vacuum is applied, the penis enlarges to fill the sheath, which is then kept in place during intercourse.

The advantage of this system is that no constriction is needed; thus penile arterial blood flow is not decreased.[6] The disadvantage is that the sheath must be worn during intercourse; the user may experience decreased sensitivity of the penis because of the thickness of the material required and his sexual partner may experience discomfort, irritation, or trauma from the sheath.

Few reports of clinical experience with the VE device have been published. In a study that included 44 patients impotent from a variety of organic causes,[14] the VE device was used successfully by 73%. Overall, 22% of the patients rated the erection obtained very good, while 63% rated it satisfactory, and 16% rated it very poor. The vagina of the partner was reported traumatized by two patients, and the major male complaint was poor sensitivity due to the thickness of the device. The investigators also reported "many complaints" about improper sizing. Another study was limited to patients with spinal cord injuries,[3] so that the question of decreased sensitivity could not be addressed.

More studies of the VE device are needed to clarify the issues of loss of sensitivity, discomfort or trauma to the partner, and problems related to proper fitting.

Constriction Rings

Several manufacturers offer constriction bands to men who can achieve, but not maintain an erection. No reports of the indications for or efficacy of these products have yet appeared in the peer-reviewed literature. Since constriction bands maintain the rigidity of a vacuum-induced erection they should be expected to maintain a physiologically normal erection and can be recommended for trial by selected patients.

Conclusions

External devices are older and less sophisticated than penile prostheses or injectable pharmacologic agents, but have only recently gained attention. Because sex is a very personal matter, no one method of treating impotence is acceptable to all couples. The low cost, safety, and wide patient and partner acceptance of the VCD recommend it for trial by almost every couple; the VCD should be considered before more costly and invasive methods of treatment are used. Men who are able to achieve, but not maintain, an adequate erection should try using a constriction band alone.

REFERENCES

1. Herman JR: Penis congesters. Urology 1977; 10(5):431–C.
2. Nadig PW, Ware JC, Blumoff R: Noninvasive device to produce and maintain an erection-like state. Urology 1986; 27:126–131.
3. Zasler ND, Katz PG: Synergist erection system in the management of impotence secondary to spinal cord injury. Arch Phys Med Rehabil 1989; 70:712–716.
4. Marmar JL, DeBenedictis TJ, Praiss DE: Penile plethysmography on impotent men using vacuum constrictor devices. Urology 1988; 32:198–203.
5. Diederichs W, Kaula NF, Lue TF, Tanagho EA: The effect of subatmospheric pressure on the simian penis. J Urol 1989; 142:1087–1089.
6. Katz PG, Haden HT, Mulligan T, Zasler ND: The effect of vacuum devices on penile hemodynamics. J Urol 1990; 143:55–56.
7. Wespes E, Schulman CC: Hemodynamic study of the effect of vacuum device on human erection. Int J Impotence Res 1990; 2, suppl. 2:337.
8. Nadig PW: Six years experience with the vacuum constriction device. Int J Impotence Res 1989; 1:55–58.
9. Sidi AA, Becher EF, Zhang G, Lewis JH: Patient acceptance of and satisfaction with an external negative pressure device for impotence. J Urol 1990; 144(5):1154–1156.
10. Meinhardt W, Kropman RF, Lycklama AAB, Nijeholt A, Zwartendijk J: Skin necrosis caused by use of negative pressure device for erectile impotence. J Urol 1990; 144(4):983.
11. Walden TB: Osbon Erec Aid (Letter). J Urol 1986; 136:689.
12. Marmar JL, DeBenedictis TJ, Praiss DE: The use of a Vacuum Constrictor device to augment a partial erection following an intracavernous injection. J Urol 1988; 140:975–979.
13. Moul JW, McLeod DG: Negative pressure devices in the explanted penile prosthesis population. J Urol 1989; 142:729–731.
14. Al-Juburi AZ, O'Donnell PD: Synergist erection system: Clinical experience. Urology 1990; 35:304–306.

ANNOTATED BIBLIOGRAPHY

Althof SE, Turner LA, Levine SB, Bodner D, Kursch ED, Resnick MI: Through the eyes of women: The sexual and psychological responses of women to their partner's treatment with self-injection or external vacuum therapy. J Urol 1992; 147(4):10024–10027.

Althof et al. (Case Western Reserve University) questioned the female partners of men using pharmacologic erection and vacuum constriction devices to learn the impact of these therapies on their psychological and sexual functioning. They point to the lack of such information in the current literature and the findings of studies after implantation of penile prostheses in which the satisfaction of the man is markedly higher than that of the woman.

The subjects were 26 women whose partners were using self-injection and 21 whose partners were using the VCD. They were followed for 12 months. During that time 43% of the men on self-injection and 20% of the men using the VCD discontinued therapy.

The women responded equally well to both treatments experiencing significant increases in their level of sexual satisfaction and arousal, and frequency of intercourse and coital orgasm. They felt more at ease in their marital relationships and they spontaneously commented on how relaxed, unhurried, assured, and enjoyable sex had become. Negative responses were the lack of spontaneity of both therapies, worry about side effects by the self-injection group, and complaints about the coldness of the penis and the need for lubricant by the VCD group.

The authors argue that sexual decisions are not solely a man's prerogative, but should be looked on as a couples issue.

As surgeons, we assume that restoration of function will lead to a happy outcome. Not always. Sex is for two people and sexual problems are many faceted. Upbringing, childhood experiences, religion, superstition, and societal norms and expectations all contribute to shaping attitudes toward sex and sexual practices. No treatment currently available is suitable for all couples and some couples find no available treatment acceptable. The high rate at which couples abandon any treatment provides ample proof.

The authors correctly point out that satisfaction of the sexual partner must be considered in evaluating the outcome of any treatment for impotence. Further, they state that the partner must be interviewed and consulted at the very onset of evaluation of the impotent man. In the case of injection and vacuum constriction therapy their study shows that many couples can have satisfying sex lives restored when offered an acceptable treatment.

The study and treatment of impotence demand not merely a knowledge of erectile physiology and the skillful selection and application of available therapies, but also an understanding of the psychological impact of the loss and subsequent restoration of erections on both individuals and on their relationship.

Diederichs W, Kaula NF, Lue TF, Tanagho EA: The effect of subatmospheric pressure on the simian penis. J Urol 1989; 142:1087–1089.

Are active mechanisms involved in the development and maintenance of penile rigidity by vacuum and constriction? Diederichs et al. (University of California, San Francisco) conclude that they are not and that the corporal distention that occurs is entirely passive. These investigators studied nine monkeys under anesthesia, measuring the cross-sectional area of the penis with a duplex scanner and recording intracavernous pressures. They found cavernous cross-sectional area increased 50% after suction compared to an 84% increase after papaverine injection. By contrast, the extratunical cross-sectional area increased 57% after suction but only 19% after papaverine. They also observed that intracavernous pressure after vacuum and constriction was similar to that after intracavernous injection of papaverine. Further, they demonstrated that partial constriction, i.e., enough to block retrograde venous flow, applied before the vacuum did not alter the effect of the vacuum and concluded that arterial inflow caused the increased penile volume. Finally, they showed that constriction of the base of the flaccid penis alone does not readily change intracavernous pressure or induce tumescence.

The evolution of the VCD was empirical. Few investigations of the underlying physiology have been published and important questions remain about the role of arterial inflow in the establishment of penile rigidity and the possibility of ischemic injury to the penis due to prolonged constriction. The fact that arterial inflow is responsible for penile engorgement under vacuum suggests that this technique might be less effective for some men with compromised arteries. Experience has not confirmed this. Experience also leads to the conclusion that ischemic injury to the penis from commercially available constricting bands must be a rare event, for no such injuries have been reported in the literature.

If constriction about the base of the flaccid penis does not appreciably increase intracavernous pressure then there is no rationale for use of commercially available rings claimed to cause an erection when applied to the base of the penis.

The possibility of applying constriction before the vacuum has led to the development of a constriction disc, which is used in conjunction with a vacuum but is applied before inducing negative pressure.

Moul JW, McLeod DG: Negative pressure devices in the explanted penile prosthesis population. J Urol 1989; 142:729–731.

Moul and McLeod (Walter Reed Army Medical Center) offered the VCD to a group of 14 patients who had had a penile prosthesis explanted for a variety of reasons, including six for whom the explantation was done because of infection. Three found the VCD unacceptable. Eleven gave the VCD a home trial.

The average follow-up period was 10.5 weeks. Eight patients described the erection as excellent or good, while one, a man with multiple sclerosis, described the erection as unsatisfactory due to sensory alteration. Eight of the partners described the erection obtained as excellent or good, two found it satisfactory, and one did not comment. Among the 11 patients, seven (64%) believed the penis to be the same length or longer than erections before implantation and eight (73%) found the circumference to be the same or greater than their previous natural erection. Overall, 10 of the 14 explant patients (71%) engaged in regular successful intercourse using the device. Five of the six patients whose explantation was due to infection reported success with the VCD.

Of the 11 users, six (55%) said that use of this device "compared much better or better" [sic] than the previous penile implant, while two believed the device was not as good as the implant, and three did not comment; six (55%) preferred the VCD to the previous penile implant, although the authors point out that this finding may be skewed because of their poor experience with the implants. All patients commented that they wished the VCD would have been available and offered as an alternative before they had received a prosthesis.

This paper illustrates the usefulness of the VCD for a difficult group of patients. Additionally, the VCD can be used to gain rigidity by men whose prosthesis is malfunctioning but who decline explantation. It can also be used by men with functioning penile prostheses but whose penile girth is still inadequate, i.e., men who have undergone urethrectomy.

The authors statement that all patients had wished the VCD had been offered to them along with the prosthesis validates the contention that at the time of initial evaluation the patient and his partner should be told about all treatment options available and be allowed to select the one that best suits them.

8 Drug-Induced Male Sexual Dysfunction

Barry J. Klyde

Progress in health care has led to a tremendous increase in the number of both physician-prescribed and nonprescription drugs taken by any one person, a situation that has also increased observed side effects and drug interactions. It is no surprise that up to 25% of impotence results from drugs.[1] Drugs for almost every affliction, both major and minor, have been found to be culprits. A study of drugs that have been implicated in causing sexual dysfunction is useful to the clinician, who can use this information to avoid drugs known to cause problems and instead choose an alternative one. It is also helpful in revealing the various factors that control normal sexual function, to point out directions for research that will improve our understanding of the mechanisms involved and lead to better therapy of sexual problems.

Review of Physiology of Male Sexual Function

The components of normal function include libido, penile erection, emission, and ejaculation. The initial component is *libido*, or sexual desire, influenced by sensory stimuli interacting with memory and fantasy and processed by the cerebral cortex and limbic system. The next component is penile *erection*. There are thought to be two neurologic centers in the spinal cord that control erections, thoracolumbar (T12–L1) and sacral (S2–S4). Erections can occur as a result of central stimuli (psychogenic), mediated via thoracolumbar sympathetic efferent nerves at T12–L1 and the hypogastric plexus.[2] Stimulation of the penis directly, as well as bladder and bowel distention, produces reflexogenic erections mediated via sacral parasympathetic outflow from S2–S4.[3] *Emission*, the deposition of semen from the prostate, seminal vesicles, and distal vasa into the posterior urethra, is followed by *ejaculation*, with semen propelled forward by rhythmic contraction of pelvic floor muscles directed by somatic efferent nerves from S2–S4 and sympathetic outflow from T12–L2.[4] Various drugs can interfere with sexual function at any of these steps.

Neuropharmacology

The penis is maintained in the detumescent state by the release of the α-adrenergic agent

Management of Impotence and Infertility, edited by Douglas Whitehead and Harris Nagler,

norepinephrine, which causes contraction of penile arteries and trabecular smooth muscle.[5] Acetylcholine relaxes the corpus cavernosum, mediated by release of factors from the endothelium, including nitric oxide, prostaglandins, and peptides, and this results in an engorgement of the penis with blood, making it rigid.[6] Numerous other substances may also play a role in initiating and maintaining erections.[5] The lacunar spaces, filled with blood because of relaxation of trabecular muscle and dilatation of cavernosal and helicine arteries, compress the plexus of subtunical veinules and thus prevent escape of blood from the turgid penis.[6] Detumescence occurs when sympathetic tone increases again, constricting arteries and reducing inflow of blood, resulting in collapse of lacunar spaces with decompression of veinules and increased venous outflow. Different drugs can alter the action of neutrotransmitters and prevent or impair erection or ejaculation as well as interfere with libido and orgasm, the initial and final components of sexual function.

Drugs Known to Cause Sexual Dysfunction

Many case reports of drug-induced male sexual dysfunction have been published, but these are mostly anecdotal: it is unusual to find a double-blind crossover study that accurately assesses a drug's potential for interfering with sexual function. A confounding variable is that men with underlying vascular or neurologic disease, hormonal imbalance, or other serious illnesses may be more likely to develop dysfunction with a particular medication. Additionally, medications used for illnesses often associated with sexual dysfunction, such as hypertension, which is a major risk factor for the development of vascular disease and subsequent impotence, are more likely to be accused of causing sexual difficulty.

Fortunately, several excellent reviews of drug-induced sexual dysfunction have been published recently. To reduce the number of references cited, I will refer to a review that provides documentation of the effects of a particular drug, rather than the individual case reports.

Psychotropic Drugs

Major Tranquilizers and Antipsychotic Drugs

Phenothiazines (e.g., chlorpromazine, or Thorazine) and butyrophenones (e.g., haloperidol, or Haldol) may diminish libido because of their sedating effects, and their antagonistic effect on dopamine receptors increases pituitary production of prolactin,[3,5,7] which results in diminished testosterone production and action. The elevated prolactin can decrease libido and impair erections (see Klyde, Chapter 9, on hormonal causes of male sexual dysfunction in this volume). The anticholinergic effects of phenothiazines are more marked than those of butyrophenones, and can also contribute to erectile difficulty. The phenothiazine drug, thoridazine (Mellaril), is the most likely one in this group to cause retarded or absent ejaculation because of inhibition of seminal emission, which results from its strong peripheral α-adrenergic blocking action.[4] This effect is seen in almost half of the men who use it. In fact, its α-adrenergic blocking effects are probably the reason why it is a rare cause of priapism, although more than 40% of men on this drug experience erectile failure,[4] probably because of the anticholinergic effects and elevated prolactin that also occur.

An additional group that can cause erectile failure and ejaculatory difficulties are the thioxanthenes, thiothixine (Navane) and chlorprothixine (Taractan).[8]

Antidepressants

Drugs used for depression that also cause increased sedation can lower libido. The anticholinergic effects of tricyclic antidepressants can impair erections, and amitriptyline (Elavil), with its greater anticholinergic activity, is the drug in this group most likely to do so.[7] Ejaculatory difficulty has also been seen with amitriptyline, and problems with both erections and ejaculations have occurred with other tricyclic antidepressants, including imipramine (Tofranil), amoxapine (Asendin), clomipramine (Anafranil), protriptyline (Vivactil), and even desipramine (Norpramin),[4] the one in this group with the least anticholinergic effects.[9] Imipramine, which is known to cause impaired ejaculation, has also been used paradoxically to treat absent seminal emission and retrograde ejaculation resulting from retroperitoneal node dissection and diabetes.[4]

Another class of antidepressants, MAO inhibitors, can diminish sexual interest and drive without causing sedation, and can occasionally cause erectile and ejaculatory difficulties.[7,8]

Lithium carbonate, used to treat bipolar depression, can also decrease libido and interfere with erections, perhaps because of decreased central dopamine activity.[4]

Trazodone (Desyrel), a nontricyclic antidepressant that has a very sedating effect,[9] can improve erectile function, perhaps because of its α-adrenoreceptor-blocking action,[5] but can also cause priapism[10] and retrograde ejaculation.[8]

Prozac, which has become a very widely used antidepressant medication, has no anticholinergic side effects, but can decrease libido and interfere with orgasm.[11]

Minor Tranquilizers and Antianxiety Agents

These include the benzodiazepines, such as diazepam (Valium), which decrease libido, probably because of their central sedative effect, although other effects on sexual function may possibly result not from the drugs, but from the underlying anxiety state being treated.[4]

Antihypertensive drugs

Almost every drug used for hypertension has been accused of interfering with erection or ejaculation, and the frequent use of drug combinations has made identification of the culprit more difficult.[3] The observation that antihypertensive medications with differing modes of action may all impair erections suggests that the common mechanism may be a reduction of perfusion pressure following lowering of systemic blood pressure.[5,6] Reduced perfusion pressure of the lacunar spaces, in patients with flow already compromised by arteriosclerosis or other factors, may result in reduced penile rigidity. In addition to the possible general effect of all antihypertensive agents, the different groups of drugs may each have specific mechanisms that produce sexual dysfunction.

α-Blockers

The α-adrenergic blocking agents phenoxybenzamine (Dibenzylene) and phentolamine (Regitine) both interfere with ejaculation while the selective α_1-adrenergic blocking agent prazosin (Minipress) generally does not.[4] Prazosin does rarely cause priapism,[8] consistent with the expected effect of α-blockade reversing norepinephrine-maintained contraction of the corpus cavernosum and penile arteries.[12] Clonidine (Catapres), an antihypertensive agent promoted as an α-blocker with central effects, is actually an α_2-agonist[6,12] and impairs erectile function,[7] as expected from the known pharmacology of penile erection. It can produce this problem in up to 40% of patients using it, and has also caused decreased libido.[4]

β-Blockers

The density of β-receptors in the corpus cavernosum and penile arteries is 10% of that of the α-receptors, suggesting that they are less important, and since the adrenergic system is thought to control contraction and keep the penis flaccid,[12] it does not seem likely that β-blockade would produce impotence. However, the observation is that the oldest β-blocker in use, the nonspecific drug propranolol (Inderal), can cause erectile dysfunction and impaired libido, which is also seen, but less frequently, with the cardiospecific β-blockers atenolol (Tenormin) and metoprolol (Lopressor).[4,8] The combined α- and β-blocker lbetolol (Trandate; Normodyne) has caused cases of impotence as well as priapism.[8]

Sympatholytics

Alphamethyldopa (Aldomet) blocks catecholamine function by its interesting mode of action of forming a false neurotransmitter, but is not often used now because of its side effects of sedation and liver disease. Additionally, erectile dysfunction is seen in 20–30% of patients, with 10% having decreased libido and impaired ejaculation.[4] In addition to its interference with autonomic function, α-methyldopa may also impair sexual function because of its effect in elevating prolactin.[3]

Reserpine blocks catecholamine reuptake and storage, both centrally and peripherally, but is no longer used much because of drug-induced depression. Up to 40% of patients have reduced erections, and diminished libido and impaired ejaculation are also often seen.[3,4] Reserpine also increases prolactin levels, which probably contributes to its interference with sexual function.[3]

Guanethidine (Ismelin), a ganglionic blocking agent little used now because of orthostatic hypotention, causes impotence and failure of ejaculation in up to one-half of patients, although some investigators considered the impaired ejaculation to be a true drug effect, and the impotence to be a secondary psychological effect.[3,4]

Vasodilators

Hydralazine (Apresoline) is a vasodilator that can cause a reflex tachycardia and is, therefore, often used together with a β-blocker. It may possibly cause cases of impotence as well as priapism.[8]

Minoxidil (Loniten) is another vasodilator not known to cause sexual dysfunction, but it is reserved for patients with severe hypertension unresponsive to other medication because of its side effects. Topical minoxidil (Rogaine) has become widely known because of its use in treating baldness, and has had some success in treating impotence when applied topically to the penis.[13]

Diuretics

Thiazide diuretics can impair libido, erection, and ejaculation, but the mechanism is not known.[4,7] Zinc deficiency is particularly common in patients taking diuretics, is associated with low testosterone values, and impotence in these patients is corrected by zinc supplementation as well as in patients with impotence on hemodialysis.[2] This is one possible mechanism of thiazide-induced dysfunction.

Spironolactone (Aldactone) causes erectile failure in up to 30% of patients, and produces decreased libido and gynecomastia as well.[4] This drug blocks androgen receptors, and, in fact, has now become widely used in women to treat androgen effects such as acne, hirsutism, and male pattern hair loss,[14] so its observed effects in men are not unexpected.

ACE Inhibitors

The first angiotensin-converting enzyme inhibitor, captopril (Capoten), as well as the subsequent ones, enalapril (Vasotec) and lisinopril (Zestril; Prinivil), are not known to cause sexual dysfunction, both in my experience and in published information, and would be good choices for patients who have experienced sexual difficulty with one medication already. Recently, many additional drugs in this class have been introduced.

Calcium Channel Blockers

The first three calcium channel blockers introduced, nifedipine (Procardia), diltiazem (Cardizem), and verapamil (Isoptin; Calan), are all potent vasodilators, but differ in their effects on cardiac conduction, with verapamil having the greatest effect and therefore also used as an antiarrhythmic agent but also having the most negative inotropic effect and thus most likely to worsen congestive heart failure.[15] All three block electrically induced contraction of trabecular smooth muscle of the corpus cavernosum[12] and should, therefore, theoretically benefit erections rather than interfere with them. My own observation is that several patients with known vascular disease and the risk factors of hypertension and diabetes developed erectile dysfunction when given verapamil, but returned to normal function when switched to nifedipine, a different calcium channel blocker with the least effect on cardiac conduction and inotropy. Verapamil-induced impotence has also been observed by others.[16] Additional drugs in this class are now available.

Cardiac Drugs

Many of the drugs used for angina, arrythmias, and congestive heart failure are also antihypertensive medications, and are discussed above.

Digoxin is associated wtih erectile failure and gynecomastia, as well as with increased estrogen and decreased testosterone, and this is thought to result from similarities between its chemical structures and that of sex steroids.[4]

The antiarrhythmic drug disopyramide (Norpace) has been associated with impotence,[7] perhaps because of its anticholinergic effects.[3]

Nitrates cause relaxation of the corpus cavernosum as well as vasodilation, and two well-controlled studies (summarized by Andersson et al.[5]) demonstrate that topical nitroglycerin therapy improved erections. Nitrates would, therefore, be a good choice for antianginal therapy in men with erectile dysfunction.

Antihistamines

Medications for allergies and colds are among the most widely used, both physician prescribed and self-selected, and most have antihistamines, which are anticholinergic. It has been stated that "any antihistamine that causes dry mouth may cause erectile problems."[7] Sedating antihistamines such as diphenhydramine (Benadryl) and hydroxyzine (Vistaril; Atarax) can decrease libido, and others can cause erectile impairment as well.[7,8]

Anticholinergic Drugs

Antispasmodics, used for irritable bowel symptoms, may cause impotence because of their anticholinergic effects. Reported ones include methantheline bromide (Banthine) and propantheline bromide (Pro-Banthine) although others in this group could potentially cause problems.[4,8]

Antiparkinsonian drugs, such as trihexyphenidyl (Artane) and benztropine (Cogentin), are anticholinergic and can impair erections,[7] but the underlying illness is also associated with erectile dysfunction. Dopamine agonists used to treat Parkinson's disease, such as L-dopa and Sinemet, are known to increase sexual activity,[4] but can interfere with ejaculation.[7]

Muscle relaxants such as orphenadrine (Norflex) and cyclobenzaprine (Flexeril) may also interfere with erections because of their anticholinergic activity.[7]

Atropine, scopolamine, and related belladonna alkaloids can cause erectile difficulty because of their ganglionic blocking properties and antimuscarinic actions.[7]

H2 Blockers

The histamine H2 receptor antagonist cimetidine (Tagamet), used to decrease gastric acid secretion, causes testicular atrophy, oligospermia, and gynecomastia, as well as diminished libido and impotence. These consequences are thought to result from the drug's antiandrogen action as well as its effect in elevating prolactin.[3,4,7] The related drug, ranitidine (Zantac), is less likely to affect sexual function and a third drug in the family, famotidine (Pepcid), has no effects on androgen receptor binding or prolactin.[8]

Metoclopramide

Metoclopramide (Reglan), used to treat esophageal reflux and diabetic gastroparesis, causes diminished libido and impaired erections, probably because of its dopamine antagonist effects producing elevated prolactin.[3,4]

Ketoconazole

Ketoconazole (Nizoral), an antifungal agent available in topical and oral forms, but taken orally for serious systemic infections, impairs erections by lowering testosterone levels.[18] This agent interferes with steroid synthesis in both the adrenal glands and testicles, in doses much larger than that recommended for therapy of fungal infections, and, in fact, is often used as therapy for cortisol excess in Cushing's syndrome.[19]

Hormonal Agents

Drugs that lower testosterone, impair gonadotropin release, or raise estrogen levels can interfere with sexual function. Antiandrogens such as flutamide and cyproterone acetate will cause sexual dysfunction by producing chemical castration. Similarly, use of gonadotropin-releasing hormone (GnRH) analogs, both agonists administered in a nonpulsatile fashion as well as antagonists, will interfere with leutinizing hormone and follicle-stimulating hormone release, testosterone synthesis, and spermatogenesis.[20] Estrogen administration for any reason will suppress leutinizing hormone release and lower testosterone. Corticosteroid excess, either endogenous or caused by administration for different conditions, will suppress gonadal function and reduce testosterone.

Miscellaneous Drugs

Numerous other agents are said to impair sexual function: baclofen (Lioresal), ε-aminocaproic acid (Amicar), disulfiram (Antabuse), and carbonic anhydrase inhibitors such as acetazolamide (Diamox), clofibrate (Atromid-S), and ethionamide (Trecator).[4,7]

Drugs of Abuse

Long-term narcotic use and physical dependence cause decreased libido, erection difficulty, and impaired ejaculation, which all persist after transfer from short-acting drugs to methadone.[3,4] Narcotic addicts often have low serum testosterone and decreased gonadotropin release and a possible mechanism may be the observation that narcotic analgesics and optiate-like CNS peptides such as enkephalins and endorphins stimulate prolactin release and lower gonadotropin levels.[3]

Cocaine is thought to have acute aphrodisiac effects, but causes erectile failure with persistent use.[4] It also causes elevated prolactin,[17] which may be one factor contributing to the resulting sexual dysfunction.

Marijuana is popularly believed to increase sexual interest, perhaps because of its disinhibiting effects, but chronic use is associated with impotence, oligospermia, and decreased testosterone levels.[3,4]

Amphetamines are said by some to intensify sexual interest, but abuse causes decreased libido and difficulty with ejaculation.[4] Fenfluramine (Pondimin), a sympathomimetic agent used for weight loss, is associated with impotence.[7]

Alcohol may initially increase libido because of its disinhibiting effects, but this may be overcome by central sedation, with resultant decreased libido, as consumption continues.[3,4] Acutely, alcohol also impairs erection, ejaculation, and orgasm, and chronic use leads to the development of alcoholic polyneuropathy, testicular damage, and liver disease, which produces increased estrogen effects.[4] These consequences of chronic alcohol use all contribute to permanent impotence.

Nicotine can acutely impair erections, perhaps because of vasoconstriction,[4] and prolonged use is well known to be a major risk factor for progression of arteriosclerosis, with subsequent permanent vascular disease as a cause for impotence.

Summary

Many different drugs can cause sexual dysfunction, but some patients are more vulnerable because of contributing factors such as vascular or neurologic disease and hormonal disorders. A knowledge of sexual side effects will help the physician to improve compliance by prescribing drugs that patients are more likely to take regularly.

REFERENCES

1. Slog MF et al: Impotence in medical clinic outpatients. JAMA 1983; 249:1736–1740.
2. Morley JE: Impotence. Am J Med 1986; 80:897–905.
3. Horowitz JD, Goble AJ: Drugs and impaired male sexual function. Drugs 1979; 18:206–217.
4. Wein AJ, Van Arsdalen KN: Drug-induced male sexual dysfunction. Urol Clin NA 1988; 15:23–31.

5. Andersson KE et al: Pharmacology. In Kirby RS et al. eds, Impotence: Diagnosis and management of male erectile dysfunction. Butterworth, Heinemann, 1991; 32–43.
6. Krane RJ et al: Impotence. N Engl J Med 1989; 321:1648–1659.
7. Abramowicz M (ed): Drugs that cause sexual dysfunction. Med Lett 1980; 22:108–110.
8. Abramowicz M (ed): Drugs that cause sexual dysfunction. Med Lett 1987; 29:65–70.
9. Richardson JW: Antidepressants: A clinical update for medical practitioners. Mayo Clin Proc 1984; 59:330–337.
10. Rakel RE: The side effect profile of Trazodone. In: Gershon S, eds. Desyrel: A compendium of three years of clinical use. Mead Johnson, 1985; 21–30.
11. Prescribing Information Update, 1992, for Prozac (Fluoxetine hydrochloride). Dista Products Company, 1992.
12. Wagner G: Neuropharmacology of penile erection in vitro. In Jonas, U et al., eds. Erectile dysfunction. Berlin: Springer-Verlag, 1991; 57–68.
13. Cavallini G: Minoxidil versus nitroglycerin: A prospective double-blind controlled trial in transcutaneous erection facilitation for organic impotence. J Urol 1991; 146:50–53.
14. Rittmaster RS: Hyperandrogenism—what is normal? N Engl J Med 1992; 327:194–196.
15. Rudd P: Utilization of calcium channel blockers in hypertension. Mod Med 1988; 56:118–127.
16. King BD et al.: Impotence during therapy with verapamil. Arch Int Med 1983; 143:1248–1249.
17. Mendelson JH et al.: Cocaine effects on pulsatile secretion of anterior pituitary, gonadal and adrenal hormones. J Clin Endocr Metab 1989; 69:1256–1260.
18. Melman A: Iatrogenic causes of erectile dysfunction. Urol Clin NA 1988; 15:33–39.
19. Loriaux DL: The treatment of Cushing's syndrome and adrenal cancer. Endocr Metab Clin NA 1991; 20:767–771.
20. Moghissi KS: Clinical applications of gonadotropin releasing hormones in reproductive disorders. Endocr Metab Clin NA 1992; 21:125–140.

9 Hormonal Causes of Male Sexual Dysfunction

Barry J. Klyde

Hypogonadism

For thousands of years, it was known that castration of domestic animals as well as men decreased sexual interest and activity, revealing the essential role of the testicles. A fascinating fact is that men with nonfunctioning testicles and low testosterone may sometimes continue to have normal desire and erections, but in most cases a drop in testosterone is accompanied by a drop in libido and performance. The extent to which less-than-optimal testosterone impairs sexual function is influenced by the state of penile blood flow and nerve conduction: a younger man in good health except for diminished testosterone may often continue to have good erections, but in older men with penile blood flow beginning to be reduced by arteriosclerosis, or nerve conduction diminished by diabetic or alcoholic neuropathy, even a moderate decrease in testosterone may interfere with erections, with improvement following supplementation.

Primary Testicular Failure

Different studies estimate that up to 30% of men with sexual dysfunction have a hormonal cause with the majority having hypogonadism.[1] The most frequent cause of hypogonadism is age-related primary testicular failure. Physical exam may reveal atrophic testicles and a prostate smaller than expected for the patient's age, but it is unusual for hypogonadism to progress, without being recognized and treated, to the point that facial hair growth is slowed, body hair is lost, and muscle mass is diminished as body fat assumes a more feminine distribution. Chemical studies reveal a typical picture of low testosterone and elevated gonadotropins, leutinizing hormone (LH) and follicle-stimulating hormone (FSH), confirming primary hypogonadism. Occasionally there is loss of only testicular ability to synthesize testosterone while spermatogenic ability persists, with decreased testosterone production causing increased LH release from the pituitary while FSH remains

Management of Impotence and Infertility, edited by Douglas Whitehead and Harris Nagler,

normal. Additional causes of testicular failure include trauma, disruption of the blood supply by torsion or rarely following inguinal hernia repair, or an infection such as mumps occurring after puberty.

Pituitary and Hypothalamic Disease

Low testosterone not accompanied by elevated gonadotropins suggests defective pituitary or hypothalamic function. The appearance of men with secondary testicular failure will be similar, with atrophic testicles and shrinkage of the prostate initially, and loss of other androgenic effects later on. The most frequent cause of secondary hypogonadism in the population of impotent men seen in our office is idiopathic LH deficit probably resulting from hypothalamic dysfunction. A hypothalamic cause is suggested, and a pituitary cause made less likely, by observing an LH rise after stimulation testing with GnRH.[2] A more serious cause is LH deficiency caused by a tumor such as a pituitary adenoma or craniopharyngioma, but this is much less frequent: during the past 10 years, 20 or more patients a year are seen in our office with hypogonadism presenting with low testosterone accompanied by low LH as the only other hormonal abnormality and none had a pituitary disease such as a tumor. In the past, after hormone blood tests, our office would do extensive evaluation, including stimulation testing with GnRH to measure pituitary LH responsiveness, and visualization of the pituitary, initially with CT scans, and more recently with MRI when this becomes available. We found that pituitary abnormalities were found only in patients with elevated prolactin or abnormal adrenal or thyroid tests. Patients with isolated LH deficiency in addition to low testosterone often had depressed LH responsiveness to GnRH and always had normal pituitary glands on CT scan or MRI. More recently, we have stopped doing further tests on hypogonadal patients with isolated LH deficiency since they were not helpful. Further discussion of elevated prolactin occurs later in this chapter.

Therapy of hypogonadism is determined by the patient's spermatogenic potential and desire for fertility. If potency is the only goal, then testosterone supplementation is the most direct way to achieve it. Testosterone administration, however, will suppress GnRH and gonadotropins and further lower an already depressed sperm count. The most effective form of testosterone supplementation presently available is the use of fat soluble esters such as testosterone enanthate or testosterone cypionate dissolved in oil, administered intramuscularly 200 mg every 2 weeks or 300 mg every 3 weeks.[3,4] Side effects include possible fluid retention with the potential for hypertension or worsening of preexisting congestive heart failure, acne, gynecomastia from conversion of the administered testosterone to estrogen, diminished HDL, and accelerated prostatic enlargement or growth of occult prostatic carcinoma. Oral medication, most frequently in the form of methyl testosterone, is not often used now because of significant hepatic toxicity resulting from a large amount of the drug passing through the liver following intestinal absorption, and suboptimal therapeutic effectiveness.[4] An alternative nonparenteral form is methyl testosterone in absorbable lozenges, which are placed in the cheek and absorbed directly into the circulation, avoiding the first pass through the liver and reducing the risk of hepatic toxicity. Effectiveness remains much less than parenteral testosterone.[4]

A new approach to testosterone replacement, not yet available, is the use of a transdermal patch.[5–7] Patches containing estradiol have been used in women for postmenopausal estrogen replacement for several years, and can be applied to the trunk and changed only twice a week, but testosterone patches required a different technology because the daily production rate of testosterone is almost 100 times greater than the amount that could be supplied by such patches.[5] A different kind of patch was developed, and applied to the scrotum each day to achieve more efficient testosterone absorption. Physiologic levels of testosterone were obtained, but levels of dihydrotestosterone (DHT) became excessive compared to normal values, probably because of the first pass through the scrotal skin, which contains large amounts of the 5α-reductase enzyme that converts testosterone to DHT.[5–7] Much interest is now focused on newly available drugs that inhibit 5α-reductase, so there is more awareness of the adverse effects of DHT.[8] It is possible that many of the side effects blamed on testosterone result from DHT.[8] Potential serious effects include more rapid progression of prostatic hypertrophy, and decreased HDL with resulting increased risk of arteriosclerotic disease. Less serious effects include accelerated male pattern baldness and acne.[8]

An additional form of testosterone replacement, still investigational, is the use of biodegradable microcapsules containing testosterone that are injected intramuscularly, are released at a steady rate over 10 weeks to provide a constant, physiologic blood level, and do not cause an excess rise in DHT or estradiol.[9]

In patients who desire fertility and have secondary hypogonadism resulting from hypothalamic or pituitary disease rather than primary testicular failure, it is possible to stimulate the dormant testicles to increase endogenous testosterone production, and thus increase spermatogenesis as well.[4] This can be done with hCG, which has LH activity, with 2,000 U injected intramuscularly three times a week. After 3 to 6 months, if sperm count is not sufficiently improved, hMG, containing FSH, is added. An additional method of testicular stimulation is the pulsatile administration of GnRH via a pump. More convenient treatment of hypothalamic impotence, if pituitary LH and FSH production is preserved, is use of clomiphene, an oral antiestrogen that stimulates LH and FSH release.[2] Guay et al.[2] administered clomiphene for one week as a diagnostic agent, but for therapy it may be more appropriate to give 25 mg each day, for 25 days a month.[10]

Estrogen Excess

Estrogen excess causing LH suppression with resulting diminished testosterone production is most often seen in obese men. This is probably a result of adipose tissue conversion of testosterone to estrogen.[11] Chronic liver disease can also produce estrogen excess both because of hepatic aromatization of testosterone to estrogen, and because of increased sex hormone binding globulin, which can result in a reduced amount of active testosterone in the circulation.[12] Causes of liver disease include chronic hepatitis, cirrhosis resulting from different etiologies, and alcohol abuse.

A rarer cause is excess production of an adrenal androgen, DHEA, which is also converted to estrogen in the liver as well as adipose tissue.[13] These men may have gynecomastia and feminine fat distribution, and blood tests reveal low testosterone and LH accompanied by elevated total estrogen (estrone + estradiol). Measurement of estradiol alone is not sufficient since much of the estrogen in men is in the form of estrone.

Treatment includes weight loss in obese men and suppression of adrenal DHEA production, if elevated, with glucocorticoid administration.[13] An additional therapeutic option, which is often helpful if the altered estrogen–testosterone balance is the only cause of impotence, is supplemental therapy with testosterone.

Hyperprolactinemia

Women with amenorrhea accompanied by galactorrhea were first described almost one and a half centuries ago,[14] and the development of an assay for prolactin revealed that these women had inappropriate increased production of this pituitary hormone, resulting in anovulation and infertility.[15] More recently, it was recognized that prolactin excess in men impairs libido and potency,[16] presumably because of its known effects on both central hypothalamic and pituitary regulation of gonadotropin production and on gonadal function.[17] Studies of the cause of elevated prolactin have been done in women because it is a much more frequent problem in them. Perhaps it is less often found in men because cessation of periods is a dramatic event that often brings a woman to a physician, while gradual waning of desire and erections is not as likely to cause a man to see his doctor. Almost half the patients with elevated prolactin have no demonstrable pituitary abnormality or other cause, and are termed idiopathic. One-third have a pituitary tumor, and the remainder have miscellaneous causes such as medication effects,[18,19] hypothyroidism,[20,21] or systemic illness such as renal failure or cirrhosis.[22] More than two-thirds of pituitary adenomas produce prolactin, and are termed prolactinomas. Prolactin is the only pituitary hormone whose level is controlled by an inhibiting factor from the hypothalamus rather than a stimulating one, so interference with transport of prolactin inhibiting factor down the pituitary stalk by either stalk section, pressure from a nonhormone producing tumor, such as a craniopharyngioma, or by cystic enlargement within an "empty sella" can cause a rise in prolactin and subsequent sexual dysfunction. The highest prolactin levels are seen with a prolactinoma: 50% of patients with a prolactin level of 100 ng/ml have a tumor while levels above 200 ng/ml are almost always caused by a tumor.[17] An additional, more recently recognized cause of elevated prolactin is temporal lobe epilepsy,[23] which is easily overlooked by patients, families, and physicians, is not corrected by bromocriptine, and requires appropriate anticonvulsant medication to restore normal sexual function.

Men with prolactin excess first come to attention because of sexual dysfunction, although occasionally the mass effects of an enlarging pituitary tumor cause visual field decrease, headaches, and other endocrine disorders that bring the man to a physician. Testosterone is often low, sometimes accompanied by low gonadotropins, but testosterone supplementation does not correct the low libido or impaired erections of these patients because the elevated prolactin interferes with end organ responsiveness.[16] In one study, the initial group of male patients presenting with elevated prolactin and sexual dysfunction all had large pituitary tumors as a cause,[16] but subsequent male patients, both in the experience of others[1] as well as myself, resembled women in that the largest group of hyperprolactinemic patients had no demonstrable tumor, the next largest group had pituitary tumors and a small number had other causes of elevated prolactin as described. Distinction between those patients with an idiopathic cause of elevated prolactin and those having a tumor was made by performing a visualization procedure: in recent years contrast enhanced magnetic resonance imaging (MRI) of the sella, and in past years computed tomography (CT).

Therapy of Hyperprolactinemia

Use of dopaminergic drugs such as bromocriptine is considered the therapy of choice for prolactinomas.[15] Dopamine is believed to be the prolactin-inhibiting factor produced in the hypothalamus and transported down the pituitary stalk[15] and bromocriptine therapy has successfully lowered prolactin in patients with either idiopathic elevation or prolactinomas.[15] Dopaminergic drugs such as bromocriptine and lisuride were found to significantly reduce the size of macroadenomas (tumors greater than 1 cm) in up to two-thirds of patients and lessened visual field defects caused by tumor compression of the optic chiasm.[24] Hyperprolactinemia was found to recur after transsphenoidal surgery in half of patients with microadenomas and most patients with macroadenomas,[25] making surgery less desirable as a therapeutic option. Bromocriptine was able to reduce the recurrent elevated prolactin in all patients in which it was used,[25] suggesting that even macroadenomas are best treated with medication rather than surgery. Therapy with bromocriptine in men having hyperprolactinemia has been helpful in restoring libido and potency and improving sperm count and sperm quality.[16]

Thyroid Disease

Thyroid hormone excess, resulting from increased endogenous production caused by hyperthyroidism, or from an excessive dose of a thyroid supplement such as Synthroid, can impair potency. The mechanism is thought to be an increase in the binding protein for testosterone.[1] Appropriate therapy corrects the thyroid problem and restores normal sexual function, confirming the cause.

Hypothyroidism also impairs both libido and potency, probably because of the generalized metabolic slowing which results. If impotence persists after thyroid hormone replacement, then further study is warranted.

Adrenal Disease

Overproduction of adrenal corticosteroids in patients with Cushing's syndrome can suppress gonadal function in both sexes and can thus interfere with both libido and erections. Adrenal insufficiency causes generalized debility, which interferes with sexual function. The clinical presentations of Cushing's syndrome and adrenal insufficiency are dramatic enough to suggest appropriate diagnostic tests, and these illnesses are quite rare, so routine testing of adrenal function should not be part of the suggested workup for impotence unless clues appear during the history and physical examination.

Diabetes

Diabetes is the most frequent cause of impotence and can produce sexual dysfunction in men of all ages.[26] Acute onset of impotence may result from the metabolic derangements of poorly controlled diabetes and is often transient, improving with effective therapy of the diabetes. However, men with diabetes often experience the gradual loss of erections over years as they begin to develop other complications of diabetes: neuropathy, vascular disease, nephropathy, and retinopathy. The progression of diabetic complications is now widely believed to be associated in patients with prior suboptimal control.[27] The cause of impotence in diabetic men is thought to result from both neuropathy and vascular disease, with some discussion of the relative contributions of these two processes.[28,29] Diabetic complications, including impotence, are more likely in patients with other risk factors for arteriosclerosis such as smoking, elevated cholesterol, hypertension, and a family history of vascular disease.

Psychological factors can also interfere with erections in diabetic men. These patients often "expect" to develop impotence, and may, therefore, be especially likely to turn transient dysfunction into a more persistent problem. In a recent study, almost 40% of impotent diabetic men had psychogenic impotence that improved with sex therapy,[30] so we are wrong to assume that diabetic men must have significant neuropathy and vascular disease causing their impotence. Additionally, other hormonal abnormalities such as hypogonadism or elevated prolactin should also be sought, so that an easily reversible cause is not overlooked

Suggested Evaluation for Hormonal Causes of Impotence

A complete history and physical examination should be done, with careful evaluation of hair and fat distribution, skin texture, thyroid size and consistency, gynecomastia, central and distal pulses, reflexes and vibration sensation, penis and testicles, and prostate size and consistency. Laboratory evaluation, in addition to routine urinalysis, CBC, and chemistries, should include free T4 index ($T7 = T4 \times T3$ resin uptake), TSH, testosterone, LH, FSH, and prolactin. Random glucose may not reveal diabetes and in a diabetic patient would not reveal the degree of control, so a test for glycosylated hemoglobin, which is a measure of the average glucose for the prior few months, is also recommended. This battery of tests, plus others if suggested by the history and physical, is essential to look for a hormonal disorder that may be readily reversible with medication, and would certainly be easier to correct than vascular disease or neuropathy.

REFERENCES

1. Spark RF: A new approach to impotence. Med Aspects Human Sexuality 1983; 17:228–244.
2. Guay AT et al.: Possible hypothalamic impotence: Male counterpart to hypothalamic amenorrhea. Urology 1991; 38:317–322.
3. Sokol RZ et al.: Comparison of the kinetics of injectable testosterone in engonadal and hypogonal men. Fertil Steril 1982; 37:425–430.
4. Snyder SJ: Treatment of male hypogonadism. Adv Endocr Metab 1990; 1:245–260.
5. Cunningham GR et al.: Testosterone replacement with transdermal therapeutic systems. JAMA 1989; 261:2525–2530.
6. McClure RD et al.: Hypogonadal impotence treated by transdermal testosterone. Urology 1991; 37:224–228.
7. Carey PO et al.: Transdermal testosterone treatment of hypogonadal men. J Urol 1988; 140: 76–79.
8. Tenover JS: Prostates, pates and pimples: The potential medical uses of steroid 5-alpha-reductase inhibitors. Endocr Metab Clin NA 1991; 20:893–909.
9. Bhasin S et al.: A biodegradable testosterone microcapsule formulation provides uniform

engonadal levels of testosterone for 10–11 weeks in hypogonadal men. J Clin Endocr Metab 1992; 74:75–83.
10. Homonnai ZT et al.: Clomiphene citrate treatment in oligospermia: Comparison between two regimens of low dose treatment. Fertil Steril 1988; 50:801–804.
11. Roncari DAK, Van RLR: Promotion of human adipocyte precursor replication by estradiol in culture. J Clin Invest 1977; 62:503–568.
12. Adlercreutz H: Hepatic metabolism of estrogens in health and disease. N Engl J Med 1974; 290:1081–1083.
13. Marynick SP et al.: Androgen excess in cystic acne. N Engl J Med 1983; 308:981–986.
14. Koppelman MCS et al.: Hyperprolactinemia, amenorrhea and galactorrhea. Ann Int Med 1984; 100:115–121.
15. Frantz AG: Prolactin. N Engl J Med 1978; 298:201–207.
16. Carter JN et al.: Prolactin-secreting tumors and hypogonadism in 22 men. N Engl J Med 1978; 299:847–852.
17. Blackwell RE: Hyperprolactinemia: evaluation and management. Endocr Metab Clin NA 1992; 21:105–124.
18. Kleinberg DL et al.: Galactorrhea: a study of 235 cases including 48 with pituitary tumors. N Engl J Med 1977; 296:589–600.
19. Gomez F et al.: Nonpuerperal galactorrhea and hyperprolactinemia. Am J Med 1977; 62:648–660.
20. Fish LH, Mariash CN: Hyperprolactinemia, infertility and hypothyroidism. Arch Int Med 1988; 148:709–711.
21. Olive KE, Hennessey JV: Marked hyperprolactinemia in subclinical hypothyroidism. Arch Int Med 1988; 148:2278–2279.
22. Molitch ME: Pregnancy and the hyperprolactinemic woman. N Engl J Med 1985; 312:1364–1370.
23. Spark RF: Impotence. Med Grand Rounds 1986; 4:8–19.
24. Chiodini P et al.: Size reduction of macroprolactinomas by bromocriptine or lisuride treatment. J Clin Endocr Metab 1981; 53:737–743.
25. Serri O et al.: Recurrence of hyperprolactinemia after selective transsphenoidal adenomectomy in woman with prolactinoma. N Engl J Med 1983; 309:280–283.
26. Whitehead ED, Klyde BJ: Diabetes-related impotence in the elderly. Clin Geriatric Med 1990; 6:771–795.
27. Chase HP et al.: Glucose control and the renal and retinal complications of insulin dependent diabetes. JAMA 1989; 261:1155–1160.
28. Ellenberg M: Impotence in diabetics: The neurogenic factor. Ann Int Med 1971; 75:213–219.
29. Herman A et al.: Vascular lesions associated with impotence in diabetic and nondiabetic arterial occlusive disease. Diabetes 1978; 27:975–981.
30. El-Bayoumi M et al.: Impotence in diabetics: organic versus psychogenic factors. Urology 1984; 24:459–463.

ANNOTATED BIBLIOGRAPHY

1. Pogach LM, Vaitukaitis JL: Endocrine disorders associated with erectile dysfunction. In: Krane RJ et al., eds. Male sexual dysfunction. Boston: Little Brown, 1983: 63–76.
2. Bouloux PMG, Wass JAH: Endocrinology. In: Kirby RS et al., eds. Impotence: Diagnosis and management of male erectile dysfunction. Butterworth, Heinemann, 1991: 44–54.
3. Schürmeyer TH, Hesch RD: Endocrinology of impotence. In: Jonas U et al., ed. Erectile dysfunction. Berlin: Springer-Verlag, 1991: 78–90.

These three articles are comprehensive, detailed reviews that provide additional information and other viewpoints on hormonal factors influencing male sexual function.

4. Leonard MP et al.: Hyperprolactinemia and impotence: Why, when, and how to investigate. J Urol 1989; 142:992–994.

Elevated prolactin was found in 5% of over 1200 impotent patients, indicating the value of checking for this, and the etiology and outcome after therapy are described.

10 Treatment of Priapism

Craig F. Donatucci
Tom F. Lue

Priapism is defined as the persistence of penile erection in the absence of sexual excitation, often accompanied by pain and tenderness. In the past most cases of priapism were thought to be idiopathic in origin. Hinman[1] described seven features that were common to all occurrences of idiopathic priapism: (1) previous episodes of priapism were usually related to periods of prolonged sexual excitement, (2) the corpus spongiosum was usually not involved, (3) dark (venous) blood was invariably present on aspiration, (4) after aspiration there was immediate filling of the corpora with arterial (bright red) blood, (5) aspiration was not usually successful in obtaining detumescence, (6) if the aspiration was performed late in the clinical course, it would result in nonfilling of the corpora, and (7) the usual outcome after idiopathic priapism was impotence. Hinman was the first to demonstrate that during prolonged periods of priapism, injury to the underlying corporal tissue occurred, with resultant edema that eventually would lead to fibrosis of the erectile tissue and loss of erectile capability.

The aim of therapy for priapism is to resolve the painful erection and to preserve erectile function. Unfortunately, none of the therapeutic options available at the time of Hinman's publication, including administration of spinal or general anesthesia, aspiration, anticoagulants, ganglionic blockade, and antiandrogen therapy, was particularly effective in resolving the priapism, because they failed to reestablish adequate venous drainage. Shortly thereafter, Grayhack et al.[2] introduced the saphenous–corporal bypass to effect venous drainage in the priapistic patient, and, at approximately the same time, Quackles[3] reported the first experience utilizing a spongiosal–cavernosal shunt to reduce priapism. These innovative techniques (see below) led to an improved outcome in many cases of idiopathic priapism, but it was not until recent advances in our understanding of the basic physiology of erection that therapeutic measures aimed at specific disorders causing priapism were developed.

Management of Impotence and Infertility, edited by Douglas Whitehead and Harris Nagler,

Pathophysiology of Priapism

The mechanisms responsible for the prolongation of erection in priapism are essentially the mirror images of those responsible for impotence. In the impotent patient, poor arterial inflow can lead to inadequate erectile function; in the priapistic patient, persistent high arterial inflow can lead to failure of detumescence. While excessive venous outflow may be responsible for venous leak impotence, restriction of venous drainage may also result in priapism.

Traditionally categorized as either primary (idiopathic) priapism or secondary to a known disorder, priapism can also be classified based on the predominant hemodynamic pattern: low flow (ischemic) priapism and high flow (nonischemic) priapism.[4] Of the two, restricted venous flow more commonly results in prolonged erection. Utilizing intracavernous pressure monitoring and blood gas determination on aspirated corporal blood, Lue et al. demonstrated that priapism can encompass a wide clinical spectrum, which depends upon the duration of erection, the degree of venous occlusion, and the severity of the underlying disease process.[4] High intracavernous pressures with minimal venous drainage and minimal flow through the cavernous arteries (monitored by penile duplex ultrasonography) resulted in significant ischemia, and rapid reestablishment of adequate venous drainage was critical for a successful outcome. Nonischemic priapism, representing a milder form of the disease, would be expected to be tolerated better, and this might explain why some patients have return of normal function weeks after the onset of priapism, while others are impotent after only several days.

Witt et al. recently documented several cases of high flow priapism after traumatic laceration of the cavernous arteries.[6] Using arteriography they showed that flow through the injured vessel bypassed the protective helicine arterioles and entered the lacunar spaces directly. Because the normal neurologic impulses initiating and maintaining erection were absent, the sinusoids were not in a state of complete relaxation and the venoocclusive mechanism was not fully activated. The continuous arterial flow distended the sinusoids, but the blood drained through open emissary veins, therefore ischemia did not develop. They termed this arterial priapism, in contradistinction to the low flow (ischemic priapism) state, which they termed venoocclusive priapism.

Failure of the detumescence mechanism can result from many causes: excessive release of neurotransmitters resulting in paralysis or prolonged relaxation of the intracavernous smooth muscles and blockage or inadequate drainage of blood through the subtunical venules. Persistence of intracavernous pressure at levels of 80–120 mm Hg results in a low flow ischemic state of the cavernous tissue. This high flow nonischemic state can occur as a result of penile arterial revascularization procedures that bypass normal control mechanisms or as a result of intracavernous arterial laceration as in cases of trauma. In the era of intracavernous pharmacotherpy of impotence, erections lasting several hours are not uncommon; however, any erection persisting longer than 4 to 6 hours may be considered priapistic. Typically patients with low flow (ischemic) priapism will not experience pain until 6 to 8 hours has passed. The degree of ischemia is a function of the number of emissary veins involved (roughly paralleling the rigidity) and the duration of venous occlusion.

When ischemic priapism lasts longer than 24 hours the corporeal tissue may become thickened, edematous, and eventually fibrotic. The natural history of prolonged ischemic priapism is erectile dysfunction, although some erectile ability may be maintained in the proximal crura. If operative intervention is required and occurs after 24 hours, potency rates no better than 55% can be expected.

Etiology

The causes of priapism can be multiple (Table 10-1), and the incidence of a specific cause is clearly affected by demographics. Sickle cell disease accounted for 23% of adult cases and 63% of pediatric priapism in a series reported by Nelson and Winter[7]; overall 46% of cases were idiopathic. In a later review by Pohl et al., one-third of all cases reported were idiopathic, 21% were associated with alcohol abuse or drug therapy, 12% with perineal trauma, and 11% with sickle cell anemia.[8] The following are frequently encountered causes.

Sickle Cell Disease

This condition affects 8% of African-Americans; in a review of 321 pediatric patients Tarry and Duckett reported a 6.4% incidence of priapism among their sickle cell patients.[9] Red cell sickling and later sludging of blood occur within the corpora cavernosa. This sludging occurs as a result of abnormal endothelial adherence, the relatively acidic state of the corpora cavernosa during erection, the mild acidosis accompanying hypoventilation during sleep, or mild trauma. Hydration, alkalinization, analgesia, and hypertransfusion have been effective therapy for this condition, increasing hemoglobin to greater than 10 g and reducing the hemoglobin S concentration to less than 30%. Complete flaccidity may require from several days to 2 weeks of therapy. Recovery of erectile function among the pediatric population is good but much poorer among the adults.

Table 10-1 Etiology of Priapism

Idiopathic (primary)
Secondary
Thromboembolic (sickle cell anemia)
Traumatic (perineal, genital, or surgical)
Neurogenic (spinal cord lesions, autonomic neuropathy, anesthesia)
Malignant penile infiltration
Oral medications and chemicals (alcohol, psychotropic agents, antihypertensives)
Intracavernous injection (papaverine alone or with phentolamine, prostaglandin E_1, or mixtures of all three medications)

Metastatic Neoplasms

A number of primary malignancies may metastasize to the penis with a resultant abnormal painful erection.[10,11] Partial replacement of sinusoids resulting in stasis and thrombosis in the remaining tissue, or extensive penile outflow obstruction may occur. Therapy for malignant priapism is directed at the primary malignancy, with adjunctive and palliative measures as necessary.

Trauma

Priapism may occur after perineal or genital trauma. These injuries can result in blockage of the penile venous drainage due to thrombosis, severe hemorrhage, or tissue edema at the base of the penis (low flow priapism). Laceration of the cavernous artery, from trauma or intracavernous injection, within the corpora cavernosa can also result in unregulated pooling of the blood into the sinusoidal spaces and priapism (high flow priapism).[6]

Iatrogenic Causes

Medications

Numerous oral medications employed in a myriad of conditions have been associated with priapism. Chlorpromazine and the antipsychotic drugs of the phenothiazine group have been associated with prolonged erection.[12] The antidepressant trazodone has been reported in 94 separate cases of priapism since its introduction in 1982.[13] Other commonly implicated medications are the antihypertensive drugs hydralazine, guanethidine, and prazosin.[14] The apparent action of these drugs is α-adrenergic blockade. Priapism occurs in only a small percentage of patients on antipsychotic or antihypertensive medications and is not dosage specific.

Vasodilator Injection

Diagnostic and therapeutic injections of vasoactive pharmacologic agents into the corpora cavernosa with subsequent prolonged erection is the most common iatrogenic cause of priapism, and the most likely cause of priapism to confront urologists. Junemann found an incidence of 0.4% of priapism in over 44,000 self-injections.[15] The majority of these prolonged erections occur among patients with either neurogenic or psychogenic impotence.

Cavernosography

When pharmacologic cavernosography is performed without the use of diluted contrast, hyperosmotic injury to the sinusoidal epithelium can occur with subsequent development of priapism. In this instance the injury leads to particularly severe interstitial edema, detumescence may not occur until resolution of the edema, and this condition can be mistaken for continuing priapism.

Surgical Revascularization

Procedures designed to improve arterial flow to the cavernous tissue may lead to high flow priapism. In particular, the Michal I procedure,[16] which directly anastomosed the inferior epigastric artery to the corpus cavernosum, led to initial high flow priapism before ultimate thrombosis of the anastomosis. This procedure has now been abandoned, but epigastric–dorsal vein bypass, designed to improve inflow into the corpora cavernosa, may lead to high flow priapism or glans hyperemia.

Medical Management

The traditional treatment of priapism has been diverse and nonspecific: ice packs, enemas, vigorous prostate massage, pressure dressings, analgesics, sedatives, anticoagulants, estrogens, antispasmodics, fibrinolysins, hypotensive agents, and general and caudal anesthesia.[17,18] With the recognition of the importance of sympathetic (α-mediated) stimulation in the detumescence mechanism, introduction of intracavernous injection of sympathomimetic α-adrenergic vasoconstrictors has opened a new era in the treatment of priapism.

In sickle cell priapism recurrence is more the rule than the exception. The risks of surgery and general anesthesia in the pediatric population outweigh the benefits of early operative intervention. However, a small amount of α-adrenergic agent may be injected into the corpora without anesthesia, and this may abort the priapism. Therefore it is justified to give a trial of α-adrenergic agent when a reasonable trial of conservative therapy has failed, as this may lessen the suffering and hospital cost and probably better preserve erectile tissue.

When intracavernous agents are used for

diagnostic testing, an erection lasting over 1 hour can be expected in about 10% of patients. Therefore, informed consent should include a discussion of possible aspiration or injection of an α-adrenergic agent after 1 hour. It has been our policy to intervene uniformly after 1–2 hours of rigid erection with the patient remaining on the premises during that period. If full erection lasts for more than 1–2 hours during the diagnostic study, aspiration of corporal blood and injection of α-adrenergic agent should be performed. Pain usually will ensue in the untreated patient after 6–8 hours. When treated within 24 hours, almost all patients will respond to the above therapy with minimal change of potency status. However, if therapy is delayed for more than 36–48 hours, marked hypoxic tissue injury is likely to occur and shunting procedure may be required to treat the priapism. Because tissue ischemia begins after 4–6 hours, we recommend therapeutic intervention to abort the priapism, which preferably should begin within 6 hours to minimize any possible tissue damage.

When priapism is the result of improper or overly enthusiastic self-injection of intracavernous vasodilators, appropriate treatment also will depend on the duration of erection and the patient's medical history. The initial procedure is the same, the reduction of intracavernous pressure by repeated corporal aspiration; this is the safest mode of therapy in patients with a history of severe cardiac or cerebrovascular disease. Injection of an α-adrenergic agent after aspiration is a more effective therapy in those patients without cardiac disease.[4] Aspiration can be performed through a 21-gauge scalp vein needle inserted into one of the corpora cavernosa, and injection of diluted α-adrenergic agent can follow through the same tubing if necessary. Aspiration will reduce intracavernous pressure and remove excess vasoactive agent while injection of an α-adrenergic agent will initiate sinusoidal smooth muscle contraction, thus improving venous outflow. Many α-adrenergic agents are available, including epinephrine, norepinephrine, ephedrine, and phenylephrine (Table 10-2). Alternatively, corporal aspiration can be combined with irrigation of the corpora cavernosa with diluted adrenergic solutions.

Table 10-2 Intracavernous Medications for the Management of Priapism

Drug	Usual Dose[a]
Epinephrine	10–20 μg
Phenylephrine	100–500 μg
Ephedrine	50–100 mg
Norepinephrine	10–20 μg

[a] These doses can be given repeatedly every 3–5 minutes until detumescence.

In our practice we have routinely begun with aspiration followed by injection of phenylephrine (NeoSynephrine) 100–200 μg in 1 ml of normal saline. The patients are continuously monitored for blood pressure elevation and tachycardia. The injection of phenylephrine can be repeated every 5 minutes until detumescence occurs. Utilizing this technique our complications have been relatively mild. Transient rise in blood pressure (10–20 mm Hg) occurred in about half of the patients; few reported palpitations for 1–2 minutes. Two of our patients with a history of migraine developed severe headache lasting several hours. Similar experience has recently been reported by Dittrich et al. who treated 36 priapistic patients with intracavernous injection of phenylephrine.[19] All patients were successfully detumesced, none underwent aspiration, none suffered adverse systemic effects, and all had return of potency.

Frequently the episodes of priapism will be

recurrent, as in sickle cell disease. Dreil et al. reported the use of intracavernous self-injection of epinephrine in a patient with recurrent priapism.[20] They reported no adverse effects in this single case report, but concern over potentially serious cardiac sequelae limits enthusiasm for this approach. Levine et al. reported on six patients who suffered from recurrent veno-occlusive (ischemic) priapism.[21] All six patients were successfully treated with phenylephrine injection. The recurrent episodes were painful and four of the six patients were taught to use the phenylephrine as home therapy. None of these patients suffered serious adverse effects. Dittrich et al. taught eight patients to use home phenylephrine therapy; these patients were also able to reduce their erections when necessary, and no ill effects were noted.[19]

In cases of priapism other than those induced by intracavernous injection of vasodilators, an initial trial of repeated intracavernous injection with α-adrenergic medications can also be recommended, especially if the duration of priapism is within 24 hours. If the duration is more than 36 hours, or if detumescence fails to occur after more than 10 injections of 200 μg of phenylephrine, success is unlikely and shunting procedures are recommended.

Surgical Therapy

The era of surgical therapy for priapism began in 1964 with the near simultaneous publication of the saphenocorporal bypass procedure by Grayhack, and the corporal–spongiosal bypass by Quackles. Both procedures were designed to address the primary reason for failure of therapy at that time, inadequate corporal venous drainage.

Corporal–Saphenous Vein Shunt

As described by Grayhack et al.[2] the corporal–saphenous shunt begins with exposure of the corpus cavernosum. Initially a 1-cm elliptical segment of Bucks fascia and tunica albuginea is removed. Detumescence is obtained by corporal irrigation until arterial bleeding is observed. The saphenous vein is exposed and is divided 10 cm below the point of entrance into the femoral vein. A subcutaneous tunnel is developed and the end of the saphenous vein is delivered to the point of the corporal ellipse. Next an anastomosis is fashioned between the saphenous vein and the corpus, thus establishing adequate venous drainage.

Corporal–Spongiosal Shunt

As described by Quackles,[3] a urethral sound is placed to facilitate dissection. Next an 8-cm incision is made in the perineum behind the median raphe of the scrotum and carried down to the urethral bulb. The dissection is carried up the dorsolateral side of the spongiosum. An orifice as wide as possible is created on the dorsum of the corpus spongiosum. Care must be taken not to make the opening in the spongiosum too deep so that the underlying urethra is not damaged. A ellipse of tunica albuginea is removed from the corpus cavernosum opposite the site of the spongiosal opening and the corpus is irrigated and clot removed. An anastomosis is created between the cavernosum and spongiosum using absorbable suture. In the initial publication, Quackles described the creation of a second shunt proximal to the first on the opposite side of the penis.

For the next decade after publication of these techniques, patients failing initial conservative measure underwent one or the other of these shunting procedures. Dahl and

Middleton compared the outcome of the saphenous vein shunt to that of the spongiosal–cavernosal shunt.[22] They noted that failure of the initial shunting procedure, whether saphenous–cavernosal or cavernousspongiosal shunting, did not preclude the successful use of the other procedure as a second decompression. The relative ease of the Quackles procedure argued in favor of that approach initially; however, Dahl and Middleton noted that neither procedure was as yet the ideal operation for priapism, as many patients were still left impotent after successful decompression. In addition to fibrosis as a cause of impotence in the postpriapistic patient, prolonged patency of the shunt was now recognized as a new cause for erectile dysfunction in these patients.

Dorsal Vein–Cavernosal Shunt

Barry described construction of a shunt utilizing the dorsal vein of the penis.[23] Both the superficial and deep dorsal vein are usually patent during an episode of priapism, and readily available locally. Of the two, construction of a superficial dorsal vein to cavernosum shunt is simpler. The dorsal artery and nerves are carefully dissected free of the tunica albuginea and retracted locally. The dorsal vein is ligated distally, the proximal end is spatulated, and an anastomosis is made to the ipislateral corpus cavernosum.

Glanular–Cavernosal Shunt: Winter's Procedure

In 1976 a simplified procedure to create a shunt between the tumesced cavernosa and the glans was described by Winter.[24] After aspiration and irrigation of the corpora, Winter introduced a Travenol biopsy needle through the glans penis and removed two cores of tissue from the tip of the corpora cavernosa. Detumescence was prompt as a fistula had been created between the cavernosa and the glans. Because of its simplicity and the ability to perform the procedure in an outpatient setting, the glanular–cavernosal shunt quickly gained acceptance as the initial invasive procedure used for decompression of the priapistic patient. However, a number of patients will fail after an initial positive response to the Winter shunt and will need a second decompressive procedure. This number can be minimized if, after creation of the fistula with the Travenol biopsy needle, the fistula tract is widened using a Kerrison rongeur.

Glanular–Cavernosal Shunt: El Ghorab Procedure

Under the best of circumstances the glanular–cavernosal shunt as performed by Winter will not succeed in some patients, therefore an alternative, albeit somewhat more invasive technique to create a glanular–cavernosal shunt has been described. First reported by Ebberhoj[25] in 1975, and later referred to by Ercole et al. as the El Ghorab shunt,[26] this procedure exposes the tips of the cavernosa through a transverse incision made in the dorsum of the glans penis. The tunical albuginea is incised in a circular fashion and the corpora are irrigated and drained. The glanular incision is then closed creating a glanular cavernosal fistula. Local anesthesia is sufficient, and this approach shares both simplicity and the ability to be performed in the outpatient setting.

Correction of Arterial–Venous Fistulae

High flow priapism resulting from laceration or injury to the cavernous artery is diagnosed by duplex ultrasound or arteriography. Correction of abnormal arterial flow by embolization with autologous clot or coils results in prompt cessation of priapism. Excellent residual erectile function has been reported, although the number of patients so treated is limited.[5]

When priapism is the result of penile revascularization, reoperation is usually necessary to correct the abnormal flow. Any large venous channels should be ligated, but more often than not resolution of the priapism will require ligation of the arteriovenous anastomosis with resulting failure of the initial revascularization.

Scheme for the Management of Priapism

Given the large number and variety of medical and surgical treatment modalities for priapism, clearly, no single therapy is applicable to all situations. Rather, a systematic and reasoned approach based on an understanding of the underlying pathophysiology (ischemic versus nonischemic priapism) should be employed The use of intracavernous pressure monitoring and intracavernous blood gas analysis is of great assistance in caring for these patients. When priapism is secondary to a recognized factor such as sickle cell disease or trauma, the primary condition should be immediately corrected. When the patient presents early in the episode, an initial attempt at aspiration alone or in conjunction with the injection of an α-adrenergic agent should be employed. If the patient is delayed in presentation, aspiration and α agents will only temporarily detumesce the penis as the intrinsic smooth muscle of the sinusoids and terminal arterioles have been paralyzed by the hypoxia and acidosis. Under these circumstances a surgical shunt procedure will be necessary to resolve the priapism. Initially glanular–cavernosal shunts should be created and the intracavernous pressure monitored after the procedure. A fall in the intracavernous pressure to below 40 mm Hg that is sustained for 10 minutes should lead to resolution of the priapism, if the intracavernous pressure remains elevated (greater than 50 mm Hg) or if the pressure begins to rise, larger shunts will be needed between the tip of the corpora and the glans. If this fails proximal shunting will be needed as thrombosis or tissue edema distally is likely. The corporal–spongiosal shunt described by Quackles, the saphenous–cavernous shunt of Grayhack et al., or the dorsal vein–corpora shunt of Barry will then be needed. The use of intracavernous monitoring and blood gases should enable the surgeon to distinguish persistence of the priapism from ongoing tumescence, which can occur with severe edema of the interstitial corporal tissue after injury. Failure to recognize persistence of tumescence secondary to edema may lead to unnecessary secondary shunting. On the other hand, failure to recognize recurrent priapism will lead to severe ischemia and impotence. It cannot be overemphasized that a circular penile dressing should not be applied after distal or venous shunting because it will lead to impairment of venous drainage and recurrence of priapism.

Future Perspective on Priapism

While our basic understanding of the vascular pathophysiology of priapism has increased over the last decade, the initiating events leading to idiopathic priapism remain to be identified. The discovery that sympathetic α-adrenergic stimulation is responsible for penile detumescence has advanced our ability to treat the priapistic patient. The parasympathetic neuropharmacologic impulses responsible for the initiation of erection are still under investigation. The role of nonadrenergic–noncholinergic (NANC) neurotransmitters in cavernous smooth muscle relaxation appears important in the initiation and maintenance of erection; deficiency of intermediate biochemical messengers like endothelin may later be implicated in priapism.[27] Erection is effected through this as yet incompletely understood complex biochemical pathway. A specific defect in any step of this process could result in either erectile dysfunction or persistence of erection with priapism. Pharmacologic agents that therapeutically manipulate the cavernous smooth muscle through a different biochemical pathway may represent an effective therapeutic alternative for these patients in the future.

REFERENCES

1. Hinman F Jr: Priapism, reasons for failure of therapy. J Urol 1960; 83:420.
2. Grayhack JT, McCullough W, O'Conor VJ, Trippel O: Venous bypass to control priapism. Invest Urol 1964; 1:509.
3. Quackles R: Cure of a patient suffering from priapism by cavernospongiosa anastomosis. Acta Urol Belg 1964; 32:5.
4. Lue TF, Hellstrom W, McAninch JW, Tanagho EA: Priapism: A refined approach to diagnosis and treatment. J Urol 1986; 136:104.
5. Juenemann KP, Lue TF, Abozeid M, Hellstrom W, Tanagho EA: Blood gas analysis in drug-induced penile erection. Urol Int 1986; 41:207–211.
6. Witt MA, Goldstein I, Saenz de Tejada I, Greenfield A, Krane RJ: Traumatic laceration of intracavernosal arteries: The pathophysiology of nonischemic, high flow, arterial priapism. J Urol 1990; 143:129–132.
7. Nelson JH, Winter CC: Priapism: Evolution of management in 48 patients in a 22-year series. J Urol 1977; 117:455.
8. Pohl J, Pott B, Kleinhans G: Priapism: A three phase concept of management according to aetiology and prognosis. Br J Urol 1986; 58:113.
9. Tarry WF, Duckett JW Jr, McC Synder H III: Urological complications of sickle cell disease in a pediatric population. J Urol 1987; 138:592.
10. Juenemann KP, Lue TF, Abozeid M, Hellstrom W, Tanagho EA: Blood gas analysis in drug-induced penile erection. Urol Int 1986; 41:207–211.
11. Van Arsdale K, Chen JW, Smith MJ: Vernon: Penile erections complicating transurethral surgery. J Urol 1983; 129:374.
12. Dorman BW, Schmidt JD: Association of priapism in phenothiazine therapy. J Urol 1976; 116:51.
13. Priapism with trazodone (desyrel): Med Lett Drugs Ther 1984; 26(658):35.
14. Rubin SO: Priapism as a probable sequel to medication. Scand J Urol Nephrol 1968; 2:81.
15. Junemann KP: Pharmacotherapy of impotence: Where are we going? In: Lue TF, ed. World book on impotence research: Basic and clinical. Smith-Gordon, London, 1992; 181–198.
16. Michal V, Kramar R, Pospichal J, Hejhal L: Direct arterial anastomosis to the cavernous body in treatment of erectile impotence. Rozhl Chir 1973; 52:587.
17. Maraluz JN, Sullivan JW: Priapism: Review of 34 cases. Urology 1985; 26(3):233–236.
18. Warmer JM, Carrion HM, Mekraos F, Politano VA: Evaluation and treatment of priapism. J Urol 1981; 125:204–207.
19. Dittrich A, Albrecht K, Bar-Moshe O, Vandendris M: Treatment of pharmacological priapism with phenylephrine. J Urol 1991; 146:323–324.
20. Driel MF, Joosten EAHM, Mensink HJA: Intra-

corporeal self-injection with epinephrine as treatment for idiopathic recurrent priapism. Eur Urol 1990; 17:95–96.
21. Levine FJ, Saenz de Tejada I, Payton TR, Goldstein I: Recurrent prolonged erections and priapism as a sequela of priapism: Pathophysiology and management. J Urol 1990; 1145:764–767.
22. Dahl DS, Middleton RG: Comparison between cavernosaphenous and cavernospongiosum shunting in the treatment of idiopathic priapism: A report of 5 operations. J Urol 1974; 112:614–615.
23. Barry J: Priapism: Treatment with corpus cavernosum to dorsal vein of penis shunt. J Urol 1976; 116:754.
24. Winter CC: Priapism cured by creation of fistulas between glans penis and corpora cavernosa. J Urol 1978; 119:227.
25. Ebberhoj J: A new operation for priapism. Scand J Plast Reconstr Surg 1975; 8(3):241–242.
26. Ercole CJJ, Pontes JE, Pierce JM: Changing surgical concepts in the treatment of priapism. J Urol 1981; 125:210–211.
27. Andersson KE, Holmquist FN: Mechanisms for contraction and relaxation of human penile smooth muscle. Int J Impotence Res 1990; 2:209–225.

ANNOTATED BIBLIOGRAPHY

Hinman F Jr: Priapism, reasons for failure of therapy. J Urol 1960; 83:420.

In this classic article on priapism the author summarizes the clinical course of a typical idiopathic episode, reviews then current concepts of erectile function, and explores the pathophysiologic consequences of priapism. The study of seven patients with priapism led the author to enumerate seven features that appear to be common to all cases: (1) previous episodes of priapism, (2) erection of the corpora cavernosa alone, (3) presence of dark thick nonclotting blood within the corpora, (4) refilling of the corpora if aspiration was performed early in the course of the episode, (5) limited detumescence after aspiration, (6) eventual nonfilling after aspiration, and (7) partial or complete impotence as the final result. The author stresses the importance of abnormal venous occlusion as a contributing factor and documents the edema and fibrosis that occur with resolution of the priapism. The importance of the autonomic nervous system and, in particular, the parasympathetic nervous system for normal erectile function is explored. However, this article appeared well before the introduction of venous shunt procedures or pharmacologic manipulation of the erectile process, and therapeutic efforts as reported here were of little benefit.

Lue TF, Hellstrom W, McAninch JW, Tanagho EA: Priapism: A refined approach to diagnosis and treatment. J Urol 1986; 136:104.

Contemporary management of priapism based on fundamental advances in our understanding of the physiology of erection and the pathophysiology of priapism are introduced in this article. The impact of intracavernous pharmacotherapy is explored. Priapism is seen as a spectrum ranging from severe low flow (ischemic) to high flow (nonischemic) states. A flow diagram is provided that utilizes intracavernous pressure monitoring and corporal blood gas aspiration to determine the degree of ischemia present. Nonischemic patients respond to α-adrenergic agents, mildly ischemic patients undergo aspiration and irrigation initially to restore blood gases, and severely ischemic patients underwent shunt procedures. This basic schema with modifications remains clinically useful today.

Nelson JH, Winter CC: Priapism: Evolution of management in 48 patients in a 22-year series. J Urol 1977; 117:455.

This article reports the authors 22 year experience in the management of patients with priapism. The period covered began before the first venous drainage procedures were introduced and serves as an example of the therapeutic results one could expect before the current era of intracavernous pharmacotherapy. The authors document the evolution in their treatment, which resulted in 100% resolution of the priapismic episodes, and maintenance in potency in 50%.

Witt MA, Goldstein I, Saenz de Tejada I, Greenfield A, Krane RJ: Traumatic laceration of intracavernosal arteries: The pathophysiology of nonischemic, high flow, arterial priapism. J Urol 1990; 143:129–132.

The pathophysiology of high flow priapism is explored in this article. The authors review two cases of nonischemic priapism, both of which failed repeated conservative attempts at management by aspiration and instillation of α-adrenergic agents. In one case a straddle injury was the initiating event, while intracavernous injection of papaverine led to the onset of priapism in the second case. Each patient underwent arteriography, and a lacerated branch of the cavernous artery was discovered in both. Embolization of the injured branch led to prompt resolution of priapism for both patients, and potency was maintained. The underlying pathologic event in high flow priapism is felt to be the unregulated inflow of arterial blood into the corpora, and the authors introduce a therapeutic algorithm for management.

11

Treatment of Peyronie's Disease

Steven M. Schlossberg
Charles J. Devine, Jr.

Peyronie's disease is not rare. It has been present in a little over 1% of two small groups of physicians with which we are familiar. It is most frequent in middle aged men, though it is not unusual in sexually active older men. We have seen no patients under 19 years of age and very few blacks or orientals. In Peyronie's disease an inelastic scar (plaque) in the compliant tunica albuginea of the corpora cavernosa shortens the involved aspect of the erect penis causing a bend. Though trauma in a susceptible individual, possibly during sexual intercourse, has been associated with the occurrence of Peyronie's disease,[1–4] the cause has not been well understood. Smith[5] described its pathology and attributed the lesion to perivascular inflammation in the space he first noted between the tunica and the underlying erectile tissue. He could not define the source of this inflammation,[6] but most nonsurgical treatment of Peyronie's disease has been aimed at controlling it. Indeed, inflammation is present in this space of Smith, but it is also present in and beneath Buck's fascia, where it overlies the lesion. In our view the inflammation is a response to the process in the tunica and not the cause of it. It is not a cancer not is it an autoimmune process. In young patients there may be the possibility of a sarcoma, but a biopsy would be necessary only if the lesion is uncharacteristic.

Figure 11-1A is a diagram of a cross section in the midshaft of the penis showing the two corpora cavernosa containing the erectile tissue separated by a septum composed of strands of tissue running from the midline dorsally to the midline ventrally. Almost without exception plaques of Peyronie's disease are located in the tunica at the dorsal or ventral midline where the strands of the septum are attached. At the base of the penis the corpora become separate structures, fixed to the inferior rami of the pubis within their covering fascia.

The third erectile body, the corpus spongiosum, containing the urethra, runs in the groove on the underside of the fused corpora cavernosa separately enclosed by Buck's fascia and secured in place by lateral thickening of that

Management of Impotence and Infertility, edited by Douglas Whitehead and Harris Nagler,

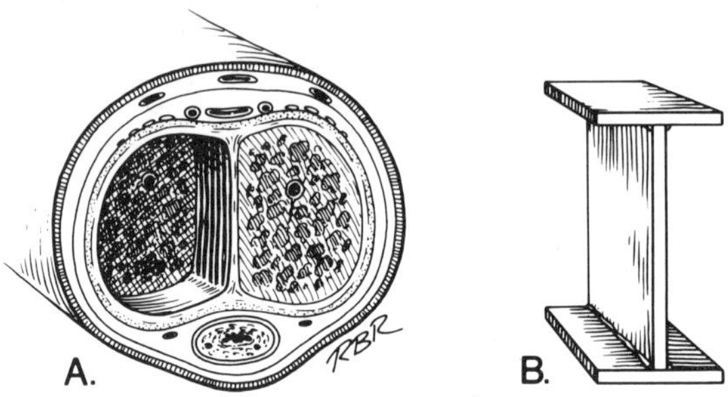

Figure 11-1 (A) Diagram of the penis as related to the occurrence of Peyronie's disease. The fibers of the septum are attached to the inner surface of the tunica albuginea of the corpora cavernosa along the dorsal and ventral midlines. Plaques of Peyronie's disease occur in the tunica albuginea at the site of attachment of the septal strands. (B) A diagram of an I-beam illustrates the configuration of the septum that is responsible for the ultimate rigidity of the penile erection. The function leads to the occurrence of Peyronie's disease. (From Devine et al.[7])

fascia adherent to the tunica of the corpora cavernosa. On the dorsal side the deep dorsal vein—which may consist of several trunks—runs in the midline with a dorsal artery on each side and a number of the fascicles of the dorsal nerve lateral to that. They are contained within and attached to the underside of Buck's fascia. Outside of Buck's fascia the loose dartos fascia allows the skin to slide easily on the shaft of the penis. Normally with erection these compliant structures of the penis expand and elongate symmetrically, resulting in a straight phallus.

There are two layers of elastic fibers in the tunica of the corpora cavernosa, the outer being longitudinal and the inner, circular. The strands of the septum are composed of similar elastic fibers. At their attachment to the tunica, the fibers of the septal strands fan out and are interwoven with the fibers of the inner layer of the tunica. During erection this septal configuration, acting like the web of an I-beam (Figure 11-1B), imparts the ultimate rigidity to the erect penis, resisting upward or downward bending of the shaft (Figure 11-2A). As in an I-beam, when the penis is bent dorsally or ventrally, as happens during intercourse, the attachments of the septal fibers to the tunica are stressed with compression on the concave side and tension on the convex side. In young men, despite the turgor of the penis and the vigor of the intercourse, the elasticity of the tissues will allow the structures to deform and rebound, but as a man ages his tissues will become less elastic and the tension caused by this same degree of penile bending may delaminate the circular fibers of the tunica where they are interlaced with the fibers of the attachment of the septum (Figure 11-2B). With this tear, there is microvascular injury with bleeding and clot formation. Many of these patients have a vivid memory of this happening, perhaps a month prior to the onset of their Peyronie's disease.

Other patients will not have had this type of acute trauma to the penis. They may have lost some of the turgor of their erection, and, though continuing to have what they and their partner consider to be satisfactory intercourse, the less rigid shaft of the penis flexes. Over time this action causes elastic tissue fatigue, further reducing the elasticity of the connections of the septal strands to the tunica, resulting in multiple tears with multiple smaller collections of blood clot (Figure 11-2C). We feel that Peyronie's disease results from this acute or chronic trauma. The clots in the tissue spaces lead to fibrin deposition. Fibrin in the tissue is associated with (1) fibroblast activation and proliferation, (2) enhanced blood vessel permeability, and (3) generation of chemotactic factors for inflammatory cells (histocytes). The fibrin is not cleared during the usual healing process in the not well-vascularized tunica. The lesion fails to resolve due to this retention of

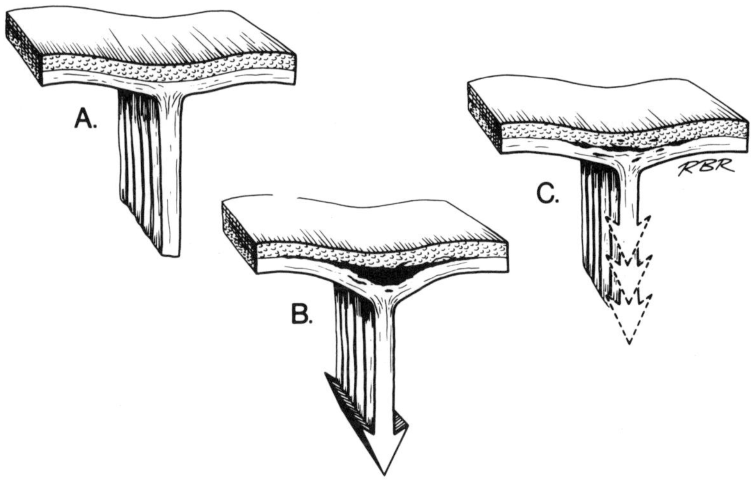

Figure 11-2 (A) Fibers of the septal strands fan out and are interwoven with the inner circular layer of fibers of the tunica albuginea. The outer layer consists of longitudinal fibers. (B) In the acute form of Peyronie's disease, bending the erect penis out of column produces tension on the strands of the septum delaminating the fibers of the tunica albuginea. Bleeding occurs, and the space fills with a clot. The scar generated by the response of the tissue to this process becomes the plaque of Peyronie's disease. (C) In the chronic form of Peyronie's disease, less turgid erections allow flexion of the penis during intercourse producing elastic tissue fatigue, further reducing the elasticity of the tissue and leading to multiple smaller ruptures of the fibers of the tunica with smaller collections of blood producing multiple scars. (From Devine et al.[7])

fibrin or the further deposition following repeated trauma. The trapped collagen produces pathologic fibrosis. This scar is the plaque.[7]

Surely, diminution of the elasticity of the aging tissues of the penis plays a major part in the pathogenesis of Peyronie's disease. There is an association with conditions involving other tissues where elasticity is important to function: Palmar fascia with Dupuytren's contracture, Plantar fascia with Ledderhose disease, ear drum with tympanosclerosis, and, indeed, with another condition involving the penis, venous occlusive incompetence. Ten percent of patients with Peyronie's disease have Dupuytren's contracture. The rapidity of this loss of erection may be genetically determined. This could account for the familial association of patient's with these conditions—male relatives having Peyronie's disease or Dupuytren's contracture or females having the latter.

There are two modes of onset. In about half of the patients we have seen the condition appears acutely with one erection being straight and the next bent with little or no further progression. In others, the onset is chronic with a slowly progressive bend eventually reaching an end point. It may be that these two presentations represent the two sets of patients—acute and chronic—described above. Pain is often thought of as a feature of Peyronie's disease, but pain has been present in only two-thirds of our patients and has persisted in only 1%.[8] Usually the plaque involves the dorsal aspect and the penis will bend upward. Sometimes, asymmetry of the dorsal plaque produces a rotational distortion (dorsal and left to right). However, if the plaque is on the ventral aspect, the penis will bend downward. At times both aspects will be involved and the plaques will balance each other with the penis having a lateral curve or being straight but shortened with a reduction of circumference in the involved area. These patients are especially bothered by the restriction of expansion caused by apposing plaques. Patients with an upward bend of 45° or less can usually continue with intercourse satisfactory to both partners. If the bend is downward or lateral, the critical angle is 30°. Patients with greater distortion can continue with sexual activity, but with the penis this far out of column, despite their ability to attain a firm erection, attempts at intromission are met with further bending and failure.

Usually patients complain of a lump or pain in the penis or simply a bend with erection. We ask each patient to bring Polaroid photographs of the erection showing the defect and have each patient fill out a questionnaire. (A copy of this questionnaire can be obtained by writing to The Devine Center for Genitourinary Reconstruction, Sentara Norfolk General Hospital, 600 Gresham Drive, Norfolk, VA 23507.) Palpation of the plaque in the shaft of the penis makes the diagnosis, though, because the plaque is confined to the tunica, palpation must be precise. A dorsoventral squeeze of the penis may locate the lesion but not define its extent. The penis must be stretched so that the edges of the plaque can be palpated between the thumb and index finger of the other hand placed laterally on the shaft. It will be easy to differentiate dorsal plaques from ventral plaques and the extent of the involved area can be defined.

When the scar has matured, there will be no further change in the bend of the penis unless the quality of the erection changes. If the patient and his partner are satisfied with their sexual function, the couple should be encouraged to persist. Though the plaque can reach maturity without becoming calcified, calcification is a sign of this end stage of the disease. We have X-rayed each of the patients whom we have seen and in one of four of these patients X-ray has disclosed calcification and in 25% of these there has actually been bone formation.

Patients with Peyronie's disease may complain of impotence. Usually a man will be able to attain erection but may lose it quickly—especially if pain is present—or may note that the penis proximal to the plaque is firm while the shaft distal to the plaque is soft. Patients presume, and may have been told by a physician, that the plaque has blocked the flow of blood into the penis. The scar of Peyronie's disease, however, involves only the tunica albuginea and does not extend into the erectile tissue. As demonstrated by doppler flow studies, arterial inflow is usually normal even beyond the plaque. Why does this happen? The tunica and supporting structures within the penis[9] must be stretched to the limit of their elasticity to maintain the rigidity of the erection. The extension of these structures attached to the inelastic tissues of the plaque is restricted and that portion of the penis cannot be made turgid by physiological arterial inflow. If impotence is associated with Peyronie's disease it will be found to be due to concurrent venoocclusive incompetence (venous leak), a minor degree of which may often have been a factor in the genesis of the disease in the patient with a chronic onset of the condition.

Two studies are used to evaluate impotence. Duplex ultrasound will record inflow vascular dynamics of the penis.[10] We use 30 μg of prostaglandin E_1 to establish a pharmacologic erection. Prior to injection there will be no diastolic flow within the cavernosal arteries. After injection, the arteries will dilate and there will be an increase in the velocity of blood flow, with diastolic flow continuous until the penis fills. Normally, as the penis becomes rigid, the increase in systolic velocity will remain but diastolic flow disappears. However, if a venous leak is present, the penis never fills to rigidity and diastolic flow will persist. In such a situation it will be necessary to do a dynamic infusion corpus cavernosogram (DICC) to identify the veins that are leaking. These may be emissary veins associated with the area of the tunica involved with the Peyronie's disease plaque but most often they are not, arising from nearby or elsewhere on the penile shaft. In these patients a pharmacologic program (PEP) may generate enough rigidity so that they can resume intercourse despite the bend in the penis.

Treatment is aimed at maintenance or reestablishment of sexual function. After having established the diagnosis we discuss the situation with the patient and his sexual partner. We explain the disease and note that this not mean the end of their sex life. There is no specific medical therapy for Peyronie's disease; our favorite medication has been vitamin E. The disease has become static or has resolved with continuing function in two-thirds of our patients taking 200 mg with each meal or 400 mg twice a day. Potaba is expensive and is not a specific cure for "the bent spike," and its 24 powders or tablets per day may be accompanied by gastric distress and sometimes bleeding. We have seen increased fibrosis and tissue atrophy following injection of steroids so we do not inject plaques. Though radiation therapy may relieve pain it will not reverse the process of scarring and it can cause damage and further fibrosis, so we do not use it routinely. However, if pain is intractable we would deliver 450 rads to the lesion using the beta beam from the linear accelerator.[11] There is no quick cure for the lesion, just slow maturation of a scar in the not well-vascularized tunica albuginea.

The active process usually does not last longer than a year to a year-and-a-half, after which the lesion may remain static or recede. Occasionally, in a very young patient, the plaque may disappear entirely, but this is rare. In 1978 and 1979 we saw 200 patients with Peyronie's disease: 75 required surgery; the rest were sent home with vitamin E therapy. In 1981 we were able to contact 105 of those patients who did not have surgery and two-thirds of them had continued to function in a satisfactory fashion. Some had improved and in four the lesion had resolved. In 11 the bend had increased and they did undergo surgery. Four of the original 125 were impotent and at resurvey this number had doubled. We inserted a penile prosthesis in three of these; the other five declined further treatment.[8] In all, only a third of the patients we have seen required surgical treatment. If the lesion is calcified or the disease has been present for a year to a year-and-a-half and there is enough distortion of the penis to preclude sex, we offer the patient surgical therapy consisting of excision of the plaque with replacement of the diseased area of the tunica with a graft from the dermal layer of the skin.[12,13]

Other surgical procedures have been described for Peyronie's. Pryor and Fitzpatrick[14] have used Nesbit's plication procedure[15] straightening the shaft by shortening the aspect of the penis opposed to the plaque. A number of others have accomplished this by reefing up the tunica with various patterns of sutures without excising elipses of tunica.[16–18] Das and Amar[19] used a graft of tunica vaginalis after

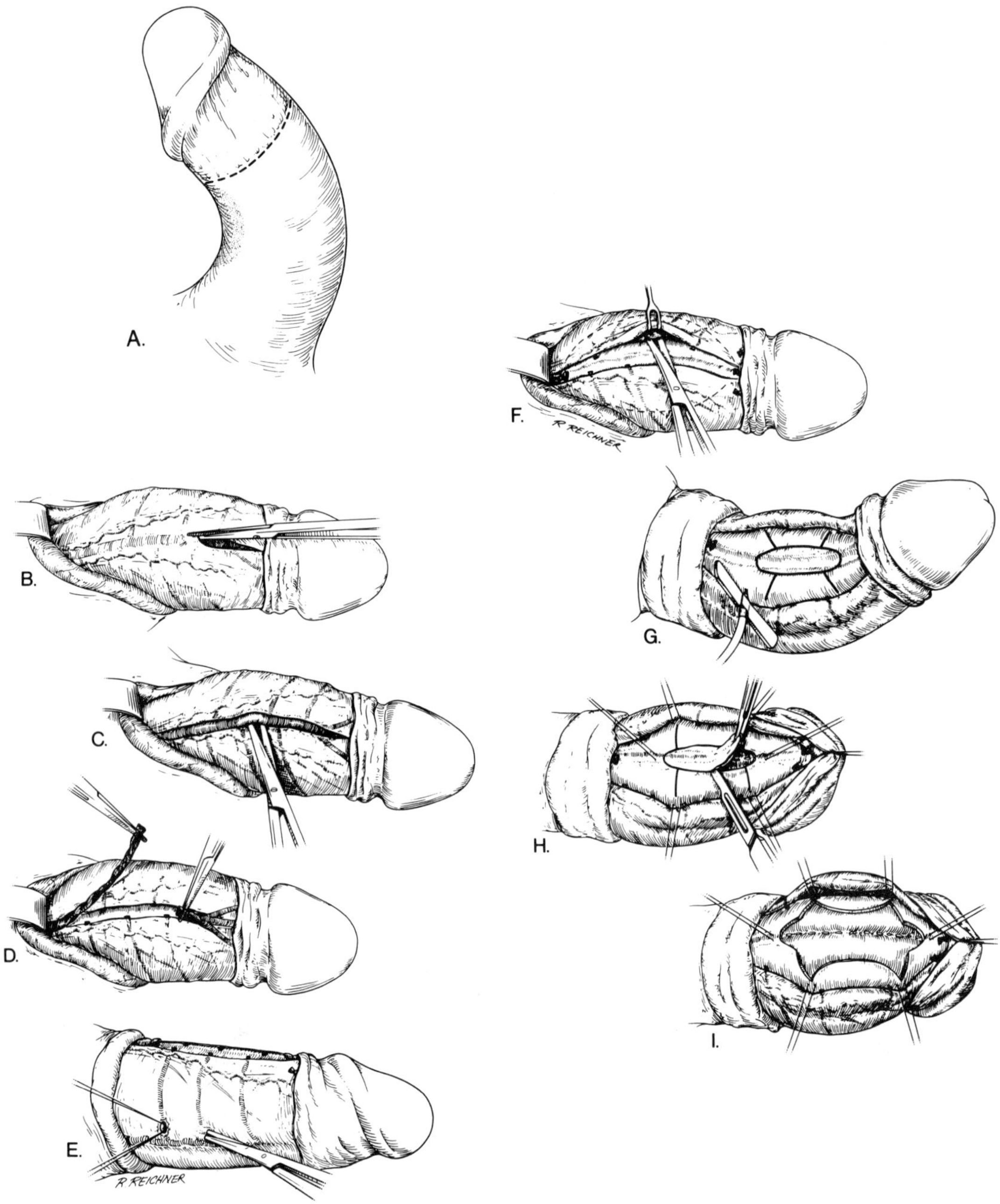
A.
F.
R REICHNER
B.
G.
C.
H.
D.
I.
E.
R REICHNER

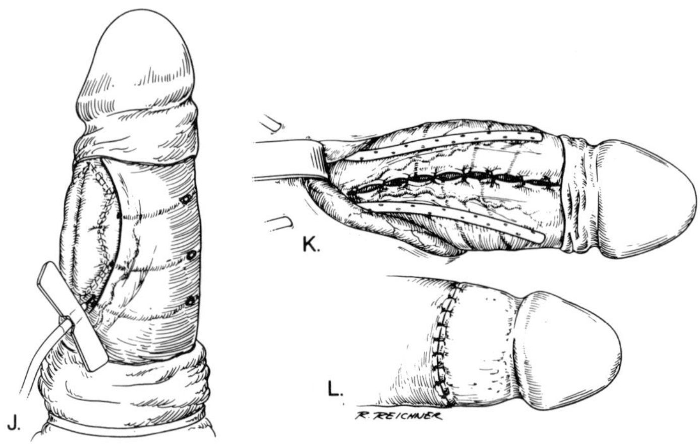

Figure 11-3 (A) An erection demonstrates the dorsal curvature of the penis caused by the inelastic scar tissue in a dorsal plaque of Peyronie's disease. The incision to be made in the scar of the previous circumcision has been marked. (B) The skin has been reflected to the base of the penis by dissecting in the layer of the dartos fascia. An incision made with scissors in the dorsal midline of Buck's fascia exposes the deep dorsal vein. The coiled dorsal arteries and the circumflex veins are demonstrated. (C) The deep dorsal vein is mobilized by dissecting beneath it with blunt-tipped iris scissors. (D) After dividing the deep dorsal vein, it is dissected proximally, dividing the emissary veins and ligating them with fine black silk sutures. Distally, the vein is mobilized and followed to the point where the veins draining the glans penis combine to form the deep dorsal vein and then dividing and ligating each of these. (E) The circumflex veins are isolated and are oversewn with sutures of 4-0 black silk on each side where they join the vein running lateral to the corpus spongiosum. (F) Using the blunt-tipped scissors, Buck's fascia is elevated from Peyronie's plaque. The area of dissection is outlined by the dashed line in the diagram, continued far enough proximally, distally, and laterally to allow excision of the plaque without distraction injury to the dorsal arteries and the nerves in Buck's fascia, which are clearly seen and avoided during this dissection. (G) An artificial erection demonstrates the curvature caused by the inelastic plaque, which has been outlined on the tunica. Stellate releasing incisions have also been marked. (H) Prolene sutures have been placed distal and proximal to the plaque and at the tip of each of the releasing incisions. Each suture has been tagged to control the tunica as the surgery progresses. An incision has been made outlining the plaque, and the tip of the plaque is grasped with forceps as it is being excised, using sharp dissection to separate it from the erectile tissue. The strands of the septum have been excised and are seen in the midline of the defect being created. (I) The plaque has been excised, and the lateral incisions have released the shortness of the dorsal aspect of the penis. This defect must now be filled with a dermal graft. To determine the size of the patch we measure the defect in the tunica while stretching it first longitudinally, then laterally. (J) The dermal graft has been obtained and applied to the defect. An artificial erection shows the penis to be straight. If there is a leak in a suture line, it is oversewn with 5-0 polydioxanone sutures. (K) Buck's fascia is loosely reapproximated in the midline with interrupted 5-0 polydioxanone sutures. One or two small suction drains are left in the space above Buck's fascia. (L) The skin closure is completed using several sutures of 5-0 Vicryl in the subcutaneous tissue and 4-0 chromic catgut to approximate the skin. A Bioclusive dressing is applied. A light pressure wrap of Kling dressing is left on for 3 to 4 hours. A 14 French catheter is placed and removed next morning. (From Devine et al.,[29] with permission.)

excision of the plaque, reasoning that it was easier for a urologist to obtain this tissue than dermis. Others have carried this one step further by applying Dacron or Gore-Tex "vascular grafts"; however, these materials are not elastic and form inflammatory collections of collagen beneath them. We have treated failures of all these procedures. Poutasse[21] made multiple incisions excising small portions of the plaque to straighten the penis and did not apply grafts to cover these; Gelbard[22] has done this in a more systematic fashion and applied grafts of temporalis fascia. Harvesting this fascia from the face seems to be an heroic effort. Lue[17] has approached the plaque through the bed of the dorsal vein, excising the vein and using it with its endothelial surface turned inward to patch multiple incisions in the involved area of the tunica. Lockhart[23] used the tunica vaginalis as a flap rather than a graft to patch the area after having excised the plaque and recently Buncke and associates[24] reported an experimental study transferring temporalis fascia as a microvascular free flap to cover the defect in the tunica. We have considered each of these but reports of the results have not shown a higher success rate than our own use of the dermal graft and we have not been persuaded to change our present technique.

As noted, only a third of the patients have required surgical treatment. Presently all of our patients who come to surgery undergo a detailed preoperative evaluation of their erectile function.[25] The association of preoperative erectile function with postoperative results is the basis for our recommendations for surgery. Criteria for normalcy in DICC studies have been developed,[26] but a man does not have to achieve these values to have sexual relations he considers satisfactory. Most patients who have been able to accumulate at least 50 mm Hg of intracorporal pressure in response to provoked pharmacologic erection have been able to have intercourse following excision of a Peyronie's plaque and application of a dermal graft. About 60% of patients able to accumulate 40–50 mm Hg of intracorporal pressure have also been able to have intercourse. Those unable to function will have a straight penis not rigid enough for intercourse. If they do not respond to PEP, they will require placement of a prosthesis as will most men not able to accumulate at least 40 mm Hg of intracorporal pressure. Though placement of a prosthesis is not complicated by the previous dermal graft, we advise men who do not achieve an adequate level of pressure to have a prosthesis placed at the time of the straightening operation.

Even in patients happy that they can function after surgery the penis is "not like it used to be." There will still be some distortion with patchy areas of hypoesthesia and the penis will not be as long as it was prior to the onset of Peyronie's disease. One will note that even in our hands, some men with Peyronie's disease will require placement of a prosthesis. Many of our patients have arrived here for further advice because their urologist has told them that all men with Peyronie's disease will need a prosthesis. This is not so and no man able to achieve his own erection should be relegated to a prosthesis because that is what his surgeon does best.

Surgical Procedures

Our approach to a Peyronie's plaque will depend on its position in the shaft of the penis. Most plaques will be on the dorsal side in the mid-portion of the shaft. If the patient has previously been circumcised, we will make another circumcising incision through the old scar (Figure 11-3) and reflect skin by releasing the dartos fascia from its deep attachments to Buck's fascia. The superficial dorsal vein will be incised and ligated. Often there may be a connection between this vein and the deep dorsal vein. If the patient has not been circumcised, we will recommend that the prepuce be removed. However, if he does not wish that this be done, we will make a circumcising incision and release the skin and Dartos fascia by dissecting in the same plane as above and, having made an incision in the scrotum lateral to the base of the penis, we deliver the shaft of the penis through this incision and lay the penile skin to the side covered with a warm sponge (Figure 11-4). This protects the skin from trauma resulting in much less edema after the surgery. We also use this incision for more proximal lesions in men who have been circumcised and when, because of leakage noted on DICC, we plan to excise the proximal part of the deep dorsal vein. At the end of the operation we replace the penile shaft within the sleeve of the skin and close the incision.

At present we are concerned that because vascular anastomoses become established on both sides of a dermal graft, venous short circuits not controlled by the normal occlusive

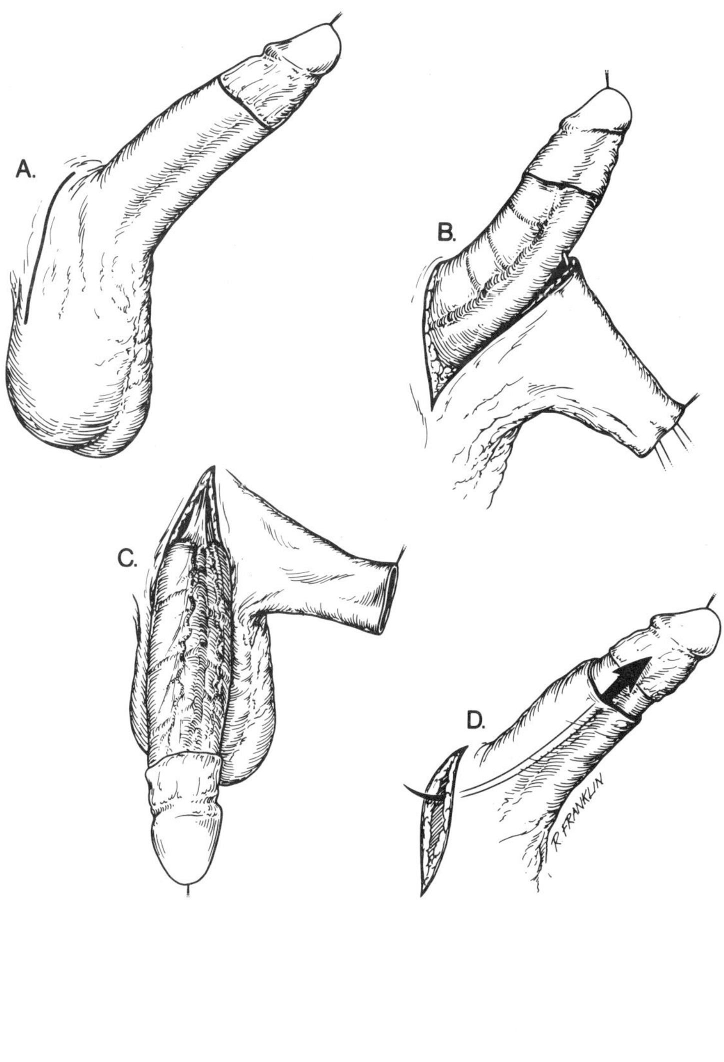

Figure 11-4 (A) When exposure of the full length of the shaft of the penis is necessary, two incisions are marked: one in the scar of the previous circumcision and the other lateral to the base of the penis and carried down into the scrotum. (B) The two incisions are completed, and the shaft of the penis is freed by dissecting close to Buck's fascia leaving most of the dartos fascia with the skin. The shaft of the penis is delivered into the scrotal incision. (C) Retraction of the penis exposes the full length of the shaft and with minimal dissection the suspensory ligaments can be visualized. With further dissection, complete resection of the dorsal vein can be accomplished. (D) At the conclusion of the surgical procedure, the shaft of the penis is replaced within the relatively untraumatized sleeve of skin. (From Devine et al.,[29] with permission.)

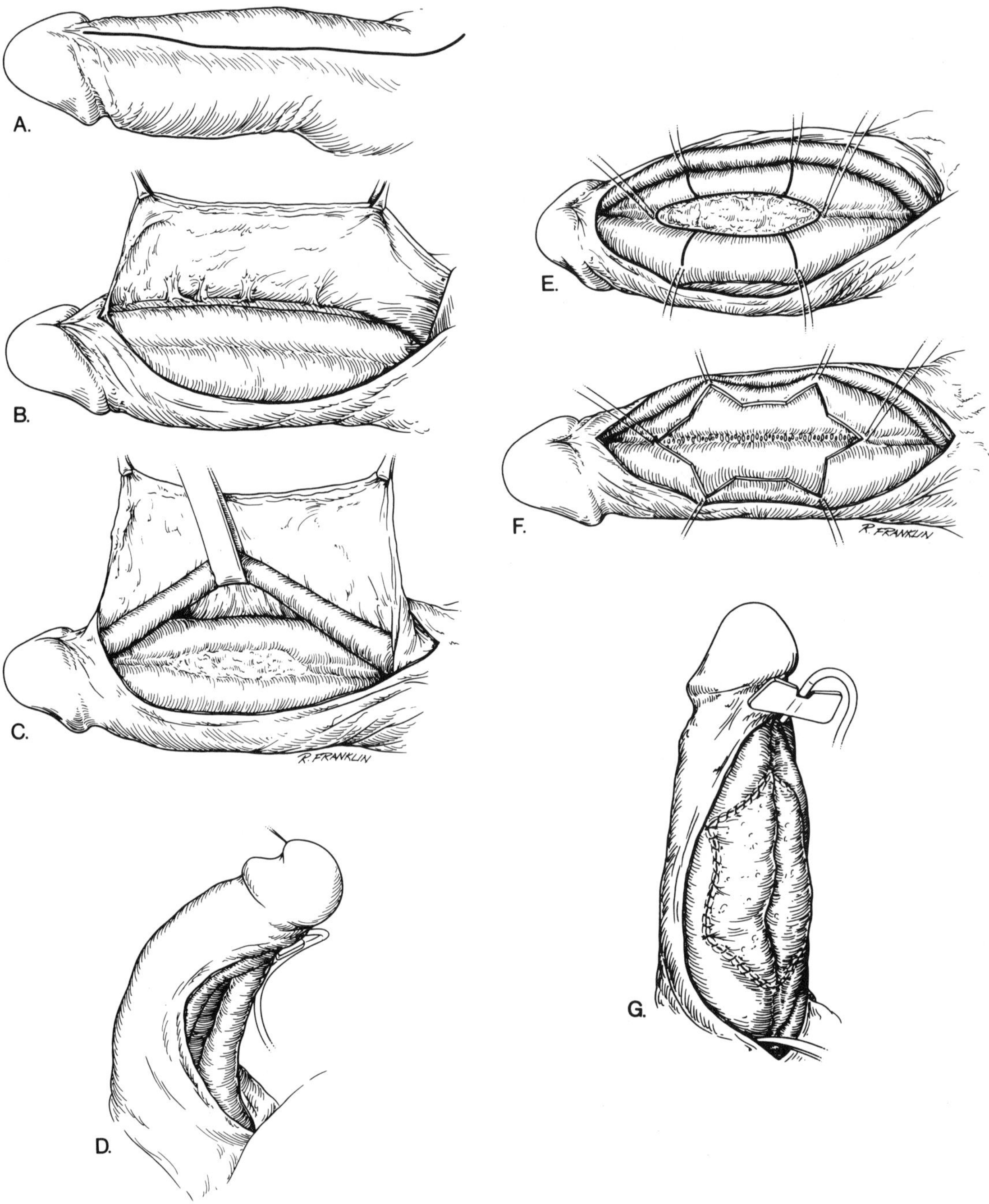
A.
B.
C.
R. FRANKLIN
D.
E.
F.
R. FRANKLIN
G.

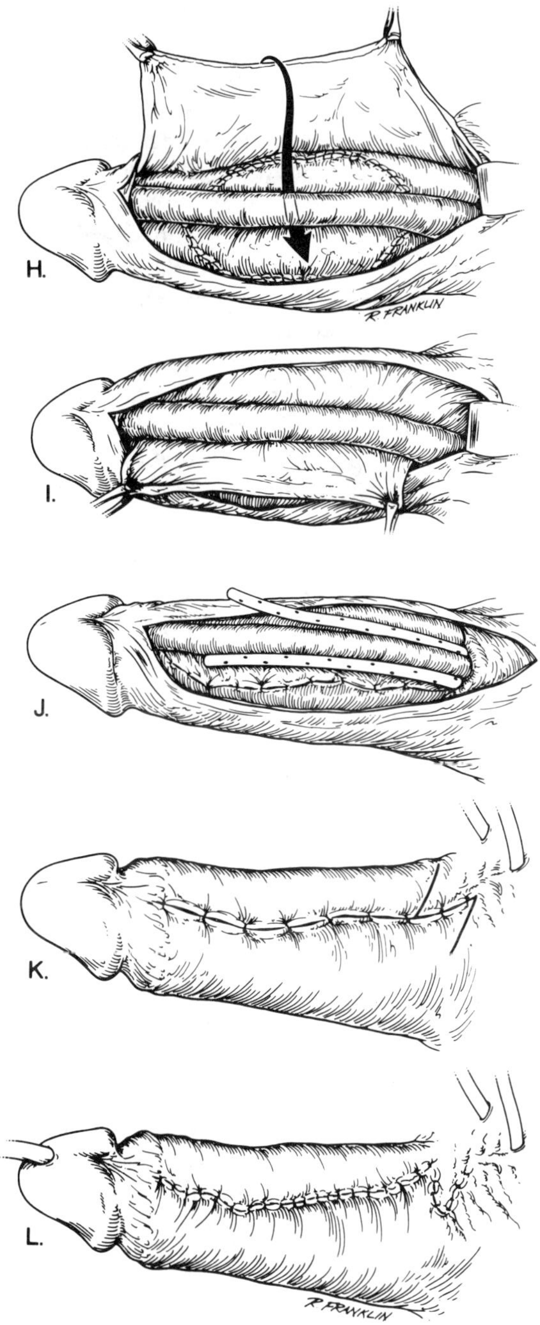

Figure 11-5 Exposure of a ventral plaque of Peyronie's disease. (A) A midline incision marked on the ventral aspect of the penis is continued into the scrotum for a more proximal plaque. This can also be extended distally by combining it with an incision in the old circumcision scar. (B) The skin is elevated with the full thickness of the dartos fascia elevated to expose the corpus spongiosum. (C) The corpus spongiosum is mobilized by incision of Buck's fascia on each side. The connections of the circumflex veins with the veins running lateral to the corpus spongiosum are ligated during this dissection. The inelastic plaque of Peyronie's disease is seen on the ventrum of the corporal bodies. (D) An artificial erection demonstrates the extent of the curvature. (E) The incision to excise the plaque and the releasing incisions have been marked. Stay sutures of Prolene are placed at the ends of the plaque and of the releasing incisions. (F) Resection of the plaque is complete. The defect is ready for the dermal graft. Note the ends of the strands of the septum in the midline of this space. (G) A dermal graft has been obtained and placed in the defect. An artificial erection shows the penis to be straight. Note that the expansion of the graft is restrained by its attachment to the strands of the septum in the midline. (H) A dartos fascial flap has been mobilized from one edge of the penile skin. It will be passed between the graft and the overlying corpus spongiosum. The edges of the layer of Buck's fascia are tacked to the tunica albuginea but are not closed over the graft. (I) The flap has been brought across the graft and will be secured to the dartos fascia on the other side. (J) Closure of the dartos fascia is complete. Two TLS suction drains are in place. (K) The skin is approximated and a Z-plasty has been marked where the incision crosses the penoscrotal junction. (L) Closure is complete. A Bioclusive dressing will be applied, and the 14 French catheter will be removed on the following morning. The patient remains in the hospital for about 3 days. (From Devine et al.,[29] with permission.)

mechanism can occur. Therefore, with dorsal plaques we remove the penile portion of the deep dorsal vein and approach the lesion by dissecting laterally beneath Buck's fascia through the bed of the vein. To obviate all of the possibilities for "short circuits" it has also been necessary to ligate the circumflex veins at their junction with the corpus spongiosum and the deep vein that is often found lateral to that structure. We approach ventral plaques by making a midline incision in the skin and mobilizing the corpus spongiosum (Figure 11-5). We do not excise the deep dorsal vein but do ligate the circumflex veins and, to prevent uncontrolled connections between the graft and the corpus spongiosum, we impose a flap of the dartos fascia between the graft and the corpus spongiosum before closing the skin over the urethra.

The inflammation in the tissue plane between Buck's fascia and the plaque makes it necessary to use sharp dissection to free up the fascia. Retracting the tunica with hooks and lifting Buck's fascia with Beazley forceps (W. Lorenz, Jacksonville, Florida) we define a sharp angle between the tissue layers allowing us to cut with blunted tipped scissors to open this space while minimizing damage to the nerves and vessels attached to the fascia. When the underlying tunica is normal, Buck's fascia is easily lifted off by spreading the tips of the scissors between the tissue layers. Mobilization must be continued proximally far enough to be sure that the dorsal nerves are not stretched as the fascia is retracted during excision of the plaque. To mobilize the corpus spongiosum for exposure of a ventral plaque we make an incision in Buck's fascia lateral to that erectile body, ligating the connections with the circumflex veins with black silk sutures. Dissecting beneath the corpus spongiosum we keep the blunted tips of the dissecting scissors against the tunica to lessen the chance of opening into the urethra. The corpus spongiosum is freed up well proximal and distal to the plaque.

With either a dorsal or a ventral plaque when the tunica has been exposed the extent of the lesion will be evident from the inelasticity of the tissue and the roughness of its surface. An artificial erection defined the curvature (Figure 11-3G). The plaque is outlined with brilliant green marking solution. Stay sutures of prolene are placed at the proximal and distal extent of the lesion and at the ends of the planned lateral releasing incisions. Following the marks, an incision is made around the plaque through the full thickness of the tunica. The tip of the plaque is elevated and, using a knife or sharp pointed scissors, it is resected (Figure 11-3H). Though the ends of the septal strands will be cut across, the disease process does not extend into the spongy erectile tissue, which must not be injured during this dissection. Matching lateral incisions into the surrounding tunica will release the tightness of the rim of the defect and expand its area by 1.5 to 2 times the area of the excised plaque (Figure 11-3I). We measure this defect stretching it laterally and longitudinally and apply a dermal graft about 30% larger than those measurements.

During this dissection it is not necessary to apply a tourniquet to control bleeding. Actually a tourniquet would get in the way. When the penis is flaccid, the helicine arteries are contracted and the erectile space contains blood at central pressure so only minimal compression is required to control bleeding. However, the level of anesthesia must remain as deep as that required for an open abdominal operation or manipulation of the penis will stimulate the erectile mechanism resulting in dilatation of the arteries with increased bleeding. Should this occur, surgery should be stopped and pressure applied to the penis while anesthesia is deepened to the proper level.

The dermal graft is outlined on the skin of the abdomen just above the iliac crest and lateral to the hairline (Figure 11-6). Though the epidermis can be removed with a dermatome, usually we make an incision around the donor site and roll back the epidermis as it is undermined free-handed with a #10 knife blade. The epidermis is discarded. An incision is made around the dermal patch leaving a few millimeters of dermis as a cuff to aide in closure of the wound. One end of the dermis is elevated and as the graft is removed the fat is excised from its underside exposing its subdermal plexus. The donor area is closed primarily, placing 5-0 Vicryl sutures in the dermal cuff tying the knots inside and a pull-out subcuticular suture of #3.0 prolene for the skin. When this suture is removed in 3 weeks, this closure leaves a linear scar that widens slightly. The epidermis must not be used as a graft to close the defect as it will leave an ugly scar; for this reason the graft should not be taken from the skin of the thigh

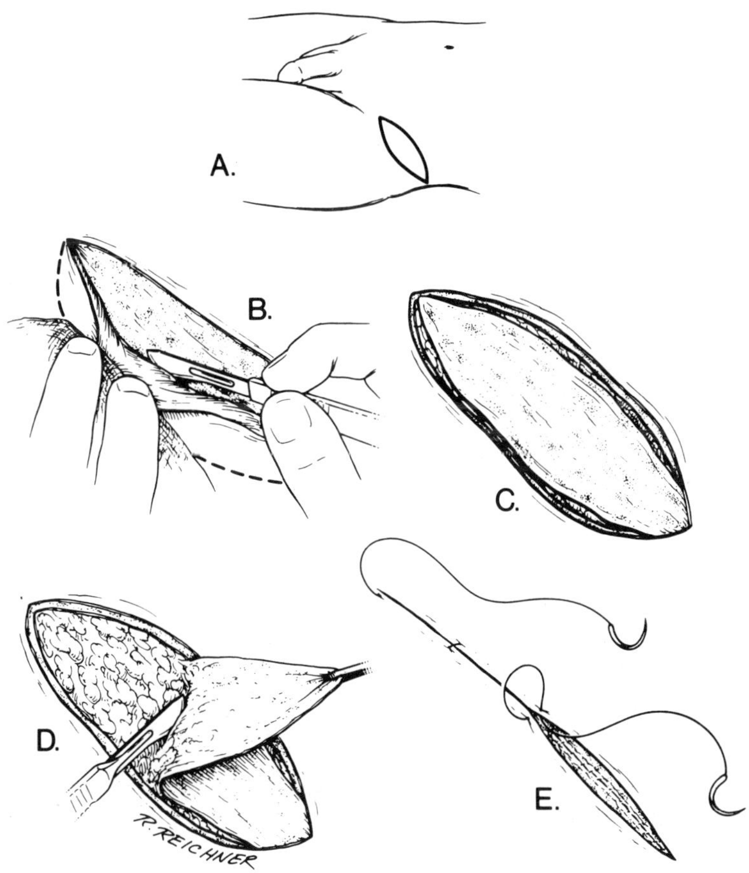

Figure 11-6 Harvesting a dermal graft. We excise a portion of dermis from the skin over the crest of the ilium lateral to the hairline. (A) The area is marked on the skin. (B) The epidermis is removed freehand with a knife. A dermatome could also be used. (C) An incision is made around the dermal graft leaving a narrow cuff of dermis to aid in closure of the skin. (D) One end of the graft is elevated while the fat is trimmed off the underside. (E) The skin is closed with dermal sutures of Vicryl and a running subcuticular double ended suture of Prolene or nylon. Closure is begun in the middle of the incision placing each needle from the outside in, leaving a loop of suture outside the wound to aid in its removal. Sewing is continued to the two ends, bringing another loop to the surface half way there. The two ends are tied together loosely and a Bioclusive dressing is applied. (From Devine et al.,[30] with permission.)

as the only way to close the defect in that area would be to reapply the epidermis as a split-thickness graft.

The graft is placed in the corporotomy defect approximating the edges of the graft to the edges of the tunica with a water-tight running suture of #5.0 PDS and fixing the midline of the graft to the midline septal strands with the same suture material (Figure 11-7). Tacking sutures of #4.0 PDS are placed at the proximal and distal midline of the defect and at the tips of the releasing incisions on one side of the opening. Then, using a cutting needle, a #5.0 running suture of PDS is applied securing the graft to the tunica with an edge-to-edge closure. When one side has been completed, the graft is folded, and after marking its midline, it is secured to the strands of the septum with another running suture of the same material. The graft is then unfolded and sewn to the other side in the same manner as the first. When this has been accomplished, another arti-

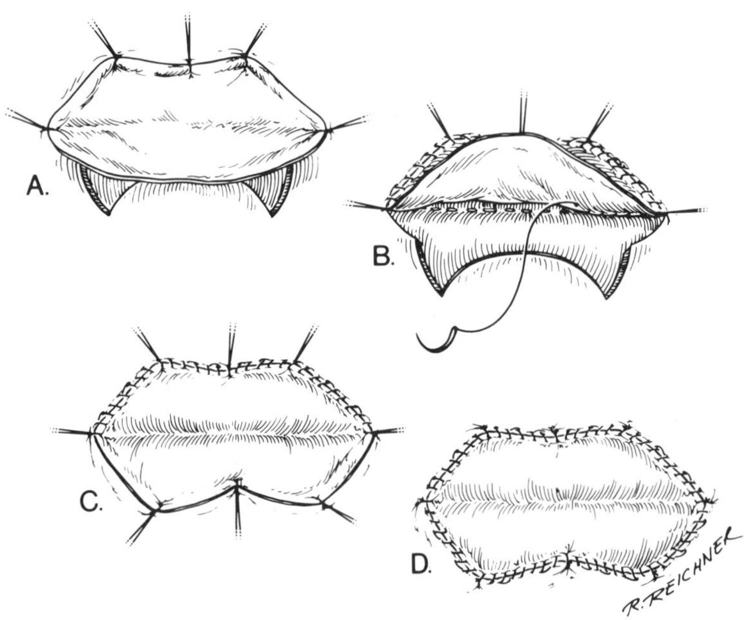

Figure 11-7 The dermal graft is placed into the defect fat side down. (A) Stay sutures of 4-0 polydioxanone are placed, securing the midline of the graft proximally and distally at the ends of the defect and at the tips of each of the releasing incisions, on just one edge of the repair. That edge of the graft will be sewn to the tunica with a running 5-0 polydioxanone suture, locking every second or third throw. (B) The graft is folded, and the midline is marked with a brilliant green solution. This midline of the graft is secured to the tips of the strands of the septum with a running 5-0 polydioxanone suture. This anastomosis will help to ensure continued function of the septum in erections subsequent to the surgery. (C) Stay sutures are applied on the opposite side. (D) The remaining edge of the graft is secured to the tunica with a running 5-0 polydioxanone suture to make a watertight anastomosis. (From Devine,[31] with permission.)

ficial erection is carried out to be sure the penis is straight and that the suture lines are watertight. Leaks are oversewn with #5.0 PDS. If the penis is not straight, the incisions in the tunica will have to be extended and further grafts applied. If the penis is straight, we close the tissue layers of the penis.

On the dorsal side (Figure 11-3K), Buck's fascia is approximated in the midline with interrupted sutures of #5.0 PDS avoiding the dorsal arteries and nerves. Small suction drains are placed superficial to Buck's fascia. The dartos fascia is closed over them also with #5.0 PDS and the skin with interrupted sutures of #5.0 chromic (Figure 11-3L). On the ventral side (Figure 11-5H,I) a flap of the dartos fascia is developed and placed between the graft and the corpus spongiosum securing it with interrupted #5.0 Vicryl sutures to the dartos fascia on the other side. Drains are placed and the skin is closed over the urethra.

We dress the penis with Bioclusive (Johnson & Johnson Products Inc., New Brunswick, NJ 98903), applying it loosely extending from the base of the penis to mid-glans. We leave a #14 Foley catheter until the patient ambulates on the first postoperative day. The suction drains are removed at 24 to 48 hours whenever they are no longer productive. Erections are suppressed with Valium and Amyl Nitrate. Patient's are discharged by the third to the fifth day.

Dermal grafts take and mature as do other grafts. At first they are hydrated and nourished by imbibition of tissue fluids from the graft bed while inosculation is taking place. Stimulated by growth factors elaborated within the graft, buds from the blood vessels in the graft bed penetrate and anastomose with the arteries and veins in the graft. By the fifth day this process has been completed and blood flow has been reestablished. The graft continues to undergo remodeling for up to a year. All grafts contract at first as they mature. In the first 3 months this may be 30% and some curvature will recur, but as remodeling progresses the graft will become more elastic and the shape will improve. For the first 2 weeks we discourage erections; for the month after that we encourage erections but without intercourse. During that time the erect penis should be manipulated to keep the skin from adhering to the deep layers of the penile shaft and to stretch the graft. To intimately involve the patient's wife or sexual partner in the patient rehabilitation we ask her to carry out this therapy. Also, this sexual activity can lead directly to intercourse when the suture line can withstand the stress. The patient continues to take vitamin E 400 mg twice a day with vitamin B_1 150 mg a day and vitamin C 500 mg twice a day.

In reviews carried out prior to our beginning to evaluate potential surgical patients with studies of erectile function, at least 75% of the patients treated with these grafts have been happy.[27] This compares well with the results of other penile surgeries.[16,28] As we continue to evaluate the results in patients who have had erectile function studies we will be able to refine our statistics still further. Patients must have reasonable expectations concerning the outcome of any surgery on the penis. In addition to our counseling, all patients with their partner are interviewed by our sex therapist colleague. He helps ensure that both individuals have proper expectations so that they may deal with the surgery and recovery of function and, in this process, he may discover problems that must be dealt with prior to the operation.[29] Most men with Peyronie's disease will be able to continue sexual function despite the curvature. About a third will need surgery and the odds are good that they will be able to function after surgery without a prosthesis.

REFERENCES

1. DeSanctis PN, Furey GA: Steroid injection therapy for Peyronie's disease: A 10-year summary and review of 38 cases. J Urol 1967; 97:224.
2. McRoberts JW: Peyronie's disease. Surg Gynecol Obstet 1969; 12:1291.
3. Godec CJ, Van Beck AL: Peyronie's disease is curable—is it also preventable? Urology 1983; 21:257.
4. Hinman F Jr: Peyronie's disease: Ethological considerations. Prog Reprod Biol Med 1983; 9:5–12.
5. Smith BH: Peyronie's disease. Am J Clin Pathol 1966; 45:670.
6. Smith BH: Subclinical Peyronie's disease. Am J Clin Pathol 1969; 52:385.
7. Devine CJ Jr, Jordan GH, Somers KD: Peyronie's disease: Cause and surgical treatment. AUA Today 1989; 2(5):1–3.
8. Snow R, Devine CJ Jr: The conservative management of Peyronie's disease. Unpublished data, 1981.
9. Goldstein I, Siroky MB, Nath RL et al.: Vasculogenic impotence: role of the pelvic steal test. J Urol 1982; 128:300–306.
10. Lue TF, Hrieak H, Marich KW, Tanagho EA: Vasculogenic impotence evaluated by high-resolution ultrasonography and pulsed Doppler spectrum analysis. Radiology 1985; 155:777.
11. El-Mahdi AM: Personal communication, 1990.
12. Devine CJ Jr, Horton CE: The surgical treatment of Peyronie's disease with a dermal graft. J Urol 1974; 111:44.
13. Horton CE, Devine CJ Jr: Peyronie's disease. Plast Reconstr Surg 1973; 52:503.
14. Pryor JP, Fitzpatrick JM: A new approach to the correction of the penile deformity in Peyronie's disease. J Urol 1979; 122:622.
15. Nesbit RM: Congenital curvature of the phallus: A report of 3 cases with description of corrective operation. J Urol 1965; 93:230.
16. Frank JD, Mor SB, Pryor JP: The surgical correction of erectile deformities of the penis of 100 men. Br J Urol 1981; 53:645.
17. Lue TF: Penile venous surgery. Urol Clin North Am 1989; 16:607–611.
18. Devine CJ Jr: Editorial Comments: on Gelbard, Martin K, and Hayden Barbara: Expanding contractures of the tunica albuginea due to Peyronie's disease with temporalis fascia free grafts. J Urol 1991; 145:772–776.
19. Das S, Amar AD: Peyronie's disease: Excision of the plaque and grafting with tunica vaginalis. Urol Clin North Am 1982; 9:1.
20. Devine, CJ, Jordan GH, Schlossberg SM: *Reoperative Urology*, Cohen, Mark S, eds. Boston: Little, Brown and Co., (in press).
21. Poutasse EF: Peyronie's disease. Transactions of the American Association of Genito-Urinary Surgeons 1971; 63:97–100.
22. Gelbard MK: Personal communication. At the Peyronie's Disease Conference, Norfolk, 1989.
23. Lockhart JG: Personal communications, 1992.
24. Stefanovic K, Clark AS, Buncke H Jr: Microsurgical temporo-parietal fascia transfer for Peyronie's disease: An experimental study. Presented at the 22nd Congress, SIU, Sevilla, Spain, 1991.
25. Jordan GH, Kodama RT, Rowe DF, Devine CJ Jr: Interpretation of penile duplex ultrasound wave forms and measurements in pharmacologically induced erections. Abstract 33. J Urol 1990; 143:197A.
26. Padma-Nathan H: Evaluation of the corporal veno-occlusive mechanism: Dynamic infusion cavernosometry and cavernosography. Sem Intervent Radiol 1989; 6:205–211.
27. Wild RM, Devine CJ Jr, Horton CE: Dermal graft repair of Peyronie's disease. Survey of 50 patients. J Urol 1979; 121:47–50.
28. Kaufman JJ, Boxer B, Quinn MC: Physical and psychological results of penile prostheses: A statistical survey. J Urol 1981; 126:173.
29. Jones WJ Jr, Horton CE, Stecker JF Jr et al: The treatment of psychogenic impotence after dermal graft repair for Peyronie's disease. J Urol 1984; 131:286.
30. Devine CJ Jr, Jordan GH, Schlossberg SM: Surgery of the penis and urethra. In: Walsh PC, Retick AB, Stamey TA, Vaughan ED Jr, eds.

Campbell's Urology, 6th ed. Philadelphia: WB Saunders, 1992: 2957–3032.

31. Devine CJ Jr: Peyronie's disease. In: Glenn JF, ed. Urologic surgery, 4th ed. Philadelphia: J. B. Lippincott, 1991: 873.

ANNOTATED BIBLIOGRAPHY

Lindsay MC, Schain DM, Grambsch P, Benson RC, Berard CM, Kurland LT: The incidence of Peyronie's disease in Rochester, Minnesota, 1950 to 1984. J Urol 1991; 146:1007–1009.

There were 101 cases of Peyronie's disease in male residents of Rochester, Minnesota, between 1950 and 1984. This is an age adjusted 25.7/100,000 men. The mean age of these patients was 53 with a range of 19 to 83. The highest incidence was in the 50–59 decade, 66/100,000. Including a decade older and one younger modifies this 2/3 of a patient per 100 men to a little less than 1/2 a patient per 100 men. We found about one patient per 100 men in two groups of physicians who were about of this age. In Rochester they found an increased incidence of arthritis, diabetes, and hypertension in the patients with Peyronie's disease but no increase in the use of β-blockers. The incidence of Peyronie's may have increased with the passage of time during this 35 years. They could make no statement as to etiology. Also, although at least half of the patients had had radiation therapy, there was no indication that this had been of any benefit.

Gelbard MK, Dorey F, James K: The natural history of Peyronie's disease. J Urol 1990; 144:1376–1379.

The authors questioned 97 men with Peyronie's disease about their symptoms: penile pain, bending, and the effects of these symptoms on their sexual function. Also, they were asked about their concept of the evolution of the situation. Most of the findings agree with what we know of the disease. Few, if any, of their patients returned to their premorbid condition and few, if any, progressed to complete sexual inability. The physical changes in the penis often did not correlate with the sexual difficulty of the patient. Because the psychological affect can be disabling, the authors felt that a survey based on physical evaluation of the lesions carries less objectivity than the response of the patient to questions about his status.

In some patients the progress of the signs and symptoms of Peyronie's disease is slow, but in others the deformity seems to appear overnight. I think that we have explained these two mechanisms of onset in this chapter: an acute tear in some of the patients versus the chronic effects of tissue fatigue leading to a similar lesion—in each incidence a slowly healing scar in the tunica albuginea of the corpora cavernosa. Early features such as pain, tenderness, and easily palpable plaque may resolve, but, when significant deformity occurs, it usually persists.

Cohen ES, Schmidt JD, Parsons CL: Peyronie's disease: Surgical experience and presentation of a proximal approach. J Urol 1989; 142:740–742.

This anecdotal report does not prove that placement of a prosthesis will guarantee a higher success rate than operations designed to preserve potency. In two patients they incised the plaque and put in some type of a graft. This is not a well-designed operation, and I would not expect that potency would have been preserved in these patients. Four of six patients (66%) returned to function after the plaque was excised and the defect was patched with a "vascular graft." One of these patients had a secondary procedure 7 years later, and despite the fact that his skin sloughed he maintained function for 2 more years before decreased erections and pain with inter course developed. The authors have inflated this minimal experience into a global indictment of all "operations designed to preserve potency." They have a selection of references to support the statement that "results with the penile prostheses have been uniformly good." One must read these studies before accepting this conclusion. The patients reported on by Raz and associates[1] are repeated and added to by Bruskewitz and Raz.[2] In a larger series of impotent patients in whom prostheses had been installed, Kaufman and associates (Kaufman was an author in reference 1) noted that only 49% were completely satisfied and 29% somewhat satisfied.[3] Subrini[4] described 69 patients, 40 of whom underwent simple implantation of a prosthesis and 29 of whom underwent transcavernosal removal of the plaque with insertion of a prosthesis. Eleven of these patients had complications requiring reoperation within 1 year. Eighty-one percent of the patients were reported to be satisfied with their sexual function. However, in a 10-year study of 137 impotent patients who received implants, Subrini reported that 73.8% believed the operation to be beneficial postoperatively, but only 55% of their partners did so.[5] The experience of the authors with prostheses includes 24 patients, 25% of whom were lost to follow-up. The statistics are based on the remaining 18 patients, six of whom were potent before the prosthesis was implanted.

Despite the inapplicability of the conclusions, we can learn from this study. Impotent patients with Peyronie's disease will need a prosthesis, and they should be evaluated before the decision is made. If the patient is potent, a properly designed procedure should be done in an attempt to straighten the penis while preserving potency. Prosthetic vascular grafts, for example polytetrafluoroethylene or monofilament knitted polypropylene, are not satisfactory as patches when the scar in the tunica has been excised, though they will work as patches when a prosthesis has been inserted. When a prosthesis is needed, the technique described in this study would be useful.

1. Raz S, deKernion JB, Kaufman JJ: Surgical treatment of Peyronie's disease: A new approach. J Urol 1977; 117:598.
2. Bruskewitz R, Raz S: Surgical considerations in treatment of Peyronie's disease. Urology 1980; 15:134.
3. Kaufman JJ, Boxer RJ, Boxer B, Quinn MC: Physical and psychological results of penile prosthesis: A statistical survey. J Urol 1981; 126:173.
4. Subrini L: Surgical treatment of Peyronie's disease using penile implants: Survey of 69 patients. J Urol 1984; 132:47.
5. Subrini L: Subrini penile implants: Surgical, sexual and psychological results. Eur Urol 1982; 8:222.

Eigner EB, Kabalin JN, Kessler R: Penile implants in the treatment of Peyronie's disease. J Urol 1991; 145:69–72.

The authors report a series of 35 patients who were treated for Peyronie's disease by insertion of a variety of prostheses.

In the abstract they state that a prosthesis is indicated in selected patients, but in the paper they do not tell us how they selected these patients. We know from the reply to our editorial comment that not every patient with Peyronie's disease received a prosthesis, but we do not know how they evaluated complaints of impotence. If I read the numbers correctly, 20% of these patients were still able to engage in intercourse while 55% were obtaining sufficiently firm erections but could not enjoy intercourse because of pain or the configuration of the penis. Only 25% of these men were impotent.

Complications of the operation were not substantially different from their entire series of inflatable prostheses.[1] Improvements in the mechanics of the prostheses hopefully should decrease the incidence of these problems in the future. The complications that the authors enumerate did not seem to have figured in the calculations of the "happiness ratio." I will not comment again on the studies they have cited that report bad results for dermal grafts or similar procedures. The latest of these was published in 1982,[2] and one must really read that paper before accepting the opinion of it that is expressed in this paper. The authors have reported our good results but not the latest ones.[3]

I have been criticized as being rigid (no pun intended) by people who believe that I do not approve of any surgery for Peyronie's disease except excision of the plaque and dermal grafting. This is not the case. In some impotent patients with Peyronie's disease, the use of a penile prosthesis is indicated; but in this day and age when injection therapy and vascular surgery are supplanting the simplistic concept of inserting a prosthesis into the penis of any man who complains of impotence, the selection process must be better designed that what I see in this study.

1. Kabalin JN, Kessler R: Penile prosthesis surgery. Monogr Urol 1989; 10:21.
2. Gangai MP, Rivera LR, Spence CR: Peyronie's plaque: excision and graft versus incision and stent. J Urol 1982; 127:55.
3. Horton CE, Sadove RC, Devine CJ Jr: Peyronie's disease. Ann Plast Surg 1987; 18:122.

Gelbard MK, Hayden B: Expanding contractures of the tunica albuginea due to Peyronie's disease with temporalis fascia free grafts. J Urol 1991; 145:772–776.

The authors discuss 12 patients with a deformity severe enough to inhibit satisfactory sexual relations, yet who were able to maintain a rigid erection. Dr. Gelbard, the urologist, exposed the plaque in a similar fashion to what we have described above while Dr. Hayden, the plastic surgeon, obtain a 4 × 5-cm patch of temporalis fascia. After generating an artificial erection with a saline injection, they marked the point of maximum distortion. Calcified areas in plaques were excised, but simply fibrotic tunica was incised full thickness to expose the erectile tissue beneath it, taking care not to injure this tissue. Extending the incisions lateral to the plaque created gaps that lengthened the affected aspect of the penis without plaque excision. These gaps were patched with segments of the fascia. According to their "limited experience, severe deformities can be corrected without resecting the tunica albuginea." Note that they are using living tissue, and we echo their concern regarding prosthetic materials as we have removed other surgeon's prosthetic grafts that have behaved exactly as the authors fear, "the capsule that forms around the material may contract and defeat the purpose of the procedure."[1] It is of interest that these authors can achieve a straight penis with this procedure. Tom Lue has also made lateral incisions through the lesion patching them by applying the opened out dorsal vein with its endothelial surface against the erectile tissue.[2] When Charlie Horton and I tried various substances for grafts in dogs, we tried vein grafts and fascia grafts in addition to the dermis grafts. The dermal grafts persisted and resulted in tissue that was very much like the normal tunica of the dog's penis, whereas both the vein and the fascia grafts scarred and contracted. Perhaps it is the thin nature of this fascia, and the application of the endothelial surface of the vein graft that has allowed these two groups to accomplish what they have.

1. Devine CJ Jr, Jordan GH, Schlossberg SM: Reoperation for Peyronie's disease. In: Cohen MS, ed. Reoperative urology. Boston, MA: Little, Brown, (in press).
2. Lue T: Personal communications.
3. Horton CE, Devine CJ Jr: Peyronie's disease. Plast Reconstr Surg 1973; 52:503–510.

12 Reconstruction after Genital Amputation Injuries

Gerald H. Jordan

Experience with amputation injuries of the genitalia is confined to individual case reports or reports of small series. State of the art management must then be gleaned from literature reviews with comparison of similarly applied therapeutic techniques.

In our culture, most cases of penile amputation result from attempts at self emasculation, in the psychotic individual, or as a sequela of felonious assault. In 1979, in the Archives of General Psychiatry, Greilhimer and Groves[5] reported a heterogeneous group of individuals with genital amputation or mutilation injuries. That series showed 87% to be psychotic at the time of the act with 51% in a decompensated schizophrenic state. The remainder consisted of individuals with severe character disorders or gender identity problems, but who were felt to be nonpsychotic. In the nonpsychotic, many were under the influence of drugs or alcohol at the time of their emasculation episodes. The psychotic individual usually had a long history of mental illness, but the act of self-mutilation occurred during an acute psychotic decompensation. There is a subset, however, of individuals who during their first acute psychotic break will attempt mutilation of their genitalia in some form. These individuals are operating under command hallucinations that order them to amputate or mutilate their genitalia. A series by Blacker and Wong[2] also described many of these individuals; and it is their feeling that the self-mutilation behavior is a form of focal suicide. In the past, and even in some centers currently, patients who had attempted genital mutilation were not considered to be candidates for replantation or reconstruction. In 1980, however, Stewart and Lowrey[13] suggested that self inflicted genital mutilation or amputation is not a contraindication to replantation. The literature attests to a high degree of successful mental rehabilitation in these patients. The dictum now would support replantation first, with psychiatric intervention to follow. In Greilschimer and Groves' review of more than 40 patients with penile amputation injuries, only one, postreplantation, attempted suicide,

Management of Impotence and Infertility, edited by Douglas Whitehead and Harris Nagler,

and only one repeated the attempt at emasculation.

In 1983, a large series of 100 genital amputation or mutilation incidents was reported from Thailand. This series has allowed us to glean a great deal of information with regards to the options for managing injuries. In the 1970s in Thailand, there was a virtual epidemic of penile amputation injuries. In a series of 100, 18 cases were managed by either microvascular or macroreplantation techniques with the remaining 92 cases treated as partial penectomies. In those 92 cases, the amputated distal portion of the penis did not accompany the patient to the treating center.

Penile Anatomy

The vasculature of the penis is totally dependent on branches of the internal pudendal artery and external pudendal arteries. For the most part, the deep structures are totally dependent on branches of the internal pudendal artery, which is the distal branches of the hypogastric artery. The internal pudendal artery courses to the perineum via Alcock's canal. In the perineum after giving off the scrotal branch, the artery becomes the common penile artery. This artery branches giving off the artery to the bulbospongiosum, the circumflex cavernosal arteries, which also go to the corpus spongiosum, the deep arteries of the corpora cavernosa, and the dorsal arteries of the penis. There are some arterial connections between the corpora cavernosa and the corpus spongiosum which exist in the "urethral groove." Quartey's work[11] has very nicely documented the superficial vascularity of the penis. He describes a dual blood supply with the skin able to survive on either the fasciocutaneous vascular supply based on the dartos fascia of the penis or the superficial cutaneous supply.

The venous drainage systems have been subcategorized into the superficial dorsal venous system, which exists superficial to the outer lamina of Buck's fascia and in the dartos layer; the deep dorsal venous system, which in many individuals is a single deep dorsal vein and in others occurs as dual dorsolateral veins; the crural vessels, which depart from the corpora cavernosa at the crus and drain into the periprostate plexus along the deep doral venous system; and the cavernosal system, which departs the corpora far proximal and can drain either laterally to the femoral system or medially to the periprostatic plexus. The deep dorsal or dorsolateral veins are contained between the inner and outer lamina of Bucks's fascia on the dorsum of the penis.

Testicular Anatomy

The testicular blood supply is dependent on 3 arteries: the internal spermatic artery, which arises from the aorta, the deferential artery, which arises from the inferior vesicle artery, and the cremasteric artery. The internal spermatic artery gives off a large branch to the globus major of the epididymis, which then arborizes to branch into the superior pole of the testis. The main spermatic vessel enters the mediastinum of the testis where it divides into terminal branches. The deferential artery, for the most part, follows the vas deferens to the globus minor where it then arborizes to anastomose freely with the internal spermatic system in the testis. The cremasteric artery arborizes to the surface of the tunica albuginea and also anastomoses via perforators with the superficial internal spermatic plexus. The venous drainage systems follow the arteries with the main drainage occurring through the internal and external spermatic veins. The scrotal skin appears to be totally dependent upon the terminal branches of the external pudendal system with some collateralization to the adjacent groin skin.

Principles of Tissue Transfer

The literature has established the fact that hypothermia prolongs ischemic survival times of all tissues. Hayhurst and associates[6] in a series looking at digital replantation with cooling of the amputated digit and hand have shown that hypothermia prolongs the ischemic times that are compatible with successful replantation and survival. The times were extended from 6 hours ischemia to 24 hours ischemia. In a rabbit flap model, it was shown that 12 hours of normothermic ischemia led, in all cases, to flap loss. However, a penile replantation 16 hours after injury, with much of that normothermic ischemic time, has been successful.

It is not surprising with microvascular replantation that the amputated portion of the penis reliably survives. It is surprising, however, to realize that without microvascular replantation and only macroreplantation, the deep structures — the corpora cavernosa and corpora spongiosum and the spongy erectile tissue of the glans penis — still survive quite reliably. It is further surprising, in both cases, to see that erectile function after replantation by microvascular or macrotechniques is often not detectably altered.

Historically macroreplantation techniques were fraught with urethral and skin complications. However, even in those older series, most patients ended up with the tips of their amputated penises intact. In the literature, authors often referred to this survival as likened to that of composite grafts. Now as the process of graft take is better understood, one realizes that the survival of the penis via macroreplantation techniques is clearly not a process of graft take.

Graft take occurs in two phases, with the first being termed imbibition and the second being termed inosculation. The two phases occur sequentially with the process of graft take requiring about 96 hours. During the phase of imbibition, there is no true blood flow into the graft. The graft is held essentially in suspended animation living by osmosis. The graft is pale and cool. During inosculation, which begins approximately 48 hours after the graft is placed, there is reestablishment of the microcirculation (angioneogenesis) in the graft. As the microcirculation is restored, the graft pinkens and its temperature approximates that of the adjacent tissues. All of the cases of "composite grafts" that dealt with penile amputation injuries describe the penis becoming pink and warm either immediately or within hours of finishing the surgical procedure. Thus there is a different process other than angioneogenesis by which the distal amputated portion survives after replantation.

New studies have looked at blood gases in the lacunar sinuses of the spongy erectile tissue of the corpora cavernosa. Impotence research suggests that the spongy erectile tissue is nothing more than controlled arteriovenous fistulas. In the flaccid state, however, the PO_2 is[16] more like venous blood than arterial blood. The survival of the deep structures and the spongy erectile tissue of the glans, however, seems to survive by flap principles. The cases of "composite graft survival" of the amputated penis describe loss of the skin of the glans and the skin of the shaft of the penis. Again, this is not surprising in that there is little communication between the deep arterial supply and the superficial arterial supply. Without microvascular reapproximation of the external pudendal system, there would be little reason to believe that the skin of the penis would become revascularized. However, the exact course of arterialization during the immediate postmacroreattachment period remains unclear. No one has ever looked at blood gases in the deep penile structures after macroattachment, and these may be approximate arterial blood. Trauma, with disruption of the deep cavernosal arteries, is clearly associated with "high flow" priapism; in these cases, the intracorporal blood is almost fully arterial.

Penile Replantation

The first successful reattachment of the penis was accomplished in 1929 and reported by Ehrich.[3] In that case, "all corpora" were reapproximated using chromic suture with urinary diversion accomplished with a urethral catheter. In this case, serendipitously, the skin of the penis had been avulsed in the accident. Hence, the penis after the deep structures were approximated was "buried" in the scrotal skin. In time the penile shaft was liberated and at 2 years, the man was reported as having a virtually normal appearing penis. He reported some shortening of his erect penis but was having erections that were adequate for intercourse. Since that report some 40 cases of penile macrovascular reattachment have been reported. Many variations in management were cited in an effort to avoid the frequently observed complication of penile shaft skin loss and glans skin slough. In 1968 McRoberts and colleagues[10] reported a literature review and personal experience of cases of penile reattachment via macrovascular techniques. A review of the cases led McRoberts to propose the following management principles: (1) the distal penile skin should be removed; (2) the anastomosed penile shaft should be buried in the scrotum with the glans protruding from the dependent portion of the scrotum; (3) the glanular epithelium should be sutured to the scrotal skin; and (4) the urine should be diverted via suprapubic catheter with either a urethral stent left or the urethral catheter removed at the end of the operation. Since that time a number of cases of corporal reapproximation and macroreattachment have been published. A number of these reports indicate that the microreplantation techniques are probably superior to the macrovascular technique, but nonetheless successful management in these cases via macrovascular techniques has been reported. The series from Thailand emphasizes the need for a technique of salvage of the amputated penis when microreplantation was not available. That series describes some minor modification of the principles proposed by McRoberts with gratifying results. Their patients had excellent cosmetic and functional results.

In 1976, Tamai and Cohen and associates[14,15] reported 2 separate cases of successful replantation of an amputated penis. These gentlemen were not co-workers and performed their successful replantations, unknown to each other, at different centers within a couple of months of each other. Both groups utilized microvascular and microneurosurgical techniques with excellent results. Since these landmark reports, a number of cases using microvascular and microneurosurgical techniques have been reported with uniformly good results. In these cases, despite microvascular replantation techniques, skin loss continues to occur in some cases. In these cases there is a clear incidence of urethral complications, either stricture or fistula; however, cosmetics and results dealing with sexual function are excellent.

Replantation of the Testis

In 1977 Evins and co-workers[4] described a patient with bilateral testicular amputation and near total penile amputation. In this case, the testicles were debrided and filleted and placed in superficial pouches. This is the first reported attempt at testicular salvage following amputation with follow-up studies in that case showing the effort to be unsuccessful. In 1976 Silber and Kelly[12] reported successful autotransplantation of a testicle (microorchiopexy). That case documents the ability, technically, to successfully replant the testicle via microvascular techniques.

In 1979 Abbou and associates[1] replanted a testicle and the penis in the same patient via microvascular/microneurosurgical techniques. A number of reports since that time continue to support the feasibility of microvascular replantation of the testicle.

Current Concepts of Microreplantation

The literature makes it clear that the amputated penis or testicle should be preserved via hypothermia. The bag within a bag technique in which the amputated part is placed on a saline-soaked gauze inside a clean or preferably sterile bag, which is sealed and then placed in a second bag, containing an ice slush, makes preservation by this modality relatively simple. The amputated part can then be transported with the patient. The remarkable resilience of the penis to ischemic injury would suggest that with cold ischemia times of greater than 24 hours, penile replantation is feasible with a successful outcome.

Microvascular/microneuroreplantation should proceed in a systematic fashion (Figure 12-1). Exploration of both blunt ends should identify the necessary structures for coaptation and reanastomosis. Debridement, if necessary, should be judiciously and conservatively accomplished (Figure 12-2). One can then proceed with a 2-layer spatulated urethral anastomosis. I prefer to anastomose the epithelium with 6-0 chromic sutures with the knots placed toward the lumen. The adventitia and spongy erectile tissue are then approximated with an absorbable monofilament suture of either 4-0 or 5-0. In very proximal shaft injuries, the deep (cavernosal) artery may be of sufficient size to be reanastomosed. If this is the case, one would need to dissect the artery within the spongy erectile tissue both for vascular control and to accomplish the microvascular anastomosis. That can be accomplished with 11-0 Prolene or nylon suture. The tunica albuginea of the corpora cavernosa is then reapproximated with monofilament absorbable suture, again 4-0 or 5-0 size.

One must then address the dorsal neurovascular structures. The 2 dorsal arteries are anastomosed with 11-0 nylon or prolene suture, and both should be reconstructed if possible. The dorsal vein or in some cases the dorsolateral veins are then reanastomosed using 9-0 or 10-0 nylon suture or prolene. Should there be a prominent superficial dorsal vein that too can be reanastomosed with 9-0 or 10-0 nylon suture. Microneural coaptation is then accomplished by reapproximating the epineurium. Only in very distal injuries where the dorsal

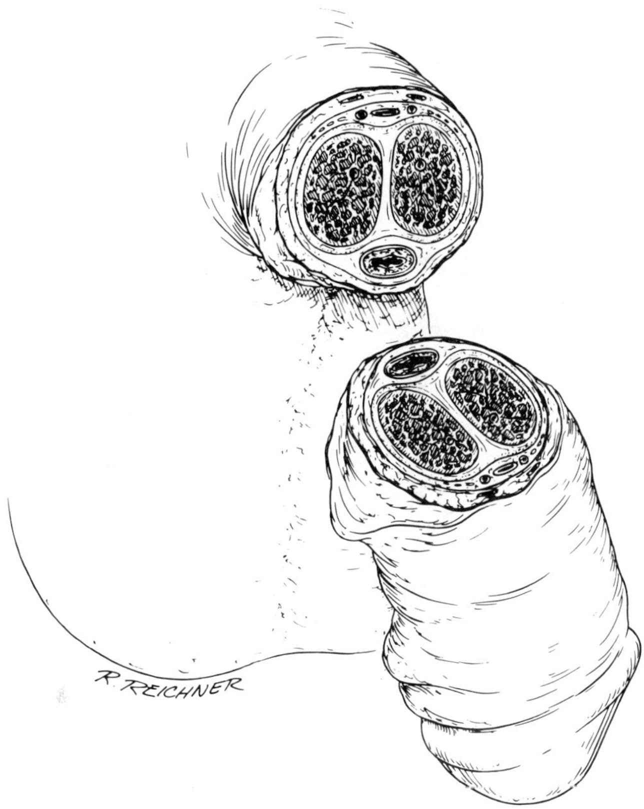

Figure 12-1 Typical amputation injury of the penis.

nerves have arborized significantly would one need to contemplate a fascicular coaptation (Figure 12-3). The dartos fascia can be reapproximated using PGA suture or monofilament absorbable suture. The skin can be approximated using chromic suture or a small sized PGA suture (Figure 12-4). A suprapubic cystostomy catheter should be placed. The urethral anastomosis can be stented with soft silicone tubing or a small soft ribbed silicone catheter. If one chooses to use a catheter, the catheter should be plugged and not placed to the drainage. Diversion should be accomplished via the suprapubic catheter.

The patient requires the same care that any other patient undergoing microvascular surgery. He must be kept well hydrated, and his body temperature must be kept normal. Heat lamps and warming of the room can be used to keep the patient peripherally vasodilated. If one employs heat lamps, care must be taken to avoid having the lamps pointed directly at the replanted part. pH monitoring and Doppler ultrasound monitoring of the replant can then be accomplished. Additionally, the replanted penile tip can be checked for blanching and capillary refill of the tissues distal to the repair. In general, the patient should be kept diverted for a period of about 21 days; however, this period can be adjusted depending on the progress of wound healing and the occurrence or lack of occurrence of penile skin loss. Voiding

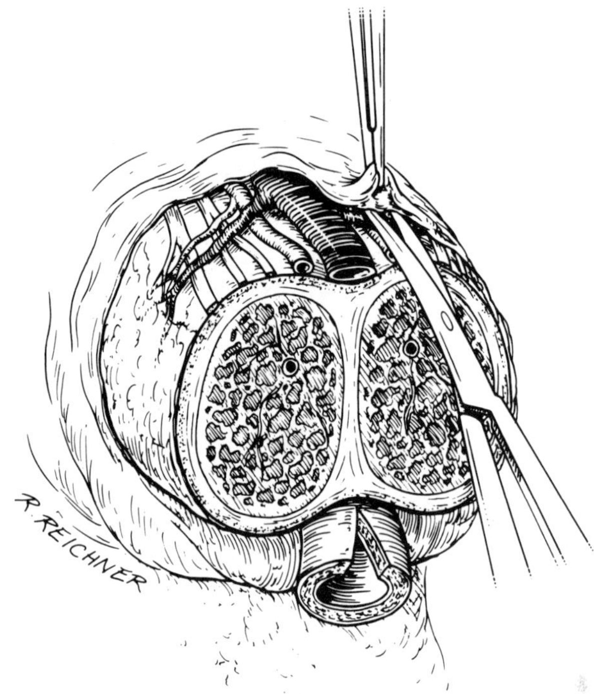

Figure 12-2 Minimal debridement must be accomplished to expose the deep dorsal neurovascular bundle. Additionally, some debridement and detachment of the corpus spongiosum must be accomplished to create a widely spatulated urethral anastomosis. Should the injury be at the base of the penis such that the cavernosal artery is of significant caliber for anastomosis, then some dissection in the spongy erectile tissue must be accomplished to allow for vascular control of that structure.

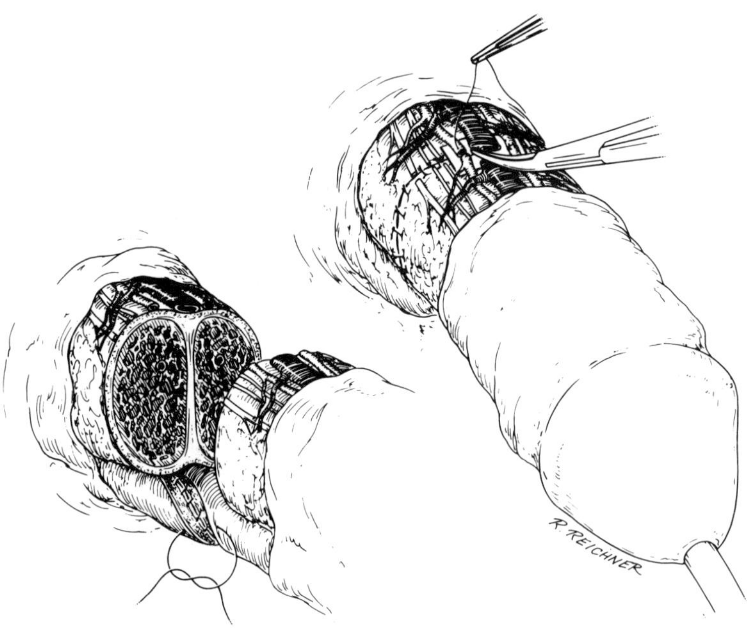

Figure 12-3 Left shows the completion of the spatulated urethral anastomosis with 6-0 chromic sutures placed to coapt the epithelium. The adventitia and spongy erectile tissue are then approximated using absorbable monofilament suture. The microvascular anastomoses are then completed, with an anastomosis of both dorsal arteries, the deep dorsal vein or dorsolateral veins, and in some cases the superficial dorsal vein. For injuries at the base of the penis, the arborization of the dorsal nerves has not occurred and an epineural coaptation is sufficient. Distally, where the arborization has occurred, a fascicular coaptation may be required.

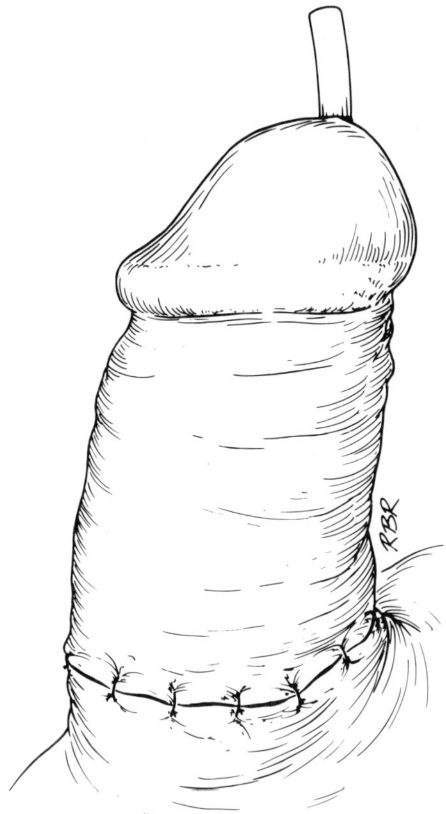

Figure 12-4 Appearance of the penis with the skin reapproximated. Note that this patient is circumcised, yet the skin between the area of amputation and the circumcision scar has not been excised. Diversion is via a suprapubic tube with a soft silicone stent.

study with contrast should be accomplished at 21 days or as adjusted, and contrast material suitable for intravascular injection should be used. The bladder is filled, and a voiding urethrogram obtained with the patient in lateral oblique position. With adequate healing of the urethral reconstruction documented, the suprapubic catheter is plugged to be pulled shortly thereafter. Urine cultures should be obtained for a baseline so that the bladder can be sterilized with culture specific antibiotics upon removing the diverting catheter. During the perioperative period, the patient should be treated with broad spectrum antibiotics in accordance with the biogram of the institution. The use of anticoagulants is controversial. Most would agree that formal heparinization is not required. Low-molecular-weight dextran is used in some centers. A daily baby aspirin is probably reasonable.

Clearly if the patient's condition allows and facilities are available, the patient should be transferred for microvascular/microneurosurgery. The literature supports a smoother course to recovery, if nothing more. If transfer to a facility is impossible or the patient's overall condition does not allow for the lengthy surgery required for microvascular/microneuroreplantation, corporal reapproximation and macrovascular penile reattachment should be done. It is clear that some of the venous structures can be reapproximated under loop magnification. The recommendations of McRoberts should be adhered to. The series from Thailand documents the success of reattachment procedures by adherence to those recommendations.

The sharply amputated testicle is likewise reliably salvageable. The cold ischemia times are probably less for successful testicular replantation. The proximal internal spermatic artery must be identified. Judicious debridement of the cord is then accomplished with reanastomosis of the spermatic arteries with 11-0 nylon or prolene suture. The distal venous stumps are identified by back bleeding. Once identified, the vigorously bleeding veins should all be reanastomosed to venous connections proximally. Depending on vessel size, the anastomosis can be accomplished with 9-0, 10-0, or 11-0 suture. One might contemplate microsuturing techniques for a couple of the venous attachments with the others coapted with one of the available microanastomotic "stapling" devices. A nonstented vasovasotomy should then be accomplished. The avulsed testicle is virtually never suitable for consideration of microvascular replantation in that the spermatic cord is stretched before finally distracting under force. The length of the endothelial injury is unpredictable and predisposes to arterial thrombotic phenomenon.

The skin of the penis, by and large, survives on the superficial blood supply; however, in some patients there must be connections to the deep vasculature. In reconstruction of the amputated penis, the penile skin should be reapproximated, not debrided. Should skin loss of the penile shaft occur in the postoperative period, debridement can be accomplished with the shaft either buried or grafted. The scrotal skin is not vascularized by the underlying deep structures. If scrotal skin is lost, ostensibly one might be able to identify a branch of the internal pudendal artery that would lend itself to microvascular reapproximation. That failing, however, the testicles can be placed in superficial thigh pouches. The testicles can then be liberated at a second procedure and either covered with a skin graft or transposed beneath inguinal flaps as described by McDougal[9] (Figure 12-5).

The patient who presents without his amputated distal part is clearly at a disadvantage. Hemorrhage should be controlled and wound management then accomplished. Often times, because of the marked elasticity of the penile skin, amputations remove more skin than actual shaft structures. In these cases, the shaft can be covered with split thickness skin as opposed to being buried. The distal urethral stump is managed as with partial penectomy with a widely spatulated neomeatus created. Many patients will have a functional organ with no further reconstruction necessary. In the patient who is left with inadequate length, delayed reconstruction can be accomplished via microvascular free transfer techniques. These techniques are covered later in this book in the chapter dealing with reconstructive surgery for the microphallus.

The patient who has suffered a penile amputation injury is not unlike the patient with a microphallus. The presence of normal corporal stumps makes subsequent prosthetic placement following phallic construction easier. Unlike the transsexual patient, who lacks corpora cavernosa, proximal corpora allows for anchoring of the devices. Distally the prosthesis is placed within vascular graft such as gortex.

A number of procedures have been described in an effort to avoid prosthetic implantation. At this center attempts at incorporation of periosteum with microvascular free transfer have not been successful nor has reliable bone growth been achieved. A number of authors describe osseocutaneous microvascular free transfer flaps. These flaps endeavor to transfer vascularized bone with the flap. Again, reliable results have not been achieved with bony reabsorption a problem. At the current time, prosthetic implantation following phallic reconstruction seems to be the best option.

Summary

Modern tissue transfer techniques have drastically modified our approach to reconstructive surgery in general. The traumatic genital amputation injury is no exception. While the unique vascular properties of the penis have allowed for astonishingly good results via macroreattachment procedures, it is certain that

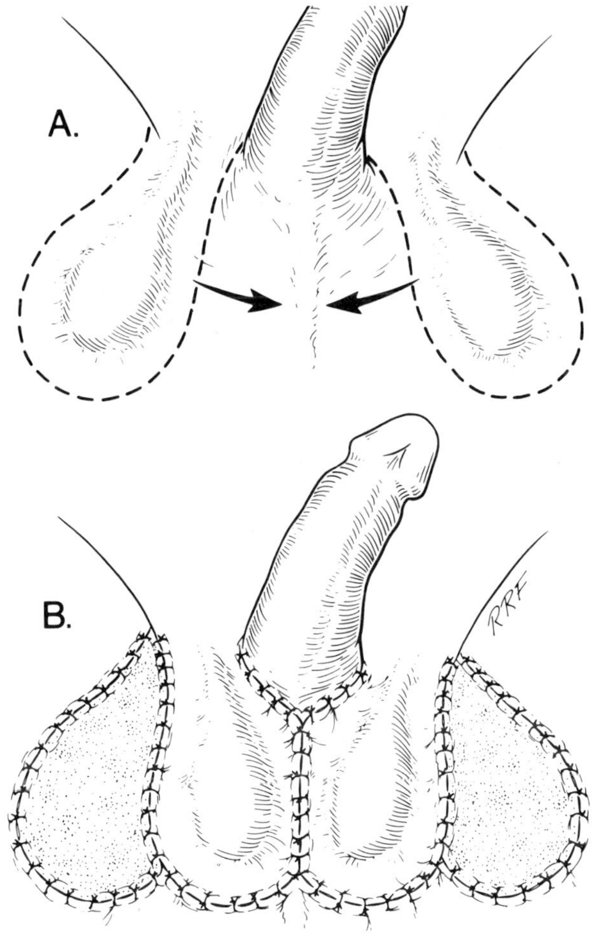

Figure 12-5 (A) Technique for the mobilization of lateral flaps commensurate with testicles in thigh pouches or lateral flaps for coverage of testicular injuries. (B) The flaps transposed to the midline with split thickness skin grafts used to close the defects laterally. (After McDougal,[9] J Urol 1983; 129.)

microreplantation procedures make for uniformly better results with a minimum of postoperative complications. After microreplantation, the literature has made it plain that the patient can be and usually is left with a penis that is cosmetically acceptable if not virtually normal in appearance and functionally normal or undetectably abnormal. It must be reemphasized, however, that no distal penile amputated part should be abandoned due to the lack of a microsurgeon. There continues to be a place for macroreattachment techniques in select patients.

REFERENCES

1. Abbou CC, Servant VM, Bennet F, et al.: Replantation du penis et des deux testicules aprs autoemasculation complete. Chirurgie 1979; 105:354.
2. Blacker KH, Wong N: Four cases of autocastration. Arch Gen Psychiat 1963; 8:189.
3. Ehrich WS: Two unusual penile injuries. J Urol 1929; 21:239.
4. Evins SC, Whittle T, Ropus SN: Self-emasculation: Review of the literature, report of a case and outline of the objectives of management. J Urol 1977; 118:775.

5. Greilheimer H, Groves JE: Male genital self-mutilation. Arch Gen Psychiat 1979; 36:441.
6. Hayhurst JW, O'Brien BM, Ishida H, et al.: Experimental digital replantation after prolonged cooling. Hand 1974; 6:134.
7. Jordan GH, Gilbert DA: Management of amputation injuries of the male genitalia. Urol Clin NA 1989; 16(2):359.
8. Breze J, Aboseif S, Lue TF: Anatomy of the penis. Atlas of the Urol Clinics of North America 1993; 1:1-8.
9. McDougal WS: Scrotal reconstruction using thigh pedicle flaps. J Urol 1983; 129:757.
10. McRoberts JW, Chapman WH, Ansell JS: Primary anastomosis of the traumatically amputated penis. Case report and summary of literature. J Urol 1988; 100:751.
11. Quartey JKM: One-stage penile/preputial cutaneous island flap urethroplasty for urethral stricture: A preliminary report. J Urol 1983; 129:284.
12. Silber SJ, Kelly J: Successful autotransplantation of an intraabdominal testis to the scrotum by microvascular techniques. J Urol 1976; 115:452.
13. Stewart DE, Lowrey MR: Replantation surgery following self-inflicted amputation. Can J Psychiat 1980; 25:143.
14. Tamai S, Nakamura Y, Motomiya Y: Microsurgical replantation of a completely amputated penis and scrotum. Plast Reconstr Surg 1977; 60:287.
15. Cohen BE, May JW, Daly JS et al.: Successful clinical replantation of an amputated penis by microneurovascular repair. Plast Reconstr Surg 1977; 59:276.
16. de Tejada IS: Personal communication, February 1992.

ANNOTATED BIBLIOGRAPHY

Tamai S, Nakamura Y, Motomiya Y: Microsurgical replantation of a completely amputated penis and scrotum. Plast Reconstr Surg 1977; 60:287.

The above two articles report the first successful replantation of an amputated penis. While Cohen's article made it in print first, Tamai's replantation was accomplished prior to Cohen's by a matter of a few weeks. Neither author was aware of the other's accomplishment at the time of their replantation.

Jordan GH, Gilbert DA: Management of amputation injuries of the male genitalia. Urol Clin NA 1989; 16(2):359.

The authors review penile anatomy in detail. The history of penile amputation injuries prior to microreplantation is reviewed followed by a literature review and history of microreplantation techniques. Current concepts of microreplantation of genital amputation injuries are then reviewed.

McRoberts JW, Chapman WH, Ansell JS: Primary anastomosis of the traumatically amputated penis. Case report and summary of literature. J Urol 1988; 100:751.

The authors report a case of a traumatic amputation of the penis. In this case, the penis was reattached. In reviewing the literature, the authors note the most frequently encountered complications of nonmicrovascular replantation. In that article, several recommendations for the successful accomplishment of a nonmicrovascular penile reattachment are made. These recommendations have persisted and stood the test of time with regards to their validity.

Quartey JKM: One-stage penile/preputial cutaneous island flap urethroplasty for urethral stricture: A preliminary report. J Urol 1983; 129:284.

Professor John Quartey, operating in Accra in Ghana, was confronted with a very difficult stricture population. He routinely saw patients with active watering pot perineum. He was forced to operate on these patients in the face of active infection and without the benefits of antibiotics. Hence, skin graft urethral reconstruction was not an option. Professor Quartey proceeded with eloquent microinjection studies that outline the cutaneous genital skin vascularity. As a product of those studies, he developed a technique of urethral reconstruction using skin islands based on dartos fascial flaps. This article and his techniques have served as a springboard for all of the flap urethral reconstruction techniques.

13

Penile Lengthening Procedures

John N. Kabalin
Inder Perkash

The Short Phallus

The short phalus may have many etiologies. At one end of the spectrum is congenital microphallus (see Chapter 12). The short phallus may also be an acquired phenomenon, with varying portions of the penile shaft lost as a result of traumatic or surgical amputation (see Chapter 11). Such cases are, fortunately, rare. Between these extreme cases are a great many men with penile lengths that would be considered within the range of "normal," but who nonetheless present to the urologist with the complaint of inadequate phallic proportion. These complaints may result from the patient's own subjective assessment of phallic length and adequacy, and although "normal" penile length in such unhappy individuals may occasionally fall well below the mean (approximately 6 inches when fully erect), such complaints are often unrelated to actual, absolute dimensions but rather to the patient's excessive expectations. These patients require reassurance that phallic length bears no relation to sexual performance or pleasure, and readjustment of their expectations in some instances; in unusual instances more in-depth psychologic counseling is necessary (see Chapter 15), and surgery is rarely, if ever, indicated.

Complaints regarding penile length may also have an objective basis, such as the man in whom the penile shaft length is inadequate to allow condom catheter management. This is most often seen in the setting of neurogenic bladder dysfunction with incontinence. Some penile shortening also occurs as a natural consequence of aging. Often, this is associated with weight gain and a concomitant increase in the mass of the prepubic fat pad, which has the effect of "burying" the penis. Except in cases of truly morbid obesity, the latter normally does not significantly affect sexual intercourse with the penis in its fully erect state. In cases where this does become problematic, weight loss may result in improved sexual function.

Management of Impotence and Infertility, edited by Douglas Whitehead and Harris Nagler,

Penile Prostheses

Penile prostheses do *not* increase the erect length of the penis. These devices provide rigidity sufficient for intercourse for the impotent man and an increase in length over the flaccid or nonerect state (see Chapter 3). However, almost every man with a penile prosthesis will report that the erection produced by the prosthetic device is somewhat less than the length of his previous normal erections, and in some cases is significantly shorter. Despite preoperative counseling regarding the capabilities and limitations of penile prostheses, some patients will be disappointed in the erect length provided and these men form a unique subset among those complaining of a short phallus. Several maneuvers are available to net some improvement in length in patients dissatisfied with the erection provided by their penile prosthesis. The three-component Scott-type inflatable penile prostheses, with separate scrotal pump and large volume intraabdominal fluid reservoir, probably provide the overall best, nearest to normal, prosthetic erections. In selected patients who are unhappy with semirigid, malleable, and mechanical and fluid hinge-type prostheses, replacement with a Scott-type three-component device may prove more satisfactory. The latest version of the Scott-type inflatable penile prosthesis, the Ultrex™ (American Medical Systems), has the added ability to expand in length as well as girth, and thus takes maximum advantage of whatever natural expansibility exists in the corporal tissues. It should be emphasized that even this device cannot duplicate the penile length of the normal erect state.

It has now been demonstrated that, over time, with prosthetic cyclinders in place the corpora cavernosa have a tendency to naturally dilate or stretch.[1] After a penile prosthesis of any type has been in place for many months or years, replacement with new cylinders will, on average, produce a net gain of 1–2 cm in corporal length. However, such an increase in length does not occur in every case, and it seems extreme to perform a surgical procedure, with its attendant potential for morbidity, to replace a perfectly functioning device only for the hope of gaining a centimeter or two in overall penile length. The Ultrex three-component inflatable penile prosthesis, with its ability to expand in length, is the only currently available device that might take advantage of such an increase in corporal length over time without requiring further surgery.

In comparison to penile prostheses, vacuum devices (see Chapter 7) more closely mimic the dimensions of the normal erect state both in length and girth, having the ability to produce spongiosal and glanular engorgement. We have used vacuum devices in selected cases to provide improved length and girth of erection for patients dissatisfied with indwelling semirigid penile prostheses who do not desire further surgery. Vacuum devices have also been used successfully after removal of a penile prosthesis.

Penile Skin Tethering

One correctable cause of acquired penile shortening is skin tethering produced by overaggressive circumcision. Prepubertal and especially neonatal circumcision rarely, if ever, produces such a problem. The residual skin of the penile shaft in the child is loose and pliant, and with normal growth and development will relax and expand to make up for all but the grossest iatrogenically induced deficiencies without tension or tethering. This is not always the case in the adult, where excessive skin removal at the time of circumcision may produce tethering, which, in effect, has the tendency to pull the penile shaft into or beneath the prepubic fat pad. Such tethering can be relieved by surgical release and plastic advancement of the prepubic skin. Figure 13-1 illustrates a simple technique to achieve prepubic skin advancement in these situations, consisting of modified Z-plasty with creation and rotational advancement of full-thickness (including subcutaneous fat) prepubic skin flaps. Placement of a closed-suction drain is optional in this procedure and its use would depend on the extent of dissection required in a given case.

In patients who have undergone placement of a penile prosthesis via a prepubic incision, resulting scar contracture may produce a similar picture of skin tethering and shortening of useful penile length. This can be largely avoided by ensuring that such incisions are never extended across the penopubic junction at the time of prosthetic implantation. Once scar contracture and skin tethering occur, it can be surgically managed with excision of the scar followed by a plastic Z-plasty procedure as described above and depicted in Figure 13-1. In less severe cases of skin tethering due to scar contracture, simple wide vertical ellipse excision of the scar with longitudinal closure may produce adequate skin advancement.

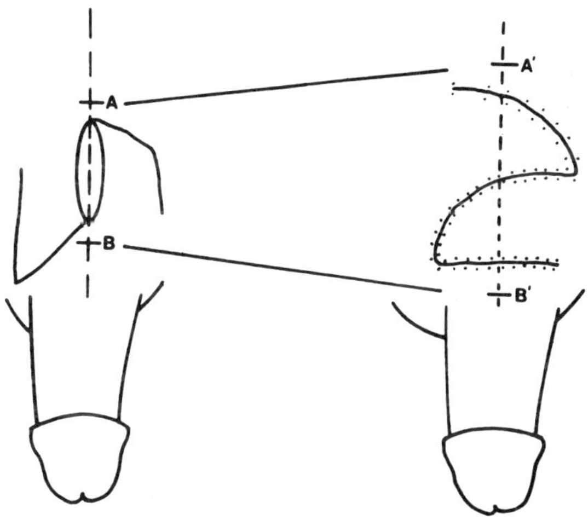

Figure 13-1 Modified Z-plasty used to advance prepubic skin and release tethering. Skin flaps should be full thickness, including subcutaneous fat. Note interval lengthening achieved from distance A–B on the left to distance A′–B′ on the right. For cases associated with contracture from a prior prepubic skin incision, the old scar can be excised with a wide vertical ellipse, as shown on the left. (Reproduced with permission from the Journal of Urology).

Corporal Advancement

In patients with neurologic dysfunction requiring external condom catheter urinary drainage for incontinence, as is the case with patients who have undergone external sphincterotomy, penile lengthening is often necessary or desirable to ensure secure condom maintenance without slippage. Most of these patients are spinal cord injured and are impotent on a neurologic basis. In such cases, the question of penile lengthening involves improvement over the flaccid state, rather than improvement of penile length in the erect state. In most, simple placement of any of a variety of semirigid or malleable penile prostheses will produce sufficient penile length and rigidity for condom catheter maintenance. Because constant rigidity is required to maintain a condom catheter, a semirigid or malleable penile prosthesis is preferred to an inflatable device in such patients.

These surgical implantation procedures have been well described elsewhere.[2]

In a few spinal cord-injured patients, simple placement of a semirigid or malleable penile prosthesis proves insufficient to maintain a condom catheter securely in position. Obesity with an increase in the size of the prepubic fat pad, which often increases over time with the inactivity imposed by paralysis and confinement to a wheelchair, usually is a significant contributing factor in these men. Many are initially managed well with a penile prosthesis, but when they later gain weight the phallus tends to retract into the growing prepubic fat pad and even with a penile prosthesis they cannot adequately maintain a condom catheter on the penis. This problem is typically exaggerated when the patient assumes a sitting position, and it is when sitting that most experience condom loss (see Figure 13-2).

In an attempt to deal with such problematic patients, we have developed a procedure to (1) advance the penile shaft outward from the pubis and (2) maintain the penis in this new position.[3] This procedure involves exposure of the suspensory ligaments of the penis through a prepubic incision. The suspensory ligaments are then divided sharply. This dissection is carried down to the point where the corpora cavernosa decussate and attach to the pubic bones. The suspensory ligaments are divided against the pubis to avoid damage to the corpora or the dorsal neurovascular structures. This dissection has the effect of dropping the corpora cavernosa away from the pubis, and has produced up to 4 cm of additional forward penile shaft extension (Figure 13-3). Note that the corpora are not and cannot be lengthened, but are *advanced* away from the pubis, with the net effect of increasing usable penile shaft

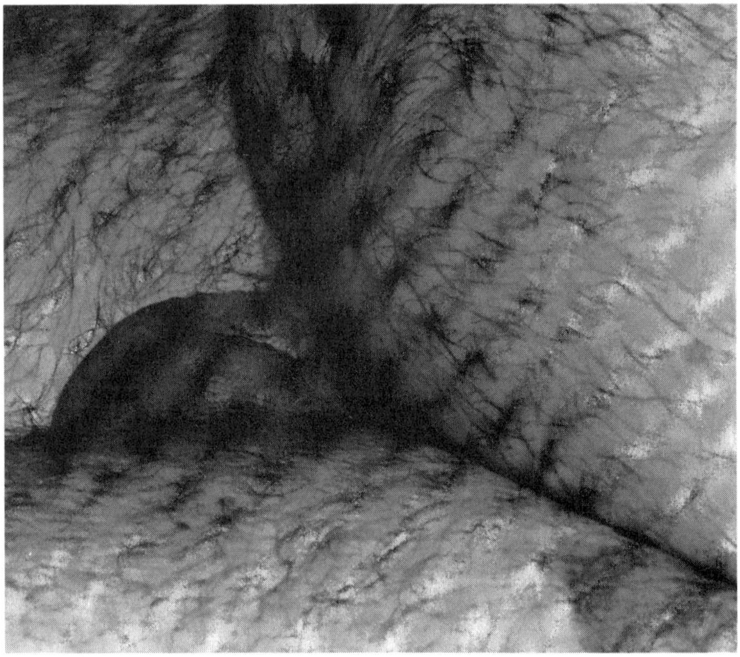

Figure 13-2 Penile retraction into the prepubic fat pad is demonstrated in this obese spinal cord-injured patient, shown here sitting upright. This patient has a semirigid penile prosthesis in place. Despite the prosthesis, because of the severity of penile retraction when sitting, he experienced loss of external condom catheter drainage whenever in his wheelchair. (Reproduced with permission from the Journal of Urology).

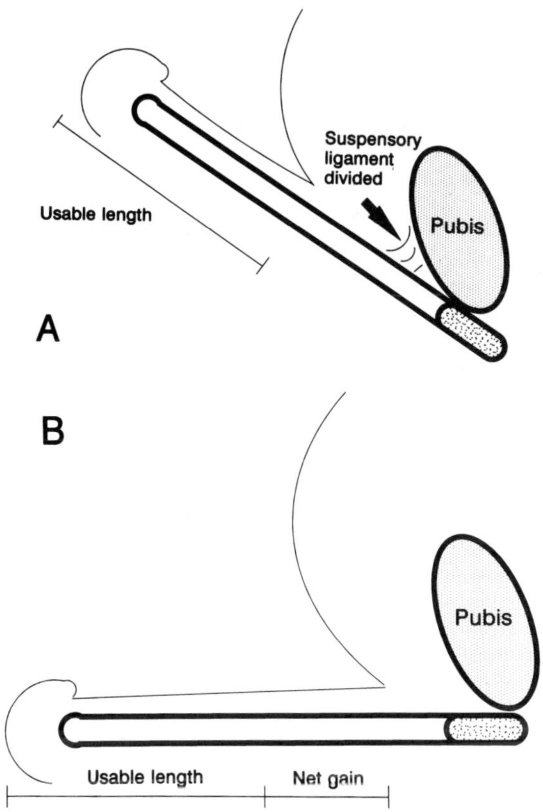

Figure 13-3 (A, B) Technique of dividing the suspensory ligament of the penis to advance the corpora cavernosa away from the pubis, thus gaining usable penile shaft length.

length. To hold the corpora away from the pubis so that they do not simply fall back to their original position, the prepubic soft tissues lateral to and above the corpora are next approximated between the corpora and the pubis. This soft tissue buttress serves to maintain the corporal advancement produced by release of the suspensory ligaments. Heavy nonabsorbable suture material is used to create this soft tissue buttress (we have used 2-0 prolene). Some care must be taken laterally to avoid including elements of the spermatic cord in these sutures. Figure 13-4 shows a spinal cord-injured patient treated with this technique, demonstrating excellent penile length and condom maintenance in the sitting position.

We have been reluctant to extend this technique for penile advancement to neurologically intact and potent patients. Although with care the dorsal neurovascular structures should be avoided during deep dissection and division of the suspensory ligaments of the penis, some damage may occur resulting in unwelcome sensory deficit. This problem may be exaggerated if electrocautery is used during the dissection. Also, division of the penile suspensory ligaments, while advancing the penis away from the pubis and providing additional usable shaft length, especially noticeable in the sitting position, tends to produce a downward rather than forward pointing erection, especially when standing. We are afraid most men would find this aesthetically displeasing.

Even further penile advancement can be obtained by division of the suspensory ligaments of the penis followed by freeing the corpora cavernosa partially or wholly from the pubic rami.[4] The freed corporal bodies are then approximated in the midline. Such procedures have mainly been utilized in the treatment of congenital penile abnormalities, in particular, those associated with the epispadias–exstrophy complex. A similar approach might also be useful in adult spinal cord-injured patients with a very short phallus and severe retraction beneath the prepubic fat pad in the sitting position. However, we have not yet seen a case so severe that it could not be corrected by the simple corporal advancement technique previously described consisting of division of the suspensory ligaments and creation of a soft tissue buttress between the corpora and pubis.

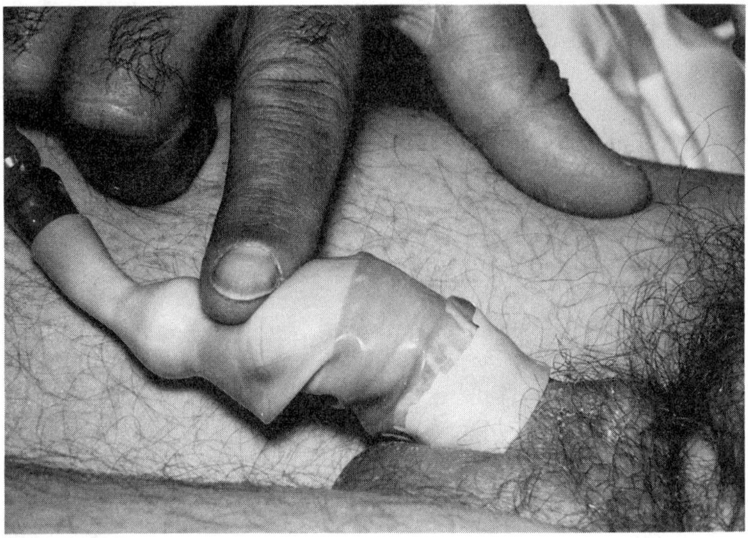

Figure 13-4 Spinal cord-injured patient who has undergone corporal advancement procedure after placement of a semirigid penile prosthesis alone failed to produce adequate penile shaft length to maintain external condom catheter drainage. He is shown sitting with condom in place. Note excellent penile shaft length even when sitting. Corporal advancement produced 4 cm of additional usable shaft in this man. (Reproduced with permission from the Journal of Urology).

Furthermore, we would be even more reluctant to extend a procedure that involved dissection of the corpora cavernosa from the pubic rami to a neurologically intact and potent man. Such a dissection produces significant downward displacement of the penile shaft, and even more of a tendency for the erect penis to point downward in an unaesthetic fashion. Of greater concern is that any dissection of the corpora from the pubic rami would interrupt the corporal branches of the nervi erigentes responsible for erection and thus produce impotence. This might happen even with partial freeing of the corpora from the pubis, and the potential for iatrogenic impotence would increase with the extent of this dissection.

Summary

In summary, the potent man with a normal but short phallus is best managed with reassurance and counseling. For the impotent man with a penile prosthesis who is displeased with the erect length of his penis, several therapeutic maneuvers are available to optimize length, but none can be expected to match the size of prior normal erections. Skin tethering due to overaggressive adult circumcision or penopubic scar contraction is a potentially correctable cause of penile shortening, easily managed with a modified Z-plasty skin advancement. In patients with neurogenic bladder dysfunction and incontinence, lengthening of the penile shaft may be desirable to allow secure maintenance of an external condom catheter. A semirigid or malleable penile prosthesis usually will provide sufficient penile length and rigidity in these individuals. Techniques to advance the corpora cavernosa forward from the pubis will provide further usable penile shaft length in selected patients. However, the latter techniques for corporal advancement are not readily applicable or advisable in the neurologically intact and potent man who simply desires a longer phallus.

REFERENCES

1. Kabalin JN, Kessler R: Penile prosthesis surgery: Review of ten-year experience and examination of reoperations. Urology 1989; 33:17.
2. Perkash I, Kabalin JN, Lennon S, Wolfe V: Penile prostheses to maintain external condom catheter drainage in spinal cord injurty patients. Paraplegia, 1992; 30:327.
3. Kabalin JN, Rosen J, Perkash I: Penile advancement and lengthening in spinal cord injury patients with retracted phallus who have failed penile prosthesis placement alone. J Urol 1990; 144:316.
4. Johnston JH: Lengthening of the congenital or acquired short penis. Br J Urol 1974; 46:685.

ANNOTATED BIBLIOGRAPHY

Kabalin JN, Rosen J, Perkash I: Penile advancement and lengthening in spinal cord injury patients with retracted phallus who have failed penile prosthesis placement alone. J Urol 1990; 144:316.

The authors describe techniques developed to maximize penile shaft length in spinal cord-injured men to ensure secure maintenance of an external condom catheter for management of urinary drainage. In the patients described, all had initially undergone placement of a semirigid penile prosthesis that alone proved inadequate for condom catheter maintenance. In all patients, the penile prosthesis was resized and replaced, usually gaining 1–2 cm in length. In two patients, significant penile skin tethering secondary to overaggressive adult circumcision was present, and a technique for modified Z-plasty to advance the prepubic skin and release the tethering is described. To provide further penile shaft length, the authors divided the suspensory ligament of the penis in all patients, thus advancing the corpora cavernosa forward from the pubis, and created a soft tissue buttress between the corpora and pubis to maintain the corporal advancement. This technique for corporal advancement produced net gains in penile shaft length of up to 4 cm. This procedure allowed all patients to maintain condom catheter drainage successfully, without slippage or urinary leakage.

14 Reconstructive Surgery in the Micropenis/Microphallus Patient

Gerald H. Jordan

Management of the young male child born with an inadequate penis has been and will continue to be a dilemma for the managing urologist. A great many people favor management of these children with gender reassignment. It is clear that when gender reassignment is selected, the evaluation must proceed quickly following birth so that, at least, gonadectomy can be effected in the immediate neonatal period. The issue of gonadal labeling of the brain remains controversial and confusing. It does appear, however, that gonadectomy must be accomplished promptly. Actual reconstruction, for children in whom gender reassignment has been elected, can be accomplished later with vaginal construction best performed at puberty.

Woodhouse recently evaluated a group of patients with micropenis for whom neither reassignment nor phallic construction was selected. These males are all now in their twenties and thirties. All were sexually active. They did report that during adolescence remarks were made by peers, babysitters, etc. However, his data shows these individuals to be well-balanced with good gender identity, and in most cases, having good sexual relationships either with spouses or (in some cases "and") significant others. His data contests both the thought that gender reassignment is in order or if not reassigned that phallic construction is an absolute necessity.

However, not all patients with microphallus who persist with their anomaly into adulthood are happy or sexually active. There remains at least a subset of patients who very properly are candidates for phallic construction for purposes of enhanced gender identity and sexual relations.

The major techniques of reconstruction of the penis were developed for patients who suffered traumatic penile amputations. The first large series was described in 1936 by Borgoraz.[1] His series dealt with the war-injured patient. In 1944, Frumkin[4] followed with another large series from the Soviet Union. Gilles[6] was aware of both Borgoraz' and Frumkin's work. In 1948, he was stationed at a major hospital on

Management of Impotence and Infertility, edited by Douglas Whitehead and Harris Nagler,

the outskirts of London and amassed a series of phallic construction patients following trauma.

All of those early procedures involved the delayed formation and transfer of tubed abdominal flaps. In the "tube within a tube" design, the inner tube allowed for placement of a baculum for rigidity during intercourse while the outer tube provided skin coverage. There was generally no attempt at urethral construction, and the patients voided through a proximal urethrostomy. These techniques of reconstruction persisted through the early 1970s. In 1972, Orticochea[10] described a technique of total reconstruction of the penis using a gracilis musculocutaneous flap. Orticochea's work required many "touch ups" from outset of reconstruction to completion. The major work was done in a single stage using the musculocutaneous flap. In 1978, Puckett[13] reported a series in which he constructed a phallus using a tubed groin flap. In his initial cases, the groin flap was delayed in its transfer to the area of the penile stump. In the latter part of his series, the tissue was transferred as a microvascular free transfer flap. Puckett's cosmetic results were exceptional. The flaps, however, were insensate, as were all of the flaps using tubed abdominal skin and gracilis musculocutaneous units.

In 1984, Chang[2] popularized the use of a forearm flap based on the radial artery for penile reconstruction and phallic construction. Biemer, in 1988, reported a modification of that forearm flap, and in 1989, Farrow and Boyd[3] reported their "cricket-bat" modification of the forearm flap. At the time of this writing, the forearm flaps are the most frequently employed tissues for penile reconstruction and total phallic construction. The forearm flap can also be elevated on the ulnar artery. There are disadvantages to the forearm flap and most relate to donor site morbidity. The donor site scar on the forearm is ugly at best. Early in the experience with the flaps, it was felt necessary to reconstruct the continuity of the artery, using a vein graft interposition. More recently, reconstruction of the artery is seldom accomplished. There is the theoretic possibility of the development of cold intolerance in the donor site arm. This, however, has not been observed in our patients in whom reconstruction of the radial artery or ulnar artery was not performed.[1]

Biemer's original description suggested the use of an osseocutaneous microvascular free transfer flap. That flap included a portion of the radius with the thoughts of creating an os penis in the new phallus. Inclusion of this bone with the flap does, in some cases, leaves the patient with some loss of function in the hand. Additionally, the inclusion of bone or periosteum has not reliably accomplished the desired rigidity.

Generally, the flap is elevated from the nondominant arm. Patients are carefully screened preoperatively for evidence of insufficiency of the forearm arteries or lack of communication distally through the superficial and deep palmar arches. Neither the radial nor the ulnar artery gives off necessary branches into the deep tissues of the forearm proper.

One screening mechanism is the Allen test. The patient makes a tight fist with the surgeon then occluding both the radial and ulnar arteries. The arteries are then released, one at a time, looking for evidence of resumption of flow to the hand as indicated by the observation of capillary refill in the palm and digits. The arteries are checked one at a time. This detects patients in whom one artery is clearly the dominant arterial supply to the hand. In such patients, the anatomy must be clearly defined, as elevation of the dominant artery with the flap or elevation of the flap on an inadequate artery both result in poor outcomes. Should doubt exist, upper extremity angiography is performed.

The forearm flap is a fasciocutaneous flap vascularized via the radial or ulnar artery with paired venae comitans. The radial artery arises as a continuation of the brachial artery. In the upper forearm, the radial artery lies beneath the belly of the brachioradialis muscle. The artery perfuses the skin via perforators to the fascial plexuses. The cutaneous vascular territory encompasses almost the entire circumference of the forearm. The lateral and medial antebrachial cutaneous nerves are included in the flap and are noted beneath the fascia. The cephalic, basilic, and medial antebrachial veins are also included in the flap. In some patients, the venae comitans are the dominant venous system, while in others, the superficial veins are dominant. At the time of flap transfer, after reestablishment of arterial continuity, it is imperative to evaluate which venous system provides runoff. By observing which veins distend or bleed, one identifies the appropriate venous outflow.

The lateral antebrachial cutaneous nerve arises at the elbow as an arborization of the musculocutaneous nerve. The lateral antebrachial cutaneous nerve provides sensation to both the volar and the dorsal radial aspects of the arm. The medial antebrachial cutaneous nerve divides distally into an interior and an ulnar branch. This nerve accomplishes similar innervation of the ulnar aspect of the forearm. The superficial branch of the radial nerve arises beneath the belly of the brachioradialis muscle and accompanies the radial artery. This nerve must not be included with the flap in that the patient is left with the potential for a painful neuroma and/or an area of anesthesia at the thenar eminence. If the nerve is inadvertently cut, primary coaptation should be accomplished.

The ulnar artery also arises as a distal continuation of the brachial artery and, like the radial artery, supplies vascular supply to the forearm fascia and skin via the fasciocutaneous plexuses. The ulnar artery cutaneous vascular territory includes, likewise, most of the circumference of the skin of the forearm. The cutaneous vascular territory is obviously rotated toward the ulnar aspect as the radial artery cutaneous vascular territory is shifted to center over the radial artery.

As mentioned, a number of modifications of the forearm flap design have been proposed. These represent, not modifications in flap elevation technique, but rather modifications in the configuration of the flap as it is sculpted into a phallus. Each of these modifications has advantages in certain situations. As described by Chang,[2] shaft coverage is accomplished by the radial aspect of the flap with a section of deepithelialized skin separating the shaft from the urethra (Figure 14-1A). The flap is a tube within a tube with the ulnar aspect (urethral aspect) tubed, and the radial aspect (shaft) wrapped around the neurethra. The deepithelialized area allows epithelial approximation of the urethral tube and epithelial approximation of the shaft. In the modification of Farrow and Boyd,[3] the flap is designed in the shape of a "cricket bat," with a wider section on the upper forearm and the urethra extending as a narrow extension, centered over the artery (either radial or ulnar respectively) (Figure 14-1B). The proximal broad portion of the flap will provide the shaft coverage. The narrow portion of the flap, (handle of the cricket bat) is tubed as the urethra. Configuration of the phallus is accomplished, transposing and inverting the urethral portion into the center of the shaft coverage. Ostensibly, the urethral portion of the flap is more reliable due to its more central location over the artery. In the "Chinese" flap (Figure 14-1A), the urethral portion is on the

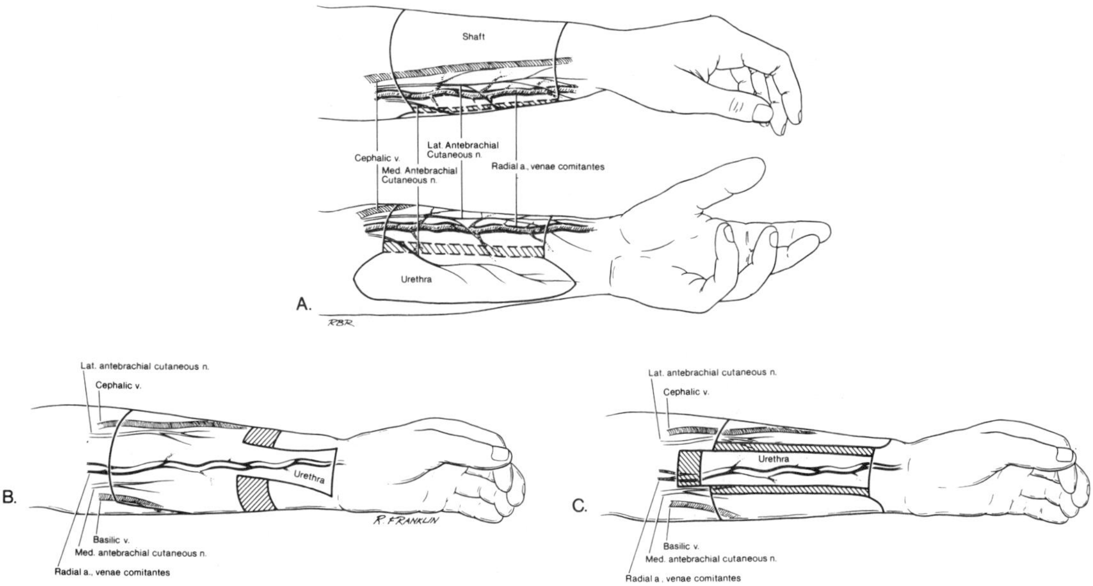

Figure 14-1 Collage depicting the various configurations of forearm flaps. (A) The radial forearm flap as described by Song and Chang outlines two areas of epithelialized islands. The urethral island, classically, is located on the ulnar aspect of the forearm with a deepithelialized strip separating it from the shaft, a portion of the flap. In general, the shaft portion of the flap is centered over the dominant artery. (B) The modification as described by Farrow and Boyd centers the urethral portion over the flap artery. The urethral portion extends as the "handle of the cricket back." The across hatch areas represent deepithelialized areas that add bulk to define the glans. The proximal broader section of the flap provides a shaft coverage. The urethra is transposed into the center of the shaft coverage during formation of the phallus. (C) Configuration as described by Biemer. In this configuration, the urethral epithelialized strip is centered over the dominant artery. Adjacent are two deepithelialized areas. This allows for epithelial apposition of the urethral strip. Shaft coverage is accomplished by the epithelialized islands adjacent to the epithelialized strips. In this configuration, with shaft coverage, there is a suture line dorsally and ventrally. As drawn, there is a deepithelialized cuff on the urethra, thus allowing for an overlapping to better anastomosis of the native urethra to the neourethra. The last two configurations have evolved in an effort to center the urethral portion of the flap over the center of the cuticular vascular territory.

lateral extent of the cutaneous vascular territory and some patients have developed ischemic stenosis of that portion of the flap. Beimer's modification (Figure 14-1C) is, likewise, aimed at centering the urethra over the forearm artery. His urethral tube is central in the flap with two deepithelialized strips adjacent. Lateral to that are two areas of skin that are approximated to form the shaft. In this modification, there are suture lines on both the dorsum and the ventrum of the phallus. All of these forearm flap designs create a neourethra that is attached to the patient's native urethra, thus allowing the patient to stand to void and also allow for a microneurocoaptation of the flap's cutaneous nerves to the recipient nerves. In the case of the patient with the micropenis, the flap's cutaneous nerves can be coapted to one or both of the dorsal nerves of the penis. If these nerves are not suitable, then the nerves can be coapted to the pudendal or the ilioinguinal nerve. Coaptation to the dorsal nerves or the pudendal nerves carries the theoretic advantage of providing not only sensibility but erogenous sensibility.

The flap is designed with every effort made to center the urethral portion in the nonhirsute forearm skin. Incisions are carried sharply to the fascia. The fascia is first incised at the base of the flap over the radial artery, as it runs in an arc beneath the edge of the belly of the brachioradilis muscle. The artery is dissected, intact, from beneath the muscle. The superficial fascia is then mobilized to include the lateral and medial antebrachial cutaneous nerves and the venae comitans. The cephalic vein will be included in the deep dissection of the flap. The flap is elevated directly off of the forearm musculature with the superficial fascia included as the deep aspect of the flap. The vascular pedicle is dissected as far as the junction of the radial artery with the brachial artery, recurrent radial artery. The ulnar artery is, likewise, dissected from the brachial or recurrent ulnar artery. Following elevation, the flap is configured into a phallus while perfusion remains intact. The recipient vessels, nerves, and native urethra must be totally prepared prior to dividing the blood supply to the flap and before transfer. A tourniquet is used during elevation. After that dissection is complete, the tourniquet is released, establishing circulation into the forearm. The flap is then configured. Warm sponges are placed about the flap while preparation of the recipient site is completed. This leaves the flap unmolested with perfusion intact on the forearm for a short period after manipulation thus limiting vasospastic phenomenon.

In some areas of China, the radial/forearm flap is elevated without the inclusion of the forearm fascia. This seems to defy our understanding of the pattern of vascularity. The author has limited experience with elevation so accomplished.

A number of vessels have been used as recipient vessels. In some patients, the deep inferior epigastric artery is elevated from beneath the rectus abdominis muscle. The artery is dissected to the level of the umbilicus, and at that level the artery branches giving off multiple perforators. The artery, a branch of the iliofemoral artery, is accompanied in most cases by one or more venae comitans. The vessels are divided at the umbilicus and passed to the base of the penis. The venous drainage of the flap is anastomosed to the epigastric venae comitans and to the saphenous veins on one or both sides. The saphenous vein is dissected in the upper leg and there divided and passed to the base of the flap. The nerves have been prepared as already described (Figure 14-2A).

As an alternative (Figure 14-2B), the recipient vessels include the saphenous veins and the femoral artery through a saphenous vein interposition graft. On the patient's nondominant side, the full length of the saphenous vein is mobilized to the level of the knee. The distal end of the saphenous vein is attached end-to-side to the femoral artery at the level of the profunda, thus creating temporarily an arteriovenous fistula that remains patent until flap transfer. On the other side, the saphenous vein is dissected as already described. Venous drainage is thus to the saphenous veins bilaterally with the donor arterial vessel being a saphenous vein interposition graft from the femoral artery. This configuration of the recipient vessels carries the theoretic disadvantages of two arterial suture lines and the inherent potential disadvantages of a vein interposition graft. A theoretic advantage of this vessel configuration

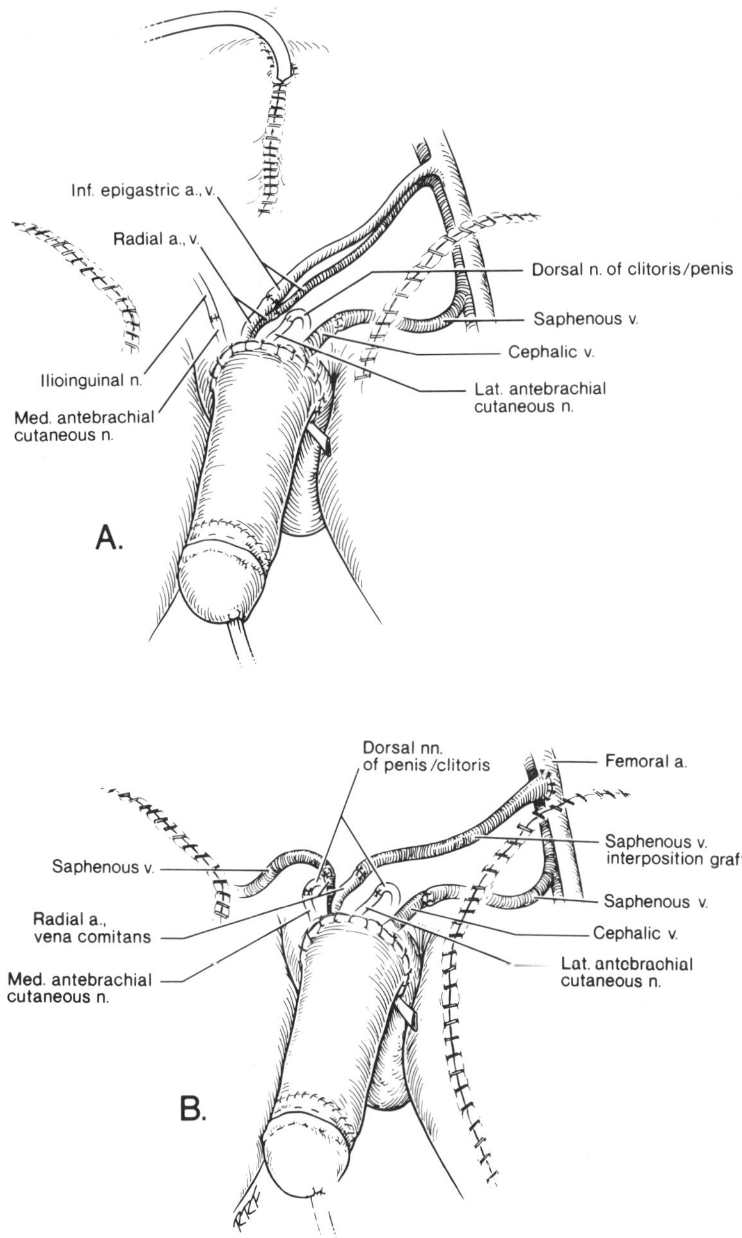

Figure 14-2 Dramatic representation of the configurations of recipient vessels for free phallic construction of the phallus. (A) The configuration utilizing the deep inferior epigastric artery as a recipient artery. The recipient veins are the saphenous veins bilaterally and the venae comitans of the deep inferior epigastric artery. The flap artery is anastomosed to the deep inferior epigastric artery. The dominant venous supply is identified and anastomosed to the saphenous veins. Additional venous anastomoses are accomplished to saphenous vein branches and/or the venae comitans of the deep inferior epigastric artery. In this configuration, both the medial and lateral antibrachial cutaneous nerves are coapted to the dorsal nerves of the penis or the pudendal nerves. (B) In this configuration the recipient vessels are the saphenous veins and the femoral artery via a saphenous vein interposition graft. An arterial venous fistula is created and then a vein interposition graft between the femoral artery and the flap artery is created. The venous drainage is accomplished as described in A. Microneurel coaptation is likewise accomplished.

is that of an end-to-side anastomosis with a high flow vessel. Ostensibly this allows the fasciocutaneous flap to autoregulate the "flow that it needs." Usually the saphenous vein can be dissected to include a number of branches for anastomosis to the flap veins.

The flap is readied for transfer by dividing and meticulously marking the nerves. The artery is then divided and marked, followed by the venae comitans and other veins. The flap is transferred to the area of the penis and the urethral anastomosis is performed in two layers. Epithelial apposition is accomplished with chromic suture with an outer buttressing layer of monofilament absorbable suture. The time necessary for this is inconsequential, and by performing the anastomosis first, exposure for the anastomosis is optimized. The operating microscope is wheeled to the field. The deep inferior epigastric artery is prepared. Alternatively, the AV fistula is divided and readied for anastomosis. The forearm vessel is anastomosed to the recipient arterial vessel. In the case of the saphenous vein interposition graft, the anastomosis is accomplished with 10-0 and in some cases 9-0 nylon or Prolene sutures. In the configuration in which the arterial anastomosis is performed to the deep inferior epigastric artery, the anastomosis uses 10-0 or 11-0 nylon or Prolene sutures.

Arterial circulation is reestablished and the veins then carefully inspected. Distention indicates the dominant venous drainage. The dominant veins are then anastomosed to the largest of the recipient venous branches. In general, at least three venous anastomoses are accomplished. The flap is now carefully inspected for capillary refill and dermal skin edge bleeding. The Doppler is used to confirm flow in the major vessels. The flap is again wrapped in warm saline sponges and allowed to sit. The neurocoaptations can be accomplished after the flap has stabilized.

Further suturing of the phallus is then undertaken. If the flap demonstrates good revascularization without signs of vasospasm, then glans definition is undertaken. The flap designs allow for some definition of the glans, including bulk with deepithelialization areas or by widening the flap in the area of the glans. Additionally, the coronal groove is made by incising the flap skin (Figure 14-3). A split-thickness skin graft or a genital full-thickness skin graft is tubed over a small catheter. Genital skin is preferred because of the difference in color between graft and flap, further enhancing the definition of the "coronal groove." The tubed graft is buried in the groove of the flap and at a second stage, approximately 4 to 6 weeks later, the groove is opened leaving an indented color "mismatched" area.

Donor sites are closed with split-thickness skin grafts and meticulously bolstered and splinted. The flap is continuously monitored via Doppler for gross signs of vascularization. The patient's temperature is kept as close to normal as possible. We recently have also had the use of a pH monitoring device in which a probe is implanted in the flap and flap tissue pH monitored. In this system, absolute pH values are not important, but rather, a change to a more acidotic state being felt to be significant. The pH measurements must be compared and assessed simultaneously with Doppler findings. The patient is kept in an intensive care setting, in a warm room, for a period of 24 to 48 hours. The flap is continuously monitored. For about 7 days the patient is kept at bed rest in an air or air sand type bed. Anticoagulation is not routinely used with the exception of a baby aspirin a day.

A suprapubic cystostomy tube provides uri-

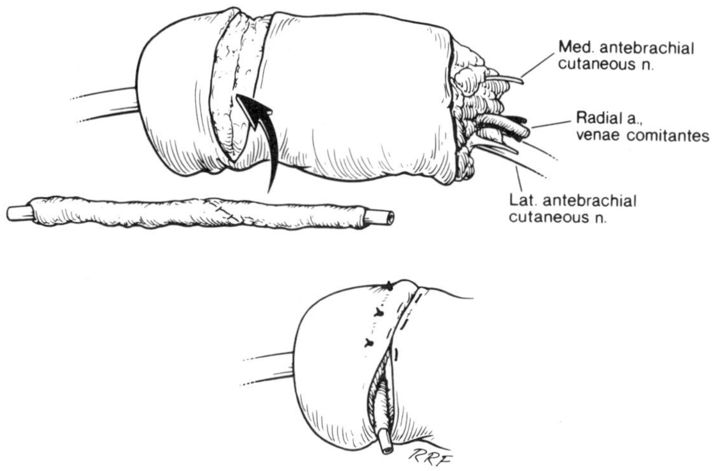

Figure 14-3 Illustration depicting the technique of definition of the coronal sulcus. A groove is cut into the flap adipose tissue. A split-thickness skin graft (preferably and genital split-thickness skin graft) is then tubed about a catheter and buried in the groove. The groove is closed. At an interval (6–8 weeks) the groove is opened, thus leaving an indented coronal groove, which is further defined by a color mismatch.

nary diversion. The urethra is stented with a soft ribbed silicone 14 French catheter. Voiding trial with contrast is undertaken between 21 and 28 days postoperatively. Fistula at the site of the urethral anastomosis has been a problem; however, internal closure is generally readily performed. Reconstruction, as described, is identical to the reconstruction that would be accomplished in the patient who has suffered a traumatic amputation injury of the penis in which replantation/reattachment was not done.

It is the feeling of this Center that prosthetic implantation should be undertaken only after the phallus is well healed and sensibility has occurred, and the urethra is proven to be adequate and a durable entity.

We have used all categories of prostheses from simple rod, malleable, articulated to multiple component hydraulic. At implantation, the stump of the penis or micropenis is exposed via a suprapubic incision that is carried down to the periosteum of the pubis. The skin is then elevated exposing the penile stump. The corporal bodies of the micropenis or amputated penis are opened at their distal extent and dilated with sounds. In some cases the Otis urethrotome can be helpful for dilatation in the case of the patient with the micropenis. The Otis is used as a dilating tool and not a cutting tool. The proximal ends of the prostheses are seated into the proximal corpora with distal corporal reconstruction using Gore-Tex (product info). The vascular graft houses the distal portion of the prosthesis. The Gore-Tex is modified with "struts" of the Gor-Tex connecting the proximal cuff to the distal tip in an attempt to limit the avascular interface between graft and prosthesis and to limit the opportunity for serous or serosanguineous collections. These patients are all treated with broad spectrum parenteral antibiotics for 72 hours and then discharged on oral cephalosporins for an additional 14 days. A Foley catheter is placed for a period of 24 to 48 hours with removal dependent on the degree of flap edema. Patients are generally kept at bed rest for a period of 24 to 48 hours. Closed drains are essential in all of these patients with removal of the drains at 48 hours. The routine use of broad spectrum perioperative intravenous antibiotics in association with drains has favorably altered our incidence of infectious complications in these patients.

We have successfully implanted prostheses in both the micropenis patient and in patients posttraumatic penile amputation. The longest followup that we have in a patient with micropenis is 6 years. The longest followup in a patient following traumatic amputation is 7 years. To date, in both subsets of patients, we have not had any infections or erosions. In our early experience with the transsexual population, we had significant problems with both erosion and/or infection. However, the combination of antibiotics and closed suction drainage has altered that experience.

In the patient in whom gender reassignment was accomplished in infancy, vaginal construction would be considered near the time of puberty. Graft techniques do not work well in this patient population. The need for bolsters and constant stenting is incompatible with the development of a healthy gender identification and sexuality. In these cases, we favor the use of bowel for vaginal construction and have used both small bowel and sigmoid colon. The techniques of vaginal construction that employ musculocutaneous flaps, by and large, are not used in this patient population. Those techniques are useful in the patient who has had exenteration and in whom one desires to accomplish two purposes: (1) vaginal reconstruction, and (2) placement of bulky vascular tissue in the exenteration defect. In the intersex patient, the dissection of the vaginal vault is limited because of the android pelvis and bowel techniques seem to provide the best long-term results.

Summary

Woodhouse's data might suggest that a great many patients with micropenis/microphallus will go on to live very productive and sexually fulfilling lives without ever having phallic construction. His data clearly make one seriously contemplate the place of gender reassignment in these patients. The success with the microvascular free transfer techniques for phallic construction likewise makes one strongly reevaluate the subject of gender reassignment in the microphallus/micropenis patient. In the patient who has suffered traumatic penile amputation, gender reassignment is not a consideration. In the microphallus/micropenis patient, during counselling of the parents in the immediate neonatal period, it is essential to emphasize the advantages and disadvantages of the options. In presenting gender reassignment, it is essential that the parents be made aware that there are now a number of cases in which gender reassignment was accomplished for the inadequate penis in the neonatal period in which the patient upon reaching puberty has demanded reassignment to a phenotypic state that matches the genotype. On the positive side, however, is the fact that surgical procedures involved with gender reassignment are technically much simpler and the end result requires fewer procedures.

With regards to the counselling concerning phallic construction, either in the pubertal or transpubertal period, it can be stated to the parents that with a number of stages of reconstruction that their child will eventually have "adequate genitalia." However, this statement must be tempered by the many unknowns concerning the long-term effects of phallic construction in the child, the multiplicity of surgeries required to eventually accomplish reconstruction, and the very true occurrence of complications with each of these surgical procedures.

REFERENCES

1. Biemer E: Penile construction by the radial arm flap. Clin Plast Surg 1988; 15:425.
2. Bogoraz NA: Plastic restoration of the penis. Sovet Khir No 1936; 8:303–307.
3. Chang TS, Hwang WY: Forearm flap in one-stage reconstruction of the penis. Plast Reconstr Surg 1984; 74:251.
4. Farrow GA, Boyd JB, Semple JL: Total reconstruction of the penis employing the "cricket bat flap" single stage forearm free graft. AUA Today 1990; 3(2).
5. Frumkin AP: Reconstruction of male genitalia. Am Rev Sov Med 1944; 2:14–21.
6. Gilbert DA: Radial forearm flap for phallic reconstruction. In: Strauch B, Vasconez LO, Hall-Findlay J, eds. Grabb's encyclopedia of flaps. Boston: Little, Brown, 1990: 1515–1520.
7. Gilles HD, Harrison RH: Congenital absense of the penis. Br J Plast Surg 1948; 1:8–28.
8. Jordan H, Schlossberg M, McCraw JB: Tissue transfer techniques for genitourinary reconstructive surgery. Part I–III. AUA Update Series, Lesson 9-12, Volume VII, 1988.
9. McCraw JB, Arnold PG: McCraw and Arnold's atlas of muscle and musculocutaneous flaps. Norfolk: Hampton Press, 1986: 265–294.
10. McDougal WS: Scrotal reconstruction using thigh pedicle flaps. J Urol 1983; 129:757–759.
11. Orticochea M: Musculo-cutaneous flap method: Immediate and heroic substitute for the method of delay. Br J Plast Surg 1972; 25:106.
12. Ortiocochea M: New method of total reconstruction of the penis. Br J Plast Surg 1972; 25:347.
13. Ponten B: The fascio-cutaneous flap: Its use in soft tissue defects of the lower leg. Br J Plast Surg 1981; 34:215.
14. Puckett CL, Montie JE: Construction of male genitalia in the transsexual using a tubed groin flap for the penis and a hydraulic inflation device. Plast Reconstr Surg 1978; 61:523.
15. Puckett CL, Reinisch JF, Montie JE: Free flap phalloplasty. J Urol 1982; 128:294.
16. Quartey JKM: One-stage penile/preputial cutaneous island flap urethroplasty for urethral stricture: A preliminary report. J Uro 1983; 129:284.
17. Schonfeld WA, Beebe GW: Normal growth and variation in the male genitalia from birth to maturity. Am J Dis Child 1942; 64:759.
18. Song R, Gao Y, Song Y, Yu Y, Song Y: The forearm flap. Clin Plast Surg 1982; 9:21.

ANNOTATED BIBLIOGRAPHY

As just mentioned, the Chinese forearm flap has had some problems owing to difficulties with body habitus in the Caucasian patients. Professor Biemer described a modification of the forearm flap. His modification provides for centralization of the urethral portion of the flap. In the Chinese flap, many times the laterally placed urethral portion is at the limits of the cutaneous vascular territory. The urethra has been a problem in the Caucasian population. Professor Biemer's modification has all of the advantages of the Chinese flap but further offers the advantage of a centralized urethral tube, hence placing that in the "most reliable" portion of the flap. Professor Biemer additionally describes the inclusion of a vascularized bone segment with the flap for rigidity. Others attempting this maneuver have had less than optimal results.

Chang TS, Hwang WY: Forearm flap in one-stage reconstruction of the penis. Plast Reconstr Surg 1984; 74:251.

The authors describe a modification of the forearm flap originally described by Song. It should be mentioned that also about this time Kao described a very similar modification. This modification of the forearm flap was an epic development in phallic construction. While the forearm flap in this country has not been the panacea that it has been in China, it is not the fault of the flap but rather the fault of the body habitus of the patient population with which we deal. Nonetheless, this modification allowed the creation of a cosmetically acceptable looking phallus with a vascularized neourethra and for the ability to give the patient erogenous sensibility.

Farrow GA, Boyd JB, Semple JL: Total reconstruction of the penis employing the "cricket bat flap" single stage forearm free graft. AUA Today 1990; 3(2).

The Canadians have described a further modification of the forearm flap. In this modification, the flap is shaped as in a cricket bat or paddle. There is a narrow "handle" section with a broader paddle section. The broad section provides the shaft coverage with the narrow section being the neourethral tube. This modification likewise allows for centralization of the urethral portion, thus making it more reliable. This particular modification has been of great use in the trauma patient or the micropenis patient in that this modification allows for precise tailoring with regards to length of the neourethra. This modification allows all the advantages of the Chinese designed forearm flap, while offering the additional advantage of centralization of the urethral portion of the flap.

McCraw JB, Arnold PG: McCraw and Arnold's atlas of muscle and musculocutaneous flaps. Norfolk: Hampton Press, 1986.

This textbook is a must for reconstructive surgeons. McCraw and Arnold have taken their years of experience and years of photos and compiled an atlas of musculocutaneous flaps that is hereto unequalled.

15 The Psychological Treatment of Erectile Dysfunction

Shirley Zussman

For almost all men in our society, sexuality is a central focus of their self-image and self-esteem. Their sexual functioning is a measure of their adequacy as a man. As a result, a considerable blow to their masculinity occurs when any inhibition or impairment of sexual functioning occurs. This is particularly true when the impairment takes the form of difficulty in getting or maintaining an erection. Difficulty in getting an erection is experienced occasionally by most men. There are some men who can take this occasional failure in stride, particularly if they or their partner attribute it to stress, fatigue, or alcohol. Men who react in this way, however, are far outnumbered by those who experience a degree of anxiety often close to panic, even at the time of their first experience with erectile failure. They quickly fear that they are impotent, nor are they immediately concerned with the cause, or whether the problem is psychological or organic. To test themselves they and often their partner will put pressure on themselves to perform, with concomitant anxiety that almost guarantees failure. Some men withdraw from any sexual activity because of the fear of failure; others, instead of abandoning themselves to the pleasure of the encounter, become monitors of their penile activity (or lack of it), and become spectators rather than participants in the sexual experience. This spectator role, identified in 1970 by Masters and Johnson, plays an important role in psychogenic erectile difficulties and serves also to interfere with the remaining erectile capacity of patients with organic conditions.[1]

As described by Kaplan,[11] for example, the patient who is partially impotent because of a mild circulatory deficiency frequently reacts to this diminished erectile capacity with panic, thereby worsening the physical disability. For this reason, the psychological aspects of an erectile problem should be evaluated in all cases of erectile difficulty, even when the cause is organic.[2] A trial of sex therapy often can avoid a long and expensive diagnostic study. As stated by Perelman,[3] in our zest to pursue technological innovation and surgery, it is critical not to lose sight of the mind and body's ability

Management of Impotence and Infertility, edited by Douglas Whitehead and Harris Nagler,

to compensate successfully for its own deficits. The trend toward "medicalization" must be tempered by the recognition that sex therapy may still be the treatment of choice for some impotent men with documented organic deficits.

With the passage of time, the term *impotence* is no longer the preferred term among many sexologists, because of its pejorative implications and its basic inaccuracy, because impotence is rarely global. For the same reasons, the term *frigidity* has been almost completely discarded in the case of women.

The new nomenclature reflects the fact that erectile difficulties are not regarded as a complete lack of function but viewed as a mixture of desire and arousal problems that are experienced as a partial or complete inability to obtain or maintain an erection sufficient for penetration. In recognition of this point of view the diagnostic criteria for male erectile disorder (302.72) DSM-III is as follows:

1. Persistent or recurrent or complete failure in a male to obtain or maintain an erection until completion of the sexual activity.
2. Persistent or recurrent lack of a subjective sense of sexual excitement or pleasure in a male during sexual activity.[4]

Psychological erectile dysfunction can be either primary and lifelong or secondary. Primary dysfunction means the man has never had an erection sufficient for penetration, and secondary dysfunction erectile means that there have been successful episodes over time (ranging from once to 20 or 30 years). Secondary impotence has been reported as being far more prevalent than primary impotence. Renshaw[5] reported that 3.5% of men seeking treatment for erectile disorders received a diagnosis of primary erectile dysfunction, compared to 48% of the sample, who received a secondary diagnosis.

Those who suffer from primary erectile difficulty do not fit into any specific diagnostic category but do have in common a sense of shame and humiliation, and rarely discuss their situation, even with a physician. Often, they have fantasies of injuring or being injured during the sexual act or they have a history of sexual abuse or trauma. Others have deep fears of closeness and intimacy and avoid social as well as sexual relationships. There is sometimes confusion about their sexual orientation or gender identity. In general, the management of these patients is best served by individual therapy (unless of course they present with a partner in an unconsummated marriage).

Premature ejaculation is not a form of impotency, although it is sometimes erroneously classified as such. Most men without ejaculatory control do not also experience difficulty getting erections, but some men have both problems. Erections are difficult to get and ejaculations are usually quick. Since many of the exercises for developing control require an erection, men with both problems should not attempt to work on gaining ejaculatory control until the erection problem is resolved.[6] In some instances, after years of ejaculatory problems, erectile problems develop.

Similarly, retarded ejaculation is not a form of impotency. On the contrary, a man with this problem has good erections but is unable to ejaculate, either inside the vagina, in the presence of a partner, or (rarely) at all.

Secondary erectile dysfunction, when it is psychological, manifests itself in many diverse ways. Rarely a man may not get an erection under any circumstances. More commonly, he will get an erection, and then lose it when he attempts penetration, or shortly thereafter. He may have good morning and nocturnal erections, and have no problem with masturbation or in his response to erotic visual stimulation. He may be successful with one partner and not another, as, for example, with an extramarital partner, but not his wife, or the opposite. He may be able to function only with a partner of his own sex.

There are special circumstances under which a man might not be able to function, although, in general, he has no erectile difficulty.

The Aging Male

For example, in the aging male, normal age-related changes sometimes are mistaken for erectile dysfunction—an error that can be made by the physician who does not make a thorough assessment of the problem presented. It takes the male over age 50 longer to obtain an erection. He does not respond as he did at an earlier age to visual stimulation but requires much more direct, intense genital stimulation. He does not ejaculate with each encounter, and his refractory period is longer. Frequency of intercourse is often reduced, although this varies, as do all these changes, from one individual to another. Desire may wane over time, but it can also be strong for some men until late into old age. If these changes are not understood by the man and his partner, and his physician, they can be interpreted as sexual dysfunction.

Management

The first step after the physician's careful history taking and medical examination is to inform the man and his partner (when one is available) of the normal effects of aging on sexuality. For this kind of situation, seen frequently in the sex therapist's office, the main task of the therapist is educational and supportive. In addition, the female partner's attitude needs to be taken into consideration. She may not be aware that the normal changes that occur with aging do not translate into impotence. She needs to be helped to offer the direct genital stimulation that is necessary and may be inhibited about offering this because of her own background and sexual attitudes. She may be focusing only on her partner's "impotence" and feel angry or contemptuous toward him. Unless her own feelings are explored and dealt with, she is not very likely to be able to help her partner regain potency. She also may be anxious about her own sexual functioning at this stage of life. All these interconnected issues need to be attended to, to help the aging couple. Both need to learn that at an older age, just as at any age, erection, insertion, and ejaculation are not the only way of giving and receiving pleasure, and that oral and manual stimulation can expand sexual horizons and be a source of gratification for many years to come.

Erectile Difficulties due to Infertility

During the period when a couple is trying to conceive, erectile problems may emerge, often for the first time. Usually, pressure is put on the man to perform on demand either by himself or his partner, possibly both. He may not be in the mood, may feel tired or stressed, or may be angry at his wife. He feels their sexual activity involves doing a job, not making love, and he cannot respond with the required erection. For some men, ambivalence about parenthood may also precipitate erectile failure.

When conception does not take place after several years of "trying," the couple's sexuality is subject to question not only by the couple themselves, but by family and friends. During the fertility work-up their sex life is put under minute scrutiny by strangers. Whatever the nature of their sexual life, questions arise within the couple themselves as to their sexual behavior and relating and examining every detail are both humiliating and anxiety producing. They begin to question "What kind of woman am I," and "Am I a normal man that I can't produce a child." Erectile difficulties frequently develop during this period. Many men lose their erection even at the anticipation of sex on demand. Temperature taking often adds to the pressure to perform.

As reported by Amelar and Dubin,[7] in a significant percentage of cases of male infertility the problem is found to be inadequate sexual performance, a factor often overlooked in male infertility. In the group they studied, the most frequent cause of the inadequate sexual performance was impotence. The authors report that in one group, intercourse was ordinarily adequate, but the husband experienced either erectile or retarded ejaculation, or both during the fertile period of his wife's cycle.

Management

For men, the double stigma of erectile failure and infertility leads to feelings of depression, anger, and isolation. In the infertility work-up, recognition of the man's feelings and of the woman's intense frustration and offering an opportunity to ventilate these feelings may help to minimize the stress and any possible iatrogenic sexual or emotional problems that arise during the work-up.

The couple can be encouraged to take a vacation from having intercourse only on "the right days" and in the "right positions." Many fertility specialists recommend having intercourse because of desire, regardless of ovulation. Another recommendation when the male is having erectile problems is for the female to minimize the information she gives him about her time of ovulation, so that hopefully he will have less anxiety about the approaching task.

They can have lovemaking sessions that do not involve intercourse from time to time, so that sex becomes a loving experience rather than only a job. The male will often get a good erection from oral or manual stimulation and ejaculate outside the vagina, helping to restore his confidence as well as giving him sexual pleasure.[8]

Two other special circumstances under which a potent male may be unable to function are the madonna–whore syndrome and the unconsummated marriage.

The Madonna–Whore Syndrome

In 1912, Freud pointed out that there are some men who are sexually aroused only or chiefly with women who are of a lower social class than they are, whom they regard as outside their social milieu, somewhat degraded, and, in essence, different from their mothers and sisters, hence the madonna–whore category.[9]

This is often experienced by these men after they become engaged or married, or when the wife becomes a mother. Sexually potent before these times, they can no longer function with their wife, but are potent with partners outside of the marriage, whom they view especially as cheap or exotic. It is as if a wife or mother is too pure for sexual activity, even though feelings of love and tenderness are present. The deep-seated, unconscious aspects of this does not yield significantly to sex therapy but requires more intensive individual treatment.

The Unconsummated Marriage

It is estimated that about 10% of couples who seek sex therapy have an unconsummated marriage.[10] They have never had intercourse, although some are orgasmic with oral and genital stimulation, but there has never been penetration. Others avoid sexual activity after having failed many times at their attempts to consummate the marriage. Often, many of these couples are ignorant about sexual anatomy, not even knowing exactly where the vagina is located, despite the fact that many are educated and successful people. They may have a good relationship in other aspects of their life together, but feel a sense of shame and difference from other couples. Usually, it is only because of desperation about having a child that they seek help. Frequently, their complaint is that the male partner is impotent. Careful assessment and physical examination usually reveals that the woman has vaginismus, causing an impenetrable barrier, which makes penetration impossible.

Management

The success of the treatment of the unconsummated relationship is highly dependent on seeing the couple together. Each one has to become aware of his or her contribution to the problem. Usually, they share a lack of sexual experience, ignorance about sexual anatomy and physiology, and a concept of sex as forbidden, often based on early parental and religious admonitions. They may have fantasies that sex is dangerous and that they can injure or be injured. Each partner needs to get accurate information, and become knowledgeable about their own bodies and that of their partner. The latter can be effectively achieved by the couple's being examined in front of each other by the gynecologist or the internist. The vaginismus demonstrated to the male helps him to realize that his inability to penetrate is not solely his problem, because he sees what happens when the speculum cannot be inserted because of the woman's tightening her pubococcygeal muscle. She too then becomes aware of her contribution to the problem. Learning about her vaginal anatomy also helps the man in dealing with the problem of nonconsummation.

Also their fantasies about injury are often dispelled when they learn more about their sexual anatomy. The success rate of the treatment of the unconsummated marriage is high.

Widower's Syndrome

Another special circumstance when erectile failure may surface for the first time is when a man begins a relationship with a new sexual partner after the death of his spouse. It is such a common occurrence that it has been dubbed by Masters and Johnson[1] "the widower's syndrome." Guilty about his being the survivor and seeking sexual pleasure with another partner often serves to inhibit a satisfactory sexual response. He may feel anxious about her finding him desirable. Divorced men may experience the same problem with new partners. In both situations, there may be some degree of shame about the inappropriateness of the partner, who is often a much younger woman. Added to this is the pressure he puts on himself to please the partner, at the same time that he feels inadequate as a lover. He may feel humiliated that he cannot perform at a level more characteristic of a younger man or in the way he did 20 or 30 years before.

An opportunity to verbalize his fears and anxieties, reassurance, and giving him permission to have pleasure again help to deal with his guilt feelings and often are sufficient for his potency to be restored, particularly if he is advised not to see sex as a performance and to focus on himself rather than on pleasing his partner in the initial stages of their relationship. Often, the female partner puts pressure on the male because of her need to arouse desire in the widower who is showing interest in her. Another contributing factor to the widowed or divorced male's erectile difficulty that needs to be investigated is the possibility that the female partner, if she is middle-aged or older and has not been sexually active recently, may have some fear of penetration because of discomfort caused by an atrophic vagina, which results in a degree of vaginismus, making penetration difficult and causing the male to lose his erection. An atropic vagina can be successfully treated by a gynecologist.

Other special circumstances that may cause erectile problems are illness of the male or the illness of his partner, particularly a serious illness or a chronic ongoing condition that dulls sexual desire of both partners. The loss of a job, or the fear of losing a job, can also play a role in erectile difficulties.

Depression is often the accompaniment of an erectile problem. To plan effective management of an erectile dysfunction, it is necessary to assess whether the depression is an expected consequence of the problem or is the depression a causal factor. If a clinical depression is present, it needs to be treated before sex therapy is undertaken.

Treatment Strategies

There is no universal treatment modality that is appropriate for all cases of psychogenic erectile difficulty. Each man has a unique history; his problem presents itself in a unique way and is influenced by his psychological state, the degree or absence of physical contributions, and the complications of his relationship with his partner or the absence of one.

Not only is each patient different, but therapists differ markedly in their experience, their skill, and their theoretical orientation.

Prior to Masters and Johnson's important contribution to the treatment of sexual dysfunction in Human Sexual Inadequacy,[1] all sexual problems, including erectile difficulties, were considered to be due to deep-seated psychological conflicts and psychoanalysis was regarded as the treatment of choice. Masters and Johnson postulated that simpler causes, less deeply rooted, accounted for many sexual difficulties with which people struggled. They considered performance anxiety, fear of failure, overconcern with pleasing their partner, anger, poor communication, and ignorance about sexual anatomy and physiology major immediate causes of erectile problems.

Their form of treatment differed in two major ways from most other forms of therapy—a time-limited format (originally 2 weeks but now often as long as 6 months) and the assignment of specific, graduated erotic exercises to be carried out at home and discussed in subsequent therapy sessions. Emphasis in the early stages of treatment is on a non-demand, non-goal-oriented approach with intercourse prohibited during this period.

Although there have been adaptations and enhancements of the treatment of psychological erectile dysfunction, all approaches owe an enormous debt to Masters and Johnson[1] and contain many elements of their therapeutic principles. The most important subsequent development was the work of Kaplan[11] in The New Sex Therapy, who agreed with Masters and Johnson's focus on immediate causes but also placed emphasis on psychological contributions and theorized that there were also unconscious determinants of erectile problems that existed in many cases from mild conditions such as anger, guilt over sexual activity and pleasure, and performance anxiety to deeper sources, such as severe relationship problems, castration anxiety, oedipal conflicts, incest taboos, and severe psychiatric conditions.

Some of these more serious conditions are not considered suitable for brief sex therapy. However, experience has demonstrated that it is possible in some instances, with proper assessment and sufficient therapeutic skill, to "bypass" some of the underlying problems and help a patient recover his potency without resolving major problems.

Some Contradictions to Sex Therapy

Some contraindications to sex therapy include clinical depression, severe physical illness, substance abuse, major active psychopathology, and severe hostility in a couple's interaction.

Performance anxiety seems to be the path that leads to impotence, no matter what the nature of the contributing factors. Once a man becomes concerned as to whether he will be able to achieve an erection, the fear permeates his mind, so that he cannot respond to the sexual stimulation he is receiving. His thought process goes over and over the questions of whether or not he will have an erection this time, what if he fails again, what is she going to think, and what if I'm "over the hill."

The powerful treatment strategy that Masters and Johnson developed, still basic to many therapeutic approaches to erectile dysfunction, was labeled *sensate focus.* The words exquisitely define the purpose of the experience—to focus on sensations. To the man troubled by performance anxiety and the fear of another failure, and to his troubled partner, when there is one, afraid and uncertain as to how to approach him, it offers a nondemand, nonthreatening experience with its sole purpose the attention to the pleasure of touching and being touched, giving and receiving pleasure, without any expectation of performance, or the achievement of an erection, insertion, and orgasm.

The patient is encouraged to be "selfish," to focus on his own sensations rather than to be preoccupied with his partner's responses.

Sensate focus exercises need to be individually designed. For example, a couple who has not had any physical contact for months or even years and who may not even share the same bed will need to have considerable help before taking the first step toward becoming intimate again. The communication that is opened up in this process has in itself curative power.

This nondemanding, non-goal-oriented experience can be extremely pleasurable. However, there are responses sometimes that are negative and therefore the experience needs to be discussed fully in the following therapy session. These negative responses may arise from the hostile relationship of the couple, the individual psychological problems of one or the other such as fear of intimacy, anxiety about becoming involved physically again, etc. These negative reactions need to be resolved before treatment can continue, and dealing with these resistances is often the core of the treatment process.

The next exercise involves genital touching—gentle, teasing, and nondemanding. Its purpose is to produce arousal, not necessarily an erection. Since arousal is often impeded in the male with erectile problems by the fear of failure, this exercise emphasizes playfulness and demonstrates two important factors to the man worrying about his erectile ability:

1. His erectile capacity is unimpaired under nonpressured circumstances.
2. Erections can come and go. If they subside, they can return if stimulation continues and panic does not set in. This is a normal process in lovemaking.

The next exercise is a continuation of the same principle.

The female partner brings the man to an erection with oral or genital stimulation. She is advised to move to other parts of his body and to let the erection subside somewhat, returning again to penile stimulation. This erect-and-subside play is repeated several times and helps to convince both of them that the male can regain an erection, even if it subsides. This exercise can also be tried by the single man while he is masturbating.

When the male has gained more confidence from these nondemanding experiences, when there is a partner, she is advised to take the "on top" position. Her knees should be at the level of his nipple line (lower if she is shorter). When an erection occurs, she is to bend forward, slide down on the penis, and insert it into her vagina. The male should concentrate on his pleasurable sensations with little concern about the state of the erection. At this stage, vigorous thrusting to orgasm is discouraged; rather, each partner should focus on sensation.

The move toward coitus may produce some initial anxiety. The man is given the option of continuing the same play as in the previous exercise or ejaculating in the vagina if he chooses to. He is encouraged once more to be "selfish" at this stage, to choose the position, the pace, and the rhythm best for him and to employ whatever fantasy is most arousing for him. As he gains more security, his partner's needs and desires are given more attention.

Because it has been so publicized as an integral part of sex therapy, the erotic exercises are sometimes regarded as all of sex therapy. Some men do regain their sexual potency as a result of the experiences and the handling of the anxieties and resistances by a skilled therapist. Other men's anxieties are not overcome by these exercises without considerable working through of intrapsychic and interpersonal issues. Sometimes treatment is sabotaged by a hostile partner or a partner who may feel threatened by the restored potency of her mate, whether this is achieved by psychotherapy, an implant, or an injection.

With patients who have some degree of organic pathology, "overcoming initial fears of failure can be more profound." Men with organic deficits are more likely to lose erections periodically and are more likely to have intermittent difficulty with potency even with successful treatment.[3]

Growing out of an awareness that reduction of performance anxiety was not always successful and a greater awareness of the complexity of psychological erectile failure, many therapists have begun to integrate the treatment of erectile failure into their particular therapeutic approach. Brief summaries of other approaches can be found in Rosen and Lieblum[12] and elsewhere.

Cognitive–Behavioral Therapy

Within the field of sex therapy the cognitive–behavioral approach led to an emphasis on the patient's thinking about sex. The emphasis grew out of the recognition that reduction of anxiety did not always result in success. Erectile failure could also be the result of the patient's cognitions about sex—unrealistic expectations, negative self-images, distortions of the opposite sex's needs or requirements, and tendencies toward catastrophic thinking. These, then, are the major foci of cognitive–behavioral therapy.[12]

Hypnotherapy

Hypnosis is another method that is used in the treatment of erectile disorders. Not included in the training and experience of most sex therapists, these are therapists with special training and skill in the use of hypnotic interventions. Hypnosis is generally defined as a focused state of awareness called "trance," usually but not always induced by relaxation techniques. In a trance state, the mind is more receptive to suggestions, provided that they are value consistent. A variety of techniques are used.

Those who practice hypnotherapy often give their patients tapes to use at home.

Group Therapy

When practical concerns, particularly of financial limitations and lack of a partner are present, a group approach is often used and can be of special value to single men.

Considerations

In the past few decades, much progress has been made in helping people accept their sexuality as a natural function to be enjoyed beyond its reproductive purpose. Freud[13] threw light on its importance as a central focus of men and women's mental health from infancy to old age and revolutionized our whole concept of sexuality. Kinsey[14] gave us statistics on the sexual behavior of men and women for the first time. Masters and Johnson[1] described sexual anatomy and physiology as previous researchers had described almost every other system of the human body; they were pioneers in giving "permission" to enjoy sex and pioneered in the treatment of human sexual inadequacy. Then came the medicalization of male sexual problems—an attempt to "fix the apparatus." Again, great strides have been made in that direction, promising even more effective ways of making erectile functioning effective under every circumstance. New ways of handling lack of sexual desire are being studied in research laboratories across the country.

Future treatment methods need to reduce the dichotomy between biogenic and psychological factors. Experts in the field, no matter which discipline, need to move away from the concept that sex is a performance rather than the most intimate form of communication between two people.

In our increasing awareness of the complexity of the operative factors and possible etiologies of the problem of erectile dysfunction, we need to place greater emphasis on the value of a multidisciplinary approach in our treatment format. As described by Whitehead,[15] "At any one point in time in a particular patient the impotence may be due to one organic etiology, more than one organic etiology, one psychogenic etiology, more than one psychogenic etiology or any combination of the preceding."

REFERENCES

1. Masters WH, Johnson VE: Human sexual inadequacy. Boston: Little, Brown, 1970.
2. Kaplan HS: The evaluation of sexual disorders: Psychological and medical aspects. New York: Brunner–Mazel, 1983: 229–231.
3. Perelman MA: Rehabilitative sex therapy for organic impotence. In: Segraves T, Haeberle E, eds. Emerging dimensions of sexology. New York: Praeger, 1984.
4. Diagnostic and Statistical Manual of Mental Disorders (DSM-III-R), American Psychiatric Association, 1987: 94.
5. Renshaw DC: Profile of 2,376 patients treated at Loyola Sex Clinic between 1972 and 1987. Sex Marital Ther, 1988; 3:111–117.
6. Zilbergeld B: The new male sexuality. New York: Bantam Books, 1992: 411–412.
7. Amelar RD, Dubin L: When Male Sexual Disfunction Causes Infertility. Cont OB/GYN 1974; 4:85.
8. Golden GH: Psychosexual problems in infertility: A preventive model. J Sex Education Ther. 1983, 9:1; 19–22.
9. Freud S: On the universal tendency to debasement in the sphere of love. In: Strachey J, ed. The standard edition of the complete works of Sigmund Freud. Vol. XL. London: The Hogarth Press, 1957: 177–190.
10. Masters W: Personal communication.
11. Kaplan HS: The new sex therapy. New York: Brunner/Mazel, 1974.
12. Rosen RE, Lieblum SR, eds. Erectile disorders: Assessment and treatment. New York: Guilford Press, 1922; 175.
13. Freud S: Three essays on the theory of sexuality (1905). In: Strachey J, ed. The standard edition of the complete works of Sigmund Freud. Vol XI. London: The Hogarth Press, 1957.
14. Kinsey A, et al.: Sexual behavior in the human male. Philadelphia: WB Saunders, 1953.
15. Whitehead ED: The need for cooperative professional relationships in diagnosing and treating male sexual dysfunction. NY State J Med 1991; 91(2).

ANNOTATED BIBLIOGRAPHY

LoPiccolo J: Postmodern sex therapy for erectile failure. In: Rosen RC, Liebrum SR, eds. Erectile disorders, assessment and treatment. New York: Guilford Press, 1992.

In a chapter on what he terms "Postmodern Sex Therapy," LoPiccolo notes that three elements are particularly involved in a new approach to sex therapy: the functional analysis of the positive value that the erectile problem may have for the couple and the individual partners, the diagnosis of both the physical and the psychological contributions to the erectile problem, and the actual sexual behavior patterns engaged in by the couple. He postulates that this new approach has developed out of a concern that the Masters and Johnson mode may not be as effective currently due to the more complex cases presenting for therapy today.

McCarthy BW: Erectile dysfunction and inhibited sexual desire. J Sex Education Ther 1992; 18(1) 22–34.

When secondary erectile dysfunction is accompanied by secondary inhibited desire, cognitive–behavioral strategies and techniques are prescribed and well illustrated in this article. Cognitions about being an intimate team, accepting variability in individual and couple self-expression, and setting realistic expectations are emphasized.

16 The Role of the Psychiatrist in the Diagnosis and Treatment of Male Sexual Dysfunction

Paul Salkin

Background

Only in the past generation have sexual dysfunctions become amenable to proper diagnosis and treatment. Psychiatric intervention was generally ineffectual prior to the pioneering and classic work of Masters and Johnson.[1] Their research clarifies crucial aspects of the sexual feelings, arousal–excitation mechanisms, and orgasm in both men and women. It was especially in the woman that illumination and clarification were necessary and innovative. And, in this later respect, symptoms of disorder in the man, and the need for treatment, became apparent as a factor in many cases of dysfunction in the woman.[2]

Current Concepts

The Diagnostic Manual of the American Psychiatric Association (DSM 111-R) defines sexual dysfunction as "an inhibition in the appetitive or psychophysiological changes that characterize the complete sexual response cycle."[3] Although the manual goes on to state that the diagnosis is not made if the sexual dysfunction is attributed entirely to organic factors (such as a physical disorder or medications) this is unduly restrictive. It is now estimated that a majority of cases of the male sexual dysfunction are in fact of organic etiology (approximately 70%), as opposed to the reverse ratio (30%) in studies of a generation ago.[4]

The Manual's categories of sexual dysfunction offer an excellent means of conceptualizing and organizing diagnostic and therapeutic approaches. The opportunity therefore should not be lost in using the categories to differentiate the dysfunctions. The issue of etiology should be clarified in the diagnostic evaluation, determining the presence or absence of organic factors.

Masters and Johnson divided the male and female sexual response into four stages. In the

Management of Impotence and Infertility, edited by Douglas Whitehead and Harris Nagler,

male the stages proceed in this sequence:

1. Excitement: There is onset of erotic feelings and onset of erection, the scrotum thickens, and the testes elevate.
2. Plateau: This occurs prior to orgasm. Erection is firm and the penile shaft is extended to maximum size. Drops of mucoid fluid appear.
3. Orgasm: There are two components: the sensation of "ejaculatory inevitability" followed by the orgasm proper: three to seven spurts of semen at 0.8 second intervals.
4. Resolution: The body returns to its resting stage, the testes and penis detumesce, and in the male a refractory period of sexual stimulation sets in.

Kaplan has more recently described the sexual response as having an additional component. This conceptualization adds to the understanding and classification of the sexual dysfunctions. She adds the component of sexual desire to the more obvious phases of excitation–plateau and orgasm–resolution. The various sexual dysfunctions can be viewed as impairments of one of the two phases, and of inhibited sexual desire. Lief has reported that 40% of patients applying for help with sexual problems suffer from inhibited sexual desire.[5]

Desire phase inhibition produces low sexual drive and diminished libido. Arousal–excitement phase inhibition leads to erectile dysfunction and orgasm phase disruption produces premature and retarded ejaculation.[5]

Diagnosis

The American Psychiatric Association Manual recognizes five sexual dysfunctions in the male—two in the desire phase, one in the arousal–excitation phase, and two in the orgasm phase. The numbers refer to the diagnostic codes.[3]

Sexual Desire Disorders

302.71—Hypoactive Sexual Desire Disorder: Persistent or recurrently deficient or absent sexual fantasies and desire for sexual activity. The judgment of deficiency or absence is made by the clinician, taking into account factors that affect sexual functioning, such as age, sex, and the context of the person's life.

302.79—Sexual Aversion Disorder: Persistent or recurrent extreme aversion to, and avoidance of, all, or almost all, genital sexual contact with a sexual partner.

Sexual Arousal Disorders

302.72—Male Erectile Disorder:[1] Persistent or recurrent partial or complete failure in a male to attain or maintain erection until completion of the sexual activity.[2] Persistent or recurrent lack of a subjective sense of sexual excitement and pleasure in a male during sexual activity.

Orgasm Disorders

302.74—Inhibited Male Orgasm: Persistent or recurrent delay in, or absence of, orgasm in a male following a normal sexual excitement phase during sexual activity that the clinician, taking into account the person's age, judges to be adequate in focus, intensity, and duration. The failure to achieve orgasm is usually restricted to an inability to reach orgasm in the vagina, with orgasm possible with other types of stimulation, such as masturbation.

302.75—Premature Ejaculation: Persistent or recurrent ejaculation with minimal sexual stimulation, or before, on, or shortly after penetration and before the person wishes it. The clinician must take into account factors that affect duration of the excitement phase such as age, novelty of the sexual partner or situation, and frequency of sexual activity.

Diagnosis and treatment of sexual dysfunctions require training and experience. Clearly the sex therapist who is credentialled and/or certified in the field will have this training. The psychiatrist may have had elective training in the residency period, or may seek training at a later point. The establishment of sex therapy training programs in residency would go a long way to enabling the average psychiatrist to treat these common clinical disorders to best effect, as would the establishment of a Council on Human Sexuality and Treatment in the American Psychiatric Association.

The Patient

The patient may present to the sex therapist/psychiatrist in one of these ways:

1. The presence of a dysfunction may become apparent in the psychotherapy or psychiatric management of the patient for another condition (depression, anxiety, psychosis, personality disorder, marital disorder, or general problems in living).
2. The individual with a dysfunction may be self-referred—or referred by another professional—with no adequate sexual dysfunction diagnostic workup.
3. The individual with a dysfunction has had an adequate diagnostic workup and is referred for specific sexual therapy and/or concomitant treatment of an emotional disorder that may contribute to sexual dysfunction, such as anxiety or depression.

In this latter case, diagnostic workup has been performed. But in the first two instances a thorough workup is necessary to determine whether organic factors are present, as they, in fact, are in 70% of men presenting with sexual dysfunction. The psychiatrist should be familiar with all aspects of the medical workup.[4,6]

History

A medical, psychological, and sexual history should be taken. The presence of the sexual partner is highly desirable as crucial details may be overlooked or repressed by the patient.

The chief complaint should be identified and note made of abrupt or gradual onset, intermittency, persistence, and progression. The erections should be graded on a scale of 1–10 (no erection to normal, rigid turgid erection). Fantasies, objects of desire, and sexual experiences and infidelities should be elicited, and this is usually best done in a private session with each partner.

Medical history may reveal organic risk factors: arteriosclerosis, heart disease, vascular disease, diabetes, hypertension, and hypercholesterolemia. Cigarette smoke and alcohol abuse are risk factors. Medications must all be listed as many impair sexual function.

Psychological and psychosexual history should also be taken. All details of early childhood experiences, sexual molestation, assault, and incestuous and homosexual experiences, should be obtained. A history of sexually transmitted disease is crucial.

The therapist should be aware of the details of the physical examination and laboratory studies—which may be done by the internist or urologist. Ideally the internist and urologist should have experience with sexual dysfunctions and their proper workup. The physical examination should emphasize urologic, vascular, endocrine, and neurologic evaluation. The findings and their implications must be known by the therapist. This is best accomplished by discussion with the examining physician and regular follow-up rather than by simply reading the reports. Laboratory tests include urinalysis, CBC, SMA-26 with coronary risk profile, testosterone, prolactin, FSH, estrogen, LH, T3, T4, and TSH. In all cases in which a suspicion of organic factors is present, a nocturnal penile tumescence study is essential.

The clinical psychiatric evaluation is essential to diagnose a concomitant psychiatric disorder. Thus history of present illness, family history, medical history, and mental status examination are performed. A diagnosis is made using the five axes of the DSM-111 Diagnostic Schema. Axis I evaluates the clinical syndrome, axis II evaluates the personality disorder (or developmental disorder), and axis III lists physical disorders and conditions. These three axes represent the official APA diagnostic assessment. Axis IV assesses the severity of psychosocial stressors from one to catastrophic (1 to 9). Axis V is a global assessment of functioning scale from absent symptoms to persistent danger of severe harm to self and/or others (90 to 1).[3]

Treatment of Sexual Disorders

The modern treatment of sexual dysfunctions began with the work of Masters and Johnson in the 1950s and 1960s. Efforts in the past through psychoanalysis and psychotherapy were usually not helpful in the treatment of these disorders. Masters and Johnson made this treatment a reality and also helped to define the variety of sexual dysfunctions that we find in our patients. The name that Masters and Johnson gave to their treatment program is *Sensate Focus.* This term defines a series of exercises that are presented by the sex therapist to the couple in a progressive manner over the course of several weeks of treatment. These exercises are the backbone of our treatment and each specific disorder will require some degree of modification in the specific application to the therapy of each condition. But, in general, the program will have a profound effect on the couple, enhancing intimacy, reducing anxiety related to performance, and helping the maturation of the mutual relationship. These exercises were first described in the classic work Human Sexual Inadequacies.[2] The essential features of this exercise program are a reduction of performance anxiety by initially prohibiting genital stimulation and genital sexual activity. There is a gradual progression over the course of several weeks. Thorough discussion of the exercise steps and any problems that may arise in the couple is done with the therapist in weekly sessions. Sessions start with caressing of all parts of the body first by one partner, then the other, excluding the genital areas. The sessions then progress through to the experience of genital stimulation and ultimately intromission culminating in actual coital activity. The first stage or Sensate Focus I is nongenital stimulation on a mutual basis on the part of one partner and then the other. All parts of the body are caressed and stimulated sensually but the genitals and the breasts are off limits. This prohibition goes a long way to reducing sexual performance anxiety and bringing the couple into a more intimate, warm and loving, and mutually satisfying situation. When the therapist believes that this stage has been adequately mastered by the couple they move on to Sensate Focus II with genital stimulation. Since there is no actual penetration, sexual performance anxiety continues to remain subdued and when this stage is adequately experienced and the couple feels ready the next stage is introduced, namely the stage of vaginal containment with insertion of the penis but with no movement.

Finally stage IV, vaginal containment with movement, is introduced when the therapist feels this is appropriate, and often the couple themselves come to this stage with some degree of spontaneity. There is no doubt that training in sex therapy and experience on the part of the sex therapist are necessary for the competent treatment of a couple in this manner. These exercises represent homework assignments that the therapist gives to the couple during weekly therapy sessions for the couple to take home with them. They are to be performed at least three times a week with a report on their progress in subsequent sessions. Effective treatment will take place with 10–20 sessions. Helen Kaplan[7] has introduced a second parameter in sex therapy, namely the addition of a psychodynamic approach that appears to be of considerable help in those conditions where the simple behavior modification aspects of the Sensate Focus program are not sufficient to bring about positive results. Dr. Kaplan's approach achieves a synthesis of behavior modification with a solid foundation in dynamic psychology for a fuller understanding of the patient and the meaning of their conflicts and symptoms. This leads to an understanding on the part of the patient that solidifies positive results. Thus a combination of the classic Masters and Johnson's Sensate Focus techniques with psychodynamic psychotherapy forms the basis of the treatment of most of the disorders that will be described.

Treatment of Specific Disorders

Inhibited Sexual Desire

The treatment of this disorder often requires many more sessions than the treatment of the other conditions.[5] The basis of the treatment is the Sensate Focus exercise program. Treatment is usually not brief and marital and individual therapy may often be necessary for each of the partners. A trial of a few sessions of sex therapy can be useful because it will help to focus on the specific difficulties that exist in either partner. A trial treatment experience can be an excellent diagnostic tool as well as a prognosticator of future results. It is in this condition that a synthesis of sex therapy and behavior modification with psychodynamic therapy is most indicated. The tasks of sex therapy in a progressive and graduated approach are discussed in great detail during the therapy sessions. Attempts are made also to discuss the inner significance of the symptoms often through the use of dream analysis and analysis of the symptoms themselves. It may with time become clear that the inhibited sexual desire is a reflection of a phobic avoidance mechanism. When this becomes apparent a therapeutic approach to relieve the phobia can be helpful in combination with the use of medication such as a tricyclic antidepressant, or one of the anxiety-relieving medications of the benzodiazepine class. The latter medications protect the patient from anticipatory anxiety while the former antidepressant medication class can significantly relieve the actual phobia and panic attack that is the basis of many of these disorders.

One more approach should be mentioned, which at this point must be considered to be investigational. That would be the use for this disorder for self-injection therapy with papaverine or prostaglandin E[1] and sometimes with phentolamine. While this approach has been used for the treatment of organic dysfunction of the erectile process with considerable success, more recently attempts have been made to utilize this treatment modality in certain of the erectile dysfunctions that are purely psychogenic in nature. The almost certain predictable and spontaneous erection that occurs following injection and that is influenced to a minimal extent by anxiety and emotional conflict can be utilized in the man, but actually for the couple, to reduce the uncertainty that frequently plagues their sexual experience. Through this the male has a reduction of performance anxiety and develops a considerable degree of confidence in his erectile functioning. The state of certainty regarding the erection can contribute greatly to a reduction in the woman's anxiety levels and consequent inhibition of her own feelings. By bringing about a certain and predictable erection through this self-injection technique the therapist can continue to work with the couple in a productive way regarding the hypoactive sexual desire with gradual reduction in the inhibitory state in the man and the development of his basic and natural potential for sexual arousal and enjoyment.

When inhibited sexual desire or hypoactive sexual desire is a function of an underlying depression, which it commonly is, antidepressant medication would be indicated. However, the majority of antidepressant medications can in fact cause diminution of sexual desire and sexual drive. One class of antidepressants, however, the dopamine-enhancing antidepressants, has been found to have no negative effects on sexuality in males treated for depression. The antidepressant bupropion (Wellbutrin) can be used quite effectively in this regard.[9] In selected cases where there would be no contraindications because of its cardiac effects, the drug yohimbine can be used as an aphrodisiac to stimulate hypoactive sexual desire. When the hypoactive sexual desire is a function of a continuing posttraumatic stress disorder, appropriate treatment with tricyclic medication to control the anxiety and depression symptoms of this disorder can be helpful to relieve the inhibited sexual desire that is so frequently an accompaniment of this disorder.

Sexual Aversion Disorder

This condition presents a great challenge to the couple as well as to the sex therapist. The treatment modalities utilized for the therapy of hypoactive sexual desire can all be utilized, but psychodynamic exploration of the roots of the aversion in the man must very definitely be pursued. Often this will be done best in individual therapy, and when some of these conflicts have begun to be worked through the combined conjoint therapy with the couple may proceed.

Male Erectile Disorder

The treatment of this disorder also has as its foundation the basic sex therapy approach of Sensate Focus progressive behavioral modification. The couple should be seen jointly. Reduction of anticipatory anxiety and phobic symptoms will be achieved through these exercises. The use of antianxiety agents and antipanic agents can be helpful. When antidepressants are used consideration should be given to those antidepressants such as bupropron that have minimal effect on sexuality. The use of self-injection therapy for the pharmacologic achievement of erection has become an important treatment modality. The certainty that an erection will be achieved has a profound anxiety-reducing effect in the couple, often leading to what has been described as the "jump-start effect." This refers to the finding that many men once they realize that they can have a predictable and satisfactory erection, can often go on to experience erections on their own without the necessity for continued use of the self-injection technique. Often male erectile dysfunction is a result of an underlying condition of premature ejaculation, which has caused anxiety in the male to such an extent that the actual erectile process itself becomes gradually interfered with. This situation is a common finding when men with an erectile disorder are studied. Therefore introducing a treatment modality that will ultimately help premature ejaculation can go far to alleviating the disorder of erectile dysfunction.

Premature Ejaculation

Two classic techniques have been employed for the treatment of this disorder. Masters and Johnson devised the squeeze technique, which can inhibit the excitatory state just prior to orgasm if a squeeze of sufficient firmness and pressure is applied either by the man or his partner to the erect penis. Perhaps a more satisfactory technique was devised by James Semans.[10] This is known as the stop–start technique. This can be practiced by the man alone without the partner present, utilizing self-stimulation to erection, allowing the erection to subside to approximately 50% of its full erectile state, continuing again with self-stimulation to the point of near orgasm, then stopping as described above. This is done three times, and on the fourth self-stimulatory trial full orgasm and ejaculation are permitted. When these exercises are done by the man on a regular basis he can usually achieve satisfactory control of his orgasm within a period of a month or so. Naturally this should be combined with appropriate sex therapy sessions for best results.

A very successful treatment approach for premature ejaculation has recently developed from the findings that certain antidepressant medications (specific serotonin reuptake inhibitors) such as fluoxetine (Prozac) have an inhibitory effect on orgasm both in the male and the female. The effect in the male of retarding the orgasmic state can thus be used often quite effectively in cases of premature ejaculation. Small doses of the antidepressant on a daily basis or use of the medication some hours prior to intercourse may be quite effective. The addition of trazadone (Desyrel) can be synergistic in bringing about the desired effect of prolonging the erectile state and facilitating orgasmic control.

Inhibited Male Orgasm or Retarded Ejaculation

The treatment of this disorder also is best done when sex therapy behavior modification techniques are combined with psychodynamic therapy. The aim of the treatment of this disorder is to achieve ejaculation in the man by whatever method is appropriate and successful for the couple when the two are in fact together in the same room rather than apart. Eventually ejaculation may be achieved through penile stimulation in close proximity to the vaginal entrance. Ultimately the penis is introduced into the vagina just prior to ejaculation. This treatment is described in The New Sex Therapy.[7]

Recently certain serotonin agents such as the antihistamine cyproheptadine (Periactin) have been used with success to bring about ejaculation in the male who suffers from inhibited orgasm. This drug can be used either on a regular basis or during the day in which sexual relations are to take place.

The treatment of the sexual disorders as described above can achieve considerable success in resolving difficulties both in the male and between the couple that a generation ago were doomed to failure. One cautionary note, however, must be presented.[4] These dysfunctions frequently have organic factors present. It is now recognized that the majority of these disorders have, to a greater or lesser degree, a significant organic component. Therefore it is essential that the sex therapist work in tandem with frequent consultation with a urologist who is familiar with the treatment and evaluation of the sexual disorders. They will clarify diagnosis and also put treatment on a rational basis. Furthermore, it will frequently lead to a combined approach utilizing modern pharmacological methods of treatment in combination with the psychological approach of behavior modification and psychodynamic psychotherapy.[8]

The Future of Sex Therapy and Psychiatry

It is ironic that the specialty of psychiatry, which owes so much to the discoveries of Sigmund Freud, has in the past decade shown a diminishing involvement in the field of sexuality and sex therapy. This is manifested by the absence in recent years of courses in human sexuality and sex therapy at the annual American Psychiatric Association meetings, as well as the rarity of relevant papers and contributions at the meetings and in psychiatric journals such as the American Journal of Psychiatry. The situation was quite different in the decade of the 1970s following the landmark studies of Masters and Johnson.

It is difficult to explain this progressive decline of interest by the profession, especially in view of recent advances in psychopharmacological treatments, which can be remarkably effective for the classic symptoms of male sexual dysfunction such as premature ejaculation, retarded ejaculation, and erectile disorders. It becomes all the more important for psychiatry to reinvolve itself in the field of sexual dysfunction because it is now more clear than in the past that the majority of disorders in the male have significant organic factors.

There are ways in which this situation can be corrected: First, the institution of a required period of training in psychiatric residency programs for sex therapy and studies in human sexuality can go a long way to emphasize the importance of the field to the psychiatrists in training. It would present the psychiatric resident with a time-limited course of treatment that can be used with a reasonable expectation of success. It would combine dynamic psychotherapy, behavior modification treatment, and the use of psychopharmacological treatment as well as appropriate consultation and liaison with departments of urology, neurology, internal medicine, and endocrinology. Furthermore, this will help the psychiatric resident become involved in the treatment of dysfunctions that are often neglected and overlooked, and that are the causes of considerable emotional suffering. It could also help the psychiatrist-in-training become more comfortable with and capable of managing sexualized transference and countertransference problems that are so frequent in the patient population that we treat. Second, it will be important to develop a committee within the Council on Psychiatric Services of the American Psychiatric Association that will focus on human sexuality and sex therapy. It is remarkable that such a committee does not exist at this time. The establishment of this committee would go a long way to reconnecting psychiatry with the field of human sexuality and sex therapy.

REFERENCES

1. Masters WH, Johnson V: The human sexual response. Boston: Little, Brown, 1966.
2. Masters WH, Johnson V: Human sexual inadequacy. Boston: Little, Brown, 1970.

3. Diagnostic and statistical manual, 3rd ed., revised. Washington, DC: American psychiatric association. 1987: 290–294.
4. Whitehead ED et al.: Diagnostic evaluation of impotence. Postgraduate Medicine, 1990: 88:123–136.
5. Kaplan HS: Disorders of sexual desire. New York: Brunner/Mazel, 1979: 55–77.
6. Kaplan HS: The evaluation of sexual disorders. New York: Brunner/Mazel, 1983.
7. Kaplan HS: The new sex therapy. New York: Brunner/Mazel, 1974.
8. Whitehead ED et al.: Treatment alternatives for impotence. Postgraduate Medicine, 1990: 80:139–152.
9. Karasu B, ed.: Treatments of psychiatric disorders Vol. 3. Washington DC: American Psychiatric Association, 1989: 2343–2359.
10. Kaplan HS: The illustrated manual of sex therapy, 2nd ed. New York: Brunner/Mazel, 1987: 153.

ANNOTATED BIBLIOGRAPHY

Diagnostic and statistical manual of mental disorders, 3rd ed., revised. Washington, DC: American Psychiatric Association, 1987.

This volume has had an enormous influence throughout the world on the diagnostic categories and nomenclature of mental dysfunction. In the category of sexual dysfunctions there is a concise description of the four phases of the sexual response cycle. The phases of sexual dysfunctions themselves are categorized in such a manner that the treatment of each dysfunction can be specific and rational. The sexual disorders in the male are conceptualized in three significant categories: the sexual desire disorders, the sexual arousal disorders, and the orgasm disorders. The fourth edition of this work is expected within the next 2 to 3 years, but at this time this book can be considered as close to authoritative as any other in the field of psychiatric diagnosis.

Kaplan HS: The illustrated manual of sex therapy, 2nd ed. New York: Brunner/Mazel, 1987.

There is no doubt that this book is a classic in the field. It is useful for training in the field of sex therapy and is referred to frequently by therapists with considerable experience. Furthermore, it has great usefulness as a book that can be recommended to patients who are in the process of sex therapy. While studying it cannot be recommended as a substitute for sex therapy, it can be used with considerable profit by the couple in sex therapy who require a book for support and encouragement during the course of their treatment. The illustrations are an essential part of this work and can enable the therapist to describe graphically aspects of the sexual encounter.

Rosen RC, Leibium SR, eds: Erectile disorders. New York: Guilford Press, 1992.

An up to date and wide ranging textbook that covers the field with great clarity both from a psychological as well as from a medical and physiological point of view. Modern diagnostic procedures on the modalities of neurophysiological studies, endocrine and vascular work-up, and nocturnal penile tumescence diagnostic methods are covered in a thorough manner. Treatment methods are reviewed in detail, with excellent discussions of sex therapy and conjoint therapy techniques as well as modern psychopharmacologic, urologic, surgical, and self-injection therapy approaches. This book can be considered an authoritative textbook in the area of male sexual dysfunction.

Whitehead ED, et al.: Diagnostic evaluation of impotence: Treatments alternatives for impotence. Postgraduate Medicine, 1990: 88(2).

These articles present a rapid introduction to the field of male sexual dysfunction with a review of diagnostic procedures. Emphasis is on the variety of medical disorders which contribute to this dysfunction, as well as a listing of a large number of medications that are significant contributors to male sexual dysfunction. There is a review of modern treatment technique including classic sex therapy and psychotherapy approaches as well as pharmacologic management and urologic surgical procedures. A good introduction for the medical practitioner and a basis for further reading and studies.

Part II
Infertility

17 Medical Treatment for Male Infertility

Christina Wang
Ronald S. Swerdloff

Infertility is defined as the failure of a couple to achieve a pregnancy after at least 1 year of unprotected sexual intercourse. Female predominant factors account for about 30% and male predominant causes account for another 30% of infertile couples. In the remainder, factors may be present in both partners or no apparent cause can be identified (unexplained infertility). Since infertility is a problem of the couple, both the male and female partners should be assessed and managed simultaneously. In a report from a tertiary referral male infertility clinic[1] more than one-third of the female partners of the infertile men had conditions such as ovulatory problems, endometriosis, or unilateral tubal disease. Correction of these problems can lead to achievement of pregnancy even though the male factor has not been treated. The couple ideally should be managed in a multidisciplinary specialized infertility or reproductive medicine center. When this is not possible, the endocrinologist, andrologist, or urologist managing the male partner should work with the reproductive endocrinologist or gynecologist attending the female partner.

Since management of male infertility requires an understanding of the process of spermatogenesis, regulation of sperm maturation, the basic evaluation of an infertile patient and the possible etiologic causes of male infertility, these topics will be briefly described. Discussion on the difficulties and problems specific to the medical management of male infertility will follow. The chapter ends with our recommended algorithmic approach to the management of male infertility.

Regulation of Spermatogenesis

Spermatogenesis is the process of maturation of male germ cells from the spermatogonia, through the stages of primary and secondary

Management of Impotence and Infertility, edited by Douglas Whitehead and Harris Nagler,

spermatocytes, spermatids to the mature spermatozoa. It involves the processes of mitotic division, first and second meiotic divisions, and spermiogenesis.[2] In the human, it takes about 72 days for an immature spermatogonia to develop into a mature spermatozoon. The spermatozoa are then released into the lumen of the seminiferous tubules by spermiation and pass through the efferent ducts to the epididymis and ultimately to the vas deferens. During transit through the epididymis, the spermatozoa undergo maturation, become motile, and acquire fertilizing capacity. This may be accomplished by the coating of sperm surface by macromolecules, secreted by the epididymis. The seminal vesicles and the prostate secrete fluid that contribute to the volume of the ejaculate. The passage of spermatozoa through the epididymis, vas deferens, and ejaculatory ducts takes about 14 days in humans. After ejaculation into the female reproductive tract, the spermatozoa undergo the maturation process called capacitation. This is characterized by the spermatozoa undergoing the acrosome reaction and the development of hyperactivated motility. These maturation processes in human spermatozoa are prerequisite to penetration through the egg vestments, binding to the zona pellucida, and fertilization of the oocyte.

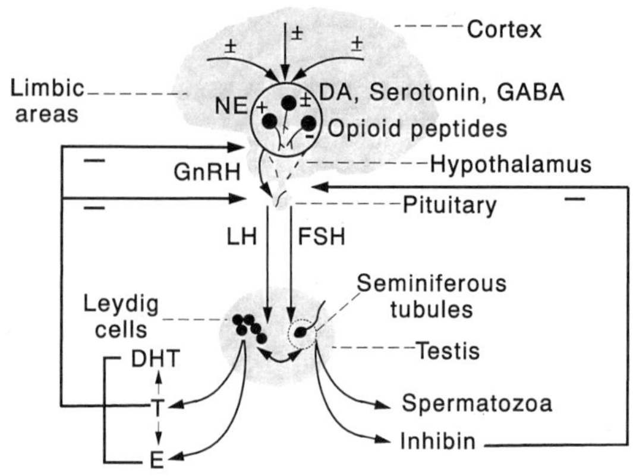

Figure 17-1 The hypothalamic–pituitary–testicular axis in the male. The hypothalamus is the integrating center for central nervous system (CNS) regulation of gonadotropin-releasing hormone (GnRH). Extrahypothalamic CNS input has both inhibitory and stimulatory influences on GnRH secretion. Neurotransmitters such as noradrenalin (norepinephrine, NE), dopamine (DA), opioid peptides, γ-aminobutyric acid (GABA), serotonin, and melatonin serve as regulators of GnRH synthesis and release from the hypothalamus. The human testis is a dual organ with endocrine and reproductive functions. Testicular function is regulated by a series of closed loop feedback systems involving the higher centers in the CNS, the hypothalamus, the pituitary, and the testicular endocrine and germinal compartments. T, testosterone; DHT, 5α-dihydrotestosterone; E, estrogen. (From Wang and Swerdloff,[4] with permission.)

Spermatogenesis is under the tight endocrine control of the hypothalamic pituitary axis (Figure 17-1). The secretion of luteinizing hormone (LH) and follicle-stimulating hormone (FSH) from the pituitary is regulated by the pulsatile release of gonadotropin-releasing hormone (GnRH) from the mediobasal hypothalamus. GnRH secretion is regulated by a number of neurotransmitters and is modulated by the negative feedback actions of gonadal steroids (Figure 17-1). In the human initiation of spermatogenesis requires both LH and FSH. LH stimulates the Leydig cells of the testis to produce testosterone (T) and high intratesticular levels of T are required for the initiation and maintenance of spermatogenesis. In adult men, it appears that either LH or FSH can maintain qualitatively normal spermatogenesis, but both gonadotropins are required to sustain quantitatively normal sperm production. The specific site or mechanism of action of FSH in germ cell maturation is not known. FSH stimulates the Sertoli cells in the seminiferous tubules to produce macromolecules including inhibin, activin, and a number of other growth factors. The exact role of the intratesticular paracrine or autocrine mediators and regulators on spermatogenesis is not clearly defined, but they are probably required to ensure the orderly progression of spermatogenesis from one stage to the next. Thus, these intragonadal peptides may regulate spermatogenesis directly or indirectly through their interactions with the gonadotropins within the testis. Testicular secretions serve to regulate the production and secretion of LH and FSH by the pituitary gland. Testosterone, directly or through its conversion to 5α-dihydrotestosterone and estradiol, exerts a major negative feedback role on the secretion of both LH and FSH. Inhibin has been shown to inhibit the production of FSH by the pituitary. In patients with severe damage to the germinal epithelium, Sertoli cell function may be abnormal, leading possibly to a decrease in secretion of inhibin and a consequent isolated elevation of serum FSH.

Basic Evaluation of the Infertile Male

The basic evaluation of the infertile male includes medical history, physical examination, semen analyses, and hormonal measurements.[3,4]

Briefly, the history includes a detailed assessment of the female partner including the menstrual history, previous fertility history, contraceptive use, history of pelvic inflammatory disease, previous investigations (including ascertainment of occurrence of ovulation and patency of the fallopian tubes), and treatment. In the male, the history includes past medical illnesses, surgery or infections, in particular of the genitourinary tract, sexually transmitted disease, cryptorchidism, vasectomy, trauma, or injury. Chronic respiratory symptoms may indicate the presence of immotile cilia syndrome, Young's syndrome, or cystic fibrosis. Abnormal pubertal development or regression of secondary sex characteristics may point to androgen deficiency. Exposure to drugs and toxins and irradiation can lead to impaired spermatogenesis. Excessive alcohol intake, heavy tobacco smoking, and chronic exposure of the scrotum to increased temperature may be associated with abnormal semen parameters. The previous fertility history, investigation, and treatment may allow the physician to assess the patient's potential fertilizing capacity. Usually a long duration of infertility is associated with poor prognosis. Sexual history including assessment of libido, frequency of intercourse, potency, or ejaculatory dysfunction must be ascertained.

The physical examination includes a general physical examination with particular emphasis to exclude clinical features of hypogonadism such as loss of body, axillary, and pubic hair, poor muscular development, eunochoidal proportions, gynecomastia, and assessment of adequate pubertal development. Testes size can be estimated with the Prader orchidometer. A testis volume of less than 15 ml in a Caucasian man is considered small and usually indicates significant seminiferous tubule dysfunction. Examination of the scrotum should include palpation for the vas and epididymis. The presence of varicocele should further be determined with the patient standing and performing a Valsalva maneuver. A rectal examination is indicated in patients with symptoms of prostatitis or when androgen replacement is considered.

The basic laboratory investigations should include semen analyses. Because of the marked intrasubject variation, at least two and preferably three semen samples should be collected at 1 or 2 weeks apart. To allow comparison within and between laboratories, semen analyses should be performed using standardized methods.[5] Routine semen analyses include assessment of volume, sperm count, motility, and morphology. Specialized sperm function tests may be required if semen analyses showed normal results or mild abnormalities, e.g., sperm count <20 but $>10 \times 10^6$/ml, sperm motility <50 and $>20\%$, and normal sperm morphology <50 and $>20\%$. Sperm autoimmunity should be excluded by testing for sperm surface antibodies by the immunobead test and the cervical mucus sperm interaction tests.[5] Other tests of sperm function such as computer-aided sperm movement analyses, assessment of acrosome reaction, hyperactivated motility, zona free hamster oocyte penetration tests, human zona pellucida sperm binding tests, and biochemical tests can be performed when indicated. Each of these tests assesses a different stage of maturation of the spermatozoa and a detailed discussion is beyond the scope of this chapter, but has been recently reviewed.[6]

In patients with azoospermia or severe oligozoospermia, basal serum levels of FSH, LH, and T should be measured. Elevations of serum FSH indicate severe seminiferous tubule dysfunction and are usually associated with poor potential fertility. Measurement of serum T together with LH will identify the presence of androgen deficiency and will help to determine whether the hypogonadism is due to a testicular or hypothalamic–pituitary disorder.[6]

Algorithmic Approach to the Diagnosis of Male Infertility

The most probable etiologic diagnosis of male infertility can be derived from an algorithm based on the information obtained from the history, physical examination, semen analyses, and hormone measurements[3] (Figure 17-2). If repeated semen analyses are normal and the female partner has no apparent cause of infertility, specialized sperm function tests should be considered and the diagnosis for the couple is "unexplained infertility." The presence of small testes, azoospermia, and low levels of gonadotropins and T point to the diagnosis of hypogonadotropic hypogonadism. Serum prolactin level should be assayed to exclude hyperprolactinemia. Appropriate radiological examination, usually magnetic resonance imaging (MRI), may be necessary to exclude a structural lesion in the region of the hypothalamus or pituitary. Elevated levels of FSH and/or LH in association with small testes, azoospermia, or severe oligozoospermia lead to the diagnosis of primary testicular failure, i.e., failure of Leydig cells to produce T as well as seminiferous tubule damage. Isolated elevation of FSH, in the presence of severe oligozoospermia or azoospermia, indicates severe germinal epithelium damage. Elevated levels of LH together with elevated circulating T levels suggest that the pituitary is not sensitive to the negative feedback by androgens and indicate androgen resistance syndrome. The diagnosis can be confirmed by measuring androgen receptor levels in cultured skin fibroblasts. Presence of normal testis size and azoospermia in association with normal hormone levels suggest obstructive azoospermia. A low semen volume and pH together with low or absent fructose in seminal plasma suggest the diagnosis of congenital absence of the vas, retrograde ejaculation, or ejaculatory duct obstruction. A postejaculation urine should be examined to exclude retrograde ejaculation. If seminal fructose level is normal, exploration during microsurgery may identify distention of the epididymis proximal to the obstruction and help to identify the site

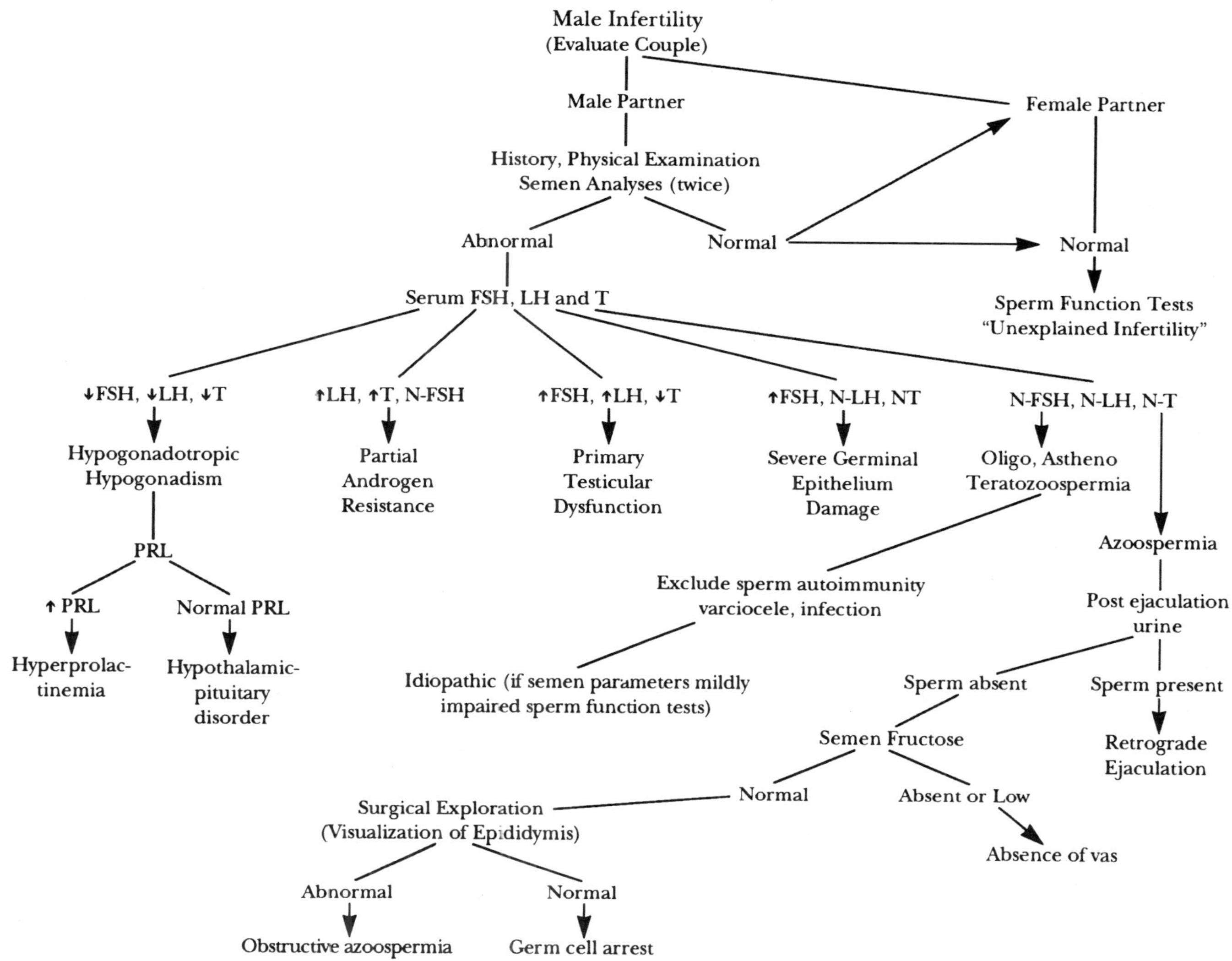

Figure 17-2 Algorithmic approach to the diagnosis of male infertility. n, normal; ↑, increase; FSH, follicle-stimulating hormone; LH, luteinizing hormone; T, testosterone; PRL, prolactin.

of obstruction. If exploration shows normal findings then testicular biopsy may be performed to exclude the diagnosis of germ cell arrest in a small group of patients with normal testis size and azoospermia. In patients with oligo-, astheno-, or teratozoospermia and normal hormone levels, the diagnosis of varicocele, sperm autoimmunity, and genital tract infection should be excluded before assigning these patients to the group called idiopathic male infertility. In patients with idiopathic infertility, if semen parameters are mildly impaired, sperm function tests may help to delineate the specific defect in the maturational processes leading to acquisition of fertilizing capacity of the spermatozoa.

Table 17-1 Common Causes of Male Infertility[a]

Cause	Frequency (%)
Primary pantesticular failure (including chromosomal disorders, cryptorchidism, orchitis, drugs, irradiation)	10 to 13
Hypothalamic–pituitary disorders	1 to 2
Genital tract obstruction	8 to 10
Sperm autoimmunity	4 to 6
Drugs, toxins, stress, illness	?
Ejaculation or erection problems	1
Varicocele	15 to 35
Genital tract infection	?
Idiopathic azoospermia, normospermia, oligo-, astheno-, or teratozoospermia	70 to 75

[a] Adapted from Baker and Burger (1986) and Burger and Baker.[29]

Diagnosis of Male Infertility

The male patient with infertility can be classified into one of the commoner diagnosis based on etiology. The common etiologic diagnoses of patients attending a specialized infertility center are listed in Table 17-1. As illustrated in this table, the pathogenic cause of male infertility in the majority of patients remains unknown (the idiopathic group). Included in the category of idiopathic male infertility is a group of patients in whom no identifiable abnormality can be detected in both the male and female partner, i.e., "unexplained infertility." The diagnosis based on etiology does not give adequate information about the probable prognosis and whether treatment is available or possible. For management purposes, we can classify male infertility into different treatment categories as in Table 17-2. The treatment of specific endocrine abnormalities such as hypogonadotrophic hypogonadism will be discussed in Chapter 29, sperm autoimmunity in Chapter 32, and infections in Chapter 30. The surgical treatment of varicocele, obstructive azoospermia, and the treatment for retrograde ejaculation, and ejaculatory and erectile abnormalities will be discussed in the section on Impotence and in Chapters 18 to 27. The application of assisted reproductive technologies including micromanipulation of gametes will be discussed in Chapter 28. In this chapter we will focus on the general approach to the management of infertile men and the nonspecific or empirical medical management of idiopathic male infertility.

Table 17-2 Treatment Category of Male Infertility[a]

Category	Treatment	Chapter
No known treatment for infertility		
Primary testicular disorder	Androgen replacement if necessary	29
Androgen resistance syndrome	High dose androgens	29
Specific treatment available		
Hypogonadotropic hypogonadism	hCG/hMG (GnRH)	29
Hyperprolactinemia	Bromocriptine	29
Potentially helpful treatment		
Sperm autoimmunity	Glucocorticoids IVF/ZIFT	32
Varicocele	Varicocele ligation or embolization	18–20
Ejaculatory/Erectile problems	Psycological counselling, electroejaculation, IUI	Part I and 25–28
Obstructive azoospermia	Vaso- or epididymovasostomy	21, 22
	Ejaculatory duct surgery	23
	Microsurgical aspiration of epididymal spermatozoa and IVF	22
Infection	Antibiotics	30
Value of treatment controversial	Empirical, nonspecific medical treatment	Present
Idiopathic		
	IUI, IVF/ZIFT, micromanipulation	28

[a] GnRH, gonadotropin-releasing hormone; hCG, human chorionic gonadotropin; hMG, human menopausal gonadotropin; IVF, *in vitro* fertilization; ZIFT, zygote intrafallopian transfer; IUI, intrauterine insemination with male partner's spermatozoa.

Nonspecific or Empirical Medical Management of Male Infertility

Before discussing the treatment of idiopathic male infertility, it must be emphasized that hormonal replacement with testosterone preparations is available for patients with androgen deficiency. While the infertility in some of these patients cannot be remedied, replacement with androgens will prevent sexual dysfunction, loss of bone and muscle mass, and low hematocrit levels in these hypogonadal subjects. In patients with hypogonadotropic hypogonadism, treatment with gonadotropins (or GnRh) results in initiation and maintenance of spermatogenesis. In contrast to other causes of male infertility, this specific therapy leads to high pregnancy rates in the female partners. Similarly, in patients with hyperprolactinemia, bromocriptine treatment will lower prolactin levels. While many subjects with prolactin-induced hypogonadotropic hypogonadism may respond to dopamine agonists with increase LH and testosterone secretion, additional androgen replacement may be required for hypogonadism or gonadotropin therapy for infertility. In the very rare patient with partial androgen resistance syndrome, infertility may be irreversible, but high dose androgen therapy may result in some benefit. In the majority of the patients with male infertility, such specific therapy is not available.

Problems Associated with Clinical Trials of Agents to Treat Male Infertility

In most of the patients (over 70%) with male infertility, the pathogenesis is not clear. Without a definite diagnosis, the patients are heterogeneous with different etiological causes resulting in varying degrees of damage to the germinal epithelium. The duration of the injury may also be variable and probably long standing. For these reasons, there is no specific therapy for idiopathic male infertility.

Another major problem with the treatment of male infertility is the duration required for the treatment to become effective. Since spermatogenesis and transport of the spermatozoa through the male reproductive tract often require over 80 days, the minimum duration of treatment for any potentially useful drug will be 90 days. These therapeutic regimes may stimulate very early stages of spermatogenesis; therefore the medical therapy must be administered for at least 12 weeks and preferably for 24 weeks before their effects can be adequately assessed.

The third problem is the requirement for placebo-controlled trials. Semen parameters showed large intrasubject variability. Regression toward the mean occurs whenever subjects with extreme values of the variables are entered into clinical trials. On repeat measurements, the results tend to be closer to the mean of the original population. This regression toward the mean was observed in many clinical trials for male infertility. In a placebo-controlled trial, assessing the effectiveness of erythromycin to improve low sperm motility, there was significant increases in sperm motility after both placebo and erythromycin treatment. The selection of patients was based on a very low sperm motility in the entry sample.[7] Because of the marked inherent variability in sperm counts, motility and morphology, and the phenomenon of regression toward the mean, placebo-controlled trials are required for testing any probable treatment regimen for male infertility. Baker[8] suggested that the requirements of male infertility clinical trials should include the following criteria: the prospective treatment should be promising, the subjects as well as the female partners should be as clearly defined as possible, information on prognostic factors should be obtained, the subjects must be randomized into placebo or treatment group, adequate sample size must be enrolled to allow meaningful statistical analyses, and cumulative pregnancy rates rather than pregnancies should be calculated.

Because of these problems, many clinical trials of empirical methods of treatment of male infertility have doubtful value. Most of the reports in the literature are based on uncontrolled, poorly designed clinical trials. We will briefly discuss some of the medical treatment of male infertility based on results obtained from the more recently reported, placebo-controlled clinical trials.

Medical Management

Table 17-3 provides a list of the nonspecific therapy for male infertility.[4,9,10] Therapeutic use of some of these agents in idiopathic male infertility has no rational basis and questionable therapeutic actions such as zinc, antiinflammatory agents, angiotensin-converting enzyme inhibitors, and many others. Others,

Table 17-3 Drugs Used for the Treatment of Idiopathic Male Infertility[a]

Hormones	Others
GnRH	Antibiotics Phosphodiesterase inhibitor pentoxifylline
Gonadotropins	
hCG	Kinins
hMG	Kallikrein
pure FSH	Vitamin E
Androgens	
Testosterone esters	Zinc (?)[a]
Mesterolone	Antiinflammatory agents (?)[a]
Antiestrogens	
Clomiphene citrate	
Tamoxifen	Angiotensin-converting enzyme inhibitors (?)[a]
Aromatase inhibitors	
Testolactone	α-Adrenergic agents (?)[a]

[a] ?, questionable therapeutic action; GnRH, gonadotropin-releasing hormone; hCG, human chorionic gonadotropin; hMC, human menopausal gonadotropin; FSH, follicle-stimulating hormone.

like the kinins, e.g., kallikrein, improve sperm motility *in vitro.* However, when used *in vivo,* placebo-controlled trials showed that kallikrein has no significant effect on sperm motility or pregnancy rates. Vitamin E, because of its antioxidant properties, improves sperm fertilizing capacity as assessed by penetration into zona free hamster oocytes. This drug, like many others listed in Table 17-3, has not been shown to be effective in placebo-controlled clinical trials.

GnRH

In patients with severe oligozoospermia or azoospermia associated with monotropic increase in serum FSH, short-term pulsatile infusion of GnRH led to a progressive decrease in FSH levels. This suggests that abnormalities in GnRH secretion could have resulted in abnormal FSH and LH secretion leading to the defects in spermatogenesis. Based on this observation, Matsumoto et al.[28] treated men with idiopathic azoo- or severe oligozoospermia and elevated FSH with pulsatile GnRH. Despite the decrease in FSH levels, the sperm concentration in these patients showed no change after GnRH therapy and there were no pregnancies. This suggests that the abnormality in secretion of GnRH and of the gonadotropins may be a manifestation of seminiferous tubule damage rather than its cause. Thus, GnRH is not recommended for the treatment of idiopathic male infertility.

Gonadotropins

Based on the observation that patients with hypothalamic–pituitary disorders respond to human chorionic gonadotropin (hCG) and human menopausal gonadotropin (hMG) therapy with highly successful outcomes, patients with idiopathic infertility have been treated with various combinations of gonadotropins.[4,9] In a recent placebo-controlled trial,[11] both the control and the gonadotropin (hCG and hMG)-treated groups of patients showed improvement in sperm concentration. The treatment was started at the nadir of sperm concentration. The increases in sperm counts observed in both treatment groups were another example of the phenomenon of regression toward the mean. A multicenter trial using pure FSH in the treatment of idiopathic oligozoospermia is in progress in Europe. At present, hCG/hMG or pure FSH is not recommended routinely for idiopathic male infertility until additional results from placebo-controlled trials become available. Recently, pure FSH has been used to treat male partners with severe oligozoospermia in an *in vitro* fertilization

(IVF) program.[12] This uncontrolled study showed that fertilization *in vitro* was improved in the FSH-treated group. The inclusion of a placebo group and increasing the number of subjects in further trials are required before it can be concluded whether FSH treatment is beneficial in this special clinical setting.

Androgens

Testosterone enanthate when administered to oligozoospermic men led to suppression of spermatogenesis. Discontinuation of testosterone administration was followed by recovery and in some reports a rebound of sperm concentration to above the pretreatment level. However, in a placebo-controlled clinical trial, there was no significant increase in sperm count or motility or pregnancy in the treated compared to the placebo group.[13] Other testosterone esters such as testosterone undecanoate have been shown to have no effect on improvement of spermatogenesis in placebo-controlled trials. Mesterolone, an orally active weak androgen, has been used in Europe and Asia for the treatment of idiopathic male infertility. A recent multicenter, double-blind, randomized study using two doses of mesterolone (74 and 150 mg per day) and placebo in 157 couples[14] showed that sperm concentration rose in all three groups with treatment. The cumulative pregnancy rates were not significantly different between the mesterolone-treated and the placebo groups. From these studies, it is unlikely that androgens have any beneficial effect on idiopathic male infertility.

Antiestrogens

Low dose (25 or 50 mg per day) clomiphene citrate has been widely used for the treatment of idiopathic oligozoospermia. The antiestrogenic property of clomiphene results in a decrease in negative feedback by estrogens mainly on the hypothalamus. Administration of clomiphene citrate leads to increases in the levels of gonadotropins and endogenous secretion of T. Numerous uncontrolled studies have shown that clomiphene citrate may increase sperm counts and pregnancy rates.[9] In recent placebo-controlled studies, clomiphene citrate did not significantly improve sperm count or pregnancy rates.[15,16] It is possible that some patients may be more responsive to one or more of the empirical treatments. Unfortunately, it is not possible to identify those patients who may respond to clomiphene citrate therapy. Tamoxifen, another antiestrogen, when tested in placebo-controlled trials, had no significant effect on sperm count, motility, *in vitro* fertilizing capacity, or pregnancy rates.[17] Thus both antiestrogens cannot be recommended for routine use in men with idiopathic oligozoospermia.

Aromatase Inhibitors

Since high levels of estrogens, in nonhuman experimental studies, are toxic to the germinal epithelium, and elevated circulatory estrogen levels will inhibit LH and FSH secretion, it has been suggested that aromatase inhibitors by decreasing estradiol production may improve spermatogenesis. When testolactone (an aromatase inhibitor) was tested in a placebo-controlled trial, no improvement in sperm concentration, motility, or morphology was observed. No pregnancies occurred in either the placebo or testolactone group. Thus aromatase inhibitors such as testolactone cannot be recommended for treatment of idiopathic oligozoospermia.[18]

Phosphodiesterase Inhibitors

Because phosphodiesterase inhibitors increase intracellular cyclic AMP levels, these agents have been demonstrated to improve sperm motility *in vitro*. However, when administered to men in a placebo-controlled clinical trial, the phosphodiesterase inhibitor, pentoxifylline, had no effect on sperm parameters or fertility in patients with idiopathic oligozoospermia.[13] The use of these agents, *in vitro*, to prepare spermatozoa for IVF is currently being tested in a number of laboratories.

Thus, in summary, none of the medical treatments tested in placebo-controlled clinical trials is of definite beneficial value in the treatment of idiopathic male infertility.

Assisted Reproductive Technologies (also see Chapter 28)

Intrauterine inseminations (IUI) with sperm prepared by methods such as swim-up and percoll gradient centrifugation are frequently recommended for couples with male factor infertility. The rationale for this therapy is the ability to separate and concentrate the more motile spermatozoa in a small volume of culture medium and to introduce the prepared spermatozoa directly into the uterus of the female partner. Samples with very severe oligozoospermia and very poor motility and morphology are not suitable for preparation for IUI. Although initial results were promising, subsequent studies showed that IUI had no advantage over natural intercourse in couples with male factor infertility.[19] To enhance fertility rates in couples with male factor infertility, controlled ovarian hyperstimulation with human menopausal gonadotropin in the female partner has been combined with IUI. These techniques have not been assessed in large-scale controlled clinical trials of male factor infertility and should be considered experimental.

The use of *in vitro* fertilization (IVF) or zygote intrafallopian transfer (ZIFT) for male factor infertility is based on the rationale that much fewer motile and normal spermatozoa are required for fertilization *in vitro*.[20,21] There are no controlled clinical trials to demonstrate that IVF/ZIFT are clearly superior to no treatment. However, fertilization *in vitro* has been shown to occur with spermatozoa obtained from men with idiopathic infertility that failed other modalities of treatment. The fertilization rates are significantly reduced only when the patient has combined sperm defects, such as decreases in count, motility, and morphology.[22] When sperm morphology is grossly abnormal, the success rate in IVF procedures is also demonstrated to be markedly reduced.[23] Once fertilization has occurred, there is no evidence of a lower implantation, pregnancy, or delivery rate in *in vitro* fertilization initiated by spermatozoa from patients with male factor infertility. There is also no increase in abortion rate in the group with male factor infertility.[22] For many of these patients techniques such as IVF/ZIFT offer the only possibility of achieving fertilization *in vitro* and pregnancy *in vivo* in the female partner. Moreover, by selecting the appropriate patients and modifying the semen sample preparation procedure, sperm recovery and subsequent fertilization may be improved.

Patients with marked impairment of semen parameters, e.g., sperm count less than 5×10^6/ml, motility less than 10%, and morphology less than 10% normal would have markedly reduced fertilization rates *in vitro*, resulting in unacceptably low pregnancy rates. For these patients the newly developed techniques of micromanipulation of gametes may be considered. Partial zona dissection may be offered to patients with less severe sperm abnormalities.[24,25] Microinjection of spermatozoa into the perivitelline space has made fertilization possible in a small number of patients with very few spermatozoa in the ejaculate.[26,27] It must be emphasized that all these techniques are experimental. In these micromanipulation techniques some oocytes should be reserved for conventional IVF to serve as controls for the more invasive techniques. The development and continued improvement of these techniques may allow the possibility of achieving fertilization and pregnancy in couples considered sterile in the past. The alternatives of donor insemination (DI) and adoption should always be discussed in conjunction with these stressful, costly, and more invasive state-of-the-art experimental procedures.

Recommended Approach to the Management of a Patient with Male Infertility

Based on the above discussions, we have developed an algorithmic approach to the management of the patient with male factor infertility. If the patient has azoospermia (Figure 17-3), measurement of serum hormone levels will determine the etiology and site of the disorder. If hyponadotropic hypogonadism is diagnosed,

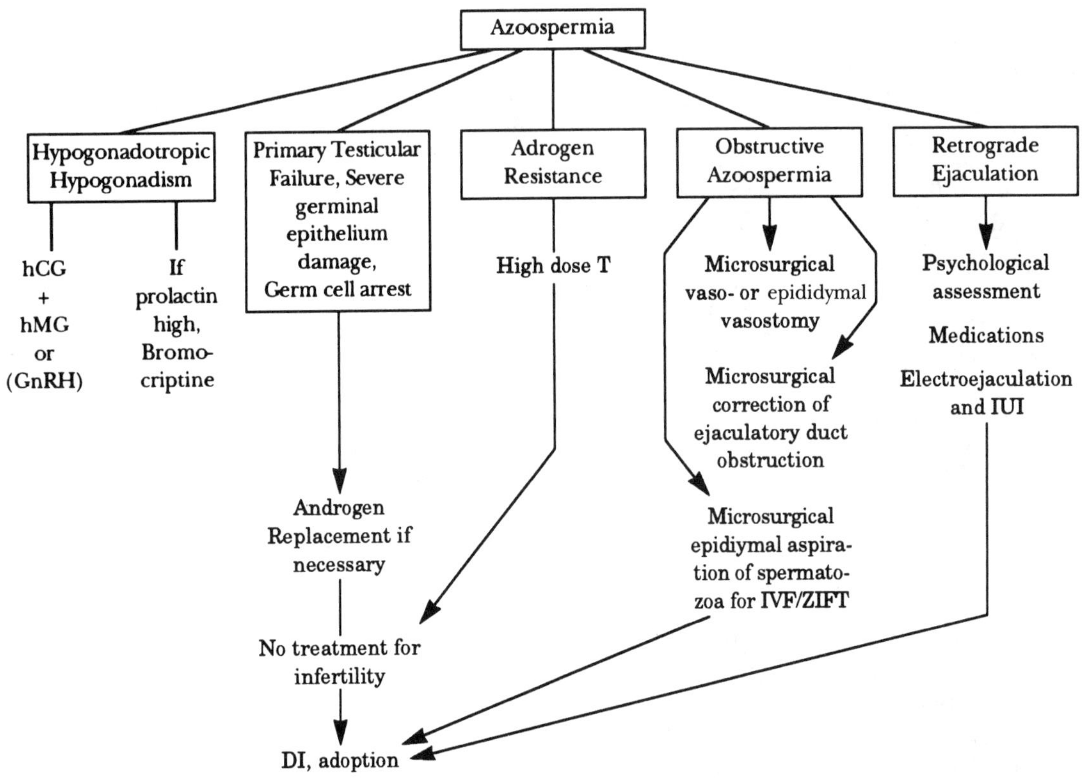

Figure 17-3 Algorithmic approach to the management of azoospermia. hCG, human chorionic gonadotropin; hMG, human menopausal gonadotropin; GnRH, gonadotropin-releasing hormone; T, testosterone; IUI, intrauterine insemination; IVF, *in vitro* fertilization; ZIFT, zygote intrafallopian transfer; DI, donor insemination.

testosterone replacement is given until fertility is desired. The patient can then be treated with gonadotropins (or GnRH) for induction of spermatogenesis with a high likelihood of successful fertility. In the patient with germinal epithelium failure or germ cell arrest, no treatment for their infertility is currently available. Alternatives such as donor insemination (DI) or adoption should be considered. In the unusual patient with partial androgen resistance, very high dose T may correct some of their clinical features but will not improve their infertility. Patients with obstructive azoospermia are assessed to determine whether they have congenital absence of the vas, obstruction at the epididymis, vas, or ejaculatory duct. Appropriate microsurgical anastomoses or corrections or microsurgical epididymal aspiration of spermatozoa followed by IVF or ZIFT are advised. If the patient has retrograde ejaculation, neurological and psychological assessment is required before medications, electroejaculation, and IUI with male partner's spermatozoa are contemplated.

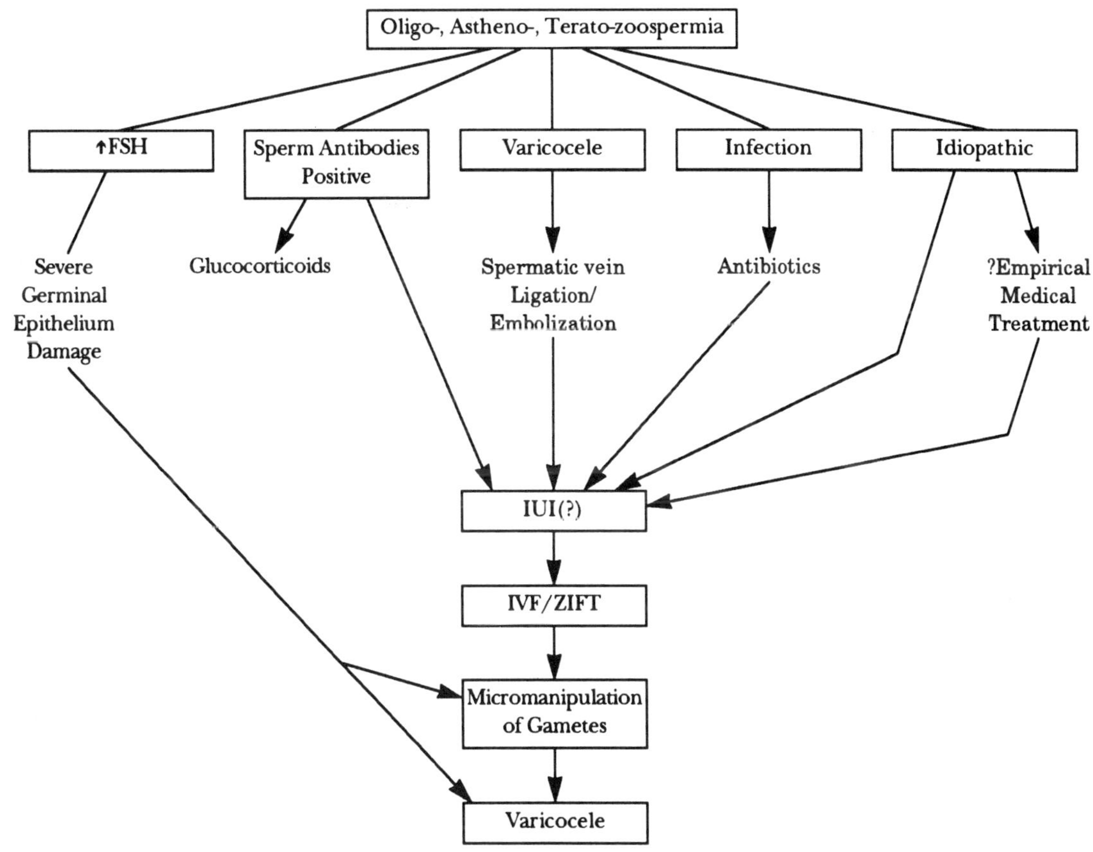

Figure 17-4 Algorithmic approach to the management of oligozoospermia (same as Figure 17-3).

In a patient with oligozoospermia (Figure 17-4) and elevated FSH, the prognosis in general is poor. The patient should be advised on the alternative procedures on donor insemination (DI) or adoption. The couple should be informed of the new procedures of micromanipulation including microinjection of spermatozoa into the perivitelline space. The lack of experience in large numbers of patients and the relatively poor outcome of these new techniques in patients with severe impairment of semen parameters should be discussed with the couple. Patients with sperm autoimmunity can be offered the choice of glucocorticoid therapy or directly referred for IUI followed by IVF/ZIFT. Patients with clinical varicocele can be advised to have spermatic vein ligation or embolization. The benefits of such therapy have been widely debated and some andrologists would prefer to consider such patients for management by assisted reproductive technologies. Patients with clear evidence of genital tract infections should be treated with antibiotics. In the majority of patients where no identifiable cause can be defined, the problems and lack of beneficial effects of nonspecific medical therapy should be discussed. In these patients, as in those who did not achieve success with potentially treatable causes, the rationale of IVF or ZIFT should be explained to the couple. It is important for the patients to recognize that unless underlying mechanism leading to impaired spermatogenesis can be identified, the treatment of male infertility, in most instance, remains nonspecific. In many circumstances, treatment is directed toward the female partner. By using controlled ovarian hyperstimulation and superovulation, the clinician hopes to compensate the defects in sperm development or maturation by increasing the availability of more than one oocyte for fertilization *in vitro.* Micromanipulation techniques may achieve fertilization in selected patients by removing some of the barriers to fertilization. At all stages of the management of male infertility, the physician should discuss with the couple all alternative treatment options including the availability of donor insemination and adoption.

REFERENCES

1. Wang C, Chan SYW, Ng M, et al: Diagnostic value of sperm function tests and routine semen analysis in fertile and infertile men. J Androl 1988; 9:384–389.
2. Heller CG, Clermont Y: Kinetics of the germinal epithelium in man. Recent Hormone Res 1964; 20:545–571.
3. Swerdloff RS, Wang C, Kandeel FC: Evaluation of the infertile couple. Endocrinol Metab Clinics North Am 1988; 17:301–331.
4. Wang C, Swerdloff RS: Male infertility: Overview of current therapy. In: Boutaleb Y, Gzouli A, eds. The Treatment of Infertility. Carnforth: Parthenon, 1991:19–24.
5. World Health Organization: Laboratory manual for the examination of semen and sperm-cervical mucus interaction, 3rd ed. Cambridge: Cambridge University Press, in press, 1992.
6. Wang C, Swerdloff RS: Evaluation of testicular function. In: de Kretser DM, ed. Bailliere's clinical endocrinology and metabolism. "The Testis". London: Bailliere Tindall, in press, 1992.
7. Baker HWG, Stratton WGE, McGowan MP, Burger HG, de Kretser DM, Hudson B: A controlled trial of erythromycin for asthenospermia. Int J Androl 1984; 7:383–388.
8. Baker HWG: Development of clinical trials in male infertility research. In: Serio M, ed. Perspectives in andrology. New York: Raven Press, 1989; 367–374.
9. Sigman M, Vance ML: Medical treatment of idiopathic infertility. Urol Clin North Am 1987; 14:459–469.

10. Haidl G, Schill WB: Guidelines for drug treatment of male infertility. Drugs 1991; 41:60–68.
11. Knuth VA, Honigl W, Bals-Pratsch M, Schleicher G, Nieschlag E: Treatment of severe oligospermia with human chorionic gonadotropin/ human menopausal gonadotropin: A placebo-controlled, double blind trial. J Clin Endocrinol Metab 1987; 65:1081–1087.
12. Acosta AA, Oehninger S, Ertunc H, Philput C: Possible role of pure human follicle stimulating hormone in the treatment of severe male factor infertility by assisted reproduction: Preliminary report. Fertil Steril 1991; 55:1150–1156.
13. Wang C, Chan CW, Wong KK, Yeung KK: Comparison of the effectiveness of placebo, clomiphene citrate, mesterolone, pentoxifylline and testosterone rebound therapy for the treatment of idiopathic oligospermia. Fertil Steril 1983; 40:358–365.
14. World Health Organization Task Force on the Diagnosis and Treatment of Infertility. Mesterolone and idiopathic male infertility: A double-blind study. Int J Androl 1989; 12:254–264.
15. Sokol RZ, Steiner BS, Bustillo M, Petersen G, Swerdloff RS: A controlled comparison of the efficacy of clomiphene citrate in male infertility. Fertil Steril 1988; 49:865–870.
16. World Health Organization: Special Programme of Research, Development and Research Training in Human Reproduction Annual Technical Report 1990. Geneva: World Health Organization 1991:146–147.
17. Torok L: Treatment of oligozoospermia with tamoxifen; open and controlled studies. Andrologia 1985; 17:497–501.
18. Clark RV, Sherins RJ: Treatment of men with idiopathic oligozoospermic infertility using the aromatase inhibitor, testolactone. Results of a double-blinded randomized placebo-controlled trial with crossover. J Androl 1989; 10:240–247.
19. Ho PC, Poon IML, Chan SYW, Wang C: Intrauterine insemination is not useful in oligoasthenospermia. Fertil Steril 1989; 51:682–684.
20. Mahadevan MM, Trouson AO, Leeton JF: The relationship of tubal blockage, infertility of unknown cause, suspected male infertility, and endometriosis to success of in-vitro fertilization and embryo transfer. Fertil Steril 1983; 40:755–762.
21. Cohen J, Edwards RG, Fehilly C, Fishel S, Hewitt J, Purdy J, Rowland G, Steptoe P, Webster J: In vitro fertilization: A treatment for male infertility. Fertil Steril 1985; 43:422–433.
22. Yates CA, Trounsen AO, de Kretser DM: Male factor infertility and in-vitro fertilization. In: Serio M, ed. IV International congress of andrology: Miniposters (Serono Symposium Review). Rome: Areserono; 1989:263.
23. Oehninger S, Acosta AA, Morshedi M, Veeck L, Swanson RJ, Simmons K, Rosenwaks ZJ: Corrective measures and pregnancy outcome in vitro fertilization in patients with severe sperm morphology abnormalities. Fertil Steril 1988; 50:283–287.
24. Cohen J, Malter H, Fehilly C, Wright G, Elsner C, Kort H, Massey J: Implantation of embryos after partial opening of oocyte zona pellucida to facilitate sperm penetration. Lancet 1988; 2:1&2.
25. Malter HE, Cohen J: Partial zona dissection of the human oocyte: A nontraumatic method using micromanipulation to assist zona pellucida penetration. Fertil Steril 1989; 51:139–148.
26. Ng SC, Bongso A, Sathananthan H, Ratnam SS: Micromanipulation: Its relevance to human in-vitro fertilization. Fertil Steril 1990; 53:203–219.
27. Fishel S, Jackson P, Antinoni S, Johnson J, Grossi S, Versaci C: Subzonal insemination for alleviation of infertility. Fertil Steril 1990; 54:828–835.
28. Matsumoto AM, Gross KM, Sheckter CB, Bremner WJ: The luteinizing hormone-releasing hormone pulse generator in men: Abnormalities and clinical management. Am J Obstet Gynecol 1990; 163:1743–1752.
29. Burger HG, Baker HWG: The treatment of infertility: In Greger WP, Coggins CH, Hancock EW. Annual review of medicine. Palo Alto: Annual Review, 1987; 38:29–46.

ANNOTATED BIBLIOGRAPHY

Baker HWG: Development of clinical trials in male infertility research. In: Serio M, ed. Perspectives in andrology. New York: Raven Press, 1989:367–374.

This is a review of the important elements and problems associated with clinical trials of therapy for male infertility. As there is no established medical treatment for male infertility, putative useful treatments have to be tested against placebo. The special problems associated with controlled trials of male infertility including variable fertility in the females and pregnancies can occur without treatment; the end point "pregnancy" occurs infrequently requiring large clinical trials and the variability of semen analyses. The author defines the basic requirements of therapeutic clinical trials in male infertility.

Knuth VA, Honigl W, Bals-Pratsch M, Schleicher G, Nieschlag E: Treatment of severe oligospermia with human chorionic gonadotropin/human menopausal gonadotropin: A placebo-controlled, double-blind trial. J Clin Endocrinol Metab 1987; 65:1081–1087.

Thirty men with idiopathic oligospermia were randomly allocated to treatment with 2500 IU human chorionic gonadotropin (hCG) twice a week plus 150 IU human menopausal gonadotropin (hMG) three times a week or placebo (saline) injections for 13 weeks. The men were followed for 12 weeks after stopping treatment. Sperm count, motility, and morphology were similar in the two groups at all times. There were two pregnancies in the gonadotropin-treated group and none in the placebo group. The pregnancy rate in the gonadotropin-treated group was within the limits of chance and not significantly different from the zero rate observed in the placebo group. The authors concluded that in a well-designed, placebo-controlled, double-blind trial hCG/hMG treatment was not useful in idiopathic male infertility.

Sigman M, Vance ML: Medical treatment of idiopathic infertility. Uro Clin North Am 1987; 14:459–469.

This is a comprehensive review of the different types of medical therapies used for idiopathic male infertility including antiestrogens (clomiphene citrate and tamoxifen), aromatase inhibitors, gonadotropins, gonadotropin-releasing hormone, testosterone, kallikrein, and phosphodiesterase inhibitors. Reviews of the results of each type of treatment were given in tables detailing the response in sperm count/motility, pregnancies, and whether the trial was placebo controlled. The authors concluded that no medical regimen had proved to be consistently effective in the treatment of idiopathic male infertility.

World Health Organization Task Force on the Diagnosis and Treatment of Infertility: Mesterolone and idiopathic infertility: A double blind study. Int J Androl 1989; 12:254–264.

This multicenter study was a carefully designed, randomized double-blind study to assess the effect of 6 months treatment with mesterolone (a synthetic androgen) on male infertility. The study was performed in seven centers in seven countries involving 157 infertile couples coordinated by the World Health Organization (WHO). All subjects were investigated according to a standardized protocol. The men were randomly assigned to treatment with placebo or 150 or 75 mg mesterolone daily. There was an increase in sperm concentration 3 months after treatment in all three treatment groups. This increase was not sustained throughout the study. The increase in sperm count was due to substantial increase among those with the lowest initial sperm concentration. The increases in sperm count were not significantly different between mesterolone and placebo groups. The cumulative life table pregnancy rates 8 months after start of treatment were 11, 12 and 19% in the placebo, 75 and 150 mg groups respectively. The differences in the pregnancy rates were not significant amongst the groups. Only a small number of pregnancies were achieved in the study. There were no correlations between treatment, pregnancy and semen analysis. The conclusion of the study was that mesterolone was not efficacious for the treatment of idiopathic oligozoospermia.

18

Surgical Treatment for Varicocele

Harris M. Nagler
Joseph N. Biase

The varicocele is thought to be the most common treatable cause of male infertility.[1] Although the incidence of varicocele in the general population has been reported to be as high as 15%, varicoceles are discovered in approximately one-third (19–41%) of subfertile men.[2,3] Therefore, while not all men with varicoceles will be infertile, a significant percentage of infertile men will have a varicocele. The beneficial effects of varicocelectomy in the treatment of the infertile male has been well documented by many authors.[4–7] Improvement has been observed in seminal parameters,[5–8] testicular size,[9,10] and testicular histology.[11,12] Several large series encompassing thousands of infertile patients who had undergone varicocelectomy demonstrate that 50% to 80% of patients experienced an improvement in semen parameters; 30% to 40% of patients initiated a pregnancy.[2] This chapter reviews the history, diagnosis, and current concepts regarding the surgical treatment of the varicocele.

Historical Perspective

In 1889, Bennett performed bilateral varicocelectomy in a patient who experienced subsequent improvement in semen quality.[13] In 1929, Macomber and Sanders, in a report in the *New England Journal of Medicine*, described an oligospermic subfertile patient who underwent varicocele ligation and became normospermic and fertile.[14]

Varicocelectomy attained its current importance in the treatment of male infertility in the early 1950s when Tulloch reported his series of varicocelectomies in infertile men.[15,16] Since then, numerous uncontrolled studies have demonstrated improved semen quality and pregnancy following varicocelectomy.[5,17,18]

Diagnosis

Physical Exam

Diagnosis of the scrotal varicocele rests on an accurate physical examination. A grading

Management of Impotence and Infertility, edited by Douglas Whitehead and Harris Nagler,

system for assessing varicocele size has been proposed.[19] The "small" (grade I) varicoceles are palpable only with a concurrent Valsalva maneuver. "Moderate" (grade II) varicoceles are easily palpable without a Valsalva maneuver. "Large" (grade III) varicoceles are visible through the scrotal skin. The distended veins have been described by Dubin and Amelar as a "bag of worms".[19] Classically, varicoceles have been described as isolated left-side lesions in 70–90%[3,17]; bilateral varicoceles had been observed in approximately 10% of patients.[3] More recent data indicate that varicoceles are far more common bilaterally then had been previously reported.[20]

Adjunctive Diagnostic Tests

Doppler Examination

The clinical impression of a varicocele may be confirmed with the use of a pencil-probe Doppler (9 MHz) stethoscope with conducting gel applied to the upper aspect of the scrotum and with the patient in the upright position. A venous "rush" is auscultated with Valsalva when a varicocele is present. The Doppler should only be used to confirm physical findings consistent with a varicocele. The Doppler should not be utilized to screen subfertile patients with oligospermia in search of "subclinical" varicoceles.

Venography

Regarded as the most sensitive technique for the diagnosis of the scrotal varicocele, the specificity of spermatic venography remains controversial. Reflux is demonstrated in almost 100% of subfertile patients with palpable varicoceles,[21] although Netto et al. reported venographic reflux in 58% of men with varicoceles and abnormal semen, in 58% of men with varicoceles and normal semen, and in 33% of normal controls.[22] Venography should not be used routinely to diagnose varicoceles in the oligospermic patients given the invasive nature of the procedure and the controversy regarding the significance of venographic reflux. The most appropriate indication for venography is in the diagnosis and treatment of a persistent varicocele in the postsurgical patient. Venoocclusion can be accomplished with the use of sclerosing agents,[23] coils,[24] or balloons.[25]

Thermography

Scrotal contact thermography has been used to detect the elevated temperatures associated with the varicocele. However, Mieusset et al. reported that increased scrotal temperatures are seen in infertile men with abnormal spermatogenesis without varicoceles.[26] We do not utilize this technique.

Surgical Treatment

The cornerstone of varicocele therapy is surgical varicocelectomy. The goal of surgery is complete disruption of the internal spermatic venous drainage and the external cremasteric system while preserving the internal spermatic artery, vas deferens with its blood supply, and spermatic cord lymphatics. Several surgical approaches have been proposed. These include the scrotal approach, an inguinal approach (modified Ivanissevich), or the retroperitoneal approach (modified Palomo). Recently, laparoscopic varicocelectomy has attracted some interest.

Scrotal Approach

The scrotal approach is rarely used and is mentioned only for historical review. The complexity of the rich anastomotic network of the pampiniform plexus within the scrotum makes this approach exceedingly time consuming and lends itself to failure. Additionally, because of the multiple sites of division and ligation, damage to the testicular artery and resulting testicular ischemia are more likely. This approach is best avoided because of the high rate of failure and complication.

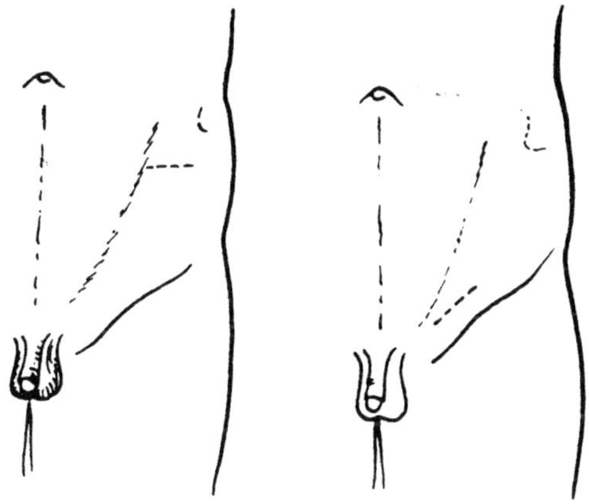

(A) (B)

Figure 18-1 (A) Location of incision for retroperitoneal approach. (B) Location of incision for inguinal approach.

Inguinal Approach/Modified Ivanissevich

The inguinal approach exposes the internal spermatic vessels within the inguinal canal. As noted by Ivanissevich,[27] this approach has several advantages over the retroperitoneal approach. First, the urologic surgeon is quite comfortable with the anatomy within the inguinal canal. As the spermatic vein approaches the internal inguinal ring, it will coalesce to form fewer and larger vessels. This approach will also allow for identification of large external cremasteric vessels that may contribute to the varicocele.

Either an oblique or a transverse incision may be used (Figure 18-1). The medial aspect of the incision should be approximately two-finger breadths above the symphysis pubis at the lateral edge of the scrotum. Before the incision is made, the exact location of the external ring should be noted by invaginating the scrotal skin. The external oblique aponeurosis is exposed and incised in the direction of its fibers. Care is taken to avoid injury to the underlying ilioinguinal nerve. This procedure can be safely carried out by making a small stab through the fascia. The Metzenbaum scissors are then passed down to the external ring with the tips of the scissors elevated against the undersurface of the fascia. The scissors are rotated 90° to expose a groove between the two blades; this is then used as a guide for the knife incising the fascia. The spermatic cord is then mobilized at the level of the pubic tubercle. A Penrose drain is passed beneath the cord, elevating it from the canal. The Penrose drain is also used to exclude the ilioinguinal nerve from the operative field. Optical loupe magnification is used during the dissection to aid in the identification of the spermatic artery.

When the cremasteric fascia is incised, one should attempt to identify the artery by visual inspection and intraoperative Doppler ultrasound.[28] When identified, a vessiloop tape is utilized to isolate the artery from the area of further dissection. With the artery protected, all venous channels are isolated and ligated with a nonabsorbable suture. A representative segment is excised. Great care is taken to identify even small venous channels. These may be cauterized with bipolar forceps. The vas deferens is identified and its vasculature preserved. At this point, attention is redirected to the artery and surrounding veins encircled by the vessiloop. Meticulous dissection allows the surgeon to remove the rich anastomotic network of veins surrounding the spermatic artery, which is identified throughout the dissection visually and by the Doppler examination. Topical application of papaverine will cause arterial dilatation and may aid in the identification of the artery. When the artery has been cleared of the surrounding veins, its pulsations are readily apparent. After the spermatic cord has been fully explored, gentle traction is applied to the previously placed Penrose drain, elevating the cord out of the inguinal canal. The external cremasteric veins perforate the floor of the canal to drain into the pudendal vein, and ultimately, the saphenous vein. These veins should be identified since they may contribute to recurrent varices in a small proportion of patients.[29] The external oblique is closed with a continuous 2-0 chromic suture, and the subcutaneous layer is approximated with interrupted 3-0 plain catgut. A subcuticular absorbable closure with 4-0 Dexon is used.

Retroperitoneal Approach/Modified Palomo

The retroperitoneal approach or modified Palomo technique exposes the internal spermatic vein within the retroperitoneum after it exits the inguinal canal. A transverse abdominal incision is made just medial to the anterior superior iliac spine at the level of the internal ring (Figure 18-1). The external oblique fascia is incised in the direction of the fibers; the internal oblique muscle is incised and retracted cephalad; this exposes the dilated internal spermatic vein, which is ligated and divided. The dissection proceeds cephalad toward the renal vein to identify the collateral vessels. Although Palomo described ligating the internal spermatic artery and veins,[30] the artery should be preserved. The theoretical advantage of this technique is that retroperitoneal ligation of the internal spermatic vein reduces the number of veins contributing to the varicocele, and thus minimizes the potential for recurrence of the varicocele. Cockett et al.[4] advocate this approach on the premise that spermatic venous communications may occur between the left and right varicoceles at a level above the internal ring. A disadvantage of this technique is that it does not allow identification and ligation of the external cremasteric vessels. These vessels have been implicated as a cause of recurrent and persistent varicoceles following varicocelectomy.[25,31] This technique is advantageous in patients with previous inguinal surgery because it minimizes incidental injury to the testicular artery and ilioinguinal nerve. We utilize the retroperitoneal technique in patients with previous inguinal surgery who refuse venographic occlusion.

Laparoscopic Ligation

The explosion of interest in laparoscopic surgery has led to laparoscopic varicocelectomy. Proponents of laparoscopic varicocelectomy suggest that it offers lower morbidity, allows for microscopic dissection with preservation of the internal spermatic artery, and is amenable to bilateral ligation without a second incision.[32,33] A preliminary report by Hagoed et al. showed resolution of the varicocele in all patients without any associated morbidity; all patients resumed normal activity within 2 days.[32] Matsuda et al. were equally effective on

12 patients and claimed that the success rate of laparoscopic varicocelectomy appears to be as good as that of conventional, open high ligation.[33]

Although good initial results have been documented by several groups, the long-term risk–benefit ratio for this procedure is not known. Critics of the technique argue that an extraperitoneal procedure that can be performed in a short period on an ambulatory basis has been transformed into an intraabdominal operation with its attendant morbidity.[34] In their review of 329 laparoscopic pelvic lymph node dissections, Kavoussi et al.[35] found a complication rate of 15%.[35] In 10 of the 48 complications, a laparotomy was necessary for resolution of the problem.[35]

Limited follow-up since the advent of the laparoscopic ligation precludes evaluation of significant recurrence rates. However, it seems that laparoscopic ligations would tend to have a higher recurrence rate since this approach may fail to identify external spermatic veins.

Nonsurgical Treatment of Varicocele

Percutaneous Venous Occlusion

Various materials have been used to achieve transvenous occlusion of varicoceles. These include the use of detachable balloons,[25] Gianturco coils, sclerotherapy,[22] or a combination thereof. All these techniques share common advantages and disadvantages.[24,36] They can all be performed on an outpatient basis using only intravenous sedation. They provide a nonoperative approach to what historically has been treated surgically, and, therefore, recuperative time is minimized.

Either a femoral or jugular approach is used. The jugular approach allows easier access to the right internal spermatic vein. Although venoocclusion is nonoperative, it is often difficult and more time consuming than varicocelectomy. Although the exposure in experienced hands is minimal, many infertility patients are unhappy about receiving any radiation exposure. The success rate for this procedure, taking into account both the occlusion rate (73%) and the nonrecurrence rate (95%), is only 69%.[2]

Embolization is generally utilized only for the treatment of surgical failures of varicocelectomy or in patients with other previous inguinal surgery. With the increased safety of local and regional anesthesia, and in addition to the greater "reliability" and efficacy of the operative procedure, varicocelectomy remains the procedure of choice for the primary varicocele.

Complications of Surgical Varicocelectomy

Recurrence or persistence of varicoceles after surgical varicocelectomy is probably the most common as well as the most disturbing "complication" of therapy. A recurrence rate between 0 and 20% has been reported after surgical therapy.[2]

Most urologic surgeons have extensive operating experience within the inguinal canal. Surgical repair may be accompanied by ilioinguinal nerve injury (<1%), hydrocele formation

(3%),[19] epididymitis (<1%), and, rarely, wound infections.

Results of Varicocelectomy

Pryor and Howard assembled 15 publications evaluating the success of varicocele surgery. This review encompassed 2466 varicocelectomies. The overall rate of improvement in semen quality was 66% (range 51–78%). The overall reported pregnancy rate was 43% (range 24–53%).[2] Dubin and Amelar found higher pregnancy rates postoperatively in patients with preoperative sperm densities greater than 10 million per milliliter.[17] Brown reported similar findings.[37] On the other hand, Cockett and associates reported an increased pregnancy rate in patients with sperm concentrations less than 10 million per milliliter.[4] In an attempt to identify prognostic factors predicting postoperative pregnancies, Marks et al. showed four preoperative parameters to be of value.[38] The absence of testicular atrophy was found to indicate a good prognosis; 56% of patients with normal testicular size established pregnancies compared with a 33% pregnancy rate in patients with testicular atrophy. Patients with initial sperm counts of 50 million or more per ejaculate were significantly more likely to establish pregnancies after varicocelectomy. Thirty percent of patients with preoperative sperm motility of <60% initiated pregnancies postoperatively, whereas 60% of those with normal preoperative motility produced pregnancies. Elevation of FSH was, as expected, a poor prognostic indicator. Only 25% of patients whose FSH was above 300 (normal <300 ng/ml) achieved pregnancies, whereas 46% of patients with normal FSH levels initiated pregnancies.

Although numerous series describe improved semen quality and pregnancy rates following varicocelectomy, there also have been reports showing no significant effect or an adverse effect of varicocelectomy.[39–41] There have been many uncontrolled publications demonstrating the "effect" of varicocelectomy on infertility, but there have been only six controlled studies. Unfortunately, these are not prospective, blinded, or randomized studies. The studies of Rodriques-Netto et al.,[2] Newton et al.,[5] and Cockett et al.[8] demonstrated improved seminal parameters and pregnancy rates in patients treated with varicocelectomy as compared with those not receiving varicocelectomy. However, the studies of Baker et al.[39] and Vermeulen et al.[28] did not demonstrate a beneficial effect. Furthermore, Nilsson et al.[40] indicated that varicocelectomy had a deleterious effect on fertility. The design of this study has been criticized for bias.

Standard semen analysis is limited in its ability to differentiate fertile from infertile males. Thus, pregnancies attributed to alterations in semen parameters may, in fact, be unrelated. Rogers and associates attempts to demonstrate functional improvement following varicocelectomy using the sperm penetration assay.[42] In their study, 70% of those who achieved a pregnancy demonstrated improvement in the sperm penetration assay.

Nagler et al. recently reported improved Kruger morphologic assessment in men after varicocelectomy.[41] Kruger's strict criteria have been demonstrated to correlate with fertilization rates by standard *in vitro* fertilization.[41]

Varicocelectomy remains a significant and effective treatment of male infertility. The clinician treating the infertile couple should evaluate men with subfertile semen parameters for the presence of a varicocele and render treatment when appropriate.

REFERENCES

1. Nagler HM, Zippe CD: The varicocele. Current concepts and treatment. In: Lipshultz LI, Howards SS, eds. Infertility in the male, 2nd ed. Philadelphia: W.B. Saunders, 1991; 313–336.
2. Pryor JL, Howards SS: Varicocele. Urol Clin North Am 1987; 14:499.
3. Saypol DC, Lipshultz LI, Howards SS: Varicocele. In: Lipshultz LI, Howards SS, eds. Infertility in the male. New York: Churchill Livingstone, 1983.
4. Cockett ATK, Takihara H, Cosentino MJ: The varicocele. Fertil Steril 1984; 41:1.
5. Newton R, Schinfeld JS, Schiff I: The effect of varicocelectomy on sperm count, motility, and conception rate. Fertil Steril 1980; 34:250.
6. Rodriques-Netto N Jr, Fahiani EP, Lemos GC: Varicocele: Clinical or surgical treatment? Int J Fertil 1984; 29:164.
7. Steward BH: Varicocele in infertility: Incidence and results of surgical therapy. J Urol 1974; 112–222.
8. Cockett ATK, Urry RL, Dougherty KA: The varicocele and semen characteristics. J Urol 1979; 121:435.
9. Kass EJ, Belman AB: Reversal of testicular growth by varicocele ligation. J Urol 1987; 137:475.
10. Lyon RP, Marshall S, Scott MP: Variococele in childhood and adolescence: Implication in adulthood infertility? Urology 1982; 6:641.
11. Agger P, Johnsen SG. Quantitative evaluation of testicular biopsics in varicocele. Fertil Steril 1978; 19:52.
12. Lewis RW, Harrison RM: Contact scrotal thermograph: Application to problems of fertility. J Urol 1979; 122:40.
13. Bennett WH: Varicocele, particularly with reference to its radical cure. Lancet 1889; 1:261.
14. Macomber D, Sanders MB: The spermatozoa count: Its value in the diagnosis, prognosis and treatment of sterility. N Engl J Med 1929; 200:981.
15. Tulloch WS: A consideration of sterility factors in the light of subsequent pregnancies. Subfertility in the male. Trans Edinburg Obstet Soc 1952; 59:29.
16. Tulloch WS: Varicocele in subfertility, results of treatment. Br Med J 1955; 2:356.
17. Dubin L, Amelar RD: Varicocelectomy; 986 cases in a 12-year study. Urology 1977; 10:446.
18. Greenberg SH, Lipshultz LI, Wein AJ: Experience with 425 subfertile male patients. J Urol 1978; 119:507.
19. Dubin L, Amelar RD: The varicocele and infertility in: Amelar RD, Dubin L, Walsh PC (eds): Male Infertility. Philadelphia: WB Saunders Co., 1977.
20. Kupeli S, Arikan N, Aydos K, Aytac S: Mo hiparametric evaluation of testicular atrophy due to varicocele. Urol Int 1991; 46:189–192.
21. Ahlberg NE, Bartley O, Chidekel N, et al: Phlebograph in varicocele scroti. Acta Radiol Diagn Stockh 1966; 4:517.
22. Netto NR Jr, Lerner JS, Paolini RM, et al: Varicocele: The value of reflux in the spermatic vein. Int J Fertil 1980; 25:71.
23. Seyferth W, Jecht E, Zeitler E: Percutaneous sclerotherapy of varicoceles. Radiology 1981; 139:335.
24. Morag B, Rubenstein ZJ, Goldwasser B, et al: Percutaneous venography and occlusion in the management of spermatic varicoceles. Am J Radiol 1984; 143:635.
25. Murry RR Jr, Mitchell SE, Kadir S, et al: Comparison of recurrent varicocele anatomy following surgery and percutaneous balloon occlusion. J Urol 1986; 135:286.
26. Mieusset R, Bujan L, Mondinat LA, et al: Association of scrotal hyperthermia with impaired spermatogenesis in infertile men. Fertil Steril 1987; 48:10006.
27. Ivanissevich O: Left varicocele due to reflux; Experience with 4,470 cases in 42 years. J Int Coll Surg 1960; 34:742.
28. Vermeulen A, Vanderweghe M, Deslypere JP: Prognosis of subfertility in men with corrected or uncorrected varicocele. J Androl 1986; 7:147.
29. Chehval MJ, Purcell MH: Varicocelectomy: Incidence of external spermatic vein involvement

in the clinical caricocele. Urology 1992; 39:573–575.
30. Palomo A: Radical cure of varicocele by a new technique: Preliminary report. J Urol 1969; 61:604.
31. Coolsaet BL: The varicocele syndrome: Venography determining the optimal level for surgical management. J Urol 1980; 124:833.
32. Hagood PG, et al: Laparoscopic varicocelectomy: Preliminary report of a new technique. J Urol 1992; 147:73–76.
33. Matsuda T, et al: Laparoscopic varicocelectomy: A simple technique for clip ligation of the spermatic vessels. J Urol 1992; 147:636–638.
34. Sosa RE, Poppas DP, Schlegel PN, Lyons JM: Laparoscopic surgery in urology. In: Walsh PC, Retik AB, Stamey TA, Vaughan ED, eds. Campbell's urology—Updated, 6th ed. Philadelphia: W. B. Saunders, 1992:1–18.
35. Kavoussi LR, Loughlin K, Chandhoke PJ, et al: Complications of laparoscopic pelvic lymph node dissection. J Urol 1992; 147:451A.
36. Halden W, White RI Jr: Outpatient embolotherapy of varicocele. Urol Clin North Am 1987; 13:137.
37. Brown JS: Varicocelectomy in the subfertile male: A ten year experience with 295 cases. Fertil Steril 1976; 27:1046.
38. Marks JL, McMahon R, Lipshultz LI: Predictive parameters of successful varicocele repair. J Urol 1986; 136–609.
39. Baker HWG, Burger HG, Dekrester DM: Testicular vein ligation and fertility in men with varicoceles. Br Med J 1985; 291:1678.
40. Nilsson S, Edvinsson A, Nilsson B: Improvement of semen and pregnancy rate after ligation and division of the internal spermatic vein: Fact or fiction? Br J Urol 1979; 51:591.
41. Vazquez-Levin M, Chaparro CA, Medley NE, Nagler HM: Response of critical morphologic assessment to therapeutic varicocelectomy. American Fertility Society, 48th Annual Meeting, New Orleans, October 31, 1992.
42. Rogers BJ, Mygatt GG, Soderdahl DW, et al: Monitoring of suspected infertile men with varicocele by the sperm penetration assay. Fertil Steril 1985; 44:800.
43. Wosnitzer M, Roth JA: Optical magnification and Doppler ultrasound probe for varicolectomy. Urology 1983; 22:24.

ANNOTATED BIBLIOGRAPHY

Coolsaet BL: The varicocele syndrome: Venography determining the optimal level for surgical management. J Urol 1980; 124:833.

This is a review of 67 patients with left-sided varicocele who underwent pre-operative venography of the renal, internal spermatic, and common iliac vein with the aim of determining possible causes of varicocele. From the venographic findings, three forms of varicocele were able to be differentiated: group 1, where the etiologic factor arises in the internal spermatic vein itself, with or without an associated proximal nutcracker phenomenon; group 2, where the cause is obstruction of the common iliac vein, a distal nutcracker phenomenon; or group 3, where both of the above mechanisms exist. The author suggests that routine preoperative venography is essential to establish the etiology of the varicocele and its proper management.

Kass EJ, Belman AB: Reversal of testicular growth by varicocele ligation. J Urol 1987; 137:475.

Twenty patients ages 11 through 19 years with grade 2 or 3 varicocele associated with volume loss underwent ligation of the varicocele. Preoperatively, the average relative volume of the left testis in 20 patients was 70%. Following variococelectomy, the average relative volume increased to 91%. A statistically significant increase in testicular volume occurred in 16 of the 20 patients. The results of this study suggest that a moderate to large varicocele can be responsible for testicular growth retardation and that early ligation of the varicocele potentially can reverse this process.

Mieusset R, Bujan L, Mondinat LA, et al: Association of scrotal hyperthermia with impaired spermatogenesis in infertile men. Fertil Steril 1987; 48:10006.

This is a review of 150 infertile nonazoospermic men systematically studied observing scrotal temperatures, testicular volumes, and sperm characteristics looking for the existence of scrotal hyperthermia. A control group was made up of 37 men with proven fertility. The mean scrotal temperature values of the infertile men were significantly greater than those observed in the fertile men. In addition, it was found that the higher the scrotal temperature in the infertile men, the more altered the sperm characteristics. Moreover, the testicular volumes were significantly smaller in the infertile population. Although the scrotal temperatures of the infertile men with varicocele were significantly higher than those of the fertile men, they did not significantly differ from those of the infertile men without varicocele.

Nagler HM, Zippe CD: The varicocele. Current concepts and treatment. In: Lipshultz LI, Howards SS, eds. Infertility in the male, 2nd ed. Philadelphia: W.B. Saunders, 313–336.

This is a comprehensive review of current concepts and ongoing controversies regarding pathophysiology, diagnosis, and treatment of the varicocele. Also included are timely topics of subclinical varicocele, the adolescent varicocele, and surgical and percutaneous treatment of the varicocele.

19 Radiologic Management of Varicoceles Using Embolotherapy

Robert I. White, Jr.

Surgical management of varicoceles utilizing inguinal, direct scrotal, and laparoscopic approaches has been discussed in some detail in previous chapters. The inguinal approach for varicocelectomy produces excellent results and is the standard by which other techniques are measured.[1,2]

Radiological occlusion techniques using sclerosants for managing varicocele were described in 1977 and 1978.[3,4] In Europe, these techniques have predominated, while in the United States, outpatient management of varicocele has largely been performed utilizing detachable balloons or stainless-steel coils.[5,6] Most recently, results of transvenous sclerosis of the internal spermatic vein (ISV) using hot contrast media have been described.[7]

Since developing the technique for outpatient management of varicoceles with detachable balloons, very few modifications have occurred in our approach.[5,8] We favor this approach because of patient comfort, durability of occlusion, and long-term results.[9]

Table 19-1 Indications for Transcatheter Embolotherapy of Varicocele

1. Patient with varicocele and associated infertility or pain
2. Adolescent patient with large varicocele predisposed to testicular atrophy
3. Patient with varicocele and prior inguinal herniorrhaphy
4. Patient with surgical persistence or recurrence of varicocele

Indications—Preprocedure Workup

Table 19-1 outlines our current indications for transvenous radiologic management of varicocele. Our preoperative evaluation includes discussion of the patients' past history with the referring urologist, discussion with the patient regarding pertinent medical history that may modify the procedure, i.e., bleeding tendency or previous reaction to contrast media, and brief history directly from the patient on the morning of the procedure or at an earlier time

Management of Impotence and Infertility, edited by Douglas Whitehead and Harris Nagler,

in our interventional radiology clinic. Tests to evaluate clotting and renal function are not obtained unless the patient's prior medical history indicates a clotting or metabolic abnormality.

Noninvasive Radiological Assessment

While venography remains the gold standard for diagnosis of varicocele, duplex and color doppler evaluation of the scrotum may be performed for assessment of varicocele when the physical exam is uncertain.[10,11] These techniques are useful for documenting persistence of varicocele after surgical or radiological repair. When there is clinical uncertainty about the presence of a subclinical left- or right-sided varicocele, ultrasound evaluation is very useful.

Procedural Considerations—Embolotherapy

All varicocele occlusions are performed on an outpatient basis with discharge the same day. Our technique has evolved over the past 14 years and was described in detail previously.[9] During the 60–90 minutes required for a tailored occlusion of unilateral or bilateral varicoceles, sedation results from the intravenous administration of small increments of 0.5 mg fentanyl citrate (Elkins-Sinn, Cherry Hill, NJ) and midazolam hydrochloride (Versed; Roche Pharmaceuticals, Nutley, NJ). After the procedure, patients remain at bedrest for 3 hours and are ambulated gradually over the remaining hour. During the recovery time, intravenous ringer's lactate and oral fluids are administered. Patients are not given food over the 4-hour recovery as there appears to be a correlation between eating and nausea (5%) and vomiting (1%) when patients are first ambulated after recovery. Upon discharge, patients are not permitted to drive alone or resume normal activities until the next day. A family member drives them home or to a hotel to rest through the reminder of the day. The next morning they resume all normal activities. The cardiovascular radiology nurse or physician assistant routinely calls the next morning to inquire if they have questions or concerns. Each patient is given a pertinent set of representative radiographs for their permanent record and to share with the referring urologist at their 3-month follow-up examination.

Technical Considerations—Embolotherapy

The right femoral vein is used for catheterization and occlusion of all left and right varicoceles. The jugular vein approach is used by some radiologists, but we believe the more standard femoral vein approach is more comfortable for the patient and the radiologist. A standard 8 or 9 french indwelling vascular sheath is placed in the right femoral vein and a heparinized drip of saline is connected to it for the remainder of the procedure.

Radiation Protection

Before fluoroscopy, a lead shield is placed under the buttocks of the patient.[5] This reduces radiation exposure to the scrotum to the level approximating the dose received during a standard PA and lateral chest radiograph. The scrotal contents are never fluoroscoped or radiographed during the procedure.

Catheters

Standard 7.3 french, nontapered, special curved catheters (Cook, Inc., Bloomington, IN) are used to gain entry into the left or right ISV (Figure 19-1). For left varicocele occlusion, whether one chooses detachable balloons or

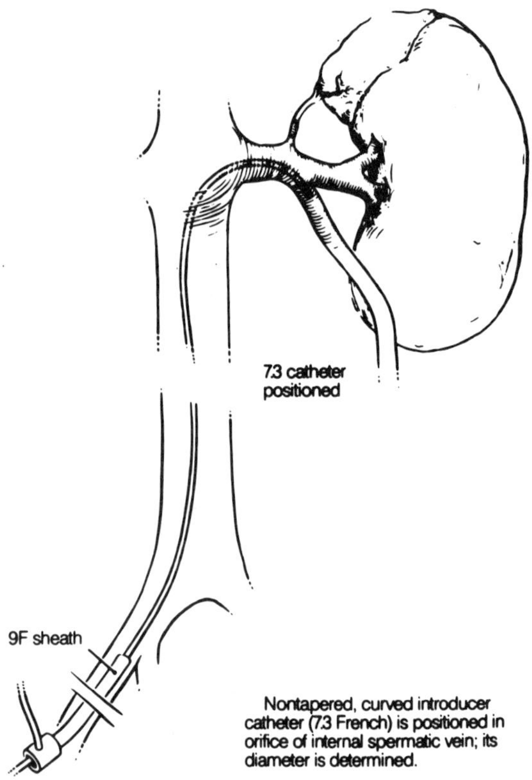

Figure 19-1 Diagram of initial catheterization procedure in all patients referred for transvenous occlusion of left varicocele. The standard 7.3 french varicocele catheter (Hopkins Curve) is placed in the orifice of the incompetent ISV through a 9 french sheath placed percutaneously in the right femoral vein. (Modified from White et al.[8])

stainless-steel coils, an additional catheter exchange is necessary after the preliminary venogram. Using an exchange "heavy duty" guidewire, the standard 7.3 nontapered, left-varicocele catheter is either exchanged for an 8 french, thin-walled polyethylene catheter (for detachable balloons) or a 5 french, thin-walled catheter (for stainless-steel coils). Catheterization techniques for management of right-sided varicoceles as well as additional details of left-sided catheterization have been described previously.[9,12]

Venography

Test injections of contrast material in the renal vein during fluoroscopy are used to identify the ISV orifice and to identify reflux down the ISV, confirming lack of or incompetent valves in the presence of a varicocele. Once the ISV is catheterized, a single 14 × 14 inch radiograph is obtained during the injection of 10 ml of contrast material into the ISV. The patient is asked to perform a Valsalva maneuver during the injection, which facilitates identification of important parallel collaterals that could be a cause for persistent or recurrent varicocele.

During placement of balloons or coils, additional test injections are monitored fluoroscopically or with a single 14 × 14 inch or 105 mm radiograph. At the end of the procedure a final radiograph is obtained.

Occlusion Techniques/Devices for Left Sided Varicocele

Sclerotherapy

In Europe, significant experience has been reported using intravascular glues (isobutyl cyanoacrylate), Varicocoid, or Aethoxylsclerol.[13,14]

These sclerosants are not approved in the United States and the experience with them experimentally is quite limited in this country. Hot contrast material has been popularized in the United States as a sclerosant by Hunter and associates.[7] Common to all sclerosants is transient pain during injection. Compression must be placed over the inguinal canal during injection to prevent penetration of the sclerosant into the pampiniform plexus, which results in phlebitis.

Embolotherapy

Detachable balloons: Silicone Miniballoons (Becton-Dickinson, Rutherford, NJ) were approved by the FDA in 1982. In June of 1990, Becton-Dickinson decided against pursuing interventional radiology products and withdrew balloons; most users of balloons switched to stainless-steel coils for occlusion of varicoceles. Subsequently, comparative testing was performed with the original silicone Miniballoon and the silicone detachable balloon developed by Hieshima (Interventional Therapeutics, Inc., South San Francisco, CA).[15] Results of these tests demonstrated equal *in vitro* efficacy of both balloons and the Hieshima balloon is now undergoing testing for cardiovascular uses. We prefer balloons over coils and are now using the Hieshima silicone balloon for all occlusions (Figure 19-2). Our balloon technique has been described previously and is essentially unchanged except for positioning of the balloons.[8,9]

For occlusion of varicocele by detachable balloon, an 8 french introducer catheter (Interventional Therapeutics, South San Francisco, CA) is positioned proximally in the ISV and a detachable balloon is placed through the introducer catheter and down the ISV to a position preferably just proximal to the internal inguinal ring. To prevent recurrences from renal hilar or capsular collaterals, occlusion at a level below the upper one-third of the sacroiliac joint is required. Occlusion at higher levels in the ISV as was originally advocated led to a higher persistence/recurrence rate than that achieved by occluding the ISV immediately above the internal inguinal ring.[9,16]

Test occlusions at different levels are performed during injection of contrast material proximally. Often by changing the position of the balloon, a position in the distal ISV is identified below which no parallel collaterals are noted to enter. If a distal position of the first balloon does not prevent parallel collaterals from reconstituting the ISV below it, this balloon is detached in the best possible position, which occludes entry of most of the parallel collaterals.

The second balloon is placed proximally near the tip of the introducer catheter at a position above all the parallel collaterals. Before detaching the second balloon, 10 ml of a mixture of 75% glucose (Abbott Laboratories, North Chicago, IL) and 1 ml of contrast material are injected into the ISV with the patient performing a Valsalva maneuver. The second balloon is rapidly inflated, trapping the glucose in the ISV and parallel collaterals between the two balloons. We have previously referred to this approach as the "sandwich technique."

The Hieshima balloons come in sizes up to 10 mm in diameter and are equally effective when compared with the silicone Miniballoons.[15] All balloons are inflated with isosmotic contrast material that assures their inflation for 30 days or longer. Previous work has demonstrated that a normal vessel totally occluded with a device for 20 days or longer will remain permanently occluded despite resorption of an embolic particle or deflation of the device.

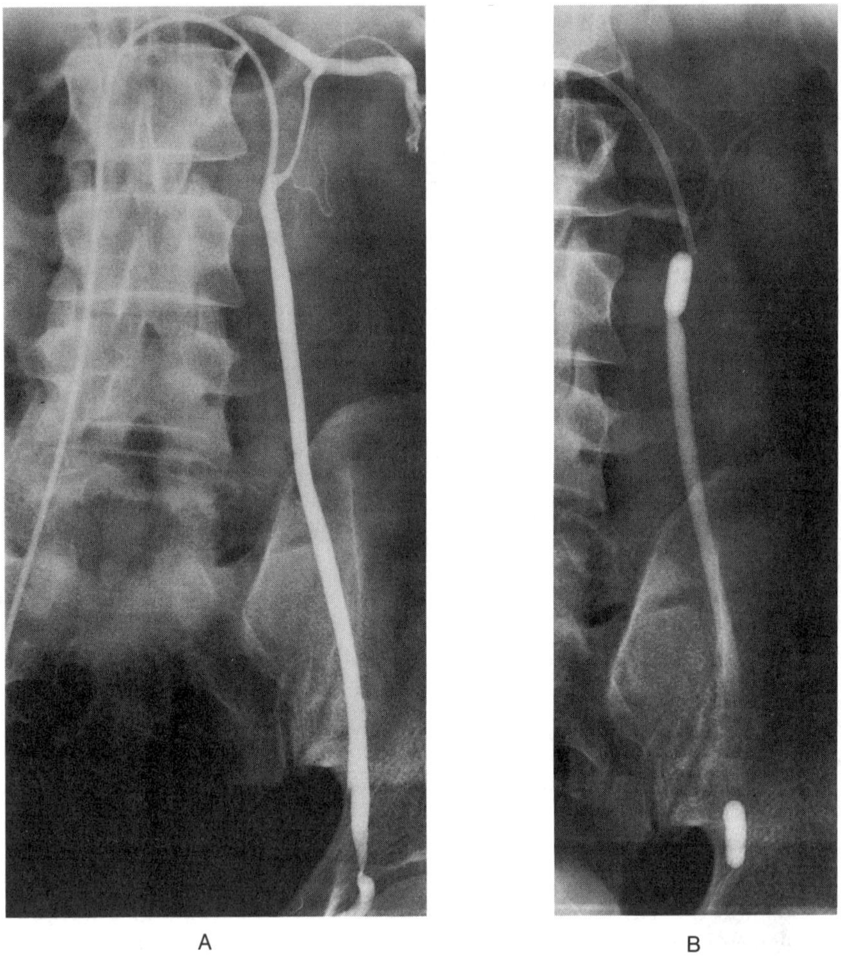

Figure 19-2 Venogram of left internal spermatic vein (ISV) before (A) and after (B) occlusion of ISV using two detachable balloons with a "sandwich" of faintly opaque 75% glucose between them. The distal balloon bridges a parallel collateral arising above the superior ramus of the pubis. The proximal balloon bridges a hilar collateral entering the ISV at the top of lumbar vertebra 3. Between the two balloons is a hypertonic mixture of 7–8 ml of 70% glucose and 1–2 ml of contrast material, which acts as a sclerosant.

Stainless-Steel Coils

Stainless-steel coils (Cook Incorporated, Bloomington, IN) developed in 1975 for vascular occlusion were available prior to the 1976 FDA device regulations. They are the mainstay of many types of embolotherapy and some interventional radiologists prefer using them over more complicated devices, such as balloons. They come in sizes ranging from 3 to 8 mm in diameter and in special order diameters up to 15 mm. Many newer versions designed to pass coaxially through catheters as small as 3 french are also available for use.

To effectively occlude the ISV and prevent persistent or recurrent varicoceles, coils must be placed low in the ISV below the point where parallel collaterals enter. Subsequently, coils are deposited along the course of the ISV in nests of three or four coils to within 3–4 cm of the ISV origin from the left renal vein (Figure 19-3). To accomplish this type of occlusion, a 5 french introducer catheter must be advanced deep into the ISV over a heavy duty exchange wire. Subsequent placement of coils while withdrawing the catheter is easily accomplished.

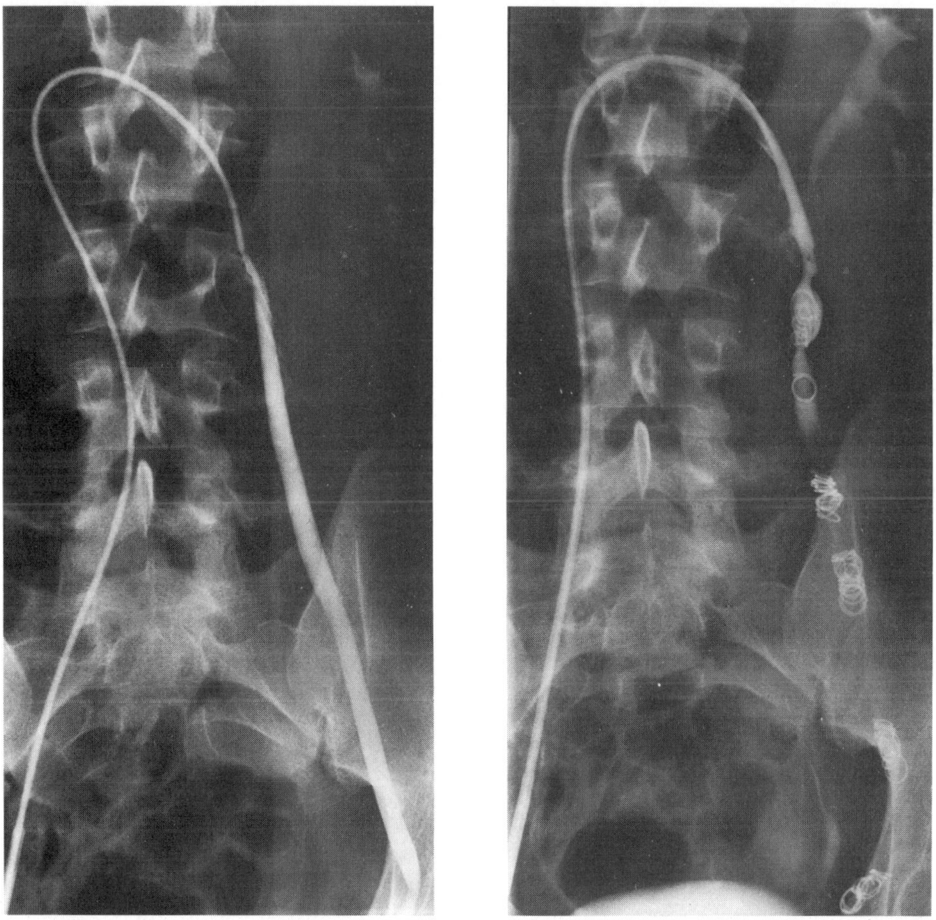

A B

Figure 19-3 Venogram of left ISV before (A) and after (B) occlusion of the ISV using segmentally placed stainless-steel coils. Note in (B) that coils are nested (three or four) from the inguinal region up to the third lumbar vertebra. At each level the coils were placed, parallel collaterals were observed to communicate with the ISV.

We have found the detachable balloon method of varicocele occlusion easier to perform than coil occlusion, but this may be because of our greater familiarity with the former method. The device expense of placing 20 coils segmentally is about the same as using two balloons. The greatest advantages of the balloon method over coils are the ease of placement of the balloon to a position low in the ISV and the ability to adjust the position of the balloon before detachment. If the test occlusion venogram obtained before balloon detachment demonstrates collaterals bypassing the balloon, the balloon can be deflated and its position adjusted.

Pitfalls

Variant Anatomy—Learning Curve

There are ample articles and monographs describing variant anatomy.[9,14] For the radiologist beginning this technique, the most important admonition is to occlude all potential collaterals. We have lowered our known varicocele persistences/recurrences from 11 to 5% between 1979 and 1985 by understanding more fully collateral pathways and adjusting balloon position accordingly.[9,16]

Some smaller series have been reported using transvenous techniques with unacceptable failure rates ranging from 20 to 30%, and these are largely due to poor understanding of the collaterals or variant anatomy, which prevented catheterization of the ISV. These failures might well have been prevented with greater training and appreciation for anatomical variations.

Palpable Varicocele with Competent ISV

In 5% of our patients, the referring urologist palpates a varicocele, but our initial catheterization demonstrates a competent ISV (a valve in the ISV prevents reflux of contrast material down the ISV (Figure 19-4). In these instances, a renal venogram is performed and will most often demonstrate a hilar collateral that joins the ISV below the competent valve at the upper border of the sacroiliac joint. To treat this variant, the origin of the ISV is catheterized and with a variety of small guidewires, the valve is crossed. Small 3 french catheters can be passed through the 7.3 french catheter over the guidewire into the ISV. The 7.3 french introducer catheter can then be removed and the larger introducer catheter passed through the valve over the 3 french catheter/guidewire combination. The occlusion can then proceed as originally planned.

Surgical/Radiological Persistence/ Recurrences

The most common cause of surgical recurrences is parallel collaterals that enlarge after surgical ligation of the main ISV, reconstituting the ISV below the point of ligation (Figure 19-5A).[17] Intraoperative postligation spermatic venography is useful for identifying parallel collaterals likely to cause persistent/recurrence when surgical repair is performed.[18] These collaterals are also identified quite easily during percutaneous ISV venography and embolization particularly during Valsalva venography with a distal balloon inflated before detachment.

Radiological persistence/recurrence usually occurs when enlarged hilar or capsular veins descend from the renal vein to join the ISV at the level of the upper one-third of the sacroiliac joint (Figure 19-5B).[17] To prevent persistent or recurrent varicoceles, a detachable balloon or nest of coils should be placed in the ISV below the level of the sacroiliac joint.

Surgical persistent/recurrent varicoceles are easily managed radiologically since the main ISV is patent and the occlusion device can be placed deep in the ISV beyond the entry point of the parallel collaterals. Radiological recurrences are more difficult to treat by transvenous occlusion techniques since hilar collaterals arising from the renal vein are more difficult to catheterize. Our results in occluding them are poor, but a renal venogram is useful before surgical repair.

Right Sided Varicocele

There is still much debate about the significance of right-sided varicocele. If the physical and/or ultrasound examinations confirm the presence of a right-sided varicocele, we will occlude it either at the time of the left-sided occlusion, or at a subsequent procedure.

Comparative Results

In most series with large numbers of patients, successful occlusion rates for managing varicoceles approximates 95% with a persistence/recurrences of 5–10%. These results compare favorably with surgical series. Unfortunately there are no prospective randomized studies comparing different radiological techniques. Similarly there are no prospective trials comparing surgical correction versus radiologic correction and our efforts to develop one 10 years ago were unsuccessful because patients with infertility were not willing to participate in randomized trials.

Complications associated with the transvenous occlusion method using coils or balloons are relatively uncommon. In experienced hands, migration of occlusion devices rarely occurs, if ever. In our earlier experience, we attempted occlusion of the proximal ISV immediately at the level of the renal vein in two patients and balloons did migrate to the lung. These patients had no sequelae and we made no attempts to retrieve the balloons. In the past 10 years, we have not experienced an episode of a balloon or coil migration to the lung. Interventional radiologists are well aware that all devices have to be placed within the ISV and not left at the orifice of the renal vein to prevent inadvertent migration from the ISV to the lung.

Between 1 and 2% of patients will have some nausea and postural hypotension during ambulation after the procedure. Intravenous hydration with Ringer's lactate and avoidance of food during recovery minimize these symptoms. Rarely patients are admitted overnight for continued hydration. In our own series of over 1000 patients treated, we have had no episodes of pampiniform phlebitis, testicular infarction, occlusion of the renal vein, or deep venous thrombosis of the femoral vein. These complications are also rare in the European experience with sclerosants and the Minnesota experience with hot contrast material, although pampiniform phlebitis and renal vein thrombosis have ben described using sclerosants.[7]

In Europe, transvenous occlusion techniques for managing varicocele are much more commonly practiced than in the United States. The results in terms of pregnancies following this technique range between 30 and 50% in the European series where pregnancy has been used as an end point.[14] In our personal series,

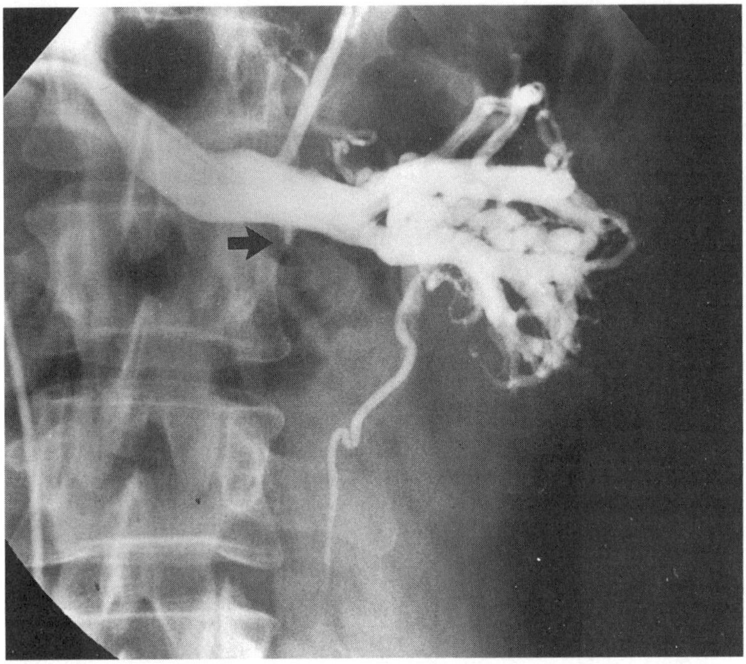

A

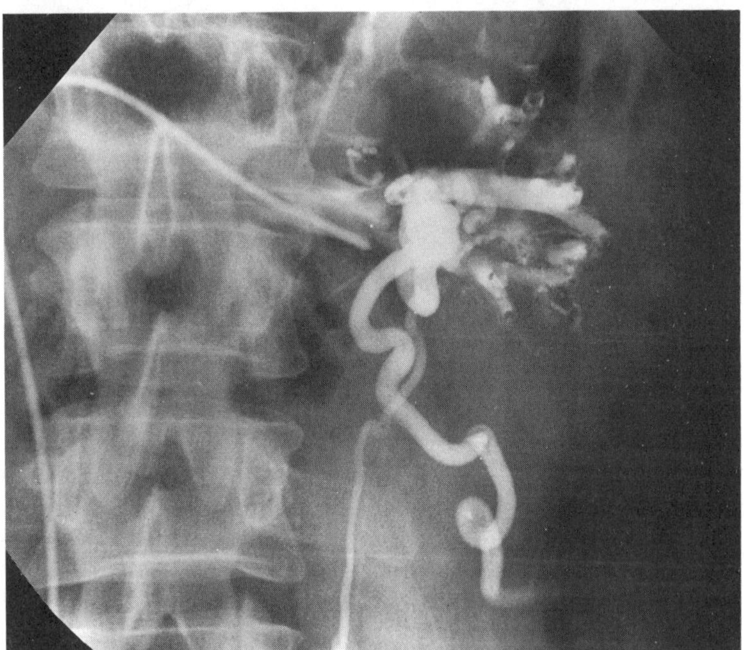

B

Figure 19-4 Early (A), mid (B), and later (C) radiographs from a left renal venogram in a patient with a large, palpable varicocele and competent internal spermatic vein. In this patient the varicocele fills primarily from a large renal hilar collateral vein that enters the ISV immediately above the sacroiliac joint (A,B,C). Immediately adjacent to the left adrenal vein, from the inferior surface of the renal vein the competent orifice (arrow) of the ISV is identified. (A) Gentle probing of the ISV orifice with fine caliber wires will usually permit crossing of a competent valve and ultimately entry into the large ISV for transvenous occlusion. It is important to know the results of physical examination and/or ultrasound examination regarding the presence of a varicocele. Because we knew that a varicocele was present, when we discovered a competent ISV, we were led to perform renal venography to identify an alternate source of venous blood entering the ISV. Renal venography is required in about 5% of patients to identify alternate sources of varicocele filling in the presence of a competent ISV.

Figure 19-4 (continued)

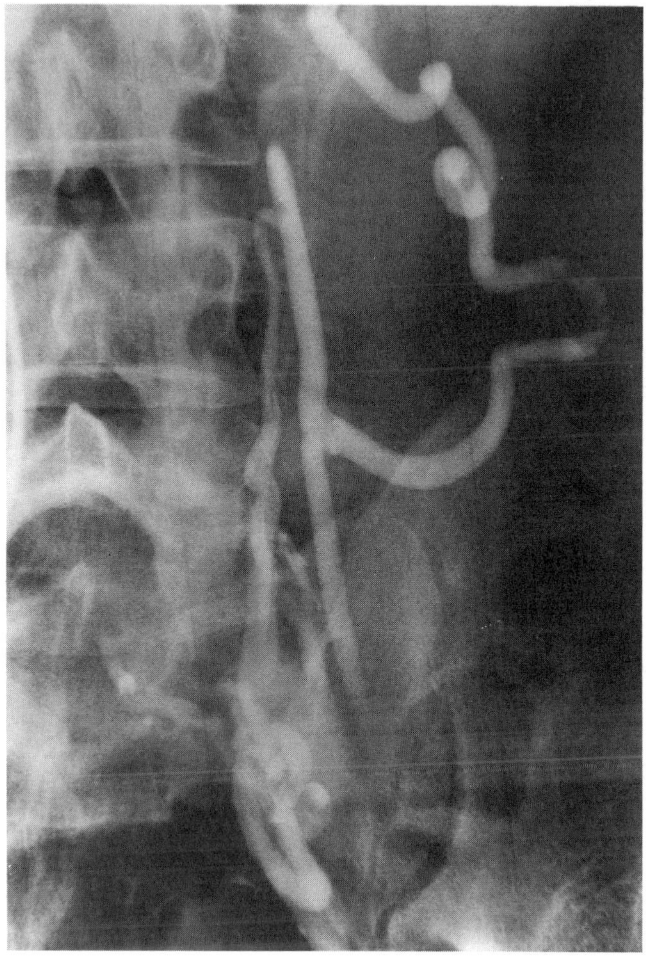

C

which has not been updated since 1987, the pregnancy rate for spouses whose husbands underwent varicocele occlusion was 36%. When those patients whose wives had some definite infertility problem were excluded, 41% of the wives became pregnant after their spouse underwent successful varicocele occlusion.[9]

Ideally, a randomized prospective trial comparing different surgical techniques with one another and with transvenous occlusion would be welcome. The transvenous occlusion technique appears to be a useful and reasonable alternative to surgery, but it is one that requires commitment and understanding by the interventional radiologist to achieve results equivalent to surgery.

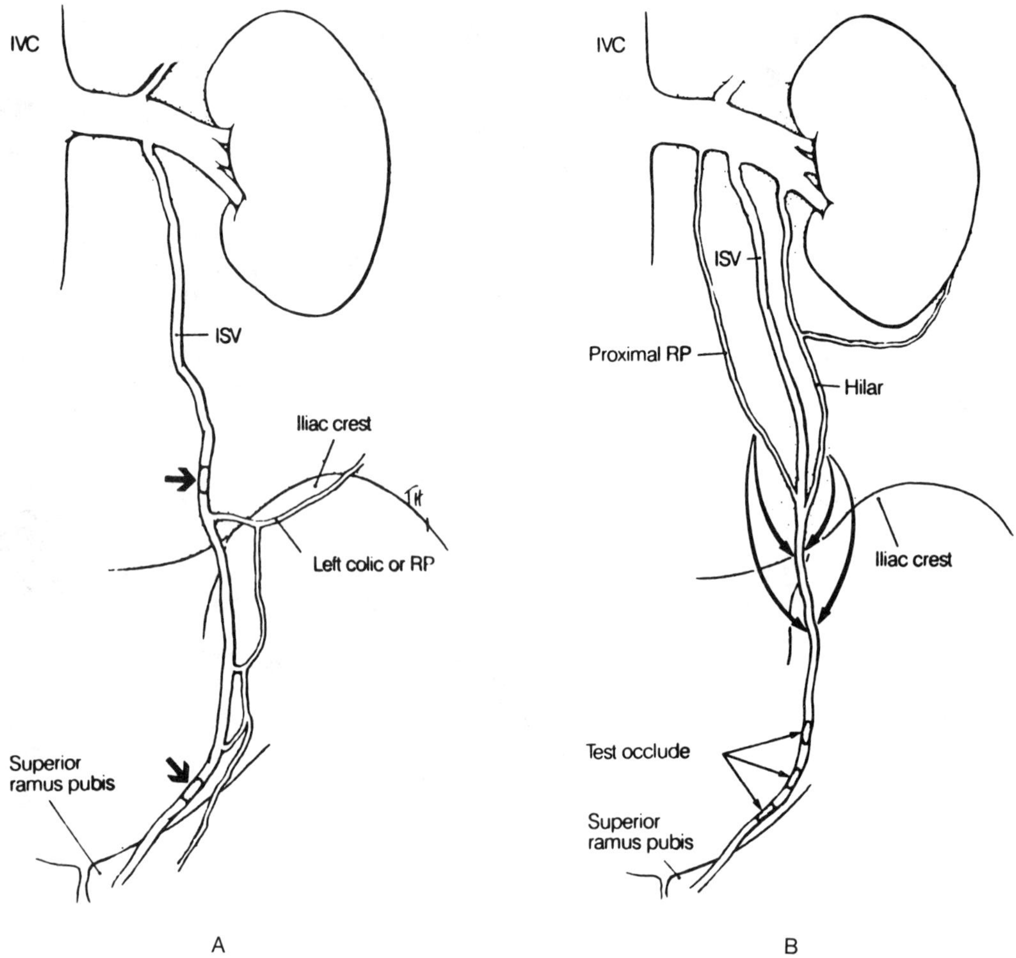

Figure 19-5 Diagrams of the important parallel (A) and hilar collateral (B) veins accounting for surgical and radiological persistent and recurrent varicocele after surgical ligation and radiological transvenous occlusion. In (A), collaterals descend parallel to the main ISV and in this instance they arise from the left colic or retroperitoneal vein. (A) The lower balloon (short arrow) is placed at the level of the superior ramus of the pubis. The upper balloon (short arrow) is placed immediately above the entry of the left colic vein. Alternatively, the upper balloon is placed bridging the entry of the left colic vein into the ISV. A "sandwich" of 75% glucose, which acts as a sclerosant, can be placed between the balloons. In (B), renal hilar and capsular collateral veins enter the ISV at the level of the upper one-third of the sacroiliac joint (curved arrows). After occluding the ISV with a balloon (long arrow), test occluded at different levels in the ISV above the superior ramus of the pubis, a second balloon would be placed bridging hilar or retroperitoneal collaterals at their entry into the ISV. As in (A), a "sandwich" of 75% glucose faintly opacified with contrast material is placed between the balloons to act as a sclerosant.

REFERENCES

1. Dubin L, Amelar RD: Varicolectomy: Twenty-five years of Experience. Int J Fertil 1988; 33:226–228, 231–235.
2. Thomas AJ Jr, Geisinger MA: Current management of varicoceles. Urol Clinic North Am 1990; 17:893–907.
3. Iaccarino V: Trattamento conservatio del varicocels. Felebografia selettiva o sclerotherapia delle uene gonadiche. Riv Radio 1977; 17:107–117.
4. Lima SS, Castro MP, Costa OF: A new method for the treatment of varicocele. Andrologia 1978; 10:103–106.
5. Walsh PC, White RI Jr: Balloon occlusion of the internal spermatic vein for the treatment of varicoceles, JAMA 1981; 246:1701–1702.
6. Weissbach L, Thelen M, Adolphs HD: Treatment of idiopathic varicoceles by transfemoral testicular vein occlusion. J Urol 1981; 126:354–360.
7. Hunter DW, King NJ, Aeppli DM, Yedlicka JW, Castenada-Zuniga WR, Hulbert JC, Kay K, Amplatz K: Spermatic vein occlusion with hot contrast material: Angiographic results. JVIR 1991; 2:507–515.
8. White RI Jr, Koffman SL, Barth KH, Kadir S, Smyth JW, Walsh PC: Occlusion of varicoceles with detachable balloons. Radiology 1981; 139:327–334.
9. Halden W, White RI Jr: Outpatient embolotherapy varicoceles. Urol Clinics North Am 1987; 14:137–144.
10. Petros JA, Andriole GL, Middleton WD: Correlation of testicular color doppler ultrasonography, physical examination and venography in the detection of left varicoceles in men with infertility. J Urol 1991; 145:785–788.
11. Demas BE, Hrihak H, McClure RD: Varicoceles, radiologic diagnosis and treatment. Radiol Clin North Am 1991; 29:619–627.
12. Shuman L, White RI Jr, Mitchell SE, Kadir S, Kaufman SL, Chang R: Right sided varicocele: Technique and clinical results of balloon embolotherapy from the femoral approach. Radiology 1986; 138:787–791.
13. Zeitler E: Selective sclerotherapy of the internal spermatic vein. Cardiovasc Intervent Radiol 1980; 3:166–169.
14. Zeitler E: Embolization of varicoceles. In: Dondelinger RF, ed. International radiology. New York: Thieme Medical Publishers, 1990; 529–536.
15. Pollak J, Lee G, Dormandy W, White RI Jr: A comparison of the mechanical properties of detachable balloons for embolotherapy. JVIR 1993; 4:91–95.
16. Kaufman SL, Kadir S, Barth KH, Smyth JW, Walsh PC, White RI Jr: Mechanisms of recurrent varicocele after balloon occlusion or surgical ligation of the internal spermatic vein. Radiology 1983; 147:435–440.
17. Murray RR Jr, Mitchell SE, Kadir S, Kaufman SL, Chang R, Kennison ML, Smyth JW, White RI Jr: Comparison of recurrent varicocele following surgery and percutaneous balloon occlusion. J Urol 1986; 135:286–289.
18. Gill B, Kogan SS, Maldonado J, Reda E, Levitt SB: Significance of intraoperative venographic patterns on the postoperative recurrence and surgical incision placement of pediatric varicocele. J Urol 1990; 144:502–505, 512–513.

ANNOTATED BIBLIOGRAPHY

Demas BE, Hrihak H, McClure RD: Varicoceles, radiologic diagnosis and treatment. Radiol Clin North Am 1991; 29:619.

Thomas AJ, Geisinger MA: Current management of varicoceles. Urol Clin North Am 1990; 17:893.

In the first paragraph of this review article, the authors discuss the relationship between varicocele and infertility. While cause and effect between varicocele and infertility has not been proven conclusively, the preponderance of evidence favors a relationship.

Beyond physical exam, the authors favor high resolution real-time scrotal ultrasound for diagnosis. Criteria for diagnosis include visualization of two or three venous channels, one of which has a diameter greater than 3 mm, and an increase in size with assumption of erect position or with the Valsalva maneuver. Sensitivity and specificity of ultrasound diagnosis of varicocele exceed 90% and are greater than physical exam, thermography, and radionuclide scrotal scanning.

Venographic techniques of diagnosis are described in detail along with the results of embolotherapy using liquid sclerosing agents, hot contrast material, coils, and detachable balloons. Success of embolotherapy is approximately the same as surgery although randomized trials are not available for comparison.

Gill B, Kogan SS, Maldonado J, Reda E, Levitt SB: Significance of intraoperative venographic patterns on the postoperative recurrence and surgical incision placement of pediatric varicocele. J Urol 1990; 144:502.

The authors describe their results of intraoperative venography to assess venous collaterals as a potential cause of recurrences after surgical correction of varicocele. Indications for surgery included enlarging varicocele and significant testicular atrophy in their 60 patients.

The authors found operative venography to be helpful in identifying proximal collateral veins to the site of ligation in 35% of cases. After additional ligation, only 7% of patients had proximal collateral veins that could account for recurrence. Pelvic collateral veins including the cremasteric, deferential, and crossover veins are rarely responsible for recurrences.

Mean follow-up of 16 months indicated a 6% incidence of recurrent/persistent varicoceles. The importance of parallel collateral veins in the etiology of recurrent varicocele is emphasized while lack of importance of the cremasteric, deferential, and pelvic crossover veins in the etiology of surgical recurrence is proven in this article.

Petros JA, Andriole GL, Middleton WD, Picus DA: Correlation of testicular color doppler ultrasonography, physical examination and venography in the detection of left varicoceles in men with infertility. J Urol 1990; 145:785.

High resolution color doppler ultrasound was used to diagnose clinical as well as subclinical varicocele. Internal spermatic venography was used as the gold standard in this study. As with standard duplex ultrasound, color doppler ultrasound was better at detecting subclinical varicocele when compared with physical examination.

Variations in hue of the color indicated velocity changes while direction of flow was determined quite easily using color doppler ultrasound. Patients with normal physical examination and normal color doppler ultrasound were not examined venographically so sensitivity/specificity and accuracy of color doppler ultrasound were not able to be assessed.

In conclusion, color doppler ultrasound as well as duplex ultrasound represent excellent noninvasive techniques for diagnosing subclinical varicocele.

20 Scrotal Hypothermia for Subfertile Semen

Adrian W. Zorgniotti

In the face of urgent demands by infertile couples, the treatment of subfertile semen is time consuming and often costly and the results are frequently disappointing. When there is success, the practitioner is rewarded with a photograph of the new baby for the office bulletin board. Because the testis'endocrine and exocrine functions are closely interrelated to the endocrine system, considerable effort has been invested in finding treatment in this area with generally disappointing outcome. The original use for *in vitro* fertilization was to bypass problems caused by disease or absence of the fallopian tubes. Extension of this technology to subfertile semen has proved expensive with a low yield of live births. The only treatment that has yielded results is varicocelectomy when a varicocele can be identified, but what about the patient with subfertile semen with increased tapering forms in whom no varicocele can be identified? Should these patients be explored surgically?

There is a vast literature showing that extrinsically applied heat can damage spermatogenesis, yet the possibility that existence of intrinsic elevation of temperature could yield yet another therapeutic modality to the vexing problem of subfertile semen has received little attention. Scrotal hypothermia was originally employed to test the hypothesis that intrinsic defect in testicular thermoregulation causes elevation of intrascrotal temperature, which results in subfertile semen.[1,2] Since then, it has become apparent that a high proportion of subfertile men have elevated intrascrotal temperature, whether or not a varicocele can be detected.[3,4] Several mechanisms have been suggested. Where varicocele is present, refluxing core temperature venous blood into the scrotal area raises temperature. Another explanation, including where varicocele is not present, is that refluxing blood in the internal spermatic vein interferes with normal countercurrent heat exchange from artery to vein within the spermatic cord, which precools arterial blood reaching the mediastinum testis. The contralateral testis becomes affected by a temperature gradient between the two scrotal compartments

Management of Impotence and Infertility, edited by Douglas Whitehead and Harris Nagler,

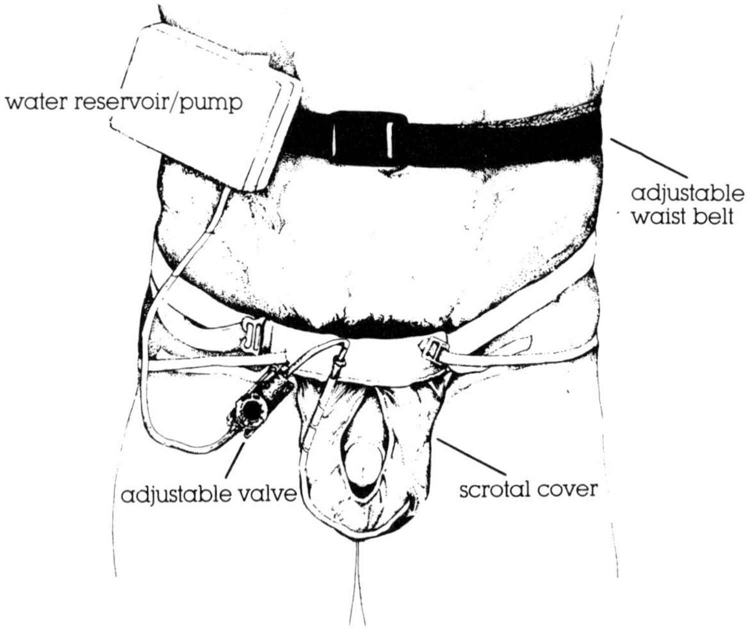

Figure 20-1 The testicular hypothermia device (THD) lowers scrotal temperature by heat of vaporization about 2°C, bringing elevated testis temperature closer to euthermic levels. Improvement in semen and pregnancies occur depending on the severity of the infertility at the time of initiation of treatment.

while scrotal wall heat loss is limited by scrotal surface size. This clinical entity has come to be referred to as Essential Testicular Hyperthermia.[5] When it was found that lowering temperature about 2°C by a prototype testicular hypothermia device (THD) could result in semen improvement and pregnancy in the wives of infertile men, a therapeutic potential was realized. The THD is a cotton scrotal covering that lowers temperature by controlled evaporation of water (Figure 20-1).

Patient Selection for the THD

Many males with subfertile semen can be treated by this noninvasive method. Couples with noncontraceptive coitus for 6 months without a pregnancy merit fertility investigation, which must include a semen analysis. Wives should be judged able to conceive on clinical impression of a gynecologist. THD suitable husbands fall into one of three clinical entities: varicocele, failed varicocelectomy, and idiopathic infertility (subclinical varicocele) with intrascrotal temperature ≥34°C. Excluded are patients with non-temperature-caused subfertile semen (e.g., endocrine, genetic, toxic, and mumps) (Table 20-1). The THD has not been approved for azoospermia as no nonobstructive patient has responded to this treatment.

Determination of Intrascrotal Temperature

To solve the problem of surveying large cohorts, a noninvasive method for intrascrotal temperature measurement was evolved. This noninvasive method employs an inexpensive water bath thermometer that is accepted by

Table 20-1 Semen and Temperature Criteria for the Male[a]

Subfertile semen in one or more parameter
Less than 20 million spermatozoa/ml
Less than 40% motile forms
Less than 60% oval forms (stained morphology)

[a] Elevated intrascrotal temperature: ≥34°C.

patients so that there is no need for patient consent in the diagnostic setting. Instrument accuracy is not in question since the thermometer measures absolute temperature and is calibrated to United States Bureau of Standards with divisions = 0.05°C. Factors that could alter the reading (scrotal skin temperature, scrotal skin circulation, and heat coefficient of the glass and mercury thermometer) are negligible. A recommended thermometer has a range of 32–40°C with division of 0.05°C (Model No. C1148: Brooklyn Thermometer Company, Farmingdale, NY). Clinical thermometers, because of a constriction in the mercury column, are not satisfactory.

The patient is placed supine without clothing over the genitalia for 6 minutes. To speed temperature estimation, the thermometer can be prewarmed to around 37°C by placing the bulb in contact with a light bulb or immersion in warm water. The mercury bulb is then placed against the scrotum over the most prominent part of the anterior testis. The scrotal skin is drawn about the bulb, invaginating it completely. Some thermometers have an "immersion line"; this should be covered by skin. When the falling mercury column reaches equilibrium, usually in <10 seconds, the intrascrotal temperature is reached. The procedure is then repeated for the contralateral testis (Figure 20-2). Measurements in men who, in cold and windy weather, present wearing cotton trousers (usually jeans) may be inaccurate owing to chilling of the testes. A long period of equilibration

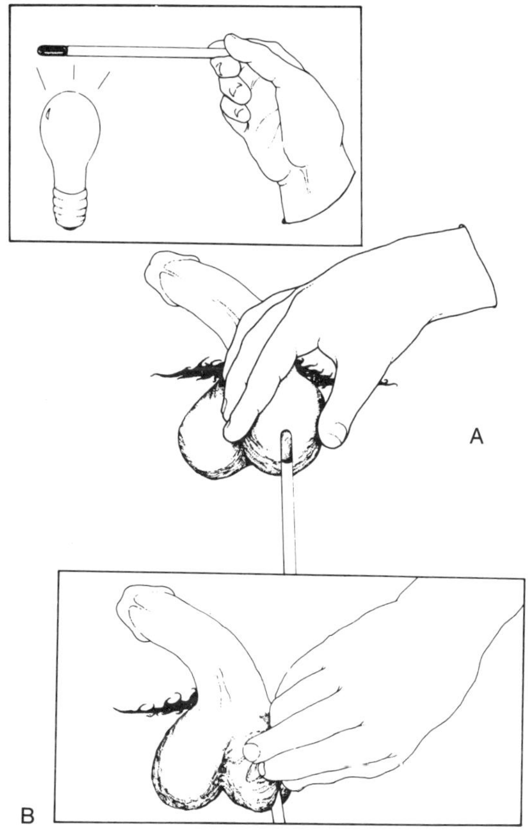

Figure 20-2 (A) Noninvasive method for intrascrotal temperature measurement. The laboratory thermometer is placed against the scrotum overlying the anterior testis. (B) The thermometer is "invaginated" by wrapping the scrotal skin around the bulb of the thermometer. When equilibrium is reached, this measures intrascrotal temperature ±0.1°C.

to indoor temperature is necessary and it is usually easier to ask the subject to return on another, milder, day wearing woollen pants.

Two recent (<6 month) semen analyses should be obtained. Semen analyses are done at 10 week intervals during treatment, included stained morphology. The patient signs a consent, following which he is fitted with the THD and instructed in its use.

Table 20-2 Decrease in Scrotal Temperature after Application of the THD

$n = 59$	Mean Decrease (°C)	Range
Right	2.0	(−0.1 to −6.2)
Left	2.3	(−0.3 to −4.9)

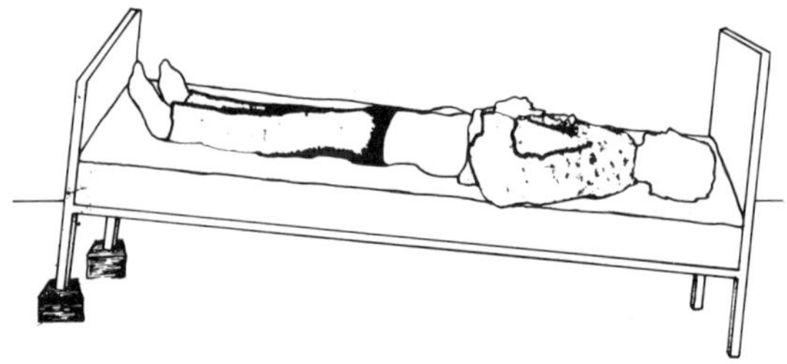

Figure 20-3 At night patients remove the THD and sleep without clothing covering the genitalia. They also have the option of sleeping in mild Trendelenberg, which helps lower intrascrotal temperature.

The hypothermic effectiveness of the device has been demonstrated by infrared thermometry. After having the patient stand for 6 minutes with genitalia exposed, an infrared thermometer (IT 4M Barnes Engineering, Stamford CT) reading of the scrotal skin over the anterior testis was made. A THD was applied and when equilibration was reached (i.e., the scrotal covering was damp), the suspensory was pulled to one side and the temperature reading repeated (Table 20-2).

The patient is required to wear the THD daily at all times while up and clothed. At night, the patient removes the THD allowing for a period of dry skin after day-long contact with the damp scrotal covering. He is asked to sleep without clothing over the genitalia; light covers are permitted. The patient may place 10-cm blocks under the legs at the foot of the bed to produce slight Trendelenburg, which also reduces intrascrotal temperature (Figure 20-3). The THD is removed for intercourse and bathing. In the event of a fever above 37.8 °C, the patient is advised to wear the THD continuously.

Results Obtained in 140 Patients

One hundred forty men met the criteria of a protocol[6] and were fitted with the THD; 76/140 did not wear the device as required or long enough. The most frequent reasons for dropping out were mechanical difficulties with the device, which have since been remedied, and discouragement over the length of wearing time required before semen improved or pregnancy occurred. A self-selected group (20 of 76) who met all criteria but never wore the THD and did not have any further infertility treatment became controls. Not conforming to the protocol were six who had nonobstructive azoospermia (having shown progressive deterioration in the semen analysis to the point of azoospermia). None of the azoospermic men showed any sperm in the ejaculate after 6+ months of hypothermia.

Sixty-four wore the THD daily for more than 16 weeks. There was improvement in semen in 42 of 64 (65.6%) and pregnancy in 16 of 64 (25.0%). The incidence of pregnancy was further refined in terms of pretreatment semen quality based on the motile oval index (MOI) (Table 20-3).

The MOI, an elaboration of the motile sperm count which takes into account morphology, has been used[7] in varicocelectomy studies and has proved useful in evaluating pregnancy rates with the THD. Semen with

Table 20-3 The Motile Oval Index (MOI)

MOI = count in millions/ml × percent motile × percent ovals, e.g., using minimum normal values (Table 20-1)
Minimum normal MOI = 20 million/ml ×40% × 60% = 4.8 million/ml

MOI of 4.8 million/ml or higher is possible when one or two parameters fall in the normal range with at least one parameter being subfertile. Striking increase in MOI and pregnancy were seen where the pretreatment MOI was 4.8 million/ml or higher (Table 20-4).

Effect of THD on Hamster Ovum Penetration

Four patients who produced a pregnancy on the THD had pretreatment hamster ovum penetration tests that were repeated at the time pregnancy was diagnosed. All four had subfertile starting semen: mean count 7.8 million/ml. At the time of conception mean count had increased to 39.4 million/ml and penetrations were also found to have increased, in two instances from zero penetrations (Figure 20-4).

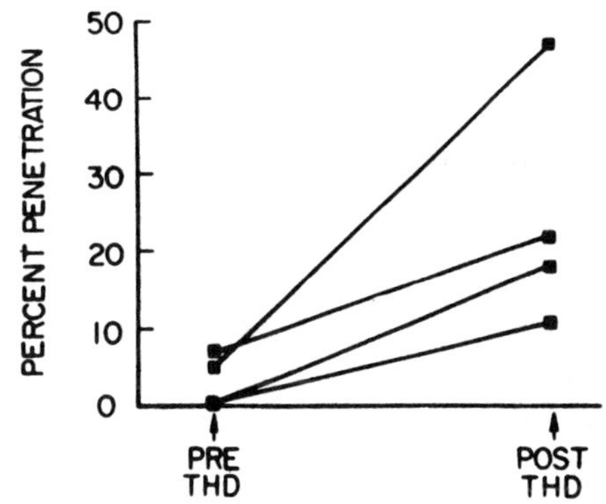

Figure 20-4 Hamster ovum penetration by spermatozoa of four men who produced a pregnancy.

Discussion

The THD removes scrotal heat by evaporation, lowering temperature about 2°C. The THD may need to be worn 4 months to a year before pregnancy occurs. The only complication noted has been exacerbation of tinea cruris, which usually responds to application of miconazole powder. Removing the THD at night allows a dry period for the scrotum and adjacent skin. While wearing and maintenance are not difficult, adherence to the wearing schedule requires considerable motivation.

The best result, in terms of pregnancy, was obtained in patients whose starting MOI was

Table 20-4 The MOI Change in Couples Achieving Pregnancy[a]

	Pregnancies	Mean MOI Increase	Range
Starting MOI <4.8 million/ml	5/43 (11.6%)	9.0	(0.8 to 22.1)
Starting MOI ≥4.8 million/ml	11/21 (52.4%)	19.9	(−1.0 to 57.0)
All patients	16/64 (25.0%)		
Untreated	1/20 (5.0%)		

[a] Mean years infertile marriage, 4.0; mean months of wearing THD to missed menses, 4.2; live births, 15 of 16.

above 4.8 mil/ml before inception of treatment. (Comparison of MOI ≥4.8 pregnancy rate with MOI <4.8 pregnancy rate is significant.) This implies that patients with better but still subfertile semen have the best chance of producing a gestation. Changes in semen parameter may be observed within 10 weeks of starting treatment. The mean THD wearing time to pregnancy was 4.2 months; in rare instances pregnancy will not occur until a year or more, so that patient motivation becomes an important factor.

Comparison with Varicocelectomy

Surgery for varicocele has been shown to produce pregnancies reported as ranging from 20 to 60%. One of the best was that of Gentile and Cockett of 57.3%.[8] The THD rates noted above are not comparable in terms of MOI. In both modalities objective studies are difficult, since adequate controls are difficult to achieve (withholding treatment, sham operation, or wearing the THD without adding water, etc). The control we were able to obtain came about by chance when 20 men who met criteria chose not to wear the device. These were surveyed and 1 of 20 (5.0%) had produced a pregnancy without further treatment. When compared to all THD patients, regardless of pretreatment MOI, significance was not achieved.

Basralian et al. noted a precipitous decline in fecundability (percentage conception rate per month) during the first 3 years of involuntary infertility.[9] Fecundability for couples "trying" less than 1 year is 4.17% and by 3 years decreased to 1.65%, and continued to decrease with the further passage of time (Figure 20-5).

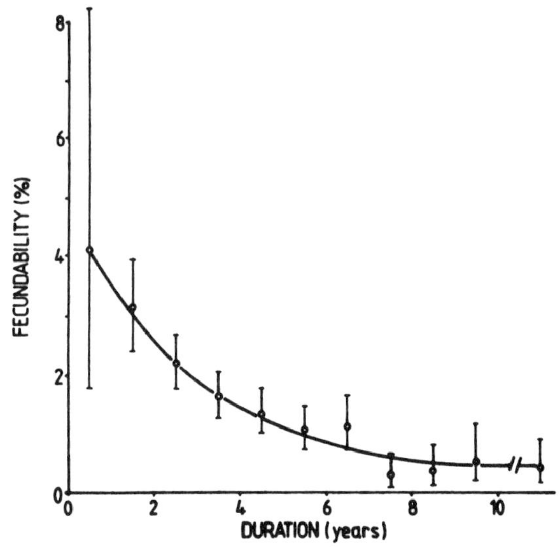

Figure 20-5 Decrease of fecundability (percentage conception rate/month) with respect to "total trying" time (involuntary infertility). In therapeutic trials for infertility, after 3 years of involuntary infertility, any success can be considered the result of the treatment rather than a spontaneous effect. (Reprinted from Basralian et al.,[9] with permission.)

The authors concluded that in clinical trials where subjects have been "trying" longer than 3 years, pregnancies that occur are no longer spontaneous but represent treatment effect. Their observation provides a useful tool for studying the results of fertility treatments including varicocelectomy and the THD. In our 16 THD patients who produced a pregnancy, the mean involuntary infertility time was 4.0 years (range: 2–10 years), with 9 of 16 "trying" for longer than 3 years. That these pregnancies occurred suggests that hypothermia offers an effective therapy (Table 20-5).

Failure of the pretreatment less than 4.8 mil/ml MOI group to do as well as the greater than 4.8 million/ml MOI group suggests that severely subfertile semen is the result

Table 20-5 Duration of Involuntary Infertility in 16 Couples Who Produced a Pregnancy with THD

Years Trying	Estimated Fecundability[a] (%)	$n = 16$
2	3.14	6
3	2.22	1
4	1.65	5
5	1.37	1
6	1.15	1
8	0.38	1
10	0.45	1

[a] From Basralian et al.,[9] with permission.

of progressive and ultimately irreversible change to the germinal epithelium. (It is further suggested that Sertoli-only finding may represent the end stage of testicular hyperthermia.) The presence of an MOI of less than 4.8 million/ml need not discourage application of the THD as improvement in semen and pregnancies do occur. Semen levels often improve to levels where *in vitro* fertilization becomes feasible and there has been one *in vivo* fertilization while awaiting an IVF appointment.

Summary

The THD provides a noninvasive first line treatment of subfertile semen associated with elevated intrascrotal temperature. Compared to surgery and gamete manipulation it is cost effective. Where prior treatment has failed (e.g., varicocelectomy, hormonal therapy, and gamete manipulation), the THD can be an important resource for the "hard core" infertile couple and should not be overlooked. The THD received approval of the United States Food and Drug administration in December 1984 and colleagues are therefore advised to include discussion of this treatment alternative in informed consent for infertility treatment where appropriate. Regrettably, the only clinical studies on the effectiveness of the THD have been published by the inventors.

The THD is available from Repromed Systems, Inc. 17 Industrial Place, Middletown, NY 10940.

REFERENCES

1. Zorgniotti AW, MacLeod J: Studies in temperature, human semen quality and varicocele. Fertil Steril 1973; 24:834.
2. Zorgniotti AW et al: Chronic scrotal hypothermia as a treatment for poor semen quality. Lancet 1980; I:904.
3. Mieusset et al: Association of scrotal hyperthermia with impaired spermatogenesis is in infertile men. Fertil. Steril. 1987; 48:1006.
4. Zorgniotti AW, Sealfon AI: Measurement of intrascrotal temperature in normal and subfertile men. J Repro Fertil 1988; 82:563.
5. Mirone V, Iacono F: Testicular hyperthermia; Physiopathology, diagnostic and therapeutical concepts. In: Zorgniotti AW, ed. Temperature and environmental effects on the testis. New York: Plenum Press, 1991:217.
6. Zorgniotti AW, et al: Chronic scrotal hypothermia: Results in 90 infertile couples. J Urol 1986; 135:944.
7. Lee HW, et al: Effect of varicocelectomy on spermatogenesis. In: Glezerman M, ed. Varicocele and male fertility II. Berlin: Springer-Verlag, 1984:100.
8. Gentile DP, Cockett ATK: Varicocelectomy effect on fertility. In: Zorgniotti AW, ed. Temperature and environmental effects on the testis. New York: Plenum Press, 1991:289.
9. Basralian KR et al: Duration of involuntary infertility and subsequent pregnancy. Urology 1987: 29:635.

21 Microsurgical Correction of Obstructive Azoospermia

Anthony J. Thomas, Jr.

Obstructive azoospermia is, in most instances, a treatable condition. The ultimate result of that treatment is dependent on the site and etiology of the blockage, the length of time that it has existed, and the skill of the surgeon in bypassing the obstruction.

A man presenting with azoospermia or severe oligospermia should be evaluated for the possibility of a complete or partial, unilateral or bilateral obstruction. Figure 21-1 presents an algorithm outlining how a patient can be quickly and efficiently assessed.

A thorough history should be taken to identify a possible cause for obstruction. In some men it is as obvious as a prior vasectomy, while in others, there may be no apparent reason for a blockage to exist. A careful physical examination is performed with particular attention to the genitalia. The testes should be measured in three dimensions or their volume determined using an orchidometer. The epididymides may feel indurated, raising the suspicion that an obstruction exists, or that one, or possibly both, vasa deferentia may be absent.

Two or three semen samples should be analyzed before making the diagnosis of azoospermia. Once azoospermia is suspected, if the semen volume is small (<1.5 ml), a postejaculatory urine sample is obtained and centrifuged. The sediment is examined for sperm to rule out retrograde ejaculation. If no sperm is found in the urine and the ejaculate is acidic in character (pH <7), there may be a congenital absence or marked hypoplasia of the seminal vesicles and ejaculatory ducts often associated with absent vasa. If the vas deferens is present on one or both sides, obstruction at the ejaculatory duct level may be present. Transrectal ultrasound (TRUS) is very useful in helping to determine if there is dilation of the seminal vesicles and proximal portions of the ejaculatory ducts. These patients are candidates for transurethral opening of the ducts. This is described in detail in Chapter 24.

When the etiology of the obstruction is known or suspected based on the patient's history (i.e., epididymitis, prior hernia repair, vasectomy, hydrocelectomy, etc.) or physical examination, appropriate planning for surgical

Management of Impotence and Infertility, edited by Douglas Whitehead and Harris Nagler,

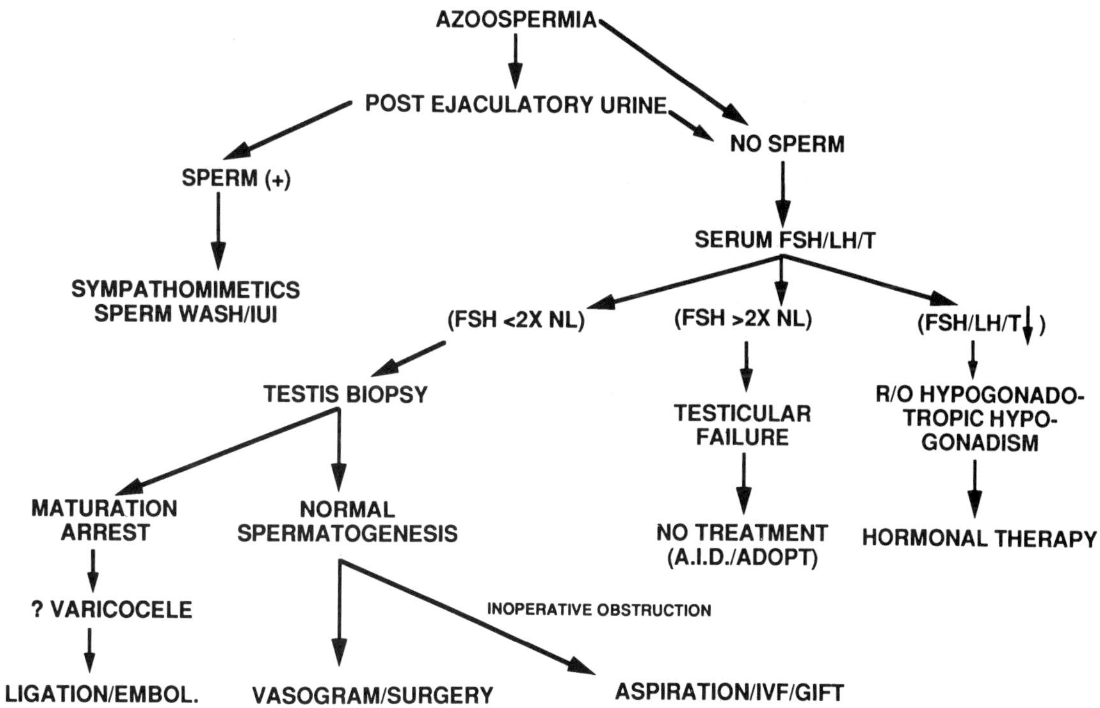

Figure 21-1 Algorithm suggested for the evaluation of the azoospermic patient. (Reproduced with permission from Falk and Thomas.[29])

correction can be more easily undertaken by both physician and patient.

The diagnosis of obstruction can be confirmed by history, by demonstrating sperm present in the efferent tubule proximal to the site of blockage, or by identifying active spermatogenesis in the testis biopsy. An individual who presents for vasectomy reversal and has previously fathered a child requires neither semen analysis nor testis biopsy unless there has been some other alteration in his reproductive status such as that caused by orchitis or significant testicular trauma. A biopsy is not necessary for the azoospermic individual who is found to have bilateral small testes (<15 cm^3) with a serum follicle-stimulating hormone (FSH) level of more than twice the upper limits of normal. This person has spermatogenic failure for which there is no effective treatment. If, however, one testis is of reasonably normal size (>20 cm^3) and the serum follicle-stimulating hormone level is less than two times the upper limits of normal, the presence of an obstruction somewhere within the efferent ductal system should be ruled out and biopsy of the larger testis considered. Spermatogenic arrest and germ cell aplasia are the histologic diagnoses that are found when obstruction is not present. Arrest of spermatogenesis is almost always associated with normal gonadotropin levels and normal size testes without evidence of epididymal induration. Germ cell aplasia (Sertoli cell-only syndrome) is often, though not always, found in association with slightly small testes and varying elevated levels of serum follicle-stimulating hormone.

Testis Biopsy

Testis biopsy can be performed as a separate operative event or, if there is a high degree of suspicion that an obstruction exists, can be the first part of the definitive surgical procedure.

Open testis biopsy is the most commonly used method to obtain tissue for histologic examination. This procedure can be done in an office or outpatient setting using a short-acting, local anesthetic. Once the anterior scrotal skin is shaved, prepared, and draped in a sterile fashion, the testis to be biopsied is grasped gently but firmly, being certain that the epididymis is held posterior to protect it from injury. To minimize discomfort to the patient, the skin should be pulled taut against the surface of the testis rather than the testis pulled up against the skin. One and one half to two milliliters of 1% lidocaine-HCl is injected just beneath the skin and a 1.5 to 2 cm incision is made through the skin to the tunica vaginalis. The tunic is lifted off the surface of the testis and opened with scissors exposing the shiny surface of the tunica albuginea. A small eyelid retractor is useful to hold the incision open and the surface of the testis can be effectively anesthetized by dripping 2–3 ml of lidocaine HCl over its surface and bathing the tunic for about 30 seconds. Using a pointed scalpel, a half centimeter incision is made in the tunic. The testis is gently compressed to express a small cluster of tubules through the incision. This cluster is cut with iris scissors and the tissue placed immediately in Bouin's or Zenker's solution for permanent fixation (Figure 21-2). If frozen section and immediate examination are to be performed, the tissue is placed on a saline moistened sponge pad and sent for processing.

A quick method for evaluating the presence

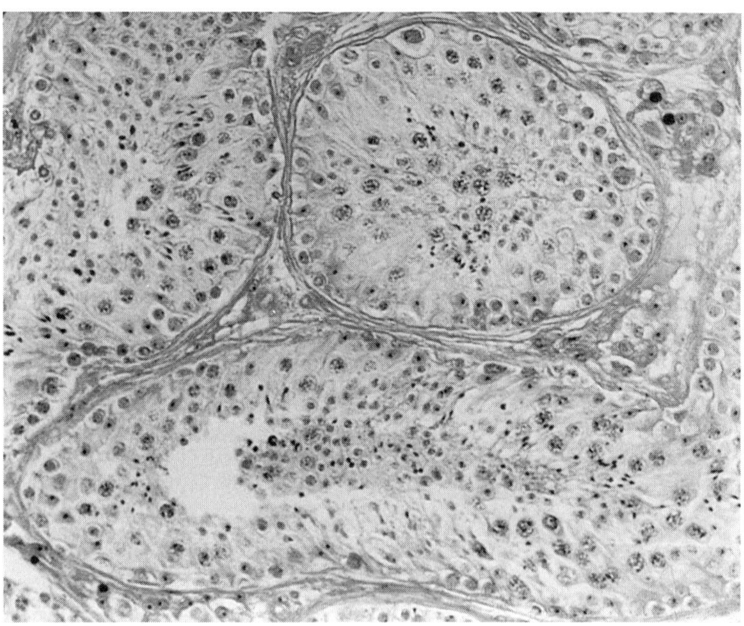

Figure 21-2 Photomicrograph of testis biopsy demonstrating active spermatogenesis is compatible with obstruction in an azoospermic man.

or absence of mature spermatids is to perform a touch preparation of the testicular tissue. Once a small piece of tissue is cut, it is grasped in a forceps and repeatedly touched against a sterile glass slide. The slide is sprayed immediately with a tissue fixative, stained, and examined for mature spermatozoa as well as their precursors (Figure 21-3).

If only the biopsy is to be done at that time, the incisions in the albuginea and vaginalis are closed with a fine chromic suture. Absorbable suture is also used to approximate dartos muscle and skin. Vasography is not carried out unless reparative surgery is to be done because of the potential to cause additional scarring and possible obstruction of the vas lumen.

Another method of obtaining testicular material for examination is with the use of a prostate biopsy needle, modified with a shorter bevel as recommended by Cohen[1] or the use of one of the newer spring loaded, disposable needles (ASAP-18, Microvasive, Boston Scientific Corp., Watertown, MA). Using these types of needles, adequate tissue can be obtained, often with a single pass. One to two milliliters of local anesthetic injected subcutaneously at the puncture site is usually sufficient to make the patient comfortable. Care must be taken so the tip of the needle does not penetrate the back wall of the testis, inadvertently injuring the epididymis or cord structures. Fine needle aspiration of the testis with immediate cytologic examination can reportedly identify sufficient cellular components to determine if an obstruction is present.[2] Unless one is dedicated to this technique, it is this author's experience that the results of fine needle aspirates vary too much to allow for a consistent histologic profile.

Obstruction of the Vas Deferens

Vasectomy is the most common cause of vasal obstruction. Millions of men have undergone

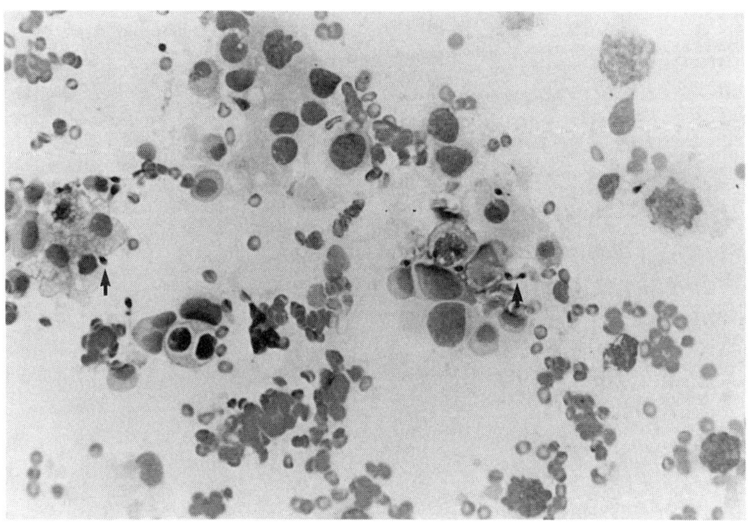

Figure 21-3 Stained touch preparation of testicular material. Arrows point to mature spermatids.

this procedure and some, for a variety of reasons, later attempt to restore their fertility by vasectomy reversal. Inadvertent transection of the vas deferens, which can occur in the course of hernia repair, hydrocelectomy, or deep pelvic surgery, may cause azoospermia if the injury is bilateral or happens on the side on which the individual may have only a single functional testis.

In 1919, Dr. Vincent O'Conor Sr. assisted Dr. William C. Quinby in a vasectomy reversal, which he later reported in 1948.[3] Quinby used silkworm gut as a stent over which the vas deferens was sewn together. The stent was removed 6–10 days after surgery. With time, materials and methods improved, but still there was only marginal success in reestablishing patency and subsequently causing a pregnancy. According to O'Conor.[3]

The results obtained were perhaps best shown in the review of two publications generated from questionnaires sent to members of the American Urological Association and ultimately published in *JAMA* in 1948[3] and in the *Journal of Urology* in 1973.[4] The first report indicated a patency rate of 38%. The second study, 25 years later described a similar patency rate with 19% of the men establishing pregnancies with their partners. Both of these studies represented the outcome of surgery done by a large number of urologists of varying skills and interest. There are other reports from surgeons who performed vasectomy reversals in relatively large numbers with greater skill, consequently with better results, but none is consistently as good as those obtained using the operating microscope.[5–8]

Microsurgical vasovasostomy as described by both Owen[9] and Silber[10] in the mid-1970s strongly influenced many urologists to learn microsurgical techniques to improve their results with vasovasostomy as well as the more technically demanding vasoepididymostomy. Various modifications for both procedures have been described, but each has certain basic principles that must be adhered to to have a reasonably good outcome: (1) adequate laboratory teaching and practice are mandatory before ever entering the operating theater; (2) the adventitia must be kept on the surface of the vas and incorporated into the outer anastomotic closure; (3) the vasal blood supply must be kept intact; and (4) there must be no tension on the anastomosis.

Techniques for Vasovasostomy

The men requesting vasectomy reversal are, for the most part, healthy. In the majority of cases, there has been a divorce and remarriage with a desire on the part of the couple to have a child. Others in their first marriage give reasons of improved economic conditions allowing them to raise and support more children. Some have experienced the tragic death of a child and have a strong desire for another. Some men who have persistent orchalgia following vasectomy will ask for a reversal in an effort to relieve that pain that may result from epididymal and vasal congestion. When the vasa were transected in the scrotum, vasovasostomy can usually be done using local anesthesia combined with intravenous sedation.

The step-by-step methods of single- and double-layer anastomoses have been described in great detail by various authors.[9–13] Figures 21-4 and 21-5 illustrate both procedures.

Results with regard to patency and pregnancy rates using the operating microscope are reported by most authors to be better than 85 and 55%, respectively. The Vasovasostomy Study Group recently compiled their data from the records of 1247 men who underwent micro-

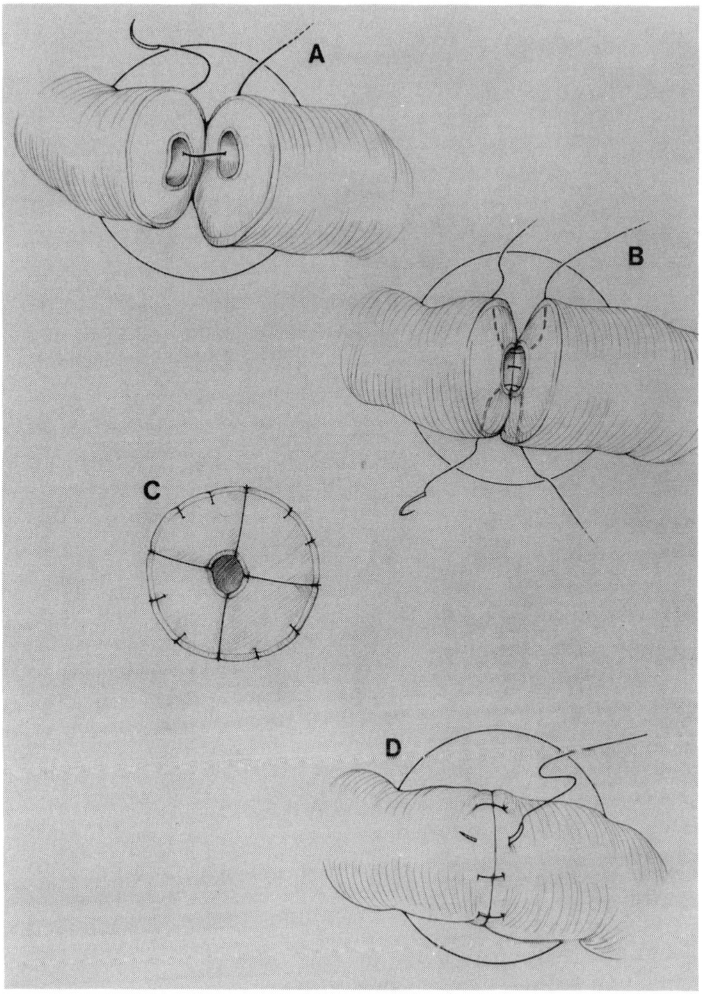

Figure 21-4 (A–D) Method of single layer microsurgical vasovasostomy. Four full thickness 9-0 nylon sutures are placed 90° from one another. Eight more 9-0 sutures are then positioned in the adventitia and muscularis, two between each full thickness suture. (Reproduced with permission from Falk and Thomas.[29])

surgical vasectomy reversal for the first time. Eighty-six percent of the 1012 men who had postoperative semen analyses had sperm present and 441 of 810 (52%) couples followed established pregnancies. Of great interest was the drop in patency and pregnancy rates with time (Table 21-1).[14]

Recently, Sharlip examined the records of his patients who had undergone reversal surgery and chose a subgroup of men who had excellent sperm quality to determine what the best pregnancy rate could be following successful surgery. In his report, 95 men were identified who had sperm counts averaging 60.4×10^6/ml with a mean motility of 65.5%. Fifty-eight (61.1%) men established pregnancies a mean of 8.5 months after surgery.[15]

At the time of vasectomy reversal, the surgeon is sometimes faced with a dilemma when fluid from the proximal vas does not contain

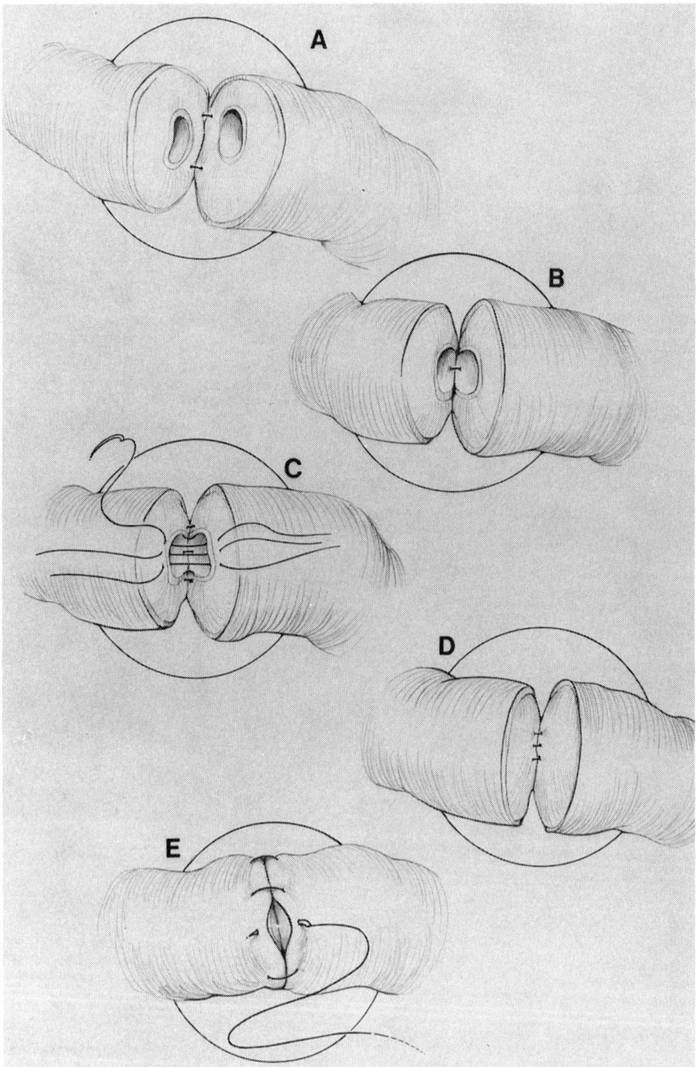

Figure 21-5 (A–E) Two layer anastomosis is begun by placing two 9-0 nylon sutures through the back wall incorporating both the adventitia and the muscularis. These sutures will stabilize the ends of the vas deferens. Six mucosal sutures of 10-0 nylon are then placed equidistant from one another to approximate the lumen. Six to eight more 9-0 sutures are then passed through the muscularis and adventitia to complete the anastomosis. (Reproduced with permission from Falk and Thomas.[29])

sperm. Should vasovasostomy or vasoepididymostomy be performed? After vasectomy, high intraluminal pressures from persistent sperm production can result in extravasation and scarring anywhere within the thin-walled epididymal tubule. These men have two sites of obstruction and need to have vasoepididymostomy performed rather than vasovasostomy.

The absence of sperm in the fluid does not *always* indicate a secondary epididymal blowout. Sharlip reported the followup of 10 men who had bilateral absence of sperm in the proximal vasa who still underwent vasovasostomy.

Table 21-1 Patency and Pregnancy Rates[a]

Obstructive Interval (Years)	Number of Men with Sperm in Semen/ Number of Men Followed (%)	Number of Wives Pregnant/Number of Couples Followed (%)
<3	86/89 (97)	56/74 (76)
3–8	525/600 (88)	253/478 (53)
9–14	205/261 (79)	92/209 (44)
≥15	32/45 (71)	11/37 (30)

[a] From Belker et al.[14]

Six had normal sperm counts within 1 year of surgery. Of the remaining four, three were reexplored and found to have patent vasal anastomoses and epididymal obstruction.[16] The Vasovasostomy Study Group, in the study previously cited, found an increase in the incidence of bilateral sperm absence associated with a longer obstructive interval. When the fluid was watery in appearance, after vasovasostomy, sperm returned to the ejaculate in 80% of men. When the fluid was opalescent, 75% returned with sperm in their ejaculate. When the fluid was thick and creamy, only 26% eventually had sperm in their semen. If one were to try and establish guidelines as to a need for epididymal exploration and possible vasoepididymostomy, it would appear that those men who have absence of sperm in vas fluid that is thick or creamy and have been obstructed more than 10 years are more likely to have ruptured the epididymal tubule than others with shorter obstructive intervals and less viscous fluid.[14]

Inguinal Vasovasostomy

Some azoospermic men will give a history of having undergone hernia repair in the past. Transection or ligation of the vas deferens during hernia repair probably occurs less often in the adult when compared to the infant due to the relative small size of the structure in the infant and the ease with which it can be cut or trapped in a suture while closing the hernia sac. If injury to the vas occurs on one side only and the contralateral testis and efferent duct are normal, the obstruction may never be noticed. If however, both sides are affected or the contralateral testis or vas is not normal, infertility will bring the patient to the urologist's attention. Physical examination of the patient will often disclose a fullness in the epididymis and proximal vas deferens. The cut end of the vas will not usually be palpable as the obstruction is often at the level of the internal inguinal ring. If the testis is of normal size and the vas and epididymis are full, one can almost guarantee the presence of normal spermatogenesis. Testicular biopsy with immediate frozen section or touch preparation can be done at the time of vasovasostomy. Once active spermatogenesis has been verified, a vasogram is appropriate to identify the distal end of the obstructed vas. It is not necessary to expose the entire testis. The same incision used for the biopsy can be slid upward to the cord structures and the vas grasped with a towel clamp and held in position for vasography. Since the vas deferens in these circumstances is generally filled with fluid (sperm), it is helpful to place the needle pointing away from the testis and aspirate back as much of the fluid as possible. This will allow space for the contrast material as well as an opportunity to examine the fluid for the presence of sperm. The area of the vas just proximal to the insertion point of the needle is pinched to compress the lumen and prevent backflow of contrast with overdistention and possible rupture of the epididymal tubule. Contrast consisting of equal amounts saline and Renografin 60 is then injected into the vas and a radiograph taken.

It is not uncommon to find the distal (abdominal) cut end of the vas deferens residing just below the level of the internal ring within the retroperitoneum. To be able to adequately mobilize both ends of the vas deferens, the inguinal incision should extend for a distance of 4–5 cm inferior and superior to the internal inguinal ring. It is necessary to incorporate the blood supply with both ends of the vas deferens. Once mobilized, this author prefers to do a single-layer anastomosis as it is technically easier when working in a deep incision as compared to the skin surface level when performing a routine transscrotal vasovasostomy.

If there is not sufficient length of vas to allow for a tension-free anastomosis, the abdominal portion of the vas along with its blood supply can be bluntly mobilized and passed beneath the floor of the inguinal canal through Hasselbach's triangle, a shorter, more direct course to the other end of the vas deferens. If no sperm is found in the fluid from the testicular side of the vas deferens, there may be a second obstruction within the epididymis and if no sperm returns in the semen within 6 months, vasography and possible vasoepididymostomy should be done if the prior anastomosis is patent.

Other Techniques of Vasovasostomy

In the past few years, some investigators have advocated the use of laser welding and, more recently, "gluing" to approximate the severed ends of the vas deferens. Rosemberg reported his experience using the CO_2 laser after placing three sutures in the mucosa to hold the ends in position. Thirteen of 14 men had sperm in their ejaculate. Three established a pregnancy.[17] In the murine model, Lowe and Poage reported very poor results using the CO_2 laser as opposed to the neodymnium-YAG laser.[18] Wilson and associates presented their experimental data comparing the results of one layer microsuturing, CO_2 laser welding, and gluing with a tissue adhesive comprised of human cryoprecipitate and thrombin. Patency was not statistically different in any of the three experimental groups, but operative time was significantly less in the adhesive group.[19] Further clinical study is needed to determine if the patency and pregnancy rates with these techniques are sufficiently better to warrant abandonment of microsurgical suturing methods for vasovasostomy.

Obstruction of the Epididymis

The epididymis is the most common site of obstructive azoospermia resulting directly from an inflammatory or congenital etiology. Inflammation with subsequent scarring and occlusion of the epididymal tubule may be a consequence of either bacterial or viral infection within the lower genital tract or a "blow-out" of the epididymal tubule caused by increased intraluminal pressure from a distal vasal blockage. A variety of congenital vasal–epididymal abnormalities have been described ranging from total absence of the distal epididymis and vas deferens to a simple nonunion of the vasa and epididymides, each of which is otherwise normal.

The presence of an epididymal obstruction is proven by demonstrating active spermatogenesis and patency of the vasa deferentia to the level of and including the ejaculatory ducts. Vasography has been the usual method by which patency was proven. Some surgeons advocate the abandonment of vasography because it can be time consuming and exposes the patient to unnecessary radiation. Instead of vasograms, it has been suggested that an indwelling catheter be inserted in the bladder and dilute indigo carmine or methylene blue be injected in the vas lumen on one side. If the liquid flows easily and shows up immediately in the catheter drainage, the vas is felt to be patent. The blue dye is then flushed through the vas with saline until the catheter return is clear or only lightly tinged with color and the same procedure performed on the other side. Some urologists simply inject 10–15 ml of saline into the lumen feeling that if flow is unimpeded, patency of the vas is presumed. While these indirect techniques are acceptable in some instances, they do not define the anatomy of the ejaculator ducts and one of the methods requires the insertion of a catheter, which can risk infection, perhaps of greater significance than the minimum dose of radiation received by taking two or three X-rays.

With very little practice, vasography, carried out at the time of reparative surgery, can be completed within 10–15 minutes. Prior to the patient being placed on the operating table, an X-ray cassette is positioned below the table pad at the level where the patient's pelvis will rest. Once the operative procedure gets underway, the vas deferens is exposed. Care is taken not to injure its blood supply. The straight portion of the vas is grasped with a towel clamp and gently pulled inferiorly to further stretch and straighten the lumen. A 30-gauge needle used for lymphangiography and attached to a 3-ml syringe filled with saline is inserted into the lumen with the needle pointed away from the testis. One or two milliliters of saline is injected into the lumen. If there is no extravasation of saline, proper position of the needle is assured. A radiograph is then taken as a scout film. A 3 ml mixture of half-strength saline and Renografin 60 is then injected and another radiograph is taken.[20] If the vas and seminal vesicle look normal and contrast is in the bladder, the needle is removed and inserted into the contralateral vas. If there is no suspicion of a contralateral abnormality other than epididymal obstruction, no X-rays need be taken on the other side. Five to ten milliliters of saline is injected and if no resistance is met, the contralateral vas deferens is presumed patent. If flow of saline is impeded, contrast can be injected and another X-ray taken. If the surgeon is uncomfortable placing a needle into the lumen or if it is not easily accomplished, an incision can be made with a small, round-tipped scalpel, halfway through the muscular wall of the vas deferens, until the lumen is exposed. The soft tubing of a 24-gauge angiocatheter is inserted into the lumen and after the injections are complete, the incision is closed with 9-0 or 10-0 nylon suture under magnification using the operating microscope.

If the vas deferens is patent and there is active spermatogenesis, there must exist an obstruction somewhere between the seminiferous tubules and the cauda epididymis. Visual inspection of the epididymis may, at times, indicate the site of the obstruction (Figure 21-6) but, ultimately, this must be determined by direct examination of the contents of the tubule beginning at the cauda and working proximally toward the caput epididymis until sperm are identified.

The method chosen to examine the epididymis is dependent on the type of vasoepididymal anastomosis to be used. If the end-to-end single tubule anastomosis described by Silber[21] is used, the epididymis is cut across as if one were slicing a loaf of bread. As each 3–5 mm slice is made, beginning at the epididymal tail, fluid from the proximal tubule is examined for sperm. Once the obstruction is passed, sperm will exude from the patent lumen though there will be other cut portions of the more distal tubule visible. Hemostasis is achieved using a bipolar cautery. When the appropriate level is identified, the proximal vas is brought to the patent epididymal tubule and the anastomosis performed as described in Figure 21-7.

This author and others found Silber's end-to-end method somewhat cumbersome, particularly when trying to identify the lumen exuding sperm and control bleeding on the cut surface of the epididymis. This single tubule end-to-end anastomosis has been modified to an end-to-side technique. This method does not require sectioning of the epididymis. Bleeding from vessels beneath the epididymal tunic is more easily controlled, and there is better visualization of the single opened tubule exuding sperm.[22] Identification of sperm is made by incising the epididymal tunic, teasing a single loop of the tubule separate from the others, and unroofing it. The fluid from the opened tubule is put on a sterile glass slide and examined immediately. This process is carried superiorly by 0.5–1 cm increments until normal appearing sperm are identified. Figure 21-8

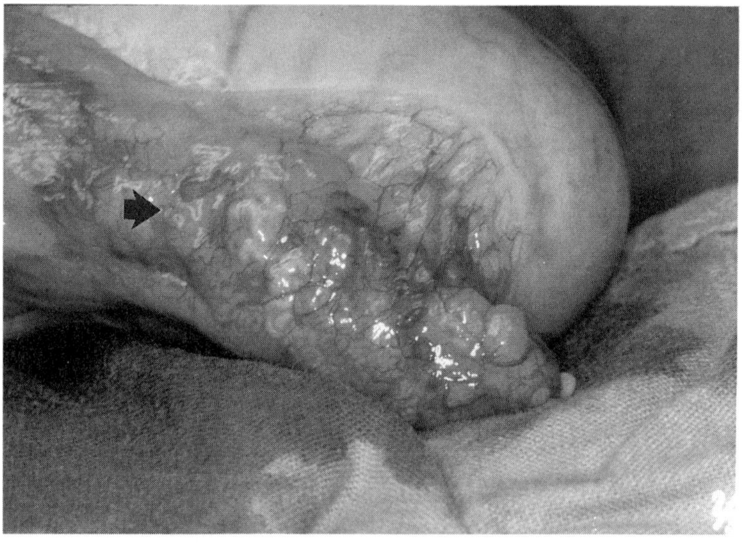

Figure 21-6 There is dilation of the proximal epididymal tubule to the point of obstruction (arrow). (Reproduced with permission from Thomas.[22])

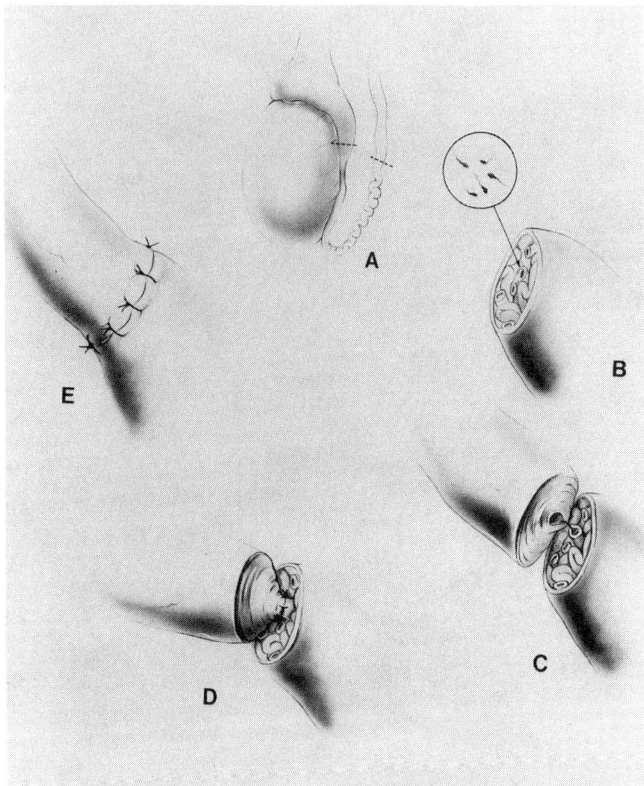

Figure 21-7 (A–E) Silber's method of vasoepididymostomy. Beginning at the distal (caudal) portion of the epididymis, progressive slices are made until sperm are identified coming from a single open end. The vas lumen is approximated to the epididymal lumen with three or four 10-0 nylon sutures. The muscularis and adventitia are then sutured to the epididymal tunic with eight or more simple interrupted sutures of 9-0 nylon. (Reproduced with permission from Thomas.[22])

depicts the basic surgical steps for the end-to-side anastomosis.

There are some caveats that can make the procedure easier:

1. The convoluted portion of the vas deferens should be used for the anastomosis if possible as it is better suited to lie more comfortably against the epididymal lumen as opposed to the more muscular straight portion of the vas.
2. The vas deferens and its attendant blood supply reside on the medial aspect of the cord. The cut end of the vas must be brought *beneath* the remainder of the cord structures and through a window created in the tunica vaginalis, close to the point of anastomosis. This will prevent compromise to the blood supply of the vas and testis and allow the tunica vaginalis to enclose the entire testis and epididymis at the completion of the operation.
3. If the cut edge of the opened epididymal tubule is difficult to visualize, a small amount of indigo carmine or methylene blue dripped over the opened lumen will stain the cut edge of the tubule for easier identification and placement of sutures.

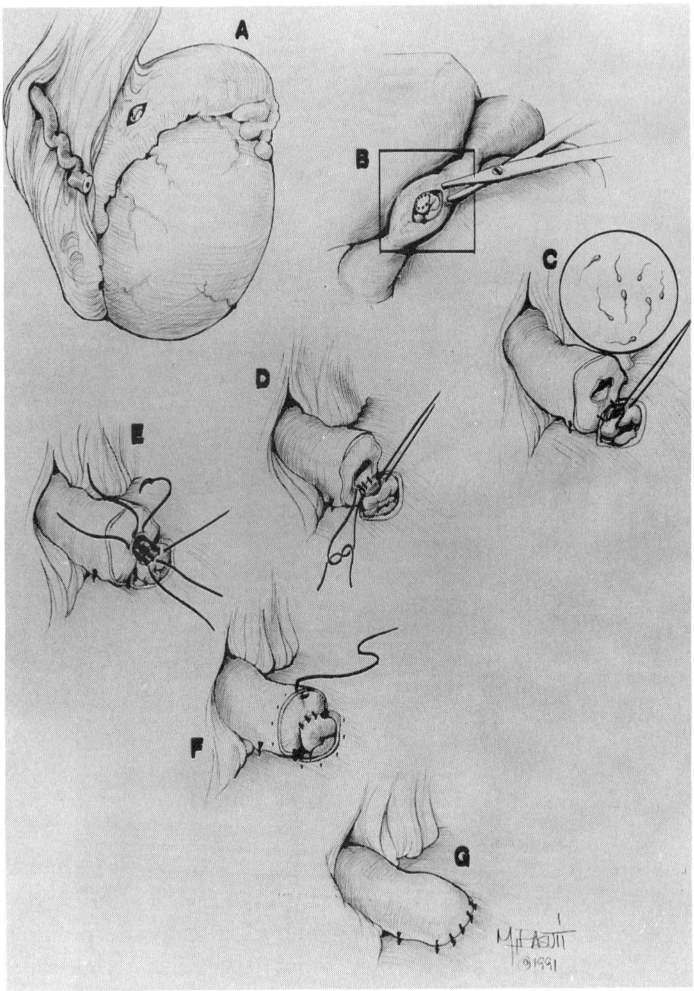

Figure 21-8 (A–G) Author's end-to-side method of vasoepididymostomy. Using this technique, the epididymal tunic is incised exposing the tortuous tubule beneath. A single loop of tubule is isolated with a small, blunt-nosed scissors and unroofed. The fluid is examined for sperm. If none is found, another incision is made 0.5–1 cm more proximal and the same procedure performed until normal appearing sperm are found. The cut end of the proximal vas is then brought beneath the cord, through the tunica vaginalis to approximate the opened epididymal tubule to which it is sutured. Four or five sutures are generally required for the mucosal anastomosis and eight to ten sutures to bring together the adventitia and muscularis to the epididymal tunic. (Reproduced with permission from Falk and Thomas.[29])

Problems Unique to the Epididymis

It has been known for almost a century that the epididymis is more than a conduit through which sperm pass. Sperm undergo a still poorly understood maturation process as they traverse the meter or so of epididymal tubule. Numerous studies have documented the fact that sperm from the caput are not as capable of fertilizing an oocyte as those in the more distal epididymis.[23–25] The tubule of the caput epididymis is more thin-walled compared to that of the corpus or cauda, making anastomosis with the vas deferens more difficult. For all these reasons, patency and pregnancy rates are not as good when the obstruction is at the level of the caput as opposed to those present at more distal levels.

In 1970, Young and associates reported a group of men with epididymal obstruction associated with pulmonary problems.[26] Twenty-eight men with obstructive azoospermia also had significant pulmonary disease (i.e., bronchitis, bronchiectasis). At the time of testicular exploration, the epididymis was found to be obstructed at the level of the caput, the tubule packed with thick, yellow material that had a paste-like consistency. Proximal to this, grossly normal appearing sperm were found. Patency and subsequent pregnancy rates in these individuals have been low. Some of these men had proven fertility prior to becoming azoospermic, which occurred with no identified inflammatory or traumatic event.

Partial obstruction of the vasa or epididymides can exist. Sperm counts are generally quite low ($<1 \times 10^6$) with poor motility. At times there may be a modest increase in concentration, but it is not sustained and there is often a history of a prior inflammatory event. Examination of the genitalia will disclose a sense of fullness in the epididymides. Testis biopsy will demonstrate normal spermatogenesis. Attempts at quantifying the mature spermatids within the seminiferous tubules to predict what the sperm count should be if the obstruction were relieved has been attempted and may be of help in determining whether exploration is worthwhile.[27,28]

Complications of Surgery for Obstructive Azoospermia

Complications associated with microsurgical correction of obstructive azoospermia should be uncommon. Meticulous hemostatis is absolutely essential. This should minimize the occurrence of any significant scrotal hematoma. Infection, in this author's experience, is rare and usually limited to the area of the skin incision and much less commonly to the epididymis. The most severe local complication that has been reported is that of testicular atrophy. This is almost always due to a compromise in the arterial blood supply. Patients who have had prior scrotal surgery where there may be extensive scarring around the cord or a large vas granuloma deeply imbedded into the cord are at greater risk for arterial injury. Granulomas may be left alone if there is any risk of injury to the testicular vessels. The proximal and distal ends of the divided vas deferens should be freed up to the point that risks entering the deep cord and cut just proximal to that point.

Care and Followup after Surgery

Postoperative instructions and surgical followup after vasovasostomy or vasoepididymostomy are essentially the same. An ice bag is applied to the scrotal area for the first 24 hours. A scrotal support is worn for a week. Showers are permitted after 3 days and baths after 7 days. Strenuous physical activity and intercourse are prohibited for 3 weeks. Work not involving heavy physical labor may be resumed as soon as the patient is comfortable, usually a day or two after surgery. If inguinal vasovasostomy was done, the recuperation is similar to that of a patient who had a hernia repair.

A semen sample is examined 4 weeks after surgery then every 3 months for the first year. Most men who had a vasovasostomy will have sperm in the semen at the initial examination, though the motility will generally be very poor.

Patients who underwent vasoepididymal anastomosis may not have sperm in their semen early on and one may need to observe the response for up to 12 months. In contrast, if no sperm appears in the semen within 6 months after vasovasostomy, the operation is considered a failure. If, in these patients, sperm was not identified coming from the proximal vas lumen at the time of vasovasostomy, it may be necessary to perform a vasoepididymostomy for these men. Patency of the prior anastomosis should be tested at the time of reexploration, injecting saline through the lumen from a point proximal to the previous anastomosis. If patent, the entire length of vas can be used for the vasoepididymostomy. If the vas is obstructed, the site of previous surgery should be excised and if sperm is not found in the proximal vas lumen at that time, the epididymis is explored for signs of obstruction and the decision made whether to perform a vasovasostomy or vasoepididymostomy.

New Technology and Obstructive Azoospermia

In the chapters that follow, the authors present new treatment modalities for patients with obstructive azoospermia who are not candidates for surgical reconstruction. Assisted reproductive technology plays a major role in these treatments and emphasizes the necessity of a coordinated effort between the couple, the urologist, and the reproductive gynecologist. Even when the obstruction is surgically correctable, the pregnancy rates are significantly less than the patency rates and some men may benefit from laboratory-assisted technology, the spectrum of treatment running from sperm washing and intrauterine insemination to *in vitro* fertilization to the more complex methods involving micromanipulation of gametes and embryo transfer.

REFERENCES

1. Cohen MS, Frye S, Warner RS, et al: Testicular needle biopsy in diagnosis of infertility. Urology 1984; 24:439–442.
2. Linsk JA, Franzen S: Aspiration biopsy of the testis. In: Clinical aspiration cytology. Philadelphia: J.B. Lippincott, 1983:267–276.
3. O'Conor VJ: Anastomosis of the vas deferens after purposeful division for sterility. JAMA 1948: 136:162–163.
4. Derrick FC, Yarbrough W, D'Agostino: Vasovasostomy: Results of questionnaire of members of the American Urological Association. J Urol 1973; 110:556–557.
5. Phadke GM, Phadke AG: Experiences in the reanastomosis of the vas deferens. J Urol 1967; 97:888–890.
6. Schmidt SS: Vas anastomosis: a return to simplicity. Br J Urol 1975; 47:309–314.
7. Middleton RG, Henderson D: Vas deferens reanastomosis with splints and without magnification. J Urol 1978; 119:763–764.
8. Lee HY: Corrective surgery of obstructive azoospermia. Arch Androl 1978; 1:115–121.
9. Owen ER: Microsurgical vasovasostomy: A reliable vasectomy reversal. Aust NZ J Surg 1977; 47:305–309.
10. Silber SJ: Perfect anatomical reconstruction of the vas deferens with a new microscopic surgical technique. Fertil Steril 1977; 28:72–77.
11. Belker AM: Microsurgery for the urologist. AUA Update Series, Volume III, Lesson 1. Houston: American Urological Association Inc., Office of Education, 1983.
12. Thomas AJ, Howards SS: Microsurgical treatment of male infertility. In Lipshultz LI,

Howards SS, eds. Infertility in the male, 2nd ed., St. Louis: Mosby Year Book, 1991:357–369.
13. Sharlip ID: Vasovasostomy: Comparison of two microsurgical techniques. Urology 1981; 17:347–352.
14. Belker AM, Thomas AJ, Fuchs EF, Konnak JW, Sharlip ID: Results of 1469 microsurgical vasectomy reversals by the vasovasostomy study group. J Urol 1991; 145:505–511.
15. Sharlip ID: What is the best pregnancy rate that may be expected from vasectomy reversal? Presented at the 86th annual meeting, American Urological Association, Toronto, Canada, June 2–6, 1991.
16. Sharlip ID: The significance of intravasal azoospermia during vasovasostomy: Answer to a surgical dilemma. Fertil Steril 1982; 38:496–498.
17. Rosemberg SK: Clinical use of carbon dioxide laser in microsurgical vasovasostomy. Urology 1987; 29(4):372–374.
18. Lowe BA, Poage MD: Vasovasostomy in the murine vas deferens: Comparison of the Nd:YAG laser at 1.06 microns and 1.318 microns to the CO_2 laser. Lasers in Surg Med 1988; 8:377–380.
19. Wilson LA, Ball RA, Steinberg J, Loughlin KR: A comparison of vasovasostomy techniques in rats utilizing suture, CO_2 laser and tissue adhesives. Presented at the 86th annual meeting, American Urological Association, Toronto, Canada, June 2–6, 1991.
20. Nagler HM, Thomas AJ: Testicular biopsy and vasography in the evaluation of male infertility. Urol Clin North Am 1987; 14(1):167–176.
21. Silber SJ: Microscopic vasoepididymostomy: Specific microanastomosis to the epididymal tubule. Fertil Steril 1978; 30:565–561.
22. Thomas AJ: Vasoepididymostomy. Urol Clin North Am 1987; 14(3):527–538.
23. Schoysman RJ, Bedford JM: The role of human epididymis in sperm maturation and sperm storage as reflected in the consequences of epididymovasostomy. Fertil Steril 1986; 46:293–299.
24. Orgebin-Crist MC: Studies on the function of the epididymis. Biol Reprod 1969; 1(Suppl):155–175.
25. Silber SJ: Vasoepididymostomy to the head of the epididymis: Recovery of normal spermatozoal motility. Fertil Steril 1980; 34:149–153.
26. Young D: Surgical treatment of male infertility. J Reprod Fertil 1970; 23:541–542.
27. Silber SJ, Rodriguez-Rigau LJ: Quantitative analysis of testicular biopsy: Determination of partial obstruction and prediction of sperm count after surgery for obstruction. Fertil Steril 1981; 36:480–485.
28. Steinberger E, Tjioe DY: A method of quantitative analysis of human seminiferous epithelium. Fertil Steril 1968; 19:959–961.
29. Falk RM, Thomas AJ: Microsurgery in male infertility. Infertil Reprod Med Clin North Am, 1992; 3(2):443-454.

ANNOTATED BIBLIOGRAPHY

Belker AM, Thomas AJ, Fuchs EF et al: Results of 1,469 microsurgical vasectomy reversals by the Vasovasostomy Study Group. J Urol 1991; 145(3):505–511.

The authors present their joint experience performing vasectomy reversal. The strength of the paper rests in the various ways that the authors evaluated their patients intraoperatively and in the postoperative period. New guidelines are established regarding expected results as related to the time of obstruction. The most significant weaknesses are the lack of any substantial experience with vasoepididymostomy ("only 14 of the 1,247 patients who underwent an initial vasectomy reversal procedure were evaluable for vasoepididymal results") and the omission of antibody data in this large number of men.

Martin E, Carnett JB, Levi JV et al: The surgical treatment of sterility due to obstruction at the epididymis. Together with a study of the morphology of human spermatozoa. Univ Pennsylvania Med Bull 1903; 15:2–15.

Dr. Martin presents his "fistula technique" for vasoepididymal anastomosis. The method was to be used by most urologists until the advent of microsurgery, more than 70 years later. Martin also defined the epididymis as a structure with specific physiologic significance and not a mere conduit for sperm. A paper worth reading for its historical and surgical significance. For further information referable to the work and writings of Dr. Martin, the article by Jequier (Jequier AM: Edward Martin (1859–1938). The founding father of modern clinical andrology. Int J Androl 1991; 14:1–10) is recommended.

Silber SJ: Microscopic vasectomy reversal. Fertil Steril 1977; 28(11):1191–1202. Dr. Silber is responsible for bringing the use of the operating microscope to the attention of many urologists. His results were consistently superior to any achieved without optical magnification. This and his description of microsurgical vasoepididymostomy offered greater hope for success for patients with regard to both patency and pregnancy.

Silber S: Microscopic vasoepididymostomy: Specific microanastomosis to the epididymal tubule. Fertil Steril 1978; 30(5):565–571. Dr. Silber details his microscopic technique for anastomosing the vas deferens to a single open epididymal tubule exuding sperm. The results reported regarding the first 14 men on whom he performed this procedure were excellent when compared to those of other investigators using the "standard" fistula technique. The concept of a single tubule anastomosis had been reported earlier by Lespinasse (JAMA 1918; 70:448 but the method was crude in contrast to that described by Silber.

Thomas AJ. Vasoepididymostomy. Urol Clin North Am 1987; 14(3):527–538.

The author has modified Silber's end-to-end technique of vasoepididymostomy. He describes an end-to-side method of single tubule anastomosis that does not necessitate resection of the epididymis and allows for clear visualization of the patent tubule to which the vas deferens is anastomosed.

22

Alloplastic Spermatocele for Treatment of Obstructive Azoospermia

Arnold M. Belker

The alloplastic or artificial spermatocele was developed to restore fertility to men who have congenital absence of the vasa deferentia. It also has been used to restore fertility to men who are born with normal vasa but who developed otherwise surgically irremediable obstruction of the male ductal system. At first, saphenous vein grafts were sutured end-to-end to the epididymal tunic.[1,2] These sperm reservoirs were then aspirated percutaneously at the time of the partner's ovulation and insemination was performed. Later, silicone caps were used for end-to-side implantation onto the epididymis. The silicone cap developed by Wagenknecht et al.[3] is aspirated directly; the silicone cap developed by Kelami et al.[4,5] is connected by silicone tubing to a subcutaneous inguinal reservoir, which is aspirated when insemination is to be performed. Conceptions were achieved first in animals and later in humans, using sperm aspirated from these silicone caps. Jimenez-Cruz[6] reported a pregnancy in the wife of a patient who had undergone end-to-end implantation of a polypropylene reservoir. He subsequently used polytetrafluoroethylene (Gore-Tex) tubing as the material for implanted alloplastic spermatoceles (Jimenez-Cruz, personal communication, 1982). The epididymal anatomy that usually is present in men who have congenitally absent vasa is shown in Figure 22-1A, and the designs of the various types of prostheses are shown in Figure 22-1B, C, and D.

Unilateral or Bilateral Implantation

Most, although not all, implanted alloplastic spermatoceles become filled with fibrous tissue ingrowth within a few months. This was shown by Hamm and Kelami[7] in experimental animals and was noted in my unpublished study of such implantations in dogs. As a result of fibrous tissue ingrowth, the lumen of the prosthesis becomes occluded. Within a few months after

Management of Impotence and Infertility, edited by Douglas Whitehead and Harris Nagler,

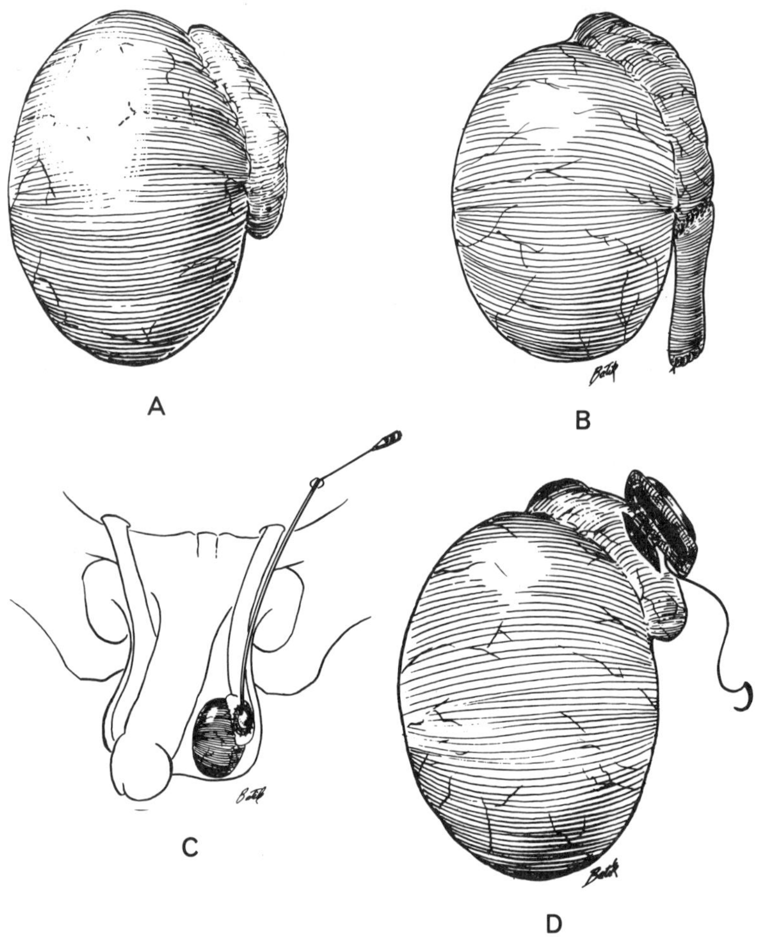

Figure 22-1 (A) The upper one-third to two-thirds of the epididymis usually is present in men who have congenital absence of the vasa deferentia. (B) Jimenez-Cruz[6] uses polypropylene or Gore-Tex tubing for the prosthesis. (C) Kelami et al.[4,5] use inguinal subcutaneous silicone reservoir attached by silicone tubing to silicone epididymal cap. (D) Wagenknecht et al.[3] use silicone cap which is aspirated directly percutaneously. (Reprinted with permission from Belker.[19])

implantation, "dry taps" result from attempted aspirations of most prostheses, although some do remain open for years.

It was theorized that this fibrous tissue ingrowth originated from the epididymal interstitial tissue surrounding the tubule. Therefore, other investigators and I (unpublished data) developed a silicone prosthesis that has an 0.5 mm diameter opening in its baseplate. This was implanted by suturing the edges of the 0.5 mm opening in the baseplate to the edges of an incised opening into the epididymal tubule. Thus, only the interior of the tubule was exposed to the lumen of the prosthesis. Nevertheless, in most instances the prosthetic lumen of this theoretically improved device was still occluded by fibrous tissue ingrowth within a few weeks to a few months after implantation in the animals.

Because of this limited time of functional

use of most alloplastic spermatoceles, it is wise to perform unilateral, and not bilateral, implantation of these devices. Unilateral implantation preserves the contralateral side for potential future use if that may become necessary.

Timing of Implantation

Considering the recent reports[8–11] of the achievement of pregnancies using sperm obtained by microsurgical epididymal aspiration combined with *in vitro* fertilization/embryo transfer (IVF/ET), gamete intrafallopian transfer (GIFT), or zygote intrafallopian transfer (ZIFT), one should consider performing such procedures at the time of implantation of alloplastic spermatoceles. The time of the implantation, therefore, should be dependent on the time of the wife's stimulated ovulation. Sperm obtained during the implantation may or may not be more optimally fertile than sperm obtained by postoperative aspirations. However, the use of sperm obtained during prosthesis implantation for IVF/ET, GIFT, or ZIFT affords the couple one more chance for conception.

Surgical Technique

Whenever foreign body material is to be implanted, the usual preoperative precautions are to be observed. Preoperative washing of the operative site with antibacterial solutions may be done the day before surgery. Systemic antibiotic coverage similar to that used when penile prostheses are inserted is advisable. The prostheses must be kept meticulously free of lint and other foreign material.

Vertical scrotal incisions are used. After the epididymis is exposed, it is transected as far caudally as possible if end-to-end implantation is to be performed. This transection will expose multiple openings of the epididymal tubule. Bipolar cautery is used for hemostasis, taking care to avoid cautery of the tubule itself. Meticulous hemostasis is advisable. The prosthesis is sutured to the circumference of the epididymal tunic with fine nylon and a routine closure of the scrotal incision is then performed.

When end-to-side implantation is performed, the epididymal tunic is incised as far caudally as is feasible on the anterolateral aspect of the epididymis for placement of the prosthesis. Most surgeons then incise across several sections of the epididymal tubule and suture the edge of the prosthesis to the epididymal tunic with fine nylon after hemostasis is accomplished. The outer circumference of the prosthesis usually is larger than the incised opening of the epididymal tunic. This necessitates suturing the edge of the prosthesis to underlying, intact, epididymal tunic. During the placement of these sutures, care must be taken to include only the epididymal tunic and not the underlying epididymal tubule to prevent occlusion of the tubule cephalad to the level of implantation.

An alternative method of end-to-side implantation is shown in Figure 22-2. This method relies on microsurgically suturing the incised edges of a single opening into the epididymal tubule to the incised edges of the epididymal tunic to keep the tubule open permanently. Although this method is theoretically appealing, it did not prevent occlusion of the prosthesis by fibrous tissue ingrowth in my experimental canine implantations.

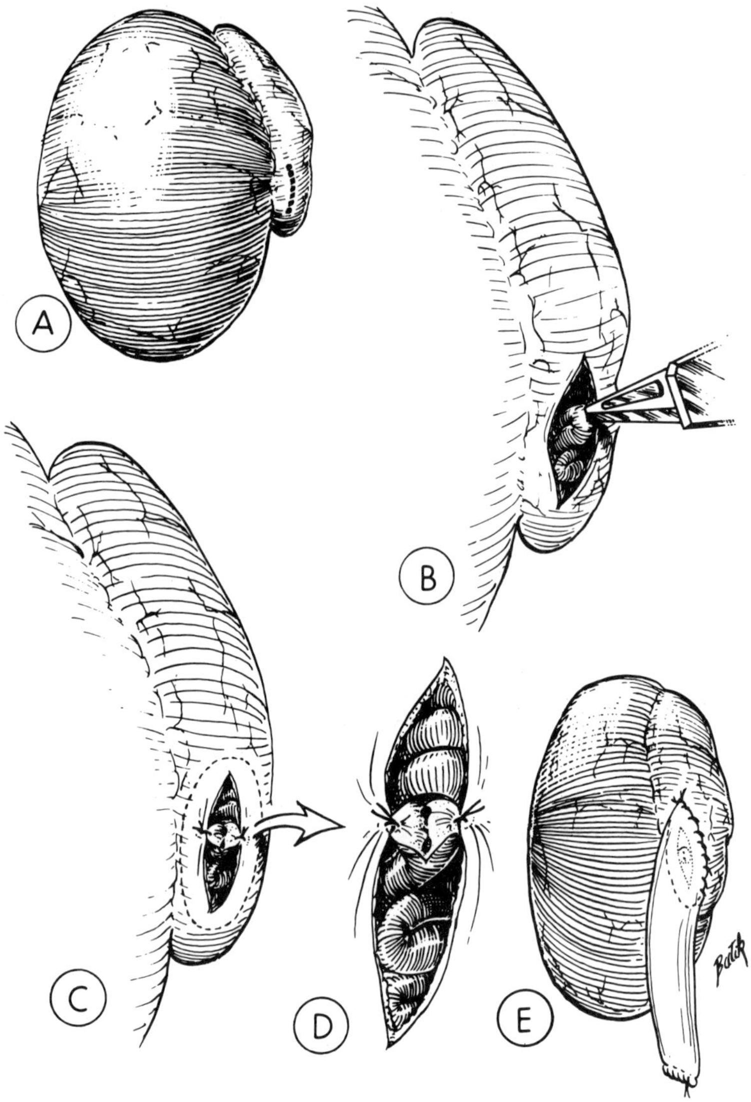

Figure 22-2 (A–E) Method of microsurgically suturing edges of opened epididymal tubule to incised edges of epididymal tunic prior to (E) implantation of overlying artificial spermatocele. (Reproduced with permission from Belker.[20])

Postoperative Care

Early postoperative care is the same as for any surgery in this area. Alloplastic spermatocele aspirations should be initiated on the day of the wife's first ovulation after implantation and performed at the time of each subsequent ovulation until pregnancy occurs or until sperm no longer can be aspirated from the prosthesis. The aspirations may be performed with local anesthesia.

An unresolved issue concerns which solution, if any, should be used to fill the prosthesis intraoperatively and immediately after each aspiration. It is quite possible that a particular sperm nutrient solution may best preserve sperm viability while simultaneously being most irritating to the epididymal tubular tissue. Until experimental evidence may indicate otherwise, Ringer's solution seems to be satisfactory for the purpose of filling the prosthesis both during implantation and immediately after each postoperative aspiration.

Results

The results of 130 (39 bilateral and 52 unilateral) alloplastic spermatocele implantations in 91 patients operated on by Jimenez-Cruz, Kelami, and Wagenknecht were reviewed by me.[12] Seven of the 91 (8%) wives subsequently became pregnant. Three of these pregnancies ended in spontaneous abortion and four progressed to full-term delivery. Thus, the "take home baby rate" after alloplastic spermatocele implantation in this series was only 4.4% (4 of 91).

There are a few isolated reports of pregnancy achieved with sperm aspirated from alloplastic spermatoceles. However, personal communication with other urologists who have implanted such devices convinces me that the pregnancy rate after alloplastic spermatocele implantation is lower than that reported in the literature.

Causes of Failure

There are numerous possible reasons that the use of sperm aspirated postoperatively from an alloplastic spermatocele may have failed to result in a pregnancy. In the past, most attempts to achieve a conception involved insemination of the wife. It is possible that the use of the new assisted reproductive technologies, such as IVF/ET, GIFT, and ZIFT, may improve pregnancy rates.

As previously mentioned, the ideal solution with which to fill the spermatocele intraoperatively and after postoperative aspirations remains to be identified. Turner[13] showed that mature rat sperm that have the capacity for motility remain quiescent in the epididymis but become motile on exposure to most physiological fluids. This also is true for human sperm. It is theoretically possible that the quiescent sperm in the epididymis are stimulated by the injected solution and that by the time another aspiration is performed, their stored energy for motility has been dissipated, rendering the sperm incapable of subsequent fertilization.

Failure to achieve a pregnancy could also result from decreased testicular production of sperm. However, as has been estimated by testicular biopsy, most men who have congenitally absent vasa appear to have normal to only slightly reduced sperm production.[14] It also is possible that epididymal function is impaired by a lifetime of epididymal obstruction. Unfortunately, clinical tests that assess epididymal function are unavailable.

The length of the interval between postoperative aspirations of the implanted spermatocele that best maintains sperm viability has not been studied. Because the aspirations are painful, they usually are performed only monthly when the wife ovulates. It is possible that more frequent aspirations are needed to maintain the fertilizing capacity of sperm. Also, there has been only one study[15] of the *in vitro* effect of the foreign material of which the alloplastic spermatocele may be constructed on the viability and motility of sperm. The ideal prosthetic material remains to be determined.

There are other possible reasons for the failure to achieve pregnancy using sperm that have been aspirated from alloplastic spermatoceles. Serum sperm agglutinating antibodies have been shown to occur in 60 to 70% of men who have congenital absence of the vasa deferentia.[16,17] It was not until very recently that investigators began to study the antibodies on the surface of epididymal sperm in such men.[18] Studies of these sperm surface antibodies may lead to an understanding of whether they impair the fertilization potential of sperm in the congenitally obstructed epididymis.

Finally, the previously mentioned ingrowth of fibrous tissue into the lumen of the prosthesis will cause obliteration of the lumen and result in "dry" aspirations. A method to prevent this problem does not appear to be available at the present time.

Present and Future Role

The alloplastic spermatocele remains an option for restoring fertility to men who have bilateral congenitally absent vasa and for those who have obstruction of the sperm conduction system that is not otherwise surgically repairable. It is possible that the future use of IVF/ET, GIFT, or ZIFT will result in pregnancy rates better than those obtained when the wife was inseminated with aspirated sperm. Future changes in prosthetic materials and in sperm nutrient solutions used to fill the prosthesis also could enhance pregnancy rates.

However, the use of microsurgically aspirated sperm from the epididymis of men who have congenitally absent vasa may offer the best chance for a pregnancy. Epididymal sperm microaspiration is considered in Chapter 23 of this book. If an alloplastic spermatocele is to be implanted, pregnancy rates may be improved by performing the implantation on the day of the wife's stimulated ovulation, so that epididymal sperm that are obtained during the implantation may be used for IVF/ET, GIFT, or ZIFT.

REFERENCES

1. Schoysman R: La creation d'un spermatocele artificial das les agenesis du conal deferent. Bull Soc R Belge Gynecol Obstet 1968; 38:307–317.
2. Schoysman R: Surgical treatments in male sterility. Andrologia 1969; 1:33–38.
3. Wagenknecht LV, Weitze KH, Hoppe LP, Krause D, Becker H, Schirren C: Microsurgery in andrologic urology. II. Alloplastic spermatocele. J Microsurg 1980; 1:428–435.
4. Kelami A, Rohloff D, Affeld K, Schroter A, Blohm B: Alloplastic spermatocele: Insemination from epididymal reservoir. Urology 1977; 10:317–319.
5. Kelami A: Kelami–Affeld alloplastic spermatocele and successful human delivery. Urol Int 1981; 36:368–372.
6. Jimenez-Cruz JF: Artificial spermatocele. J Urol 1980; 123:885–886.
7. Hamm B, Kelami A: Experimental studies on the functional capacity of the alloplastic spermatocele (Kelami–Affeld prosthesis). Urol Int 1982; 37:314–323.
8. Pryor J, Parsons J, Goswamy R, et al: In-vitro fertilisation for men with obstructive azoospermia [Letter]. Lancet 1984; 2:762.
9. Temple-Smith PD, Southwick GJ, Yates CA, et al: Human pregnancy by in Vitro fertilization (IVF) using sperm aspirated from the epididymis. J In Vitro Fert Embryo Transfer 1985; 2:119–122.
10. Silber S, Ord T, Borrero C, et al: New treatment for infertility due to congenital absence of vas deferens. Lancet 1987; 2:850–851.
11. Silber SJ, Ord T, Balmaceda J, et al: Congenital absence of the vas deferens: The fertilizing

capacity of human epididymal sperm. N Engl J Med 1990; 323:1788–1792.
12. Belker AM, Jimenez-Cruz DJF, Kelami A, Wagenknecht LV: Alloplastic spermatocele: Poor sperm motility in intraoperative epididymal fluid contraindicates prosthesis implantation. J Urol 1986; 136:408–409.
13. Turner TT: On the development and use of alloplastic spermatoceles. Fertil Steril 1988; 49:387–395.
14. Silber SJ, Patrizio P, Asch RH: Quantitative evaluation of spermatogenesis by testicular histology in men with congenital absence of the vas deferens undergoing epididymal sperm aspiration. Hum Reprod 1990; 5:89–93.
15. Turner TT, Smith CC: Alloplastic spermatocele: diffusion across the allograft material and survival of spermatozoa in vitro and in vivo. J Urol 1984; 132:591–594.
16. Amelar RD, Dubin L, Schoenfeld C: Circulating sperm-agglutinating antibodies in azoospermic men with congenital bilateral absence of the vasa deferentia. Fertil Steril 1975; 26:228–231.
17. Girgis SM, Ekladious EM, Iskander R, El-Dakkly R, Girgis FN: Sperm antibodies in serum and semen in men with bilateral congenital absence of the vas deferens. Arch Androl 1982; 8:301–305.
18. Patrizio P, Moretti-Rojas I, Ord T, et al: Low incidence of sperm antibodies in men with congenital absence of the vas deferens. Fertil Steril 1989; 52:1018–1021.
19. Belker AM: Alloplastic spermatocele: An update. In: Lipshultz LI, Howards SS, eds. Infertility in the male, 2nd ed. Chicago: Mosby Year Book, 1991:370–375.
20. Belker AM: Microsurgical repair of obstructive causes of male infertility. Sem Urol 1984; 2:91–98.

ANNOTATED BIBLIOGRAPHY

Belker AM, Jimenez-Cruz DJF, Kelami A, Wagenknecht LV. Alloplastic spermatocele: Poor sperm motility in intraoperative epididymal fluid contraindicates prosthesis implantation. J Urol 1986; 136:408–409.

The authors reported implantation of 130 alloplastic spermatoceles in 91 patients (39 bilateral and 52 unilateral). The implantations were performed for treatment of congenital abnormalities 110 times, for treatment of inflammatory obstruction in 14 instances, postoperative obstructions 4 times, and for treatment of other obstructions twice. Postoperative aspirations were performed with variable frequency, ranging over a period of several days to many months. The most common reason for termination of postoperative aspirations was the absence of sperm from one or more aspirates, which was believed to be due to cicatricial obstruction of the opening of the epididymal tubule into the prosthesis.

Without exception, the percentage of motile sperm in the postoperative aspirates closely approximated the percentage in the intraoperative epididymal fluid, until the last few aspirations, when sperm disappeared from the aspirates. A decrease in sperm concentration and motility generally appeared in two or three aspirates before the complete disappearance of sperm.

Of the 130 implantations in 91 patients, pregnancy resulted from inseminations with the aspirated sperm in seven wives. Four progressed to delivery at term and three were ended by first trimester spontaneous abortion. No pregnancy resulted when less than 20% of the intraoperative epididymal fluid sperm were motile. All seven pregnancies occurred in the wives of those patients who had congenital causes of obstructive azoospermia.

The absence of any motile sperm in the intraoperative epididymal fluid was believed to be a contraindication for implantation of an alloplastic spermatocele. Because of the relationship between the percentage of motile sperm in the intraoperative epididymal fluid and in postoperative aspirates, and since pregnancy did not result whenever less than 20% of the epididymal fluid sperm were motile, it was believed to be unwise to implant an alloplastic spermatocele if less than 20% of the epididymal sperm were motile. If these criteria had been followed during this study, implantations would not have been performed in 39 of the 91 patients (43%).

Hamm B, Kelami A: Experimental studies on the functional capacity of the alloplastic spermatocele (Kelami–Affeld prosthesis). Urol Int 1982; 37:314–323.

The authors implanted 39 alloplastic spermatoceles onto the epididymides of minipigs. Postoperative aspirations showed sperm present in 24 prostheses. When postoperative aspirates no longer contained sperm, the scrotal contents were excised and examined microscopically. Findings in the order of frequency were (1) atrophy of the sperm forming epithelium; (2) dilation of the tubules in the caput of the epididymis; (3) sperm granuloma in the interstitial tissue of the caput epididymis; and (4) fibrosis, granulation tissue, and sperm granuloma in the area at the base of the prosthesis. The testes showed impairment of spermatogenesis in 88% of the cases (reduced spermatogenesis in 60% and absent spermatogenesis in 28%). Regardless of reduced or absent testicular sperm production, sperm still were present in the tubule in the caput epididymis, thus indicating that spermatogenesis had previously taken place. In several specimens, rather extensive sperm granulomata were present in the interstices of the caput epididymis. Granulation tissue along with fresh and old blood clots were superimposed on fibrotic tissue within the prosthetic lumens.

The authors suggested that better results might be expected from experimental implantations performed with microsurgical techniques. They suggested that postoperative aspiration should be performed within the first few days following surgery to increase the possibility of obtaining the highest percentage of motile sperm. The danger of deteriorating sperm concentration and motility with the passage of time was emphasized. The timing of implantation of alloplastic spermatoceles was recommended to be synchronized with the day of the wife's ovulation.

Silber SJ, Ord T, Balmaceda J, Patrizio P, Asch RH: Congenital absence of the vas deferens: The fertilizing capacity of human epididymal sperm. N Engl J Med 1990; 323:1788–1792.

Twenty-eight men who had bilateral congenital absence of the vasa deferentia underwent microsurgical aspiration of sperm from the epididymis and/or vasa efferentia for attempted *in vitro* fertilization (IVF) of the wives'oocytes, with subsequent embryo transfer. Of 32 treatment cycles initiated, 4 were repeat cycles.

The most motile sperm were found in the very uppermost portion of the epididymis in or near the vasa efferentia. Embryos were obtained for transfer in 21 cases (66%). Ninety-three embryos resulted from 352 mature oocytes (26% rate of fertilization of oocytes). Clinical pregnancy was achieved in 10 of the 32 treatment cycles (31%). Seven women delivered normal infants and three miscarried. When fewer than 10 oocytes were retrieved from the wife, no pregnancy occurred. When 10 or more oocytes were retrieved (20 cases), the pregnancy rate was 50%. Surgical techniques, methods of ovarian stimulation and transvaginal oocyte aspiration, gamete preparation, and embryo transfer were described.

Turner TT: On the development and use of alloplastic spermatoceles. Fertil Steril 1988; 49:387–395.

The author begins by reviewing animal and human experiences with implantation of alloplastic spermatoceles. He stresses that the literature reveals that over 100 human prosthetic implantations have been performed with a reported pregnancy rate ranging between 0 and 4%. The implantation procedures that had been performed up to the time of the author's report consistently yielded poor sperm recovery and poor viability of those sperm that may have been recovered. Reasons for poor sperm recovery could be (1) occlusion of the epididymal tubule, (2) occlusion of the lumen of the spermatocele, or (3) poor sperm output by the testis. Poor sperm viability in postoperative aspirates may be a function of what happens to spermatozoa when they are in contact with an alloplastic spermatocele instead of the normal epididymal tubule.

The author investigated the effects the epididymal microenvironment and tubular epithelium on sperm motility. He found that "minimum essential medium" (MEM) maintained sperm motility as well as did intact caudal tubular epithelium. MEM is physiologically similar to epididymal tubular fluid; however, it was not possible to determine which component(s) of MEM appeared to be responsible for the maintenance of sperm motility.

The author also performed experiments regarding sperm survival in alloplastic spermatoceles. Poor sperm survival could be explained by (1) loss of the epididymal microenvironment required for sperm maturation and storage, (2) sperm dilution, and (3) loss of protection from the immune system due to absence of the blood-epididymal barrier. Experiments were conducted to examine sperm survival and the microenvironment in alloplastic spermatoceles constructed of polytetrafluoroethylene (Gore-Tex). The Gore-Tex graft material leaked electrolytes so that electrolyte concentrations in the lumen of the spermatocele were not different from concentrations in the serum, while a differential does exist between electrolyte concentrations in normal epididymal tubular fluid and serum. This was true no matter which of various diluents were used for sperm storage in the spermatocele. Although the author did not test electrolyte leakage through silicone, such experiments were planned.

It was emphasized that mature sperm that have the capacity for motility are kept quiescent in the male tract and initiate motility on exposure to most physiologic diluents. Thus, alloplastic spermatoceles that contain conventional diluents, even if the diluent constituents could be retained within the prosthesis, would initiate the motility of spermatozoa. Once motility is initiated, spermatozoa have a finite fertile life, which is around 48 hours in most species. Initiation of sperm motility within the spermatocele at the time of implantation therefore could reduce the probability that motile sperm would be recovered days or weeks after the spermatocele was implanted. The author concludes by making a plea for basic laboratory research to determine how best to maximize the fertility of sperm recovered from alloplastic spermatoceles.

23 Microscopic Epididymal Sperm Aspiration (MESA)

Mitchell B. Hollander
Michael D. Carter
Larry I. Lipshultz

In decades past, men with sterility resulting from the inability to transport sperm from the epididymis to the ejaculatory ducts because of nonreconstructible or congenitally absent ductal systems were considered untreatable. Recently, a new therapy involving the procurement of sperm using microscopic epididymal sperm aspiration (MESA) combined with either *in vitro* fertilization (IVF) or zygote intrafallopian transfer (ZIFT) has given new hope to these previously "infertile" males.

MESA, first described in 1985, is a technique for procurement of sperm from the epididymis of men with irreversible primary or secondary obstructive azoospermia.[1] Most commonly, it has been performed in the treatment of men with primary obstructive azoospermia due to congenital absence of the vas deferens. This abnormality has been reported in 1.3% of men who present for an infertility evaluation and for 11 to 50% of cases of obstructive azoospermia.[2–6] In addition, other cases of irreversible secondary azoospermia occur after failed microsurgical vasovasostomy, vasoepididymostomy, or other inflammatory processes that cannot be successfully treated with microsurgical reconstruction.

First described for the treatment of secondary obstructive azoospermia by Temple-Smith in 1985[1] and for the treatment of congenital absence of the vas deferens by Silber et al. in 1988,[7] the technique had been performed in more than 350 patients worldwide by 1991.

Patient Evaluation

Because MESA is performed in combination with either IVF or ZIFT, preliminary evaluation of both the male and female partners is necessary prior to initiation of treatment. In males, a standard medical history is obtained, including relevant information about any previous surgery that might be associated with their azoospermia. In addition, a physical examination is performed to evaluate testicular position, size, and consistency as well as to assess integrity of

Management of Impotence and Infertility, edited by Douglas Whitehead and Harris Nagler,

the cord, vas, and other peritesticular structures. In our laboratory, the serum levels of follicle-stimulating hormone (FSH) are assayed as an indirect measure of sperm production. Finally, in certain cases, ultrasonography is used as an adjunct in determining how much of the ductal system (ejaculatory duct, seminal vesicles) is present in men with suspected congenital absence of the vas.

A prerequisite to performing MESA is the presence of normal sperm production. Patients with congenital absence of the vas deferens and normal testicular size and normal FSH may still have a Sertoli-cell-only syndrome or focal atrophy (as sometimes seen many years after vasectomy). Thus, the question arises of whether to perform a testis biopsy prior to the performance of MESA.

At Baylor College of Medicine, we routinely perform testis biopsy prior to MESA. Others, however, have reported that they do not perform testis biopsies, and they base their action on reports that virtually all patients with congenital absence of the vas have normal spermatogenesis.[1,7–13] Hirsch and Choi concluded, moreover, that patients with congenital absence of the vas had a more favorable testicular histologic status than men who had undergone vasectomy. There is also a concern that a testis biopsy prior to MESA could cause scarring that might affect subsequent MESA. However, we believe that use of a "window" technique for testis biopsy results in minimal postoperative scarring that has no effect on the subsequent performance of MESA. In addition, we believe that before performing MESA, it is necessary to rule out the rare patient with congenital absence of the vas and Sertoli-cell-only or maturation arrest whose wife would thus avoid a long, time-consuming, and very expensive, needless ovulation induction process. Thus, a "window" technique testis biopsy can be performed safely in men with congenital absence of the vas without affecting subsequent MESA, and it allows one to proceed with the knowledge that sperm will be present at the time of aspiration, avoiding a possible litigious situation. Finally, in men with secondary obstructive azoospermia and normal testes on palpation, a normal FSH is enough indirect evidence to confirm normal sperm production, and one can proceed with MESA. However, if there are doubts as to the presence of normal spermatogenesis, a testis biopsy can be performed.

The female partner also undergoes a preliminary evaluation performed by a gynecologist. With this completed, the wife's ovulatory cycle is then controlled and hyperstimulated using one of many available protocols to produce numerous eggs. The cycle is monitored by ultrasonography and serum estradiol levels to optimize the time for surgical removal of the eggs. When the number and size of the follicles (usually >16 mm) are deemed sufficient by ultrasound, human chorionic gonadotropin (hCG) is injected, and approximately 34 hours later transvaginal or laparoscopic aspiration of the follicles is performed.

Whether to aspirate the male or female first is controversial. The failure to obtain eggs of adequate number and maturity seems more likely than a failure to aspirate adequate numbers of sperm from the epididymis. In addition, scarring and adhesions may preclude the future performance of aspiration and thus eliminate future hopes when the eggs are aspirated first and are of insufficient number or maturity. It is with this in mind that we recommend, as do others,[8] that aspiration of follicles be undertaken first. MESA is scheduled approximately 1 to 4 hours after the follicular aspiration is to be performed. The eggs are assessed *in vitro*, and if adequate numbers and maturity are confirmed, then MESA can proceed.

Technique

We perform MESA via two separate scrotal incisions. A longitudinal scrotal incision is carried out on the side(s) selected for epididymal aspiration. The length of the incision should allow easy delivery of the testicle and epididymis as well as other peritesticular structures [usually 3–6 cm (Figures 23-1A and B)]. The tunica vaginalis is identified and incised with subsequent delivery of the testicle and epididymis into the operative field.

At this point, the procedure is performed under the operating microscope at 10–40×

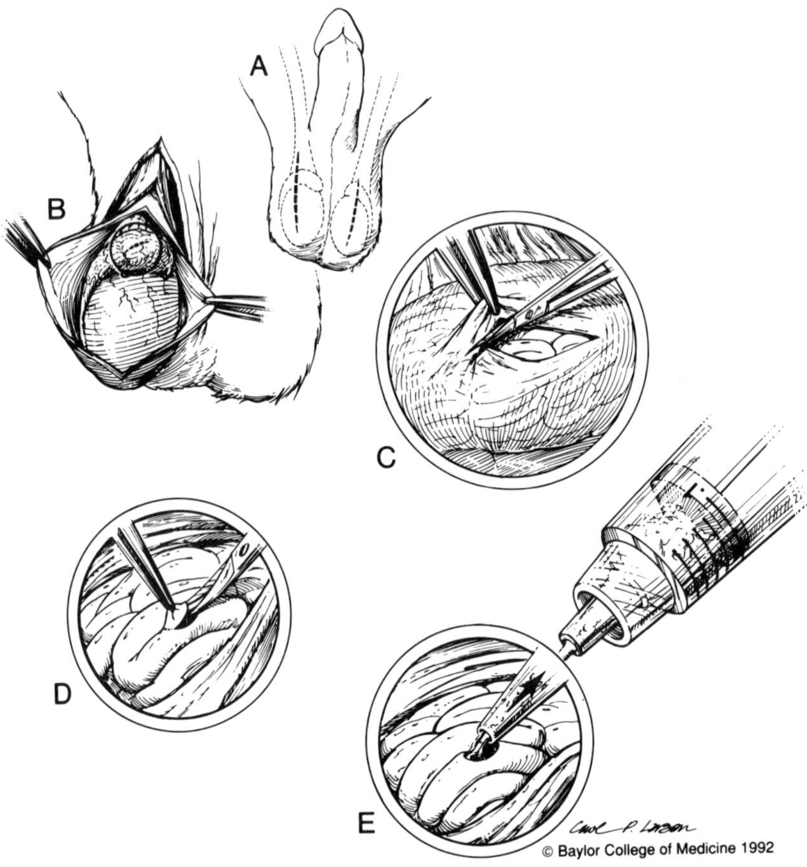

Figure 23-1 Microscopic epididymal sperm aspiration. (A) Longitudinal hemiscrotal incisions. (B) Adequate length allows easy delivery of the testicle, epididymis, and other paratesticular structures through the tunica vaginalis. (C) Tunica epididymis is incised using microforceps and microscissors to expose epididymal tubules. (D) A single epididymal tubule is isolated and incised using the microscissors. (E) Epididymal fluid is aspirated into tuberculin syringe with 25-gauge angiocatheter containing 0.1 ml of modified Hepes buffer.

magnification. The aspiration is attempted at the lowest level possible within the epididymis. The tunica epididymis is incised using microforceps and microscissors (Figure 23-1C). The epididymal tubules are now easily identified. A single tubule is isolated and incised using the microscissors (Figure 23-1D). The fluid that effluxes from the open tubule is aspirated with a tuberculin syringe containing 0.1 ml of modified Hepes buffer media and a 25-gauge angiocatheter (Figure 23-1E). The fluid is examined microscopically within the operating room for the presence of whole motile sperm. If the fluid aspirated is of a thick, creamy, paste-like quality, it usually contains no motile sperm. The microscope must be used, however, to assess the presence or absence of normal, motile sperm. If poor sperm quality is confirmed, one must select a more proximal tubule. When a tubule is found to express fluid with motile sperm confirmed under the microscope, aspiration is carried out with multiple tuberculin syringes for approximately 30–60 minutes. It is important that meticulous hemostasis be achieved prior to aspiration. This can be performed with bipolar cautery on low-voltage settings.

The epididymal fluid is transferred by the surgical nurse from the syringes into a human tubule fluid (HTF)-buffered media. A gentle pressure on the testicle and proximal epididymis assists in increasing the flow of fluid through the opening in the tubule. At the completion of the aspiration, the epididymal fluid suspended in modified HTF-buffered media is sent to the laboratory for processing and analysis.

The open tubules are then closed with 10-0 nylon sutures in an interrupted fashion. The tunica epididymis is also closed with interrupted 9-0 nylon sutures. This closure of the tubule and tunica epididymis decreases the amount of postoperative scarring and adhesions to the epididymis, thus allowing repeat MESA to take place if necessary. The closures of the tunica vaginalis, dartos, and skin are then carried out in a standard fashion.

Results

In the past, the functional ability of human epididymal sperm to fertilize an oocyte has been questioned. The evidence from animal studies shows that the maturation of spermatozoa as well as their acquisition of the ability to fertilize eggs occur as sperm traverse the epididymis.[14–18]

In the past, qualitative assessment of sperm function was difficult, since the epididymides used were from autopsy studies—frequently from old men whose fertility was unknown.[18] Recently, with the increasing use of microsurgical techniques, it has become clear that aspirated epididymal sperm from artificial spermatoceles,[12,13] epididymal cysts,[19] caput epididymides, and even *ductuli efferentes* have the capacity to fertilize eggs with subsequent pregnancies.[18,20–29] However, one can conclude that long-term occlusion of the vas, epididymis, or testicle results in physiologic changes that allow the maturation of sperm in an area where maturation normally would not take place. More studies are needed to document epididymal function in normal men with no obstruction before any further statements can be made.

MESA, although enjoying limited success at present, is a therapy that is efficacious in its use and results. Since description of the procedure by Temple-Smith et al. in 1985, well over 350 cases have been performed. A collective review by Belker and associates revealed that MESA has been performed in 284 patients at 20 centers in the United States. The fertilization rate is reported to be 33% with a pregnancy rate reported to be between 9 and 33%. Silber et al.[9] reported MESA performed on 28 men with vasal agenesis. In the original results by both Southwick and Silber, a swim-up technique was used to isolate the motile fraction of the aspirate. However, in Silber's subsequent study, a discontinuous or mini-Percoll gradient was used to process the aspirates. Thirty-two treatment cycles were performed with a fertilization rate of 60% and a clinical pregnancy rate of 40 cases in 32 cycles (31%). In these cases, the authors reported seven deliveries and three miscarriages for a live birth rate per cycle of 21.9%. Lastly, the same group reported that the number of oocytes retrieved had a significant impact on the pregnancy rate, with no pregnancies achieved when fewer than 10 eggs were retrieved.[9] It should be noted, however, that other investigators have not found these results to be reproducible.

New reports of MESA associated with an assisted reproductive technique and micromanipulation (microinjection) have shown that even epididymal sperm lacking motility have fertilizing capacity.[20] Thus, in the future, as the technology improves, so may our ability to improve on the pregnancy rates in these selected cases. Presently, one can expect pregnancy rates with MESA to be approximately 5–20%.

With pregnancy rates improving, a new concern has arisen in men with congenital absence of the vas who are undergoing MESA. Oates et al.[30] reported an association between congenital absence of the vas and cystic fibrosis in patients in whom congenital vasal agenesis is a known finding. A heterozygous (cystic fibrosis carrier) state was found in 55% of men with congenital absence of the vas compared with 4% of controls, suggesting a heritable disorder that could be transmitted to offspring following MESA. They also recommended that genetic counseling and routine screening for the cystic fibrosis gene of both the patient and spouse be undertaken prior to the performance of MESA.[30] In light of these findings, studies are in progress to further delineate this association. For these reasons, we are now referring all MESA patients and their spouses for genetic evaluation and counseling prior to scheduling of MESA.

Conclusions

In conclusion, MESA combined with IVF or ZIFT is a treatment that can be used in patients with either vasal agenesis or irreversible ductal obstruction following infection, inflammation, or surgery. The procedure will involve treating both the male and female partners, since an assisted reproductive technique is a mandatory component. As improved technology and processing techniques become available, the success rates of MESA combined with IVF or ZIFT may also improve. At present, pregnancy rates are 5–20%, which, although low, offer hope where previously there was none to this small but well-defined infertile male population.

REFERENCES

1. Temple-Smith PD, Southwick GJ, Yates CA, Trounson AO, de Kretser DM: Human pregnancy by *in vitro* fertilization (IVF) using sperm aspirated from the epididymis. J *In Vitro* Fert Embryo Transf 1985; 2(3):119–122.

2. Hirsch IH, Choi H: Quantitative testicular biopsy in congenital and acquired genital obstruction. J Urol 1990; 143:311–312.
3. Goldstein M, Schlossberg S: Men with congenital absence of the vas deferens often have seminal vesicles. J Urol 1988; 140:85.
4. Greenberg SH, Lipshultz LI, Wein AJ: Experience with 425 subfertile male patients. J Urol 1978; 119:507.
5. Hirsch IH, Lipshultz LI, Fujino A, Scardino PT: Evaluation of the accessory sex glands in azoospermic males by transrectal ultrasonography. Surg Forum 1985; 36:618.
6. El-Itreby AA, Girgis SM: Congenital absence of vas deferens in male sterility. Int J Fertil 1961; 6:409.
7. Silber SJ, Balmaceda J, Borrero C, Ord T, Asch R: Pregnancy with sperm aspiration from the proximal head of the epididymis: A new treatment for congenital absence of the vas deferens. Fertil Steril 1988; 50(3):525–528.
8. Belker A: Infertility. American Fertility Society, Course Syllabus: Scottsdale, Arizona, 1991.
9. Silber SJ, Ord T, Balmaceda J, Patrizio P, Asch RH: Congenital absence of the vas deferens. The fertilizing capacity of human epididymal sperm. N Engl J Med 1990; 323:1788–1792.
10. Schoysman R, Drouart JM: Recent progress in the surgery of male and female sterility. Acta Chir Belg 1972; 71:261–280.
11. Kelami A: Alloplastische spermatocele: Vorlanfige mitteilung. Acta Urol Belg 1976; 7:167–176.
12. Vickers MA Jr: Creation and use of a scrotal sperm bank in aplasia of the vas deferens. J Urol 1975; 114:242–245.
13. Jiminez-Cruz JF: Artificial spermatocele. J Urol 1980; 123:885–886.
14. Cooper TG: The epididymis, sperm maturation and fertilisation. Heidelberg: Springer-Verlag, 1986.
15. Amann RP: Function of the epididymis in bulls and rams. J Reprod Fertil [Suppl.] 1987; 34:115.
16. Blaquier JA, Cameo MS, Cuasnicu PS, Gonzalez Echeveria MF, Pineiro L, Tezon JG, Vazquez MH: On the role of epididymal factors in sperm fertility. Reprod Nutr Dev 1988; 28:1209.
17. Blaquier J, Cameo MS, Dawidowski A, Gonzalez Echeverria F, Sanjurjo C: On the role of epididymal factors in sperm maturation in man. In: Serio M, ed. Perspectives in andrology. New York: Raven Press, 1989:37.
18. Cooper TG: In defense of a function for the human epididymis. Fertil Steril 1990; 54(6):965–975.
19. Hanley HG: Pregnancy following artificial insemination from epididymal cyst. Proc Soc Study Fertil 1956; 8:20.
20. Olar TT, La Nasa J, Dickey RP, Taylor SN, Curole, DN: Fertilization of human oocytes by microinjection of human sperm aspirated from the caput epididymis of an individual with obstructive azoospermia. J *In Vitro* Fertil Embryo Transf 1990; 7(3):160–164.
21. Silber AJ: Vasoepididymostomy to the head of the epididymis: Recovery of normal spermatozoal motility. Fertil Steril 1980; 34:149.
22. Silber SJ: Pregnancy caused by sperm from vasa efferentia. Fertil Steril 1988; 49:373.
23. Silber SJ: Apparent fertility of human sperm from the caput epididymis. J Reprod Immunol 1988; 88:895.
24. Silber SJ: Results of microsurgical vasoepididymostomy: Role of epididymis in sperm maturation. Hum Reprod 1989; 4:298.
25. Silber SJ: Role of epididymis in sperm maturation. Urology 1989; 33:47.
26. Silber SJ: Microsurgery and andrology. In: Scrio M, Waits GMH, eds. Recent advances in andrology. Serono Symposium Review, No. 20. Rome: Ares-Serono, 1989:103.
27. Silber SJ: Apparent fertility of human spermatozoa from the caput epididymis. J Androl 1989; 10:263.
28. Silber SJ, Ord T, Borrero C, Balmaceda J, Asch R. New treatment for infertility due to congenital absence of vas deferens? Lancet 1987; 2:850.
29. Mooney JK, Horan AH, Lattimer JK: Motility of spermatozoa in the human epididymis. J Urol 1972; 108:443.
30. Oates RD, Anguiano A, Milunsky A, Amos J,

Maher T: Bilateral congenital absence of the vas (CAV) and cystic fibrosis (CF): A genetic association? 47th Annual Meeting of the American Fertility Society [Suppl.], Abstract 0-008, p. S4, 1991.

ANNOTATED BIBLIOGRAPHY

Hirsch IH, Choi H: Quantitative testicular biopsy in congenital and acquired genital obstruction. J Urol 1990; 143:311.

This is a review of 13 testicular biopsies: 8 in men who underwent vasectomies and 5 in men with bilateral congenital absence of the vas deferens. The review focuses on a comparison of the histopathologic changes seen in these two forms of genital tract obstruction.

Quantitative analysis of the seminiferous tubular and epithelial parameters demonstrated a statistically significant increase in tubular wall thickness in the vasectomized group. No significant difference was seen between the two groups comparing the mean number of late spermatids per seminiferous tubules, mean number of Sertoli cells per somniferous tubules, mean number of seminiferous tubules per field (100 times), or mean seminiferous tubular diameter.

The authors conclude that men with vasal agenesis, despite life-long obstruction of the genital tract, show a better overall testicular histologic status than vasectomized men with acquired genital tract obstruction. They suggest the use of assisted reproductive techniques as a method of treatment in men with genital tract obstruction.

Silber SJ, Balmaceda J, Borrero C, Ord T, Asch R: Pregnancy with sperm aspiration from the proximal head of the epididymis: A new treatment for congenital absence of the vas deferens. Fertil Steril 1988; 50:525.

This paper documents the first use of microsurgical aspiration of sperm and IVF from the most proximal head of the epididymis in patients with congenital absence of the vas deferens.

The authors report on two men with congenital absence of the vas deferens in whom microsurgical aspiration of sperm from the caput epididymis in conjunction with IVF produced both fertilization and pregnancies in their respective wives.

The authors conclude that (1) sperm from the caput epididymis are capable of fertilizing the human egg *in vitro*; (2) the time after emergence from the testicle may be the most important factor in sperm maturation without the absolute need for transit through the entire epididymis; and (3) microsurgical aspiration of sperm in conjunction with IVF is a useful approach in establishing pregnancies in couples when there is congenital absence of the vas deferens.

Silber SJ, Ord T, Balmaceda J, Patrizio P, Asch RH: Congenital absence of vas deferens. N Engl J Med 1990; 323:1788.

The authors report on 28 men with bilateral congenital absence of the vas deferens who were treated using microsurgical aspiration of sperm from the epididymis in conjunction with IVF in an effort to establish a pregnancy.

Interestingly, the most motile sperm were found in the proximal epididymis at or near the vasa efferentia. Embryos were obtained in 21 cases (66%). Ninety-three embryos resulted from 352 mature oocytes (fertilization rate: 26%). Clinical pregnancy was achieved in 10 of the 32 treatment cycles (31%). Seven women delivered normal infants and three miscarried. One of the seven live births was of twins. There were six girls and two boys. When fewer than 10 eggs were retrieved, no pregnancy occurred. When over nine eggs were retrieved (20%), a high pregnancy rate was seen (50%). The authors also compared motility based on the geographic site of aspiration and found an inverse pattern from normal men in that sperm with the higher motility was found in the most proximal portion of the epididymis.

The authors conclude that sperm from the proximal epididymis and vasa efferentia can fertilize the oocyte *in vitro* and result in pregnancies with live births.

24 Ejaculatory Duct Obstruction

Harris M. Nagler
Eric I. Mitchnick

Infertility is reported to affect approximately 15% of married couples.[1] In approximately 50% of these couples, male infertility is implicated.[2] It has been estimated that in 7–14% of subfertile males, ductal obstruction, congenital or acquired, exists.[1] Obstruction can occur anywhere within the ductal system including the epididymis, vas deferens, or ejaculatory ducts. Azoospermia in the eugonadotropic male is suggestive of obstruction. The diagnosis is usually confirmed with testicular biopsy.[16] The site of obstruction is usually confirmed at the time of scrotal exploration and vasography. However, obstruction secondary to ejaculatory duct abnormalities may be suggested by (1) low or negative seminal fructose and/or (2) azoospermia or severe oligospermia with a low ejaculate volume (<1 ml) in the patient with normal vas deferentia and absence of retrograde ejaculation.[3–8] Historically, vasography has been used to document ejaculatory duct obstruction, but more recently transrectal ultrasonography has become the diagnostic method used for preoperative evaluation of these patients.[4]

Anatomy

The ejaculatory ducts are formed by the confluence of the vasa deferentia and the ducts of the seminal vesicles. They pass for 1 or 2 cm downward and forward through the central zone of the prostatic glandular substance, converging as they approach their termination near the verumontanum. A neurovascular fibrous stroma surrounds each ejaculatory duct and may contribute to seminal fluid propulsion and continence. The close proximity of the two ducts and their narrow diameter allow both ducts to be obstructed by a single lesion.[17] The treatment of the infertile male with bilateral ejaculatory duct obstruction is transurethral incision or resection of the ejaculatory ducts and/or the obstructing lesion.[6,7]

Preoperative Evaluation

The diagnosis of *ejaculatory duct obstruction* is entertained when a patient is found to have a

Management of Impotence and Infertility, edited by Douglas Whitehead and Harris Nagler,

low ejaculate volume with or without azoospermia. It should be determined that the patient has normal vas deferentia on physical examination and that there is no retrograde ejaculation. If hormonal evaluation is normal (i.e., eugonadotropic), the patient should undergo transrectal ultrasonography (TRUS). The diagnosis of ejaculatory duct obstruction is definitively made only by vasography; however, TRUS in patients with ejaculatory duct obstruction may demonstrate enlarged seminal vesicles and dilation of the ejaculatory ducts to the point of obstruction.

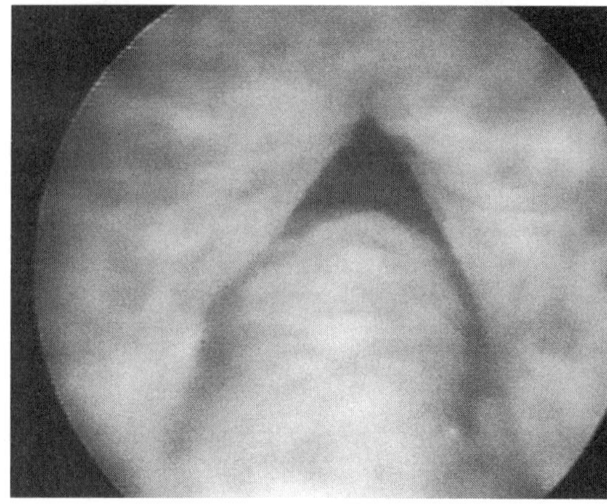

Figure 24-1 Endoscopic view of prostatic urethra demonstrating prominent verumontanum.

Procedure

The treatment of ejaculatory duct obstruction by transurethral resection has been described in the literature for almost 20 years originally by Farley and Barnes.[10] The technique involves resection of the ejaculatory ducts in the posterior portion of the prostate gland lateral to the verumontanum.

The procedure is performed under regional or general anesthesia with the patient placed in dorsal lithotomy position. An O'Connor drape is positioned in the rectum. The resection is initiated just proximal to the veru and includes the proximal most portion of the veru (Figures 24-1 and 24-2). The resection is extended toward the bladder neck and posteriorly until efflux of seminal fluid is seen (Figure 24-3). If vasography has been carried out at the time of the procedure, methylene blue instillation may be helpful to highlight the anatomy and facilitate the observation of efflux. We have found this not to be necessary when the diagnosis has been made on the basis of TRUS; however, if the diagnosis was not suspected prior to scrotal exploration and vasography, this late maneuver may be helpful. If the procedure is performed in the midline, both ducts will generally be unobstructed. If only one duct is thought to be obstructed, resection is performed only on that side. If a midline cystic structure is thought to be the cause of obstruction, simple unroofing appears to be sufficient.

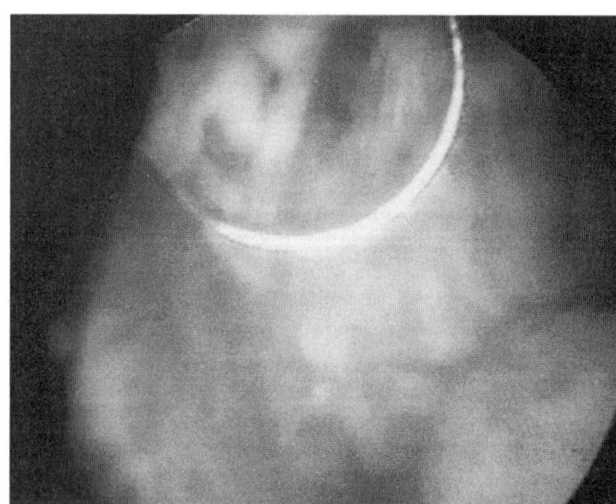

Figure 24-2 The initiation of the resection proximal to verumontanum.

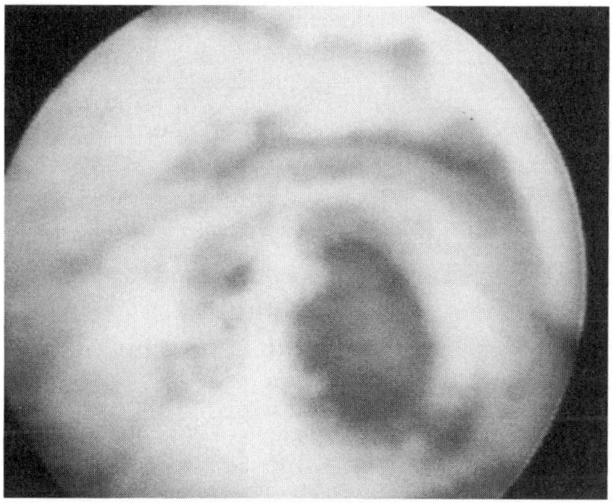

Figure 24-3 Dilated patent ejaculatory directly after resection of obstruction.

Palpation through the rectum is used to ensure the integrity of the rectum and to express seminal vesicular contents. Care is taken to (1) preserve the bladder neck to avoid retrograde ejaculation and (2) avoid the external sphincter to avoid incontinence. The rectal wall is at risk for perforation, and location of the loop must be constantly monitored during the resection of the nonhypertrophied prostate. A Foley catheter is placed after the procedure and left to gravity drainage overnight. The Foley catheter is removed on postoperative day one, and the patient is discharged home after voiding successfully. Semen analyses are performed 5 to 7 days postoperatively. We have routinely employed terazosin in the immediate postoperative period to minimize urinary retention. In our initial patients treated with TURED, the average increase in ejaculatory volume was 3.13 ml with an average increase in sperm count of 30 million/ml. Postoperatively, three of the four patients who had premature ejaculation had improvement. Two no longer have premature ejaculation, and one noted it to be infrequent compared to preoperatively. Each of these patients showed an increase in ejaculate volume postoperatively for an average increase of 340% from preoperative ejaculate volume.

Discussion

Infertility secondary to obstruction of the ejaculatory duct has previously been thought to be uncommon. However, the ability to make this diagnosis on the basis of transrectal ultrasonography has resulted in an apparent increase in the incidence of this diagnosis. Semen analysis will demonstrate azoospermia or severe oligospermia. Fructose determination has proven unreliable, and patients with ejaculatory duct abnormalities may continue to have fructose in the ejaculate. However, absence of fructose does suggest either obstruction of the ejaculatory duct, absence of the seminal vesicle, or retrograde ejaculation.[3] The postejaculate urine should be assessed for sperm to rule out the possibility of retrograde ejaculation.[8] Transrectal ultrasonography allows for assessment of the prostate, seminal vesicles, and ejaculatory ducts with relative ease and minimal patient discomfort. Patients with low ejaculate volume and large seminal vesicles by transrectal ultrasonography can be assumed to have partial or complete obstruction of the ejaculatory duct.[7] Rarely, will these seminal vesicles be palpable on rectal exam.

The causes of ejaculatory duct obstruction include inflammatory conditions, a history of indwelling catheters, prior transurethral surgery, urethral trauma, and congenital abnormalities.[5,6] Congenital abnormalities of the vasal system may be more common in patients with cystic fibrosis.[9]

We have noted that some patients with ejaculatory duct obstruction experience sexual dysfunction characterized by premature ejaculation. Relief of the obstruction of the ejaculatory duct with improved ejaculate volume resulted in improved sexual function. The correction of this dysfunction in these patients raises the specter of an organic etiology of premature ejaculation in some patients. The sympathetic innervation to the prostate and seminal vesicles is primarily from centers in the lower thoracic and lumbosacral spinal cord to the superior hypogastric plexus presynaptically acting on short adrenergic nerves postsynaptically. During emission, seminal fluid is deposited into the posterior urethra by sympathetic stimulation of the prostate. The seminal vesicles and ampulla of the vas contract; pushing sperm through the ejaculatory ducts while the bladder neck closes and the external sphincter relaxes. During ejaculation, there is rhythmic contraction of the periurethral and sphincter muscles, and seminal fluid is propelled down the urethra to the meatus. These contractions are acetylcholine-mediated through somatic nerves S2–S4. This phase of the ejaculatory process may be initiated by the presence of seminal fluid in the posterior urethra.[11,14,15] It has been shown that in some patients TURED and relief of ejaculatory duct obstruction and decompression of the seminal vesicles resulted in an improvement in ejaculatory control and premature ejaculation. The physiologic explanation for improvement in sexual function may lie in an as yet, undiscovered feedback mechanism or reflex between receptors in the seminal vesicles and the autonomic nervous system, which controls emission and ejaculation.

Transurethral resection of the ejaculatory ducts is an effective method for resolving ejaculatory duct obstruction in the infertile patient with minimal associated morbidity. Additionally, patients with ejaculatory duct obstruction and premature ejaculation may experience improved sexual function.

Ejaculatory duct obstruction can be successfully treated by transurethral resection. When the diagnosis has been accurately made, semen parameters may be reasonably expected to improve with an increase in ejaculate volume and increased sperm in the ejaculate. Some patients with ejaculatory duct obstruction may have concomitant epididymal obstruction and remain azoospermic. The patient with persistent azoospermia should be evaluated like any other patient with azoospermia. Patients with abnormalities of ejaculation and ejaculatory duct obstruction *may* obtain improved ejaculatory control after relief of ejaculatory duct obstruction. This *potential* association requires further evaluation.

REFERENCES

1. DeVere White R, Paulson D: Obstruction of the male reproductive tract. J Urol 1977; 118:266.
2. Goldwasser B, Weinerth J, Carson C: Ejaculatory duct obstruction: The case for aggressive diagnosis and treatment. J Urol 1985; 134:964.
3. Silber S: Ejaculatory duct obstruction. J Urol 1980; 124:294.
4. Belker A, Steinbock G: Transrectal ultrasonography as a diagnostic and therapeutic aid for ejaculatory duct obstruction. J Urol 1990; 144:356.
5. Carson C: Transurethral resection for ejaculatory duct stenosis and oligospermia. Fertil Steril 1984; 41(3):482–484.
6. Weintraub CM: Transurethral drainage of the seminal tract for obstruction, infection and infertility. Br J Urol 1980; 52:220–225.
7. Carter S, Shinohara K, Lipshultz L: Transrectal ultra sonography in disorders of the seminal vesicles and ejaculatory ducts. Urol Clinincs N Am 1989; 16(4):773–790.

8. Dunetz G, Krane R: Successful treatment of aspermia secondary to obstruction of ejaculatory duct. J Urol 1986; 26(8):529–530.
9. Porch P: Aspermia owing to obstruction of distal ejaculatory duct and treatment by transurethral resection. J Urol 1978; 119:141–142.
10. Farley S, Barnes R: Stenosis of ejaculatory ducts treated by endoscopic resection. J Urol 1973; 109:664–666.
11. Gillenwater J et al: Adult and pediatric urology. Chicago: Year Book Medical Publishers, 1987:1286–1287.
12. Stanley E: Sex problems in practice. Br Med J 1981; 282:1521–1524.
13. Hawton K: Erectile dysfunction and premature ejaculation. Br J Hosp Med 1988; 40(6):428–436.
14. Rajfer J: Common problems in infertility and impotence. Chicago: Year Book Medical Publishers 1990:162–163.
15. Walsh P et al: Campbell's urology, 5th ed. Philadelphia: W.B. Saunders, 1986:709–710.
16. Nagler HM, Thomas AJ: Testicular biopsy and vasography in the evaluation of male infertility. Urol Clinics North Am 1987; 14(1):167.
17. Pryor JP, Hendry WF: Ejaculatory duct obstruction in subfertile males: Analysis of 87 patients. Fertil and Steril 1991; 56(4):725–730.

ANNOTATED BIBLIOGRAPHY

Belker M, Steinbock GS: Transrectal prostate ultrasonography as a diagnostic and therapeutic aid for ejaculatory duct obstruction. J Urol 1990; 356–358.

In this case report and discussion, the authors present a patient with ejaculatory duct obstruction diagnosed by transrectal ultrasonography and then treated with transurethral resection. The patient had an excellent result with marked improvement in his semen analysis. This was the first published report of the use of transrectal ultrasonography (TRUS) to establish the diagnosis of ejaculatory duct obstruction without relying on vasography. The authors suggest that TRUS is a valuable aid for preoperative surgical planning and may also eliminate the need for vasography to confirm the diagnosis of ejaculatory duct obstruction.

Carter S St C, Shinohara K, Lipshultz LI: Transrectal ultrasonography in disorders of the seminal vesicles and ejaculatory ducts. Urol Clinics North Am 1989; 16(4):773–790.

In this review the authors review the technique of transrectal ultrasound (TRUS) of the seminal vesicles and ejaculatory ducts. The normal appearance of the seminal vesicles and ejaculatory ducts on transrectal ultrasonography including the size, location, and contour are described. Abnormal findings in their review included vasa aplasia, prostatic cysts, Müllerian duct cysts, and seminal vesicle cysts. TRUS was found to be an inexpensive, noninvasive, and reliable means of evaluating the seminal vesicles and ejaculatory ducts and may provide new diagnostic criteria to evaluate the infertile patient.

Nagler HM, Thomas AJ Jr: Testicular biopsy and vasography in the evaluation of male infertility. Urol Clinics North Am 1987; 14(1):167–176.

In this review the authors stress the importance of classification of the patient into pretesticular, testicular, and posttesticular causes of infertility. The assignment of a patient into one of these classifications is made largely on the basis of history, physical examination, semen analysis, and hormonal evaluation. Testicular biopsy is necessary for the definitive diagnosis of obstructive azoospermia in the eugonadotropic patient. The goal of testicular biopsy in the azoospermic patient is the discovery of normal spermatogenesis indicating a surgically correctable obstructive lesion. Testicular biopsy may be performed easily on an outpatient basis with excision of a small piece of seminiferous tissue using a "no-touch" technique as described by the authors. Various techniques of vasography are discussed by the authors.

25

Treatment of Retrograde Ejaculation

Mark Sigman

Abnormalities of male sexual function may involve dysfunction of the erectile process, the ejaculatory process, or both. The normal ejaculatory process requires two events: emission and ejaculation. Emission is the deposition of semen in the posterior urethra. Ejaculation involves the propulsion of this semen through the anterior urethra and out the meatus. For antegrade ejaculation to occur, the bladder neck must close during the ejaculatory process. A lack of closure of the bladder neck results in retrograde ejaculation in which semen is propelled into the bladder instead of the anterior urethra.

Physiology of Ejaculation

Antegrade ejaculation requires the coordinated contraction of both the bladder neck and external urethral sphincter. While the bladder neck is normally closed in the resting state, increased sympathetic input to the smooth muscle of the bladder neck increases bladder neck tone during ejaculation.[1] The external urethral sphincter consists of an outer striated muscle layer that is somatically innervated and an inner, smooth muscle layer that is autonomically innervated. During emission, both the bladder neck and external urethral sphincter close after deposition of semen in the posterior urethra. Pressure builds up in the posterior urethra and the external urethral sphincter opens while the bladder neck remains closed resulting in the antegrade propulsion of semen through the anterior urethra.[2] Contraction of the bulbocavernosus and ischiocavernosus muscles occurs simultaneously, aiding in the forward propulsion of semen through the urethra.[3]

Neural control of ejaculation involves both stimulatory and inhibitory central cerebral factors as well as spinal reflex arcs. Sympathetic outflow from T10 through L3 descends in the periaortic region to neuroplexes of the superior hypogastric ganglion at the aortic bifurcation. Hypogastric nerves leave the plexes to synapse in the adventitia of the end organs. Postganglionic adrenergic fibers innervate the

Management of Impotence and Infertility, edited by Douglas Whitehead and Harris Nagler,

vas, and ampulla, seminal vesicles, prostate, and bladder neck. Distention of the posterior urethra from seminal emission results in afferent sensory stimuli through the pelvic splanchnic nerves.[4] The striated pelvic floor musculature and periurethral muscles are innervated by somatic efferents via the pudendal nerve. Communication exists between cortical, brachial, lumbar, and sacral nerves.[5] The coordinated activity of the somatic and autonomic nervous system results in rhythmic contractions of the pelvic floor musculature, bulbocavernosus and spongiocavernosus musculature, as well as an intermittent relaxation of the external urethral sphincter. Contractions generally occur at 0.8 second intervals for a total of 3–7 contractions.

Table 25-1 Causes of Retrograde Ejaculation

Neurologic
Diabetes mellitus
Retroperitoneal lymphadenectomy
Colorectal surgery
Abdominal aneurismectomy
Aortoiliac bypass surgery
Spinal cord injury
Anatomic
Bladder neck surgery
Prostatectomies
Urethral strictures
Meatal stenosis
Trauma to bladder neck or posterior urethra
Extropy – epispadias
Posterior urethral valves
Ectopic ejaculatory duct
Pharmacologic
Antihypertensives
Antipsychotics
Antidepressants
Other drugs

Etiology

Any process that interferes with adequate closure of the bladder neck will result in retrograde ejaculation (Table 25-1).

Damage to the sympathetic nervous system causing incompetence of the bladder neck may result in retrograde ejaculation. Seminal emission may also be affected, resulting in lack of emission. Diabetes mellitus may affect both potency and ejaculation. Sympathetic diabetic neuropathy is responsible for the ejaculatory abnormalities. About one-third of diabetic men have evidence of ejaculatory dysfunction with retrograde ejaculation being more common than lack of emission.[6,7]

Retroperitoneal lymph node dissection remains an integral component in the treatment of nonseminomonas germ cell tumors. Traditional surgical techniques involve removal of periaortic sympathetic ganglia bilaterally. The majority of such patients have demonstrated a lack of emission with a smaller proportion demonstrating retrograde ejaculation and occasional patients retaining normal ejaculatory function. More recent surgical techniques have limited the area of dissection or spared individual sympathetic nerves. With the use of such techniques, more than 80% of patients may maintain ejaculatory function.[8,9] Other extensive retroperitoneal surgery such as colorectal surgery, abdominal aneurysmectomy, and aortoiliac bypass grafting may also interfere with ejaculation.[10]

Ejaculatory dysfunction occurs in approximately 80% of spinal cord-injured males. Almost one-third of these patients are married or subsequently marry and despite preservation of ejaculation in 20%, only 5% are able to impregnate their wives.[11] Both antegrade and retrograde ejaculation have been found in these patients.

Surgery of the bladder neck often results in retrograde ejaculation. Y-V plasties of the bladder neck were popular in the 1950s and early 1960s for males with vesicoureteral reflex.[12] It was felt that these patients had high intravesicle pressures secondary to a high resistance of the bladder neck and posterior urethra. Disruption of the normal function of the bladder neck resulted in retrograde ejaculation in a significant proportion of these patients. Elongation of the prostatic urethra during puberty may improve ejaculatory function in some patients.[13] Transurethral resections of the prostate result in retrograde ejaculation in the majority of patients. Since the majority of these patients are past the reproductive years, this is rarely of clinical significance. Open prostatectomies may also interfere with bladder neck function and result in retrograde ejaculation. Newer prostatectomy techniques such as laser-assisted prostatectomies preserve antegrade ejaculation. Urethral strictures or meatal stenosis may rarely present with retrograde ejaculation.[14] Posterior urethral and bladder neck trauma may also lead to retrograde ejaculation. Impaired antegrade ejaculation has been reported following inadequate reapproximation of bulbospongiosis muscles following urethroplasties for urethral strictures.[15] Transurethral incisions of the bladder neck preserve ejaculation in approximately three fourths of patients.[16]

Uncommon congenital causes of retrograde ejaculation include the extrophy–epispadias complex and undiagnosed posterior urethral valves. Obstruction of the ejaculatory ducts may result from inflammatory or postsurgical scarring during the repair of these lesions. Ejaculatory dysfunction may result from pharmacologic interference with the sympathetic nervous system. A sympatholytic effect is responsible for the lack of emission or retrograde ejaculation from these medications. Psychotropic and antihypertensive medications are well known agents of ejaculatory dysfunction. Offending agents should be withdrawn or alternative medications substituted if possible. Idiopathic retrograde ejaculation has been reported.[17] This diagnosis should be made by exclusion of other known causes following a thorough evaluation of the patient.

Clinical Evaluation

Any patient complaining of a dry ejaculate should be evaluated for retrograde ejaculation. Similarly, infertile patients with low volume ejaculates should also be examined. Finally, many patients present with a history of prior surgery such that the diagnosis is already known. Some patients may complain of cloudy urine following ejaculation. The diagnosis of retrograde ejaculation rests on the finding of sperm in the postejaculate urine specimen. A urine sample should be mixed thoroughly and an unspun sample may be examined under wet mount microscopy. Any sperm identified in the anejaculate patient confirms some degree of retrograde ejaculation. In patients without a known anatomical or surgical cause for retrograde ejaculation and who present with low volume semen specimens that may not necessarily be azoospermic, it is important to quantitate the number of sperm in the urine. If high concentrations of sperm are present in the unspun urine, the concentration may be determined by treating the urine as a semen specimen and performing a sperm count. In cases in which few sperm are seen in the unspun specimen, the urine may be centrifuged and the pellet resuspended in a known volume and a sperm count determined. By knowing the total volume of urine and the concentration and volume of resuspended sperm, the total number of sperm in the urine sample may be calculated. Thus, the physician is able to determine if a significant number of sperm are present in the bladder.

Table 25-2 Medications Used for the Treatment of Retrograde Ejaculation

Drug	Dose
Pseudoephedrine hydrochloride	60 mg QID
Ephedrine	25–50 mg QID
Phenylpropanolamine	75 mg BID
Imipramine hydrochloride	25 mg BID or 50 mg QHs

Therapy

There are two approaches to the treatment of retrograde ejaculation. The initial approach should be aimed at attempts to convert ejaculation from retrograde to antegrade; if this is successful the couple may conceive through normal intercourse. If the first course of action is not successful or possible, therapy is directed at sperm retrieval and attempts at conception through assisted reproductive techniques such as insemination or *in vitro* fertilization.

Both surgical and pharmacologic approaches have been used in attempts to convert ejaculation from retrograde to antegrade. In general, medical therapy is applicable in patients with an anatomically intact bladder neck. Patients with surgical destruction of the bladder neck or a congenital abnormality of the bladder neck are not amenable to medical therapy.

Medical Therapy

Various sympathomimetic agents have been used in an attempt to increase bladder neck tone to convert retrograde ejaculation to antegrade ejaculation[18,19] (see Table 25-2). Patients in whom these drugs should be tried are those with neurologic etiologies or non-bladder neck abnormalities. Medications such as pseudoephedrine hydrochloride stimulate adrenergic nerve endings resulting in an increased release of norepinephrine. Increased alpha stimulation results in increased tone of the internal urethral sphincter. Ephedrine is a direct adrenergic agonist and, therefore, similarly causes increased adrenergic tone. Phenylpropanolamine hydrochloride has a combination of effects, causing both increased release of norepinephrine and direct stimulation of adrenergic receptors. Finally, tricyclic antidepressants such as imipramine block the reuptake of norepinephrine. These medications may result in the conversion of retrograde ejaculation to antegrade ejaculation, an increase in the antegrade fraction of a patient who both antegrade and retrograde ejaculates, and may convert a patient with lack of emission into a retrograde or antegrade ejaculator.

Side effects of the sympathomimetic agents include nervousness, dizziness, or difficulty sleeping. Urinary retention may occur in patients with bladder outlet obstruction due to BPH. Tachycardia may also occur. With chronic use, tachyphylaxis may occur. Additional side effects specific for imipramine are secondary to its direct smooth muscle relaxant properties and its anticholinergic properties.

While in some cases responses may be seen within a few days, other patients do not respond to these medications until over 1 week of therapy; therefore, we place patients on a 2 week trial of medication. We will often start with medications such as pseudoephedrine. If this is unsuccessful, a trial of a medication with a different mechanism of action such as imipramine alone or in combination with the prior medication may occasionally be successful.

Reports of successful pregnancies have followed the use of other procedures. Direct voiding of postejaculate urine into the vagina has resulted in a successful conception.[20] Ejaculation with a full bladder has been reported to produce an antegrade ejaculate in two patients with retrograde ejaculation. These specimens were subsequently used for insemination. It should be noted that these two patients presented with unusual causes of retrograde ejaculation: one being due to ectopic ejaculatory ducts and the second to idiopathic retrograde ejaculation. It is unknown how well this approach would work in patients with other causes of retrograde ejaculation.[21] Neither of the above techniques has gained widespread use.

Surgical Therapy

Surgery to lengthen the posterior urethra or to tighten the bladder neck has successfully converted retrograde ejaculators to antegrade ejaculators.[22,23] With the availability of assisted reproductive techniques, these surgical procedures have not gained widespread use.

Assisted Reproductive Techniques

In many cases, it is not possible to convert a patient from retrograde to antegrade ejaculation. In these instances, sperm need to be retrieved from the bladder and subsequently used for assisted reproductive techniques. Sperm retrieval may be accomplished by noninvasive techniques wherein the patient voids the sperm out or by the use of invasive techniques where the patient is catheterized to retrieve sperm. In general, noninvasive techniques should be attempted first; if sperm of adequate quality cannot be obtained then invasive techniques should be employed. Initial attempts should involve the patient ejaculating into a bladder with urine and subsequently voiding the urine out. Since sperm will be in contact with urine, both the urine pH and osmolality need to be adjusted to physiologic ranges. Seminal plasma normally has a pH from 7.2 to 7.8. Acid pHs immobilize sperm whereas pHs above 9.0 are spermatoxic, thus attempts should be made to alkalinize urine keeping the pH roughly between 7.2 and 8.0.

Semen osmolarity ranges from 300 to 380 mosmol/liter. Hypotonic media result in an irreversible swelling of the cell membrane; therefore, it is important to attempt near physiologic urine osmolalities. This is often most easily accomplished by obtaining specimens in the morning, since a patient's breakfast habits and nighttime sleeping habits are often constant. Urine pH may be alkalinized by the administration of sodium bicarbonate, 650 milligrams qid; acetazolamide (diamox), 250 mg qid; sustained release acetazolamide, 500 mg bid; or baking soda 1–2 tablespoons in a glass of water. This is commonly begun 1–2 days prior to sperm retrieval; however, sodium bicarbonate may also be given 2–3 hours before sperm retrieval. Acetazolamide may be preferred for older patients who are on sodium-restricted diets. If the urine pH remains in the acidic range the dosage of the alkalinization agent should be increased. Similarly, urine osmolality may be changed by restricting or increasing fluid intake as needed. Once a regimen is developed that results in appropriate urine pH and osmolality, the patient is instructed to masturbate and then void into a specimen container. This is preferably done in the office, so the sperm do not remain in contact with the urine for a prolonged period of time. While some investigators recommend having an empty bladder at the time of ejaculation, others recommend having a moderately full bladder since it is the time of contact between the sperm and the urine that will be detrimental to sperm survival. The volume of urine is most likely irrelevant and the critical parameter being the time of contact between the sperm and the urine.

Immediately following voiding, sperm may be diluted in a buffered media or immediately centrifuged, the supernatant removed, and the pellet subsequently diluted with a buffered medium such as human tubule fluid. In some patients it may not be possible to accurately regulate the pH and urine osmolality or in other patients despite this regulation the quality of the sperm retrieved remains suboptimal. These patients should be catheterized prior to ejaculation, all urine drained out, and 60–200 ml of a buffered medium (such as Ham's F-10) instilled into the bladder. These patients then masturbate and void the specimen into a container. This will often result in improved sperm motility. Sperm samples may then be treated by a standard sperm wash technique involving a centrifugation at 300 *g* for 10 minutes. The supernatants are removed, the pellets resuspended, washed again, and then resuspended to 0.5 ml. While cervical inseminations may be performed, we generally feel that intrauterine inseminations are preferable. It is important to have the wife evaluated to rule out female factors. If pregnancies are not achieved by natural cycle inseminations, superovulation should be considered. Finally, in some couples, *in vitro* fertilization is required.

In many samples retrieved from the bladder, numerous epithelial cells are found in the specimen. While standard sperm washing techniques will not remove these cells, Percoll gradient separation easily removes these contaminating cells resulting in specimens of high quality that may be used for assisted reproductive techniques.[24,25] Many different buffered media have been used for sperm retrieval and there is no evidence that any one is better than the other at this point in time. We currently use human tubule fluid with 0.5% bovine serum albumin containing a Hepes buffer to maintain a neutral pH. Each case of retrograde ejaculation is unique. By having a thorough understanding of the various medical, surgical, and assisted reproductive techniques available, the urologist will be able to successfully assist these couples in achieving parenthood.

REFERENCES

1. Raezer DM, Wein AJ, Jacobowitz D, et al: Autonomic enervation of canine urinary bladder cholinergic and adrenergic contributions and the interaction of sympathetic and parasympathetic nervous systems in bladder function. Urology 1973; 2:211.
2. Gosling JA, Dixon JS, Critchley HOD, et al: Comparative study of the urinary external sphincter and periurethral levator muscle. Br J Urol 1981; 53:35.
3. Peterson I, Stones I: An electromyographical study of the striated urethral sphincter, the striated anal sphincter, and the levator ani muscle during ejaculation. Electromyography 1970; 1:23.
4. Newman HF, Reiss H, Northup JD: Physical basis

of emission, ejaculation and orgasm in the male. Urology 1982; 19:341.

5. Horne HW, Paull DP, Munro D: Fertility studies in the human male with traumatic injuries of the spinal cord and cauda equina. N Engl J Med 1948; 239:959.
6. Ellenberg M, Weber H: Retrograde ejaculation in diabetic neuropathy. Ann Entern Med 1966; 65:1237.
7. Greene LF, Kelalis PP: Retrograde ejaculation of semen due to diabetic neuropathy. J Urol 1968; 98:693.
8. Kedia KR, Markland C, Fraley EE: Sexual function following high retroperitoneal lymphadenectomy. J Urol 1975; 114:237.
9. Donohue JP, Foster RS, Rowland RG, Bihrle R, Jones J, Geier G: Nerve-sparing retroperitoneal lymphadenectomy with preservation of ejaculation. J Urol 1990; 144:287.
10. Weinstein MH, Machleder HI: Sexual function after aorto-iliac surgery. Am Surg 1975; 181:787.
11. Griffith ER, Tomko MA, Timms RJ: Sexual function in spinal cord-injured patients: A review. Arch Phys Med Rehabil 1973; 54:539.
12. Ochsner MG, Burns E, Henry HH: Incidence of retrograde ejaculation following bladder neck revision as a child. J Urol 1970; 104:596.
13. Koraitim M, Al-Ghorab M: Normal ejaculation after Y-V urethral plasty. Br J Urol 1970; 42:464.
14. Virupannavar C, Tomera F: An unusual case of retrograde ejaculation in a brief review of management. Fertil Steril 1982; 37:275.
15. Vijayan P, Sundin T: Island patch urethroplasty: Effects on urinary flow and regulation. Br J Urol 1983; 55:69.
16. Hedlund H, Ek A: Ejaculation and sexual function after endoscopic bladder neck incision. Br J Urol 1985; 57:164.
17. Sandler B: Idiopathic retrograde ejaculation. Fertil Steril 1979; 32:474.
18. Thigarajah S, Vaughan ED, Kitchin JD: Retrograde ejaculation: Successful pregnancy following combined sympathomimetic medication and insemination. Fertil Steril 1978; 30:96.
19. Stockamp K, Schreiter F, Altwein JT: Alpha-adrenergic drugs in retrograde ejaculation. Fertil Steril 1984; 25:817.
20. Schram JD: Retrograde ejaculation: A new approach to therapy. Fertil Steril 1976; 27:1216.
21. Crich JP, Jequier AM: Infertility in men with retrograde ejaculation: The action of urine on sperm motility, and a simple method for achieving antegrade ejaculation. Fertil Steril 1978; 30:572.
22. Middleton RG, Urry RL: The Young–Dees operation for the correction of retrograde ejaculation. J Urol 1986; 136:1208.
23. Abrahams JI, Solish GI, Boorjian P, Waterhouse RK: The surgical correction of retrograde ejaculation. J Urol 1975; 114:888.
24. Braude PR, Ross LD, Bolton VN, Ockenden: Retrograde ejaculation: A systematic approach to non invasive recovery of spermatozoa from post ejaculatory urine for artificial insemination. Br J Obstet Gynecol 1987; 94:76.
25. Van Der Linden PJQ, Nan PM, Te Velde ER, Van Kooy RJ: Retrograde ejaculation successful treatment with artificial insemination. Obstet Gynecol 1992: 79:126.

ANNOTATED BIBLIOGRAPHY

Benson GS, McConnell J: Erection, emission and ejaculation: Physiologic mechanisms. In: Lipshultz LI, Howards SS, eds. Infertility in the male. St. Louis: Mosby Yearbook, 1991.

This chapter is an excellent review of the physiology and neuropharmacology of emission and ejaculation.

Braude PR, Ross LD, Bolton VN, Ockenden K: Retrograde ejaculation: A systematic approach to noninvasive recovery of spermatozoa from postejaculatory urine for artificial insemination. Br J Obstet Gynecol 1987; 94:76.

The factors affecting sperm viability in urine are reviewed. Mechanism of raising urine pH are described. The effect of osmolality on sperm function and mechanisms to adjust the osmolality are explained. The authors then discuss methods of semen processing appropriate for retrograde ejaculate specimens. Two cases are discussed. The first is that of a male with retrograde ejaculation secondary to resection of the bladder neck. The patient has the pH and osmolality of his urine adjusted and a postejaculate urine specimen is processed and used for intracervical insemination. This is followed by a pregnancy and delivery of a healthy child. A second pregnancy is produced through the use of buoyant density centrifugation. A second patient with retrograde ejaculation secondary to the treatment of posterior urethral valves is discussed. Semen processing of the postejaculate urine and subsequent interuterine insemination combined with hyperovulation is performed resulting in a successful pregnancy and delivery. This article gives a very common sense approach to working through actual patient situations.

Middleton RG, Urry RL: The Young–Dees operation for the correction of retrograde ejaculation. J Urol 1986; 136:1208.

Five patients with retrograde ejaculation from various causes underwent the Young–Dees operation. Three of these subsequently induced conceptions whereas there was no follow-up on two patients. Four of the patients had normal antegrade ejaculation and in one patient retrograde ejaculation persisted. The surgical technique is described. While the authors have had success with this surgery, with the availability of modern semen processing techniques and assisted reproductive technology, it would be unusual to need to resort to this procedure in this day and age.

26

The Use of Electroejaculation for Ejaculatory Abnormalities

Dana A. Ohl

Ejaculatory dysfunction is an uncommon cause of male infertility, accounting for approximately 2% of cases. There are several types of ejaculatory dysfunction, but the most serious, anejaculation, or total absence of emission, has historically been inadequately treated. Although electroejaculation attempts in humans have been carried out since the mid-1900s,[1] the first successful human pregnancy aided by electroejaculation and artificial insemination occurred in 1975.[2] That child unfortunately had a lethal congenital cardiac malformation. The first live birth did not occur until 1978.[3] It was not until 1986 that the first pregnancy in the United States was achieved at our center.[4] Since that time the interest, research, and success of electroejaculation as a form of assisted reproductive technology have improved significantly. In this chapter I will summarize the physiology and pathophysiology of ejaculation and present our methods for incorporating electroejaculation into the treatment of ejaculatory dysfunction.

Physiology of Ejaculation

Ejaculation is a complex series of events coordinating peripheral sensory nerves, the central nervous system including the cerebral cortex, the sympathetic nervous system, and some portions of somatic fibers. While erection is primarily a parasympathetic event, ejaculatory reflex is primarily under sympathetic control.

The neuroanatomy of ejaculation has several components. Sensory input from the penis follows the dorsal nerves in the penis into the spinal cord. The cerebral cortex interprets this sensory input and integrates erotic stimulation from visual, auditory, and other sources. The final pathway of the ejaculatory reflex is initiated from sympathetic fibers arising from spinal cord levels T10 to L2. These fibers travel through the sympathetic chain ganglia at these spinal levels and merge in the hypogastric plexus, which courses anterior to the aorta below the inferior mesenteric artery. The fibers then continue distally through the pelvis to the ejaculatory organs where they synapse to short

Management of Impotence and Infertility, edited by Douglas Whitehead and Harris Nagler,

adrenergic neurons on the surface of the ejaculatory organs. Dysfunction of any of these nervous system components may result in some type of ejaculatory dysfunction.

Usually a combination of erotic stimuli processed by the cerebral cortex and sensory stimulation of the penis carried by the dorsal nerves will be integrated to initiate the ejaculatory reflex. One or the other of these types of stimuli may alone initiate the ejaculatory reflex. For example, a nocturnal emission during a dream is initiated from the cerebral cortex only. Ejaculation in a complete spinal cord-injured male in response to urethral catheterization is an example of ejaculation due to penile sensory stimulation without cerebral input. Usually, however, it is a combination of these two inputs that leads to ejaculation.

Sexual stimulation prior to ejaculation causes transport of sperm from the storage site in the tail of the epididymis into the more distal genital ducts.[5] During ejaculation, a massive sympathetic discharge causes emission and bladder neck closure. Contraction of the prostate, seminal vesicles, and vas deferens causes expulsion of seminal fluid into the posterior urethra. At the same time emission is taking place, sympathetic fibers at the bladder neck cause firm closure of this area, preventing retrograde flow of semen into the bladder.

Shortly after emission, a series of rhythmic periurethral muscle contractions initiates the phase of projectile ejaculation. This may be a reflex response to distention of the posterior urethra by the seminal fluid. Contraction of these muscles, in combination with a tightly closed bladder neck, results in rhythmic, antegrade expulsion of semen from the urethral meatus.

During emission and projectile ejaculation the feeling of orgasm takes place. This is a combination of pleasurable physical and psychological sensations. Although erection and ejaculation generally both occur during the same activity, they are separate neurologic events and may occur independently. A man may certainly have an erection without ejaculating, and some men, especially those with organic erectile dysfunction, may experience orgasm and ejaculation without achieving an erection.

Classification and Etiology of Ejaculatory Dysfunction

There are several types of ejaculatory dysfunction. Each has its own particular etiology and treatment plan.

Premature ejaculation is a condition characterized by an inability to delay ejaculation a satisfactory length of time during sexual activity. What constitutes a satisfactory length of time will vary from person to person. This is nearly always a psychogenic problem and related to delayed sexual maturation with failure to achieve control of the ejaculatory reflex. In many cases, ejaculation takes place during foreplay or at intromission. This is primarily a *sexual* dysfunction problem and not a fertility issue as a semen specimen can quite readily be obtained from a man with premature ejaculation and used for artificial insemination. This condition is best treated by qualified sex therapists (see Chapter 15).

Primary anejaculation (idiopathic anejaculation, psychogenic anejaculation) is a condition where both orgasm and ejaculation are not achieved. Patients with primary anejaculation are neurologically normal but generally have never been able to ejaculate or experience orgasm while awake. They commonly have intermittent nocturnal emissions, and many experience orgasm when awakened by a nocturnal emission. Occasionally these men can have successful orgasm and ejaculation with masturbation but not during sexual intercourse.

Primary anejaculation is also generally deemed to be a psychogenic problem. There is a great deal of correlation with sexually repressive upbringing, extreme fear of sexually transmitted diseases, etc. This condition is best initially treated by a qualified sex therapist or psychiatrist, but results of psychological treatment of this condition are not as good as in premature ejaculation. Even with extensive therapy primary anejaculation may persist and remain a fertility issue. Electroejaculation is suitable in selected cases where psychotherapy/ sex therapy has failed.

Anatomic abnormalities may result in maldirection of the ejaculate, despite a normal ejaculatory reflex. Examples would include men who have had partial loss of the penis from injury, burn, or surgery and do not have sufficient length to deposit the semen into the vagina. Men with a hypospadiac meatus may also have this problem. The problem is usually very evident to both the patient and the physician, and some men even attempt home artificial insemination with their ejaculate prior to presentation. This problem can usually be easily treated by artificial insemination and electroejaculation is not appropriate.

Retrograde ejaculation results from inadequate bladder neck closure during the ejaculatory reflex. Many of the same conditions that cause total anejaculation (see below) also cause retrograde ejaculation. In retrograde ejaculation, enough normal neurologic function may be present to produce emission but not bladder neck closure. There are also anatomic causes of retrograde ejaculation, such as prior transurethral resection of the bladder neck sphincteric mechanism. Electroejaculation is not necessary in men with retrograde ejaculation as sperm may be retrieved from the bladder following climax and used for artificial insemination. Treatment of retrograde ejaculation is discussed in detail in Chapter 25.

Anejaculation, or total absence of emission, is the most difficult form of ejaculatory dysfunction to treat. This usually presents with total absence of seminal emission, either awake or during sleep. In some cases, emission occasionally occurs, but may be so unreliable that fertility is impossible. An example would be a complete spinal cord-injured man with occasional ejaculations during urethral catheterization. Orgasm may or may not occur, depending on the patient's diagnosis. Nearly always an organic reason can be found for this condition and the cause of the problem is nearly always neurologic. As mentioned above, many of the same conditions that cause retrograde ejaculation cause total absence of ejaculation. A discussion of several of the major causes of anejaculation follows.

Spinal cord injury is the most common cause of anejaculation. Although approximately 80% of spinal cord-injured males retain the ability to have erections, only about 10% of spinal cord-injured men retain the ability to ejaculate.[6] Thus, the vast majority of men who have a spinal cord injury are unable to reproduce without medical assistance. Ejaculation is most likely to be preserved if the injury is incomplete or if the injury is at a lower level. Since most spinal cord-injured patients are young males, in whom reproductive issues may be very important, the impact of absence of ejaculation is obvious.

Retroperitoneal surgery may cause anejaculation due to surgical damage of the sympathetic ejaculatory pathways. The most common setting group is absence of ejaculation following retroperitoneal lymphadenectomy for testis cancer. In the classic bilateral radical retroperitoneal lymphadenectomy, nearly 100% of men experience ejaculatory dysfunction. Unlike the common notion that retrograde ejaculation is the problem, the vast majority of patients with ejaculatory dysfunction after this surgery experience total absence of ejaculation.[7] Orgasm is usually preserved. In testis cancer, like spinal cord injury, fertility issues are paramount, since the patient population being treated is comprised of young males, as the peak incidence of testis cancer is seen from ages 20 to 40.

Newer nerve sparing techniques have reduced the incidence of anejaculation to approximately 5–10%, but it nevertheless still occurs. The goal of nerve-sparing operations is the sparing of at least one sympathetic chain and the hypogastric plexus below the inferior mesenteric artery.

Any retroperitoneal surgery may damage the sympathetic pathways. We have treated patients for anejaculation following an aortic graft placement, staging laparotomy for Hodgkin's Disease where periaortic lymph node biopsies are taken, and perirectal surgery.

Men with *myelodysplasia* experience many of the same problems that men status post spinal cord injury experience. Erection is present in up to 92% of cases, depending on the series. Nocturnal emission has been reported in up to 73%. Despite these numbers, only one pregnancy fathered by a man with myelodysplasia has been reported in the literature.[8]

Peripheral neuropathy is a common complication of diabetes mellitus and men who experience peripheral neuropathy commonly have autonomic nerves affected quite extensively. As a result of diabetic neuropathy, the more common sexual problem diabetic men experience is erectile dysfunction, but ejaculatory dysfunction also may take place. Since these patients generally go through an evolution of progressive neuropathy, they will usually progress from normal ejaculation to partial and/or retrograde ejaculation and ultimately total absence of emission. Severe peripheral neuropathy from alcoholism and other causes may also impair ejaculation, but is seen much less commonly than diabetic neuropathy.

Patients with extensive autonomic neuropathy exhibit effects on multiple organ systems. Diabetics with advanced neuropathy may suffer gastroparesis and delayed intestinal motility, leading to increased risk of aspiration during anesthetic inductions. They may also have cardiac neuropathy, which would predispose them to arrhythmias (see below). One must keep the total patient in mind when treating fertility problems to ensure safety.

Multiple sclerosis induces widely varying nervous system dysfunction due to individual variation in the location and extent of central nervous system involvement. Again erectile dysfunction is a more well-described complication of multiple sclerosis, but we have also seen several patients who are experiencing absence of emission either as an isolated problem or in conjunction with erectile dysfunction. Many MS patients that we treat have many characteristics similar to the spinal cord-injured population due to extensive spinal cord disease.

Senile anejaculation is a new concept we would like to introduce. We have seen several neurologically normal men above age 60 who wished to impregnate their substantially younger wives, but who are unable to climax during sexual activity. Some of these men will be primarily suffering from loss of erection and treatment of this will allow intravaginal ejaculation. In others, however, ejaculation remains difficult. We consider electroejaculation an acceptable treatment in selected patients.

Brain death is an increasingly common clinical situation in which electroejaculation for retrieval of sperm is requested. Technically speaking, this procedure is not difficult and can be done successfully. The more difficult issues are ethical. Some requests we have received are from the spouse of the deceased, but in other situations, the request has come from a fiancee or girlfriend. We have even been contacted by family members of a brain dead individual wishing that sperm be collected and frozen so that the family bloodlines can be carried on via a future (but currently unidentified) artificial insemination candidate. This is certainly an example where the technological capability is far ahead of the ethical considerations.

Preliminary Evaluation and Treatment of Ejaculatory Dysfunction

The basic evaluation and treatment of a man suspected of ejaculatory dysfunction are shown in Figure 26-1.

A thorough history must be taken of all men presenting for evaluation of infertility. This should include detailed questions regarding orgasm and ejaculation, such as frequency and reliability of achieving orgasm and ejaculation, if orgasm occurs without ejaculation, whether antegrade ejaculation has ever occurred, presence and frequency of nocturnal emissions, changes in the pattern of ejaculation, presence of normal projectile phase of ejaculation, and quality of the first urine following orgasm (which may suggest the possibility of retrograde ejaculation). Questions directed at uncovering any subtle signs of neuropathy and certainly a history of the previously mentioned conditions are essential.

Inquiries regarding ejaculation must be detailed and pointed to uncover previously unexpected problems. For example, a man may report normal "ejaculation" but on detailed questioning may be found to have continual secretion of mucoid fluid from his meatus during sexual stimulation (probably bulbourethral gland secretions) but no expulsion of fluid during climax. If the patient has not previously experienced a normal ejaculation, he may feel that this situation was entirely normal. Therefore, questions such as "Do you have normal ejaculation?" may not divulge accurate information.

On physical exam there are very few clues to the presence of ejaculatory dysfunction aside from the obvious spinal cord injury, etc. Occasionally one finds an anatomic problem such as hypospadias that may affect semen deposition into the vagina. The physical exam is, however, important in determining testicular volume and presence of normal cord structures. Even though the patient may have ejaculatory dysfunction, other conditions that impair fertility may be concurrently present.

Semen analysis may give several clues that would suggest ejaculatory dysfunction. The most reliable clue is a low volume ejaculate. This is usually 1 ml or less in men with absence of antegrade ejaculation but some patients may produce more, especially if the loss of antegrade ejaculation is partial. The specimen may be entirely azoospermic or may contain low numbers of spermatozoa. If the fluid is very mucoid in appearance and does not liquefy, it may represent only bulbourethral gland secretions.

If the specimen is completely azoospermic and of small volume, or if no fluid is obtained at all, the possibility of ejaculatory duct obstruc-

Figure 26-1 Initial evaluation and treatment of patients with ejaculatory dysfunction. EEJ, electroejaculation; AIH, artificial insemination with husband sperm; TRUS, transrectal ultrasound.

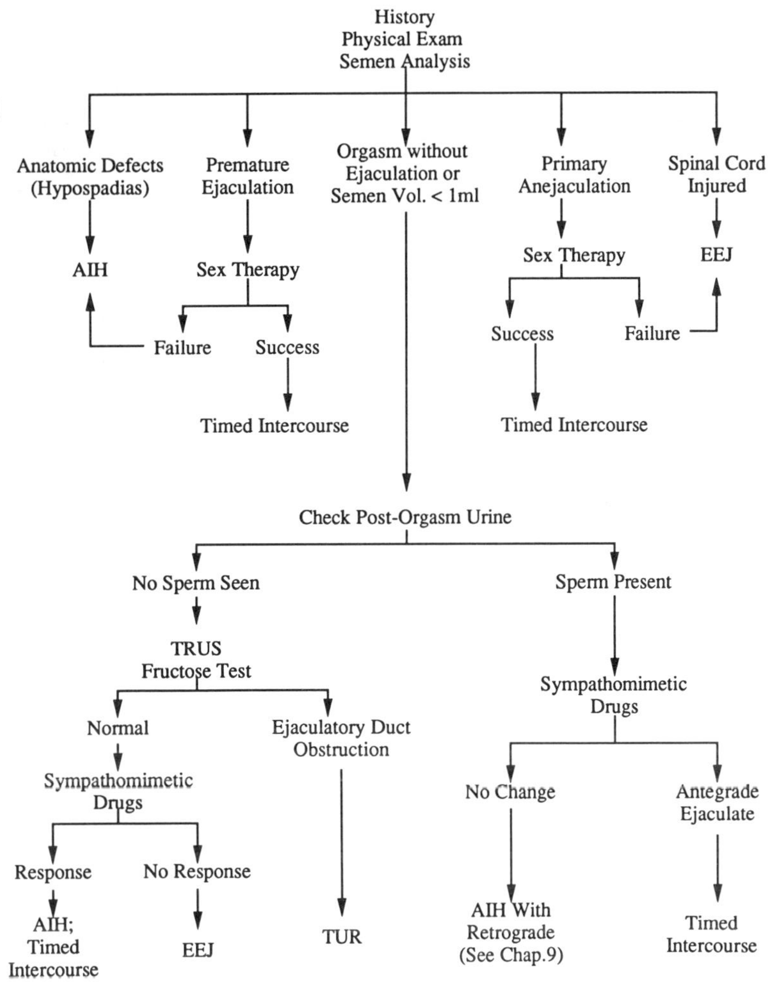

tion must be considered. This is especially true if there are no clinical factors to suggest ejaculatory dysfunction. The fructose test is generally negative in both ejaculatory duct obstruction and anejaculation and usually not helpful. Previously vasogram was the only method to accurately identify ejaculatory duct obstruction, but the success of transrectal ultrasound (TRUS) in diagnosing this condition noninvasively makes it the next best test in the evaluation.

The postejaculate urine examination is of utmost importance to document which men are suffering from retrograde ejaculation and not absence of emission. As mentioned above, identification of men with strict retrograde ejaculation can be helpful in guiding them on to assisted reproductive technology immediately and not subjecting them to electroejaculation procedures.

If all the above evaluation verifies absence of ejaculation, then treatment to induce seminal emission should be undertaken. Patients who are status post-retroperitoneal lymphadenectomy or who suffer from a partial neuropathic condition may be tried on sympathomimetic drugs in an attempt to bring about antegrade ejaculation. Drugs to try may include imipramine, phenylpropanolamine, ephedrine, and pseudoephedrine. Success from this type of treatment has varied greatly in reports in literature with some success rates in men following retroperitoneal lymphadenectomy reported as high as 50%.[9] Our experience in men at least several months out from retroperitoneal lymphadenectomy and continued absence of ejaculation is very poor. On the other hand, men in the early stages of a progressive neuropathic condition resulting in ejaculatory dysfunction, such as diabetic neuropathy, have a significant response rate. Men with a complete spinal cord injury and/or myelodysplasia uniformly do not respond to sympathomimeic drugs and it is not a worthwhile endeavor treating with this method.

These medications are generally well tolerated. Side effects consist of dry mouth, anxiety, insomnia, headaches, and hypertension. Blood pressure should be monitored frequently during treatment and the drugs discontinued if significant hypertension results.

Historical Perspective of Treatment of Anejaculation

Intrathecal injection of neostigmine was first used by Guttman in 1947 to induce ejaculation in a spinal cord-injured man. In 1971, Guttman and Walsh reported experience with this procedure in 134 patients.[10] The procedure was successful in 58% of cases in inducing ejaculations, but was not without hazard. Severe autonomic dysreflexia may occur with this technique and a death has been reported. With current options available to induce ejaculation, intrathecal neostigmine should not be used.

In an attempt to decrease the side effects of the intrathecal injection but maintaining efficacy, Chappelle et al.[11] attempted ejaculation in spinal cord men with subcutaneous physostigmine. In a study of 135 spinal cord injured men, physostigmine induced ejaculation in 75 and 15 in the group fathered children.[12]

Vibratory stimulation has been used quite successfully by several investigators to induce ejaculation in spinal cord-injured males with lesions above L2, but little success has been seen in men with lesions below L2 and patients with diagnoses other than spinal cord injury. The use of vibratory stimulation is discussed in detail in Chapter 27.

Electroejaculation has been reported for quite some time, as noted in the introduction of this chapter. The first large experience of electroejaculation of spinal cord injured men with the goal of achieving pregnancies was written by Brindley in 1984.[13] In that paper he reported experience in 154 patients with a 62% success rate in obtaining sperm and three pregnancies were achieved.

Direct aspiration of the vas deferens to retrieve sperm and implantation of alloplastic spermatoceles have been reported in the literature, but the reports are few and far between and reports of pregnancy extremely rare. With current treatments available (vibratory stimulation and electroejaculation), that are easily repeatable multiple times, these surgical options have no place in treating anejaculatory men.

Electroejaculation at the University of Michigan

Preparation for Electroejaculation

Prior to undergoing electroejaculation of our spinal cord patients, we feel it is quite important to optimize general health and particularly bladder management. Our preferred method of management of a spinal cord-injured man is suppression of reflex bladder activity and draining the bladder with intermittent self-catheterization. Results from electroejaculation would suggest that this is the optimal management for preservation of fertility also. Since many spinal cord-injured men are on multiple medications, it is important to review the medication list and stop drugs that would be detrimental. An example would be methenamine, occasionally given to suppress urinary tract infections, which would kill sperm in the bladder during electroejaculation. Since patients with myelodysplasia and multiple sclerosis have many problems similar to the spinal cord-injured patients, the same general guidelines apply. Nearly all other types of patients, i.e., retroperitoneal lymphadenectomy patients, diabetics, have a normal functioning bladder and no special attention is needed.

In preparation for electroejaculation, patients are instructed to take 1.5 g of sodium bicarbonate 12 hours prior and 2 hours prior to the electroejaculation. This is to neutralize urinary pH to which the retrograde sperm will be subjected. A fluid restriction is instituted to limit the urine output during the procedure. Men with a neurogenic bladder are instructed to begin antibiotics 5 days prior to the procedure. Antibiotics that attain high levels in the prostatic fluid are chosen such as norfloxacin, ciprofloxacin, and trimethoprim. All spinal cord-injured patients perform their usual bowel program and non-spinal cord-injured men take an enema the night before the procedure to clear the rectal vault.

Men with high spinal cord injury (i.e., above T4 level), may experience significant autonomic dysreflexia during noxious stimulation such as electroejaculation. Patients are questioned very carefully about whether this phenomenon has ever occurred in the past. If there is any history of autonomic dysreflexia, 20 mg sublingual nifedipine is given 15 minutes prior to the procedure.[14] By utilizing nifedipine, these procedures can be safely carried out in nearly all spinal cord patients without an anesthetic, in a clinic type of situation.

In men with anejaculation from diagnoses other than spinal cord injury, or in spinal cord-injured men with a great deal of sensory sparing, the procedure is too painful to be done without an anesthetic. We have performed these procedures under both spinal and general anesthesia successfully and have no convincing data at the present time to recommend one technique over another. The addition of an anesthetic raises the cost a great deal (anesthesiologist, recovery room personnel, medications, etc.) We have limited cost somewhat by performing these procedures in our recovery room area and not incurring the greater cost of an actual operating room.

We have had experience with one man with diabetic neuropathy who was undergoing general anesthesia for electroejaculation and who experienced a ventricular fibrillation cardiac arrest. After successful resuscitation, he underwent extensive cardiac evaluation. He was deemed to have autonomic neuropathy involving the heart with frequent ventricular arrhythmias. The general anesthesia and/or electrical stimulation was thought to have exacerbated the situation. Because of that experience, we now require an evaluation by a qualified cardiac electrophysiologist for all diabetic patients prior to undergoing electroejaculation.

Electroejaculation Technique (Figure 26-2)

At present we are using a Model 11 Electroejaculator (G & S Instrument Company, c/o

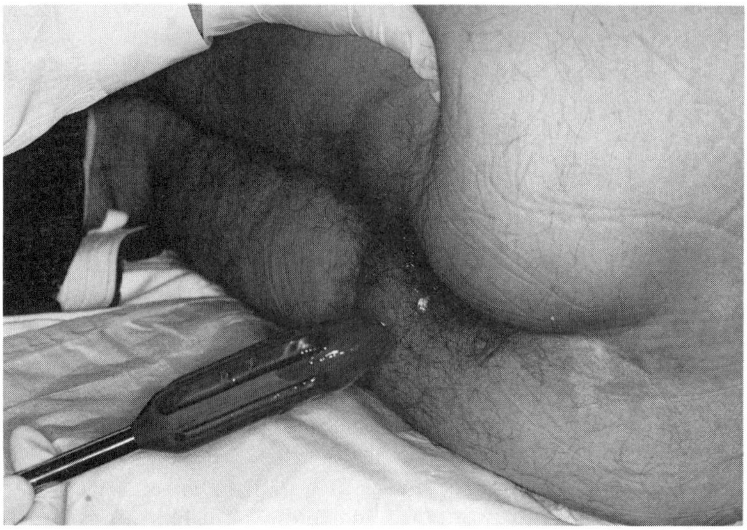

A

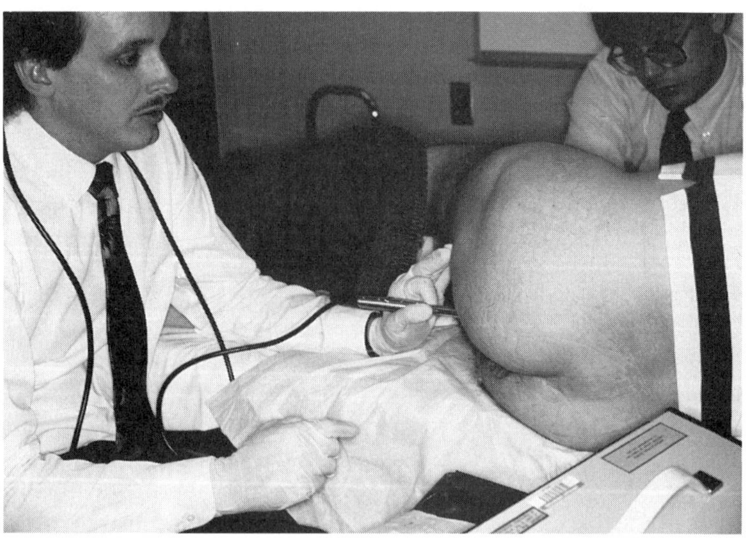

B

Figure 26-2 Electroejaculation technique. (A) Probe is lubricated and inserted into the rectum. (B) Probe held in place by operator during stimulation. (C) Assistant milks urethra throughout procedure and collects antegrade semen. (D) After stimulation, the retrograde ejaculate is retrieved from the bladder.

National Rehabilitation Hospital, Washington, D.C.) The equipment has an AC electrical generator that is controlled by a central rheostat dial. By turning the dial, the operator determines the voltage delivery. Electricity delivery is via cylindrical polyvinyl chloride probes with stainless-steel electrodes implanted into the surface. Currently the three electrodes are arranged longitudinally on the anterior surface. The probe is placed into the patient's

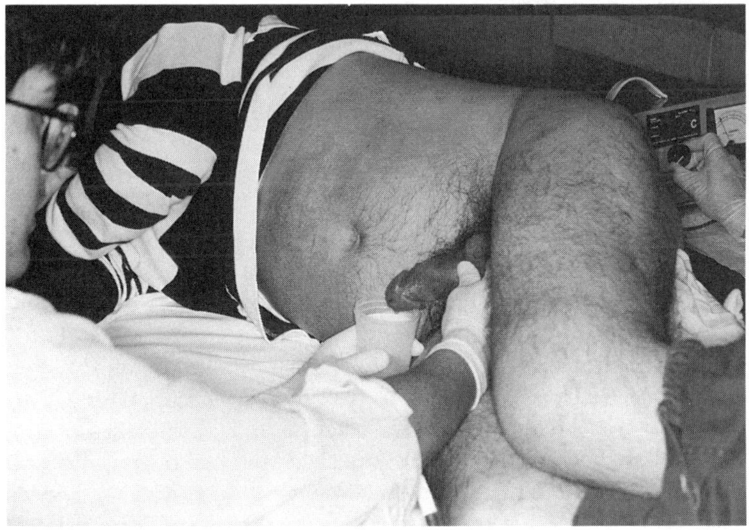

C

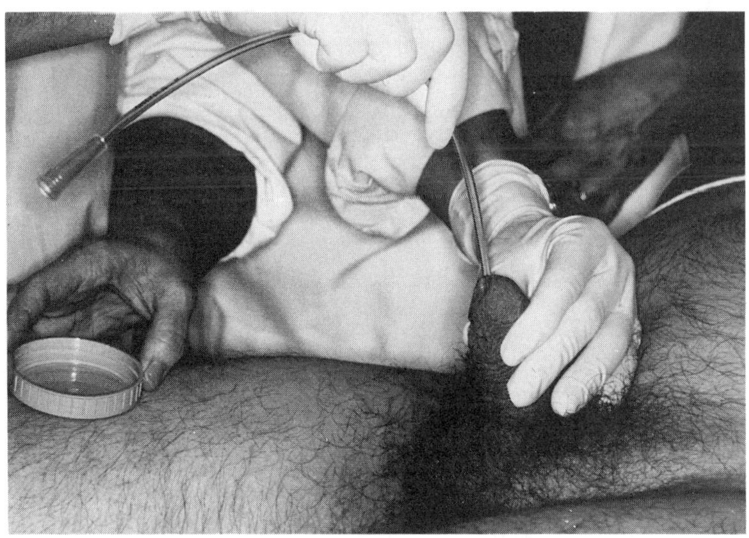

Figure 26-2 (continued)

D

rectum, bringing the electrical source in close proximity to the ejaculatory organs. The relationship between the voltage given by the operator and the patient's tissue resistance determines the actual electrical energy delivered. There is a digital temperature readout that constantly reports actual electrode temperature.

In the supine position the patient is catheterized and the bladder drained completely. The pH of the urine is measured, and if it is not between 7 and 8, 5 to 10 ml of a buffered Hams F-10 solution is instilled into the bladder. In the lateral decubitus position, a short sigmoidoscopy is carried out to approximately 12 to 15 cm to ensure that no preexisting rectal lesions are present. An appropriate size rectal probe (average 1-1/4 inch diameter) is inserted into the rectum with the electrodes facing anteriorly. Electricity is given in a progressively increasing wave-like pattern until ejaculation is deemed to be complete. The operator pays careful attention to the electrode temperature. This is of the utmost importance in avoiding thermal rectal injury.

During stimulation, an assistant milks the posterior bulbous urethra to push any ejaculate deposited into the urethra out through the meatus. Since this is not a normal ejaculatory reflex, projectile ejaculation does not occur. The milking is a necessary part of the procedure so that the operator knows precisely when emission has taken place and can tailor the procedure accordingly. This antegrade semen is collected in a sterile specimen cup.

Blood pressure is taken by a third person during stimulation and pressure is reported to the operator frequently. This is particularly important in men with autonomic dysreflexia. Despite nifedipine pretreatment, many quadriplegics still become significantly hypertensive during the procedure.

Following completion of ejaculation, the probe is removed and the sigmoidoscope is inserted again to ensure that no rectal injury has taken place. Presence or absence of blood should be noted. The rectum should be insufflated to look for any mucosal tears. The patient is then catheterized again to extract any retrograde ejaculate. The bladder is rinsed with insemination media to suspend any sperm present and sticking to the bladder wall. The post-procedure catheterization is quite important, as most patients will have a combination of antegrade and retrograde ejaculate produced.

After the procedure spinal cord patients are sent home immediately. In patients that have received nifedipine, resuming the upright position is carried out very slowly to watch for orthostatic hypotension and dizziness. In patients that have received an anesthetic a standard recovering room protocol is followed. All patients are given a short course of antibiotics following the procedure to prevent complication of cystitis or prostatitis from the electrical activity through the prostate and/or the catheterization procedures.

Risks involved with the electroejaculation procedure are minimal. Autonomic dysreflexia, as mentioned above, is a very common situation seen but very easily managed prophylactically with sublingual nifedipine. Extremity spasm and tightness in the stomach and chest in the spinal cord-injured patients occur but are usually easily tolerated.

Rectal injury is a potential complication any time foreign bodies are inserted into the rectum, and we have had one rectal injury at our center. This was with a previous model of our current equipment where the probes were much longer and had sharper ends. Since that rectal injury occurred, the probe design has been modified to become blunter and shorter, and no rectal injuries have been noted since that change in design, in approximately 1000 procedures.

There has been one documented case at

another center of thermal injury to the rectum from electroejaculation requiring colostomy when temperature monitoring was not carried out. This underscores the need for accurate temperature monitoring.

Insemination Protocol (Figure 26-3)

After an initial electroejaculation procedure has been carried out on the husband and sperm determined to be of suitable quality for artificial insemination, the spouse is evaluated by our gynecology team. An initial routine gynecologic evaluation consisting of a fertility history and pelvic exam is carried out. Basic basal body temperature charting and home ovulation predictor kits are used as evidence of ovulation and an adequate luteal phase. Because of the great deal of effort and cost involved with coordinating this type of a program, we have elected to have a hysterosalpingogram performed on all spouses beginning the insemination phase of the program. It has been very uncommon to find abnormalities on hysterosalpingogram, but if found, the problem can be treated prior to undergoing multiple cycles of insemination.

Depending on the adequacy of ovulation, the spouse is sometimes placed on clomiphene citrate to regulate ovulation. The exact time of

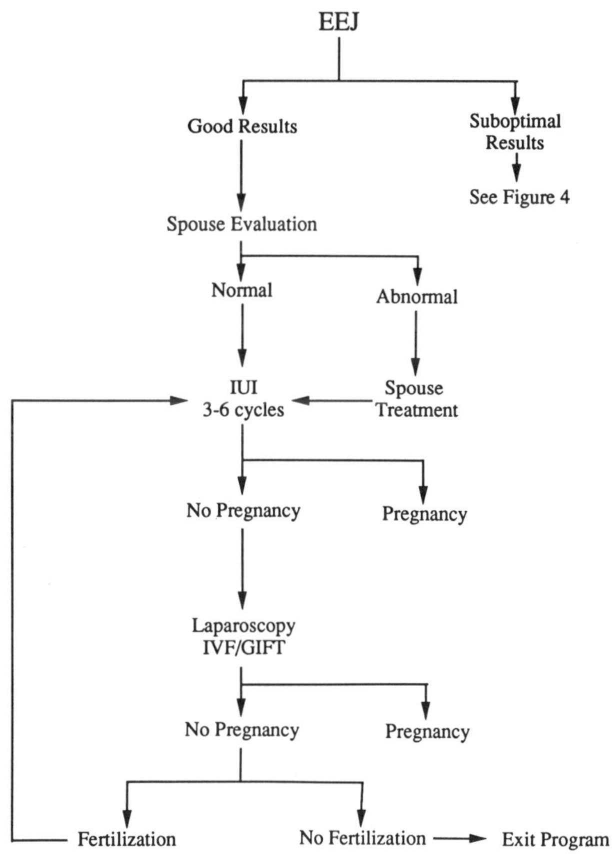

Figure 26-3 Current insemination protocol at the University of Michigan.

ovulation and, therefore, the proposed time of insemination is determined by a variety of methods such as urinary LH detection, transvaginal ultrasound of the follicles, progesterone levels, and exogenous HCG injection.

Sperm obtained from electroejaculation slated to be used for artificial insemination is processed in the laboratory by either the swim-up technique or Percoll gradient method. Since we are currently performing intrauterine insemination for these couples, it is essential to remove the seminal plasma as this cannot be injected directly into the uterus.

Intrauterine insemination (IUI) is the method used currently. Although it is controversial whether intrauterine insemination improves the chances of pregnancy in the face of male factor infertility, the only pregnancies in our program have resulted from intrauterine insemination or more technologically advanced procedures. Our early experience with vaginal and intracervical insemination resulted in no pregnancies and was abandoned after a short period of time.

Following three to six cycles of apparently well-timed intrauterine insemination that do not result in pregnancy, our couples are encouraged to proceed on to a cycle of *in vitro* fertilization and gamete intrafallopian transfer (IVF/GIFT). Our reasons for proceeding on to this level are three-fold. One, the spouse will be undergoing a laparoscopy, which is one further diagnostic technique that may give further information as to why a pregnancy has not occurred. Two, we can gain a great amount of prognostic information by observing excess eggs *in vitro* to see if the sperm–egg interaction is intact. And three, the success rate for one cycle of gamete intrafallopian transfer is substantially higher than one cycle of IUI. Certainly this level of care is substantially more expensive than IUI and for many patients the cost factor must be balanced with the advantages of proceeding on to this much more expensive procedure.

Results

It is extremely uncommon to not get an emission from all electroejaculation patients. The difficulty in electroejaculation is the quality of what is obtained in the seminal fluid. The usual result from electroejaculation is an ejaculate of quite significant volume and a very high count, but a very poor sperm quality.[15,16] It is not uncommon for sperm count to be in the billions, but motility to be in the 5–10% range. We also see very high numbers of abnormal forms.

The reason for this poor sperm quality is not entirely clear. We have performed extensive sperm function studies on specimens obtained from electroejaculation.[17] Several general conclusions have been drawn. The very low motility seen represents poor viability. There is an extremely high correlation between the sperm cell membrane integrity as measured by the eosin/nigrosin stain and sperm motility. In other words, the sperm that are not moving after an electroejaculation procedure are in fact dead. The bovine cervical mucus penetration test shows mildly defective sperm transport through the mucus by electroejaculated specimens as compared to donor sperm. We have also identified mild to moderately depressed penetrating capability of the sperm as measured by the hamster egg penetration assay. Antisperm antibodies testing was done in both the semen and the serum of electroejaculation patients and an extremely low incidence of positive tests verifies that sperm antibodies are not the cause of the poor quality semen.[18]

The above discussion gives several generalizations about sperm obtained from electroejaculation. Next I will discuss results particular to different patient groups.

Spinal Cord Injury

This is the largest group that we have treated with electroejaculation. Approximately 70% of men with anejaculation due to spinal cord injury have electroejaculation procedures that result in what we feel is adequate numbers and quality of sperm for some type of assisted reproductive technology. In general, nearly all of these men are suitable for IUI. There are very few that have total motile sperm counts in the one to two million range that we feel are probably more suited for higher technology procedures. There is very small gray zone in the middle—either patients are suitable for insemination or they are total failures either due to total lack of motility or azoospermia.

It is extremely uncommon to not get an ejaculate from these men. The problem with failure of the procedure is lack of enough motile sperm in the ejaculate. If suitable semen is obtained and patients are promoted on to the insemination phase of the program, we see a pregnancy rate of approximately 35% per couple from IUI alone. The average number of cycles to achieve a pregnancy is three.

In a paper looking at several prognostic parameters that may affect electroejaculation results in spinal cord men,[15] the best results were seen in thoracic paraplegics and in complete injuries versus incomplete injuries. These differences, however, were small. Time since injury up to 20 years was not found to a significant factor in success or failure for the procedure. At the present time we are not recommending the emergency banking of sperm in new spinal cord-injured men. Rather, we are recommending maintaining good general health with a healthy urinary tract as the best method for fertility preservation.

The most significant factor we have found to affect results of electroejaculation is the type of bladder management used. Men performing intermittent self-catheterization have a higher success rate from the procedure in obtaining useful sperm and a higher motility and total motile sperm count. Preliminary information may indicate that the pregnancy rate is significantly higher in these men also. Why men performing intermittent self-catheterization have an advantage is not clear, but this likely results from maintenance of a low pressure urinary tract where serious infections are not seen and the risk of reflux of urine into the ejaculatory ducts from high pressure voiding is minimized.

Retroperitoneal Lymphadenectomy

This group of patients is the second most numerous group we have treated. As they are neurologically normal other than absence of ejaculation, they require an anesthetic for performing electroejaculation. Again, emission is obtained in 100%. Our success rate in obtaining usable sperm from this group is 87%.[17] Of failures in this group, one man had carcinoma in his remaining testis and the other men were deemed to have testicular failure from previous chemotherapy treatment. Thus, if men with testicular failure are excluded from the data, one can expect a nearly 100% success rate in obtaining usable sperm by electroejaculation.

We had several other patients in this group who had previously been treated with cyclic chemotherapy. Two-thirds of postchemotherapy patients had successful procedures with reasonable numbers of motile sperm produced.

Two-thirds recovery of sperm production following cyclic chemotherapy for testis cancer is consistent with rates quoted in the literature.[19]

Despite somewhat higher sperm counts and somewhat better quality of the sperm in performing the procedure in men who are neurologically normal with a normal urinary tract, the pregnancy rate again is only about 30–35% per couple. The reason for this low pregnancy rate is unclear.

Other Diagnoses

The other diagnoses mentioned previously have been seen by us in too small numbers to give generalized comments. We have had successful retrieval of usable sperm from men with diabetes mellitus, multiple sclerosis, myelodysplasia, and refractory primary anejaculation. We have successfully achieved emission, but substandard specimens in patients with senile anejaculation and brain death. Pregnancy has been achieved in couples where the man suffered from multiple sclerosis,[20] primary anejaculation,[21] and myelodysplasia. We have treated three diabetic men and their spouses with electroejaculation/IUI but have not achieved a pregnancy to date.

Work-up of "Infertile" Electroejaculation Patients

Since there is a substantial failure rate for electroejaculation further evaluation and possible treatment are necessary on some patients. Figure 26-4 summarizes our algorithm for investigation of difficult subjects. As shown in Figure 26-4, work-up of these patients does not differ much from routine evaluation of male infertility problems. It is important to remember that in the general population, approximately 5–7% of males have some degree of subfertility, and, therefore, a substantial number of men in a large electroejaculation population will have additional problems that were preexisting. Also, the condition that causes the anejaculation may also impair normal sperm production and these possible problems need to be investigated.

In normal ejaculators, two or three sperm counts are obtained prior to invasive testing or therapy. In electroejaculation, the same principle needs to be followed. The only difference is that the "sperm count" in this case is done on specimens obtained from electroejaculation. Also, the length of time necessary for spermatogenesis must be remembered. Any event or therapy that affects sperm production will not be seen in the electroejaculation results for approximately 3 months.

Serum testosterone and gonadotropins are obtained in all our patients prior to electroejaculation. They are usually normal, but on occasion we have found abnormalities that can be treated with medication. Usually this is a low testosterone, and low dose clomiphene citrate is usually successful in restoring the testosterone to the normal level.

The level of follicle-stimulating hormone (FSH) is the most useful prognostic blood test in these patients. A level of more than three times the upper limit of normal is used to advise patients that they have an irreparable condition. Patients who have previously had a unilateral orchiectomy for cancer and are undergoing electroejaculation commonly have a mildly elevated serum FSH level in response to

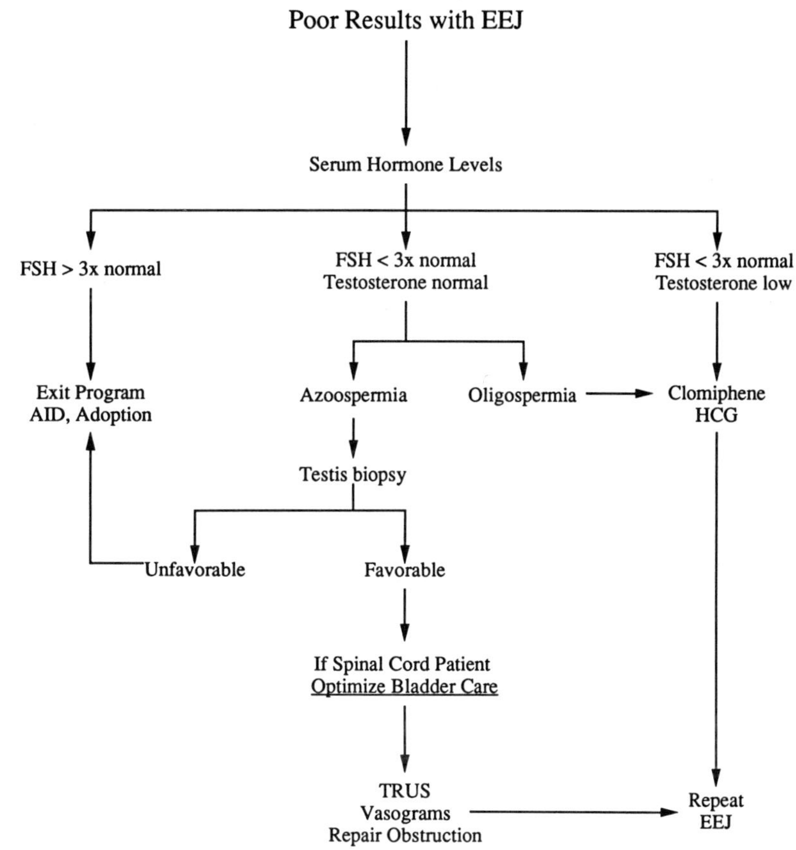

Figure 26-4 Further evaluation and treatment of difficult electroejaculation patients.

a decreased amount of testicular tissue. The FSH has always been below 2 times the upper limit of normal in patients with adequate specimens at electroejaculation.

In men who have two or three azoospermic electroejaculation procedures and normal serum hormone studies further invasive testing is indicated. Before assuming the man is truly azoospermic, however, one must be sure that the electroejaculation procedure resulted in actual emission. Usually careful visual examination of the urine pre- and postprocedure will reveal retrograde ejaculate. Fructose testing may be helpful in some cases.

Testis biopsy is performed to investigate FSH-normal azoospermia. Some urologists have recommended testis biopsy prior to beginning electroejaculation series, but we feel that with current success rates, biopsy of all patients is not a reasonable practice.

If an azoospermic subject has a favorable testis biopsy, we proceed to vasography and surgical repair of the obstruction. We have identified and successfully treated a small number of electroejaculation patients with epididymal obstruction and/or ejaculatory duct obstruction. One patient had epididymal obstruction from a previous hydrocele repair in his only remaining testis and the others were in spinal cord patients, probably the result of epididymitis/urethral irritation from the neurogenic bladder and/or bladder management (indwelling urethral catheter, high-pressure voiding, etc.) Prior to operating on a spinal cord patient for obstructive azoospermia, we feel *very* strongly that the bladder management needs to be critically examined and optimized, to avoid a postoperative recurrence of the same problem.

In men with low numbers and/or poor quality sperm from electroejaculation, but normal hormone levels, we have attempted empiric treatment with clomiphene citrate. As is seen in the general population, favorable results are very rare.

Electroejaculation and Advanced Reproductive Technology

Assisted reproductive techniques are discussed in Chapter 28. The place of higher technology and certainly more expensive reproductive techniques in conjunction with electroejaculation is not clear at the present time. The cost of more expensive procedures must balance the potential higher pregnancy rates with one cycle of these procedures.

Our experience with GIFT demonstrates that there is a significant higher pregnancy rate over that of intrauterine insemination cycles. Our initial 11 patients undergoing electroejaculation and GIFT achieved five pregnancies for a pregnancy rate of 45%. Two early spontaneous abortions occurred and three babies were delivered at term, giving a "take-home" baby rate of 27%. At our center, however, the cost for the patient and/or insurance company with one electroejaculation procedure coupled with the GIFT procedure is eight times that of the electroejaculation/IUI procedure. At present we feel that IVF and GIFT has a place in couples who undergo at least three cycles of intrauterine insemination and have not achieved pregnancy, as discussed above.

The place of newer techniques such as zygote intrafallopian transfer and micromanipulation in conjunction with electroejaculation is not clear at present. Work is currently being done in this area and we may have guidelines for use of this technology in the very near future.

Conclusion

Although ejaculatory dysfunction is an infrequent cause of male infertility, in certain groups, such as spinal cord-injured males, it is the most common cause of infertility. At present we have excellent technology to treat this problem. Electroejaculation will be successful in inducing emission in nearly 100% of patients. Nevertheless, many of these patients have inadequate quality specimens to be used for artificial insemination of the spouse. Even when seemingly adequate numbers of motile sperm are available, pregnancy rates remain low. Some of our laboratory work has defined some of the defects of electroejaculated sperm, as identified above, but much more work needs to be performed to improve these results. Hopefully, as more centers begin offering electroejaculation procedures, answers to many of these questions will be forthcoming. Perfecting techniques that may improve prospects for severe male factor infertility, such as micromanipulation, are exciting things to look forward to in the future.

The knowledge and experience in this area have increased greatly since our initial pregnancy in 1986. We look forward to the electroejaculation procedure being further improved and also becoming more widely available to anejaculatory males seeking treatment of their problem.

REFERENCES

1. Horne HW, Paull DP, Munro D: Fertility studies in the human male with traumatic injuries of the spinal cord and cauda equina. N Engl J Med 1948; 239:959–961.
2. Thomas RJ, McLeish G, McDonald IA: Electroejaculation of the paraplegic male followed by pregnancy. Med J Aust 1975; 2:798–799.
3. Francois N, Maury M, Jouannet D, David G, Vacant J: Electro-ejaculation of a complete paraplegic followed by pregnancy. Paraplegia 1978; 16:248–251.
4. Bennett CJ, Ayers JW, Randolph JJ, Seager SW, McCabe M, Moinipanah R, McGuire EJ: Electroejaculation of paraplegic males followed by pregnancies. Fertil Steril 1987; 48:1070–1072.
5. Prins G, Zaneveld L: Distribution of spermatozoa in the rabbit vas deferens. Biol Repro 1979; 21:181–185.
6. Comarr AE: Sexual function among patients with spinal cord injuries. Urol Int 1970; 25:375–378.
7. Kedia K, Markland C, Fraley E: Sexual function following high retroperitoneal lymphadenectomy. J Urol 1975; 114:237–239.
8. McGuire EJ, Denil J: Adult myelodysplasia. AUA update series 1991; 10:298–303.
9. Narayan P, Lange PH, Fraley EE: Ejaculation and fertility after extended retroperitoneal lymph node dissection for testicular cancer. J Urol 1982; 127:685–688.
10. Guttmann L, Walsh JJ: Prostigmine assessment test of fertility in spinal man. Paraplegia 1971; 9:39–51.
11. Chapelle PA, Blanquart F, Puech AJ, Held JP: Treatment of anejaculation in the total paraplegic by subcutaneous injection of physostigmine. Paraplegia 1983; 21:30–36.
12. Chapelle PA, Roby BA, Yakovleff A, Bussel B: Neurological correlations of ejaculation and testicular size in men with a complete spinal cord section. J Neurol Neurosurg Psychiatry 1988; 51:197-202.
13. Brindley GS: The fertility of men with spinal injuries. Paraplegia 1984; 22:337–348.
14. Steinberger RE, Ohl DA, Bennett CJ, McCabe M, Wang SC: Nifedipine pretreatment for autonomic dysreflexia during electroejaculation. Urology 1990; 36:228–231.
15. Ohl DA, Bennett CJ, McCabe M, Menge AC, McGuire EJ: Predictors of success in electroejaculation of spinal cord injured men. J Urol 1989; 142:1483–1486.
16. Ohl DA, Denil J, Bennett CJ, Randolph JF, Menge AC, McCabe M: Electroejaculation following retroperitoneal lymphadenectomy. J Urol 1991; 145:980–983.
17. Denil J, Ohl DA, Menge AC, McCabe M, Keller LM: Functional tests on sperm obtained from spinal cord-injured men by electroejaculation. J Am Paraplegia Soc 1991; 14:73–74.
18. Menge AC, Ohl DA, Denil J, Korte MK, Keller L, McCabe M: Absence of antisperm antibodies in anejaculatory men. J Androl 1990; 11:396–398.
19. Winfield H, Lange P: Modern concepts about fertility after treatment for nonseminomatous testicular cancer. AUA update series 1987; 6:1–7.
20. Ohl DA, Grainger R, Bennett CJ, Randolph JF, Seager SWJ, McCabe M: Successful use of electroejaculation in two multiple sclerosis patients including a report of a pregnancy utilizing intrauterine insemination. Neurourol Urodynam 1989; 8:195–198.

21. Stewart DE, Ohl DA: Idiopathic anejaculation treated by electroejaculation. Intl J Psychiat Med 1989; 19:263–268.

ANNOTATED BIBLIOGRAPHY

Bennett CJ, Seager SW, Vasher EA, McGuire EJ: Sexual dysfunction and electroejaculation in men with spinal cord injury: Review. J Urol 1988; 139:453.

This article is a review of erectile and ejaculatory dysfunction in spinal cord-injured men and of the methods used historically to treat the ejaculatory dysfunction. The authors conclude the discussion by giving the University of Michigan early experience in electroejaculation/artificial insemination.

Several series examining erectile and ejaculatory dysfunction of spinal cord-injured males ($n = 1909$) are reviewed. Erection was preserved in 1287 or 67% of patients (range 54–82%). Ejaculatory dysfunction was noted in only 203 or 10.6% (range 3–15%). Several reasons for poor sperm quality in spinal cord-injury are discussed such as hormonal changes, testicular damage, and abnormalities of testicular temperature regulation.

Following a discussion of various treatment options for anejaculation, the authors give the early experience at the University of Michigan electroejaculation program. Thirty-seven spinal cord-injured patients were treated. Fifty-nine percent of patients had an adequate ejaculate. Ejaculation was more likely with cervical and thoracic lesions as compared to lumber lesions and more common with complete lesions than incomplete lesions. Total sperm count averaged 182 million but counts to over one billion were seen. Motility averaged 22% and normal morphology averaged 21.5%.

Ten patients underwent artificial insemination with the spouses and four pregnancies were achieved. Interestingly, two of the four pregnancies achieved were in patients who had a negative sperm penetration assay, prompting questions of the accuracy of the assay in an electroejaculation population.

The authors conclude that their early experience suggests that electroejaculation is an excellent method for management of anejaculatory infertility following spinal cord injury.

Linsenmeyer TA, Perkash I: Infertility in men with spinal cord injury. Arch Phys Med Rehabil 1991; 72:747.

In this review Dr. Linsenmeyer and Perkash discuss the problem of infertility in men with spinal cord injury.

Five series of electroejaculation of spinal cord-injured men ($n = 190$) were reviewed. Only 25 patients (13%) had normal sperm concentration (>20 million/ml) and only one of 190 patients had a motility greater than 40%. Possible causes of poor semen quality after spinal cord injury were discussed in detail including stasis of prostatic fluid, testicular hyperthermia, urinary tract infections, type of bladder management, abnormal testicular histology, sperm contact with the urine, possible changes in the hypothalamic–pituitary–testicular axis, sperm antibodies, and use of various medications. Published studies both support and refute most of these purported mechanisms of poor sperm quality. The conclusion of the authors is that it is most likely that there is a combination of several factors that adversely impacts sperm quality following spinal cord injury.

In the review of ejaculatory dysfunction it is noted that of men with complete lesions, those with upper motor neuron lesions ejaculate only 5% of the time versus 18% with lower motor neuron lesions. In men with incomplete lesions, ejaculation is reported in 32% of upper motor neuron lesion patients compared to 70% of men with lower motor neuron lesions. Alternatives for sperm retrieval from spinal cord-injured men are discussed including intrathecal neostigmine, subcutaneous physostigmine, direct surgical aspiration, vibratory stimulation, and again electroejaculation.

The authors conclude by suggesting that an "SCI Reproductive Team" consisting of members from several disciplines would be the ideal way to best serve the infertility needs of spinal cord injured males.

Thomas AJ: Ejaculatory dysfunction. Fertil Steril 1983; 39:445.

This is an excellent review of the neuroanatomy and physiology of seminal emission and ejaculation.

Ejaculation is composed of two parts, seminal emission and projectile ejaculation. Seminal emission is under control of the sympathetic nervous system. Normal ejaculation requires intact lower thoracic/upper lumbar cord segments, sympathetic chains, hypogastric plexus, and pelvic autonomics coursing to the ejaculatory organs. Dysfunction of any of these levels can result in ejaculatory dysfunction.

Modern methods and results in treating ejaculatory dysfunction are not discussed in this chapter as they did not exist or were not widespread at that time. The value of this article is in its excellent review of the normal physiologic mechanisms of ejaculatory dysfunction.

27

The Use of Vibratory Stimulation for Ejaculatory Abnormalities

Robert D. Oates
Nabet G. Kasabian

Anejaculation, or the inability to ejaculate, is an uncommon cause of sexual dysfunc tion and infertility. Its etiology is most often secondary to organic pathology affecting the neuromuscular mechanisms controlling the ejaculatory sequence but psychopathology may rarely be found as the underlying cause as well. Men with spinal cord injuries (SCI) and cauda-equina syndrome comprise the vast majority of these patients. Young men with prior testicular cancer, treated with orchiectomy and subsequent retroperitoneal lymph node dissection, may be left anejaculate due to consequent damage to the paraaortic sympathetic fibers during the lymph node dissection and make up the second most common group evaluated clinically. Finally, multiple sclerosis, transverse myelitis, diabetes mellitus, current α-sympatholytic pharmacotherapy, and various idiopathic causes complete the rather diverse list of etiologies.

Anejaculation results from a pathological interruption at any neurological/muscular level of the ejaculatory process. Treatment regimens to induce ejaculation either utilize the existing or remaining neuroanatomy to their advantage or bypass it altogether. Examples of the former include *intrathecal* pharmacotherapy with α-sympathomimetic agents, e.g., neostigmine,[1] *subcutaneous* injection of α-sympathomimetic drugs, e.g., Physostigmine,[2] and penile vibratory stimulation (PVS).[3–5] All three of these techniques depend on an intact sympathetic outflow to the seminal vesicles and vasal ampullae. PVS is the paradigm around which this present discussion will revolve as it is the most straightforward and simplest of the three. However, it requires for its success a complete and intact neurological and anatomical apparatus below the level of the neurological deficit and is, therefore, most appropriate for the treatment of anejaculation secondary to spinal cord injury. Rectal probe electroejaculation (RPE) is an example of the latter, in which application of electrical current directly to the area of the seminal vesicles and terminal vasa results in their contraction, thereby bypassing, and independent of, the normal neuroanatomy that may still exist, in whole or in part.[6] Its indications, limitations, and the

Management of Impotence and Infertility, edited by Douglas Whitehead and Harris Nagler,

technique used are discussed in Chapter 26. In the treatment of the anejaculate spinal cord injured male, PVS and RPE are to be thought of as complementary and not competing procedures. When PVS is unsuccessful, RPE will often work quite well. Only a small percentage of patients will be refractory to both and, in this rare circumstance, direct microsurgical aspiration of vasal sperm may be contemplated.[7]

Neuroanatomy of the Ejaculatory Apparatus

Emission

Ejaculation consists of three distinct events (Figure 27-1). "Emission" describes the sympathetically-mediated (T10–L2) contraction of

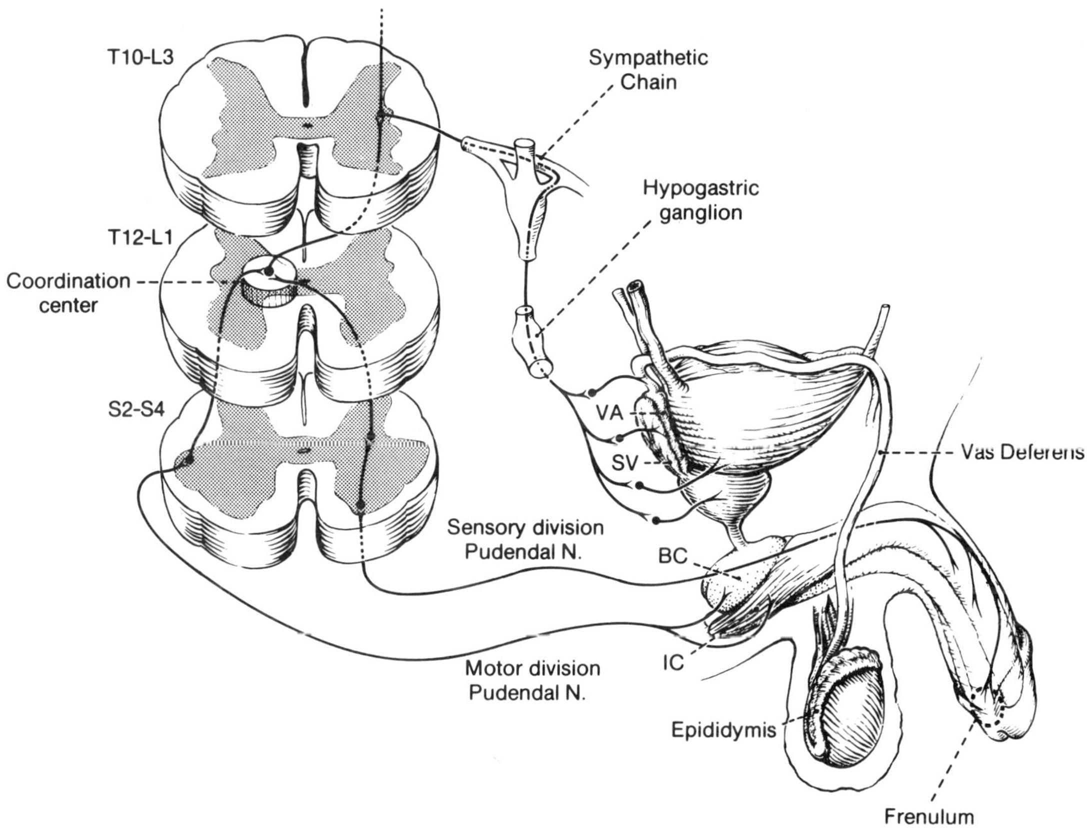

Figure 27-1 Neurophysiology of the ejaculatory spinal reflex. Genital skin sensory afferent fibers arrive at the sacral cord (S2–4) via the sensory division of the pudendal nerve. Second tier neurons travel up to the putative coordination center (T12–L1) and synapse here. Sympathetic neurons, activated in sequence by the coordination center, exit the lower thoracolumbar cord destined for the vasal ampullae (VA), seminal vesicles (SV), and bladder neck. Efferent motor fibers, also stimulated by the coordination center, leave the sacral cord within the motor division of the pudendal nerve to innervate the bulbocavernosus (BC) and ischiocavernosus (IC) muscle groups.

the seminal vesicles and vasal ampullae with resultant discharge of their contents into the posterior urethra. These sympathetic fibers arise from the lower thoracolumbar sympathetic outflow and initially travel in and around the abdominal aorta and aortic bifurcation. They soon coalesce in the hypogastric ganglion but do not synapse here as they ramify to their eventual destination in the adventitia of the seminal vesicles, vasal ampullae, ejaculatory ducts, and bladder neck. Synapsing then occurs with the second neural link, termed the "short adrenergics." These resultant neurons are responsible for the direct muscular innervation of the emission apparatus. The bladder neck, or internal sphincter mechanism, is also under sympathetic control. It closes and tightens like a constricting collar during emission to prevent retrograde flow of the seminal fluid from the posterior urethra backward into the bladder. Synchronization of these two events is usually intact in the SCI patient if no surgical disruption of the internal sphincter mechanism has taken place previously.

Antegrade Ejaculation

"Antegrade ejaculation" is the forceful propulsion of the seminal fluid entrapped in the posterior urethra in an antegrade or forward direction out the urethral meatus. This results from the rhythmic contraction of the periurethral bulbocavernosus and ischiocavernosus muscle groups, along with bladder neck closure and appropriately timed and coordinated relaxation of the external sphincter. The bulbocavernosus and ischiocavernosus are striated muscles and are innervated via the motor division of the pudendal nerve (S2–4). The external sphincter consists of an inner, autonomically innervated muscle layer and an outer, somatically innervated (S2–4) muscle group.

Integration of Emission and Antegrade Ejaculation

Tactile sensation from the glans and frenular area is transmitted to the sacral cord via the sensory division of the pudendal nerve. It appears that a neural "coordination center" exists in the region of T12–L1, which integrates tactile input, emission, and antegrade ejaculation. As ascending fibers from cord segments S2–4 deliver the message of appropriate tactile stimulation to the putative "coordination center," efferent sympathetic outflow is stimulated, resulting in the initial phases of seminal fluid deposition and emission. Coupled to this sympathetic discharge and in a rhythmic and pulsatile fashion, the "coordination center" precisely directs the activation of the descending, efferent somatic outflow through the sacral cord to the pudendal nerve, resulting in clonic contractions of the periurethral musculature and antegrade semen flow. An intact cord below and including this level is a necessary prerequisite for the success of vibration-induced ejaculation. Ejaculation can therefore be a reflex-mediated event, dependent on an intact sensory limb via the dorsal division of the pudendal nerve, unimpaired efferent motor limbs via the sympathetics and pudendal nerve and, most importantly, a complete, functioning "coordination center" in the lower thoracolumbar cord. Vibratory stimulation of ejaculation in the SCI patient takes full advantage of this reflex arc to obtain semen. The successful application of PVS requires a viable and active central and peripheral neuroaxis below the T10 level. If any part of the neural hierarchy up to the T10 level is dysfunctional, vibratory stimulation is not likely to be successful. However, since it is so simple and easy to perform, all patients deserve a trial stimulation attempt. Obviously PVS will not work in the patient left anejaculate following retroperitoneal node dissection since the sympathetics involved in emission have been surgically interrupted.

Penile Vibratory Stimulation

Technique

The patient may lie supine or be seated in a relaxed position in his chair. Patients with lesions above T6 may experience autonomic dysreflexia during ejaculation as the sympathetic system is activated during the emission phase. Usually this is not a problem since as soon as the stimulus (the vibrator) is removed, the hypertension will quickly abate. If needed, sitting the patient upright, amyl nitrate, α-sympatholytics, or calcium channel blockers may be supportive measures. All patients with lesions above T6, therefore, should have their blood pressure monitored during the first trial attempt. If dysreflexia is a persistent problem, then pretreatment with a calcium channel blocker would be appropriate. An α-blocker, as prestimulation prophylaxis, would not be recommended due to its sympatholytic effect. This may inhibit or alter the emission process, leading to total failure of the procedure or retrograde semen flow (if only bladder neck function is altered). If the patient has a significant amount of baseline lower extremity spasticity, his legs should be secured as PVS often elicits an increased level of all lower cord reflex activity.

Although Brindley[8] and others employed modified electrovibrators originally designed for industrial use, Oates et al.[5] showed that a commercially available vibrator/massager was equally successful. The patient's bladder should be emptied completely prior to stimulation. If retrograde semen flow is anticipated or has been present on prior attempts, 30 ml of a media appropriate for sperm collection is left indwelling in the bladder after urine drainage. The tip of the vibrator is placed on the undersurface of the glans penis in the frenular area. Compressing it lightly and moving it from side to side slowly, usually a "trigger" point can be found when a sudden enhancement of tumescence or an increase in abdominal or lower extremity spasticity is noted. By leaving the vibrator in this location, the "coordination center" is probably receiving adequate afferent tactile input. When a crucial level of activation is reached, the ejaculatory sequence is initiated and a concomitant final increase in corporeal tumescence and rigidity is often noted. Although the ejaculatory and erectile spinal reflexes are for the most part separate, there is probably some type of communication present to explain this erectile augmentation that occurs just prior to ejaculation. Semen propelled via the urethral meatus is collected in a sterile cup. If it is to be used for intrauterine insemination, it is placed in the incubator while liquifaction occurs prior to formal processing. If it is to be used for self-insemination at home, it may be immediately aspirated into an appropriate syringe and discharged intravaginally in and around the cervical os.

The vibrator can be removed as soon as enough volume has been collected. This usually occurs after just a few seconds of ejaculation. It is important to be more cautious when the patient experiences autonomic dysreflexia concomitant with ejaculation and to withdraw the vibratory stimulus as quickly as possible following semen recovery. If periurethral muscular contraction is apparent but no semen has been expelled, the bladder is catheterized and the fluid is microscopically surveyed for sperm to indicate whether retrograde flow of seminal fluid has occurred. After months or years of anejaculation, the first semen sample is often brownish and filled with cellular debris. This discoloration will resolve after frequent repeat ejaculations and the semen will regain its normal whitish tint. As recommended by Brindley,[8] stimulation to the penis is applied until ejaculation occurs or for 3–4 minutes. If ejaculation does not occur in this time span, a pause of 1.5 minutes follows and the cycle is then repeated. The trial is regarded as unsuccessful if no ejaculation occurs in four cycles. Most patients who show a consistent, positive response ejaculate within a short period of time, usually within the first 2 minutes of stimulation. If the first trial is unsuccessful, medications the patient is currently using should be reviewed carefully. Many will have central cord depressant effects while others may have peripheral antagonistic properties. Obviously, elimination of those that may affect the success of PVS needs to be weighed against the beneficial effects of those therapies in that individual patient.

Results of PVS in the SCI Male

Following the publication of work by Sobrero et al.[9] that focused on the technique of vibratory stimulation in men anorgasmic secondary to psychotropic medical therapy and also in normal volunteers, Schellen[10] described the use of an electrovibrator in a cohort of patients suffering from *psychogenic* ejaculatory dysfunction. Success occurred in a majority of both volunteers and patients in these two studies. Presumably, the neuroaxis was completely intact and the supranormal level of tactile stimulation to the penis was able to activate the ejaculatory reflex via the "coordination center." Comarr[11] first reported that one of his patients had used PVS to achieve ejaculation. Francois et al.[12] helped to then define the indications and refine the technique of PVS in the SCI patient.

In 1984, Brindley[8] reported the results of PVS in a group of 81 male SCI patients who had been injured for greater than 6 months. It was successful in providing semen in 48 of those patients. A number of clinical observations were made on both the technique itself and also on the prognostic factors that predict a successful result. He found that PVS fails if tried within 6 months of injury and is most likely due to the period of relative cord inactivity, "spinal shock," that occurs in the early postinjury period. The cord below the injury level must regain its uninhibited reflexive nature for PVS to activate the ejaculatory reflex. In this regard, he noted that patients in whom the hips did not flex on scratching the soles of the feet had a poor response to PVS. This would be anticipated since that maneuver tests the integrity and activity of the lower cord segments (L2–S1). Also explained by the knowledge of the neural pathways involved in the ejaculatory reflex is the fact that PVS in patients with lesions at or below T12 is almost invariably unsuccessful. Brindley's overall success rate was 59%, while in those with reflex hip flexion it was 77%. Oates et al.[5] reported that patients with cervical cord injury respond to PVS with ejaculation in 75% of cases, those with thoracic cord injuries above T12 in 62% of attempts and those below T12 did not respond at all. Beretta et al.[4] report an overall success rate of 70%. Since different vibratory units were employed in these three studies, it does not appear that the type of vibrator used is crucial, although more powerful stimulation may make the difference for an individual patient, as inferred by Brindley. Most patients will have normal antegrade flow during ejaculation but in those in whom bladder neck resection has been carried out, the flow of semen may be in a retrograde direction. Siösteen et al.[13] report that repeated PVS over the course of 4–6 months leads to improvement in the total motile sperm fraction ejaculated, implying that the patient should perform PVS on a scheduled basis to continually "drain" the ductal system and perhaps enhance the quality of sperm ejaculated.

PVS and Pregnancy Achievement

The successful application of PVS in an individual couple allows that couple to attempt conception at home, employing PVS to obtain semen and vaginal self-insemination to place it appropriately. Timing of ovulation is based on predictions using the prior onset of menses or, more accurately, at-home urinary kits that detect the luteinizing hormone surge that materializes approximately 24–36 hours prior to ovulation. If the sperm quality is poor, as reflected by a low sperm density or inadequate sperm motility, more vigorous combined therapies can be employed. These include intrauterine insemination and the advanced reproductive techniques,[14] e.g., *in vitro* fertilization. However, the semen is still collected by the couple without the need for assistance, as is requisite when electroejaculation is utilized for semen recovery. Exact pregnancy rates are difficult to calculate, as each patient may be quite different from another equally matched SCI male as regards his present testicular function and output. Spousal fertility potential is also crucial to a couple's chances and it is advisable to have a baseline fertility evaluation on all spouses performed early on.

Conclusion

Penile vibratory stimulation is a simple technique that may allow for the recovery of semen in a majority of patients with spinal cord injury. The success of the technique depends on the exact neurological situation existing in the individual patient, the higher cord lesions showing greater rates of positive results. The ejaculation is typically antegrade, completely mimicking the normal ejaculatory event. PVS activates a putative reflex "coordination center" in the lower thoracolumbar cord that precisely times and sequences the neurological outflow involved in the complex event of ejaculation. The ultimate goal is to discharge the couple from the medical environment by teaching them the steps to achieve pregnancy on their own. However, PVS may serve to simply attain semen that can then be used combined with any of a number of advanced reproductive strategies. When PVS is not able to generate a semen specimen, rectal probe electroejaculation may allow for recovery.

REFERENCES

1. Spira R: Artificial insemination after intrathecal injection of neostigmine in a paraplegic. Lancet 1956; 1:670–671.
2. Chapelle PA, Blanquart F, Peuch AJ, Held J-P: Treatment of anejaculation in the total paraplegic by subcutaneous injection of physostigmine. Paraplegia 1983; 21:30–36.
3. Brindley GS: Reflex ejaculation under vibratory stimulation in paraplegic men. Paraplegia 1981; 19:299–302.
4. Beretta G, Chelo E, Zanolla A: Reproductive aspects in spinal cord injured males. Paraplegia 1989; 27:113–118.

5. Oates RD, Staskin DR, Krane RJ: Penile vibratory stimulation in the spinal cord injured male to induce ejaculation. J Urol 1990; 143:344A.
6. Bennett CJ, Seager SW, Vasher EA, McGuire EJ: Sexual dysfunction and electroejaculation in men with spinal cord injury. A review. J Urol 1988; 139:453–457.
7. Bustillo M, Rajfer J: Pregnancy following insemination with sperm aspirated directly from the vas deferens. Fertil Steril 1986; 46:144–146.
8. Brindley GS: The fertility of men with spinal injuries. Paraplegia 1984; 22:337–348.
9. Sobrero AJ, Stearns HE, Blair HJ: Technic for the induction of ejaculation in humans. Fertil Steril 1965; 16:765–767.
10. Schellen TMCM: Induction of ejaculation by electrovibration. Fertil Steril 1968; 19:566–569.
11. Comarr AE: Sexual function among patients with spinal cord injury. Urol Int 1970; 25:134–168.
12. Francois N, Lichtenberger JM, Louannet P, Desert JF, Maury M: L'ejaculation par le vibromassage chez le paraplegique á propos de 50 cas avec 7 grossesses. Ann Med Phys 1980; 23:24.
13. Siösteen A, Forssman L, Steen Y, Sullivan L, Wickström I: Quality of semen after repeated ejaculation treatment in spinal cord injury men. Paraplegia 1990; 28:96–104.
14. Elliot S, Szasz G, Zouves C: The combined use of vibrostimulation and in-vitro fertilization: Successful pregnancy outcome from a retrograde specimen obtained from a spinal cord-injured male. J In Vitro Fertil Embryo Transf 1991; 8:348–352.

ANNOTATED BIBLIOGRAPHY

Brindley GS: The fertility of men with spinal injuries. Paraplegia 1984; 22:337–348.

Still one of the best early references documenting the successful application of penile vibratory stimulation in the spinal cord population. Many of the clinical "pearls" originally described by the author are included.

Comarr AE: Sexual function among patients with spinal cord injury. Urol Int 1970; 25:134–168.

This lengthy work details the spontaneous rates of erectile and ejaculatory ability in the spinal cord-injured male patient. The level and completeness of the lesion are taken into account and it can be readily appreciated that there is a striking degree of difference and individuality between patients. It is requisite reading for those interested in the care of the spinal cord-injured male.

Seftel AD, Oates RD, Krane RJ: Disturbed sexual function in patients with spinal cord injury. In: Woolsey RM, Young RR, eds. Neurologic clinics, Volume 9, Number 3. Philadelphia: W.B. Saunders, 1991.

Both erectile and ejaculatory disorders in the spinal cord-injured male are thoroughly reviewed. Outlined as well are the presently accepted modalities of treatment including penile vibratory stimulation.

28 Assisted Reproductive Technologies in the Treatment of Male Factor Infertility

Richard T. Scott
Daniel Navot

Abnormalities of the male reproductive system contribute to an inability to conceive in approximately 40–50% of couples presenting for initial infertility evaluation in the United States.[1] Recent advances in our understanding of the physiology of reproduction including the areas of gametogenesis, gamete transport, and the mechanisms of fertilization have provided greater insight into these disorders. This in turn has allowed a more systematic and comprehensive evaluation of male related ("male factor") infertility.[2]

Many couples with male factor infertility are able to conceive with traditional therapies. These include medical and surgical therapies for the husband, superovulation in the female with cervical and intrauterine inseminations following sperm washing, and various gradient separations and filtrations to enhance sperm viability. The combination of increased concentrations of sperm in the female genital tract and the optimization of insemination timing provided by monitoring the ovulatory cycle provides a small but real increase in fecundity.[3] Unfortunately, couples with male factor as a significant component of their infertility will commonly fail to conceive with conventional therapies and have to resort to assisted reproductive technologies (ART) for further evaluation and treatment.

All of the prevalent assisted reproductive technologies, including *in vitro* fertilization (IVF), gamete intrafallopian transfer (GIFT), and zygote intrafallopian transfer (ZIFT), have been described as being effective in the treatment of male factor infertility. Approximately 23% of the ART cycles performed in 1989 in the United States had male factor as the principal indication.[4] Although differing technically, these procedures have in common the theme of selecting the best sperm and placing them in high concentration in the immediate proximity of the oocytes. This allows the naturally occurring sperm/oocyte ratio of approximately 500/1 to increase to upward of 500,000/1 and substantially enhance the chances for fertilization.[5] For couples who fail to fertilize following IVF, recent advances in gamete micromanipula-

Management of Impotence and Infertility, edited by Douglas Whitehead and Harris Nagler,

tion have provided the means for a new group of procedures known collectively as assisted fertilization. In these procedures the zona pellucida may be breached or altered to allow sperm greater access to the oolemma, or sperm may be inserted into the perivitelline space or directly injected into the ooplasm.

With the emergence of these technologies, clinicians may be overwhelmed by the need to select the appropriate treatment modalities for each individual couple. Proper patient selection and referral are made more difficult because of inconsistencies in the definition of what constitutes severe "male factor." Furthermore, there is lack of consistency in reporting and divergent results are obtained with similar techniques in different ART programs. One must be particularly cautious in interpreting the term success. Although the ultimate goal is a healthy baby, some may consider the cycles with at least one oocyte fertilized as proof of fertilization and thus "success." Ultimately, judicious patient selection should be based upon conventional and computerized semen analysis, and tests assessing sperm fertilizing capacity. These should be considered in the context of the length of infertility and exhaustion of noninvasive clinical therapies.

Patient Selection

The majority of the information in the literature regarding minimum standards for semen analysis is derived from IVF experience. Indeed successful *in vitro* fertilization of human oocytes is the ultimate test for sperm function. The goal of the following is to set standards of conventional SA that are predictive of fertilizing capacity.

Proposed semen analysis criteria may be divided into two broad categories. The first group is *observational* and includes both the routine semen analysis parameters such as concentration, motility, and morphology and the more sophisticated measurements, usually determined through computerized digitizing systems such as velocity, linearity, curvilinear motion, and the amplitude of lateral head displacement.[6,7] The second class of tests could be categorized as *functional*, or *dynamic* and includes sperm penetration assays (SPA), hemizona assays (HZA), and possibly zona penetration testing.

Observational Tests

The initial sperm concentration in the raw ejaculate was one of the first parameters to be correlated with fertilization rates and clinical outcome. During the early clinical development of IVF, when the majority of patients had tubal disease, Mahadevan and Trounson reported that sperm concentration was unimportant for clinical success.[7] It is intuitive, however, that there must be a lower limit of sperm concentration below which inadequate numbers of sperm are available to obtain acceptable fertilization and pregnancy rates. Several authors recognized that fertilization rates declined when initial concentration were below 10–20 million/ml.[8–11] (Table 28-1).

Sperm motility was also evaluated and shown to prognosticate fertilization rates. The lower limits of motility that consistently resulted in acceptable fertilization rates ranged from 10 to 64%.[7,8,12,13] These criteria were refined by evaluating postprocessing motilities; however, the range of acceptable motility still varied from 30 to 86%. The wide range reflects in part the differences in how investigators defined acceptable fertilization rates (Table 28-1).

Table 28-1 Threshold Values of Various Sperm Parameters for Fertilization in IVF

Author and reference	Raw concentration	% Initial motility	% Swim-up motility	Swim-up (total motile fraction)	Normal morphology (%)
Mahadevan and Trounson[7]		20	30		40
Hirsch et al.[8]	10×10^6/ml		30		
Alper et al.[12]	104×10^6/ml	64	86	18×10^6/ml	
Acosta et al.[14]	10			1.5×10^6	4
Yovich and Stanger[15]				5×10^6/ml	

Although overall fertilization rates were poorer in male infertility than in tubal factor many individuals whose sperm concentrations were relatively low (10–20 million/ml) or who had less than 30% motility had excellent fertilization rates, thus limiting the predictive value of these parameters. Several investigators suggested combining concentration and motility and stated that the total number of motile sperm available for actual insemination (i.e., after processing) would have the best prognostic value.[12,14–16] The minimal accepted concentration of total motile spermatozoa for a succcssful fcrtilization varies from 1.5 to 18 million, with 5 million motile sperm as a useful threshold that carries a good chance of fertilization (Figure 28-1).

Sperm morphology is another parameter that has been shown to have great bearing on prognosis. Scvcral invcstigators havc rcportcd that fertilization rates decline significantly when the percentage of normal shaped sperm falls below 30–40%.[7,17] Although most programs continue to use the WHO criteria,[6] Kruger et al. have suggested that the use of "strict" criteria for morphology assessment may improve predictive values.[18,19] These criteria consist of narrow ranges for sperm head width and length, acrosome region, and the shape of the neck and tail. They have demonstrated significantly enhanced fertilization rates in 71 patients with >14% NL forms (88.3%) compared to 25 patients with <14% normal morphology (49.5% $p<0.001$). However, despite the better fertilization rates, pregnancy rates in

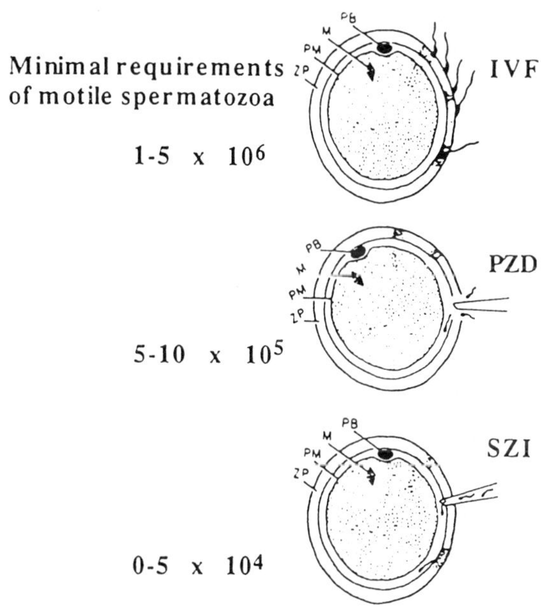

Figure 28-1 Theoretical thresholds of motile sperm counts in *in vitro* fertilization and gamete micromanipulation. Men with $<5 \times 10^6$ motile spermatozoa (Grade <3) are likely to resort to either IVF or related technologies (GIFT, ZIFT). Counts of $<1 \times 10^6$ will require either PZD or SZI depending on how compromised the total motile count is.

the poor morphology group (16%) did not differ significantly from the good morphology group (34.3%). This group has also determined that while fertilization rates may be improved by altering *in vitro* culture conditions, pregnancy rates remain poor suggesting an intrinsic deficiency in the reproductive potential of the morphologically abnormal sperm.[5] In Table 28-2 the group's definitions of poor (P pattern) morphology and good (G pattern) are depicted. It clearly illustrates the correlation between several morphology indices and fertilization rates. If further studies by other investigators confirm the reproducibility of the method and its predictive value for fertilization and pregnancy rates, then morphologic assessment using Kruger's strict criteria may become part of the routine evaluation prior to entering patients into an ART program. At the current time there is no consensus on the optimal way to assess sperm morphology. In fact, the methods used in different centers are so diverse that the Society of Assisted Reproductive Technologies eliminated morphologic criteria from their definition of male factor.

Table 28-2 Sperm Morphology as a Predictor of Human *in Vitro* Fertilization in 45 Patients with Sperm Concentration >20 Million, Motility >30%.[a]

	Low fertilization ($n = 13$) P pattern	High fertilization ($n = 32$) G pattern
Normal forms (%)	1.8 ± 2.4	7.7 ± 3.3*
Slightly amorphous (%) (head and neck)	18.0 ± 10.9	34.3 ± 6.7*
Morphology index (normal + slightly abnormal forms)	19.8 ± 11.7	42.0 ± 7.8*
Concentration (million/ml)	63.3 ± 42.8	83.3 ± 57.8
Motility (%)	45.6 ± 13.2	55.3 ± 18.6
Fertilization rate (%) (per oocyte)	7.6%	63.9%*
Number of embryos	0.4	2.6*

[a] Values are mean ±SD. Reproduced with permission from Oehninger and Hodgen.[2]
* $p < 0.0001$.

As sperm undergo capacitation, they develop a number of characteristics collectively termed as hyperactivation. These include increases in velocity, linearity, curvilinear velocity, and the amplitude of lateral head displacement. A number of techniques have been used to try and quantitatively assess these parameters and evaluate their relationship to fertilization rates. Recently, most of this research has been conducted with computer-assisted semen analysis (CASA) systems that digitalize and then analyze patterns of sperm motion. Several studies have criticized CASA systems for their inability to separate debris from immotile sperm. This may result in significant overestimation of concentration and underestimation of the percentage of motile sperm.[20,21] Nevertheless, they provide the most objective assessment of the motion patterns of the sperm that are actually moving.

Mack et al. compared the fertilization rates in patients who developed the typical characteristics of hyperactivation (increased velocity, etc.) versus those who did not.[22] They found that significantly higher fertilization and pregnancy rates occurred in the couples where hyperactivation occurred early during *in vitro* culture. Jeulin et al. found that the parameter that correlated best with fertilizing ability was the amplitude of lateral head displacement.[23] Lateral head displacement is the index that gauges the force of the flagellar motion of the tail of the sperm. Still other authors have found these parameters less helpful.[24] While these techniques appear to hold promise for the future, standardization of digitizing techniques, motion and shape parameters, and the methods of calculation of results will be required before CASA results can be used to direct treatment.

Dynamic Tests

Tests that actually assess the ability of sperm to perform one or more of the functions required for fertilization are collectively known as dynamic tests. Sperm penetration assays determine the ability of sperm to penetrate an oolemma and form pronuclei. Hemizona assays assesses the ability of sperm to tightly bind to the zona. Research into the area of *in vitro* zona penetration testing is ongoing but is unavailable for clinical use at this time.[25]

Sperm penetration assays were developed soon after Yanagimachi demonstrated that cross-species penetration was possible between human sperm and hamster oocytes after the zona pellucida had been removed.[26] Identification of penetration during a SPA confirms the ability of the sperm to undergo capacitation, the acrosome reaction, fuse with the oolemma, and be incorporated into the ooplasm. Thus a positive SPA demonstrates the capacity for the sperm to complete several of the steps necessary to achieve fertilization.

The initial clinical experience with the SPA was very favorable. Swanson et al. noted that all patients with a normal SPA (>20% oocytes penetrated in his laboratory) had fertilization at the time of IVF while none of the patients with a negative SPA achieved fertilization.[27] However, with improvements in human IVF the predictive values of the more contemporary studies are much less favorable. Auzmanas found that the predictive value of a normal SPA remained very good with 40 of 42 patients fertilizing, but that a negative result had no predictive value since all 11 patients with negative SPA's fertilized *in vitro*.[28] Margalioth et al. found a very good correlation between SPA results and subsequent human IVF in couples with unexplained infertility, while a lesser correlation was found in couples with male infertility.[29] The group from Baylor claims that penetration and head decondensation can be achieved in nearly 100% of patients irrespective of semen analysis.[13] As an alternative to SPA this group suggests a "sperm capacitation index" (SCI) that depicts the number of penetrations per ova. They found that a SCI of less than 5 defines the population of patients who will perform poorly in IVF. The role for SPA testing in evaluating patients for ART is still evolving. Better standardization of laboratory conditions and reporting will be necessary for widespread application of the technique. Until that time, clinicians must be familiar with the results of their own laboratories and the predictive values it provides within their own IVF program.

The HZA was originally described by Burkman et al. in 1988.[30] This elegant model uses the zona of a human oocyte that has been bisected to assess the binding potential of sperm from both a patient and a known fertile control. Although the potential for zona binding can vary significantly from oocyte to oocyte, using hemizonas from the same oocyte provides a natural internal control. Results are expressed as a Hemizona Index, which is defined as the percentage binding of the patient relative to the control. Early investigations with this technique have demonstrated good predictive values for fertilization when the index exceeds 35 and in some cases has had better predictive value than SPA.[31] However, specific limitations of the test and the predictive

Table 28-3 HZA Results According to Sperm Quality in Patients with Normal Semen[a] and in Male Factor Patients[b]

	Normal sperm parameters ($n = 17$)	Male factor patients ($n = 17$)
Concentration	126.0 ± 8.2	64.2 ± 17.5*
Percent motility	75.5 ± 2.5	42.9 ± 6.5**
Percent normal morphology	12.1 ± 1.2	3.1 ± 0.9**
HZA binding	72.2 ± 17.6	16.7 ± 5.0***
HZA index	124.5 ± 23.2	59.2 ± 13.0*

[a]Sperm concentration >20 million/ml, motility >50%, and >14% normal morphology.[5,6]
[b]Reproduced with permission from Oehninger et al.[31]
* $p < .05$.
** $p < .001$.
*** $p < .005$.

values in larger populations are still being defined.[32] The results of these long-term evaluations, along with an accessible and cost-effective source for human oocytes, will be required to fully evaluate the applicability of this new assay[32] (Table 28-3).

In summary, there is no testing regimen that can clearly delineate which patients will and will not fertilize in an Assisted Reproduction program. The series of test described above, when performed selectively, can provide valuable insight into the pathophysiology of a particular patient's infertility (Figure 28-2). This information may be helpful when counselling patients about their chances for conceiving through ART. At the current time, the only certain way to determine a given male's ability to fertilize oocytes is to perform IVF. *In vitro* fertilization remains the ultimate diagnostic test for male factor infertility.

Results with Assisted Reproductive Technologies

There are no prospective randomized studies evaluating the efficacy of ART in the treatment

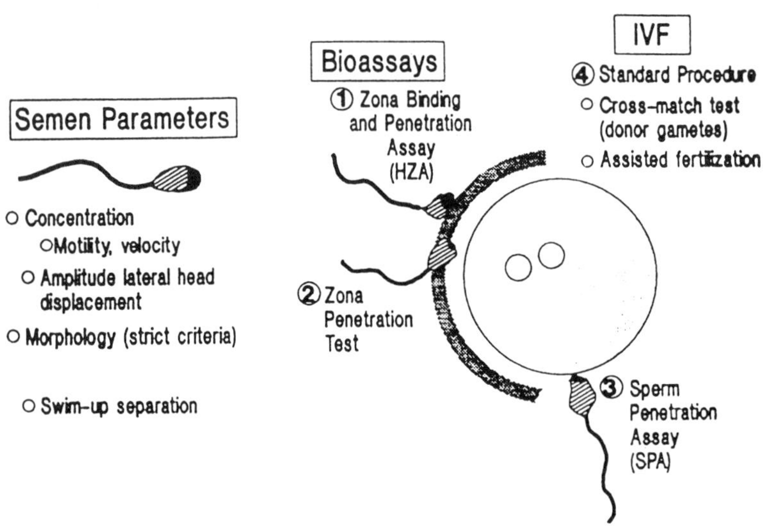

Figure 28-2 Treatment-oriented diagnostic workup of men who have failed *in vitro* fertilization. (From Oehninger and Hodgen,[2] with permission.)

of male factor infertility. Specifically, definitive studies comparing ART to the more conventional therapies or even comparing the different types of ART to each other are unavailable. Here again, the clinician is confronted with the need to make treatment decisions on the basis of inferential data.

Before selecting which of the ART procedures is best for an individual patient, the fundamental question of whether or not ART offers patients increased chances for conception must be addressed. Data regarding spontaneous pregnancy rates in couples with male factor infertility indicate that cumulative rates may reach 50%.[33] Even severely oligospermic males with sperm concentrations of <5 million achieved a 42% pregnancy rate with treatment of the female alone.[33] Even more impressive is the report by Collins et al. who reported a 35% treatment independent pregnancy rate compared to 41% who received therapy.[34] These data suggest that ART is not first line therapy for male factor infertility except in the most extreme cases. Clinically, most patients will be referred for ART after other less complex and expensive therapeutic options have been exhausted.

While direct comparisons of ART to other therapies are lacking, there are definitive data to quantitate their effectiveness in treating male factor infertility. Data from the SART registry are available for the calendar years 1988 and 1989 (Table 28-4 and 28-5). In 1988, 1785 stimulations and 1068 retrievals were performed in couples with male factor infertility. Of these, only 496 went to transfer. This indicates that an astounding 54% did not fertilize even a single oocyte. This is much greater than the 15% (320 of 2123) nontransfer rate found in tubal factor patients (Table 28-4). Furthermore, the delivery rate per retrieval (11%) was the lowest for any of the diagnostic groups.[35] There was little change in the clinical success rates between 1988 and 1989; however, the proportion of ART cases done for the indication of male factor increased by almost 50%[4] (Table 28-5). This change may reflect increased acceptance of ART as a treatment of male factor, but also altered definitions including prior failed fertilizations from couples previously thought to have fertile males.

Compared to IVF, clinical success rates of 24–31% have been reported with GIFT that are appreciably higher than the 10% described for IVF[4,35] (Table 28-6). These excellent results with GIFT may reflect the superiority of the *in*

Table 28-4 The National IVF Registry Results for Male Infertility Compared with Tubal Disease in 1988[a]

		Embryo transfers		Clinical pregnancies		Deliveries		
						Per retrieval		Per embryo transfer
	Retrievals	*N*	%	*N*	%	*N*	%	%
Tubal disease	2,123	1803	85	282	13	211	10	12
Male infertility	1,068	496	46	114	11	83	8	17

[a] Adapted with permission from the IVF Registry.[35]

Table 28-5 The National IVF Registry Results for Male Infertility Compared with Tubal Disease in 1989[a]

	Retrievals	Embryo transfers N	Embryo transfers %	Clinical pregnancies N	Clinical pregnancies %	Deliveries: Per retrieval N	Deliveries: Per retrieval %	Deliveries: Per embryo transfer %
Tubal disease	3,070	2,348	76	468	15	333	11	14
Male infertility	1,898	807	43	162	9	121	6	15

[a] Adapted with permission from the IVF-ET Registry.[4]

vivo environment, however, they are more likely to reflect a more conservative patient selection process rather than superiority of the treatment modality. Only couples with mild to moderate male infertility who have good chance of achieving fertilization are likely to have GIFT due to the diagnostic limitations. Namely, a pregnancy failure subsequent to GIFT does not allow differentiation between failure of fertilization and failure of implantation. This discrimination is crucial when making decisions regarding a couple's future therapeutic options. At the current time, GIFT for the treatment of male factor infertility is generally reserved for those couples with prior *in vivo* or *in vitro* proof of fertilization.

Another option is to combine IVF with a tubal transfer. This may be accomplished in at least two ways. First, the oocytes may be inseminated *in vitro* and then transferred to the tube after fertilization is confirmed. The technique of tubal preembryo transfers was originally

Table 28-6 The National IVF Registry Results of GIFT in Male Infertility Compared to Unexplained Infertility

	IVF Registry 1988[a]					IVF Registry 1989[b]				
	Number of cycles	Clinical pregnancies N	Clinical pregnancies %	Deliveries N	Deliveries %	Number of cycles	Clinical pregnancies N	Clinical pregnancies %	Deliveries N	Deliveries %
Unexplained infertility	180	43	24	43	24	378	126	33	99	26
Male infertility	188	46	24	38	20	578	180	31	146	25

[a] Adapted with permission from the IVF Registry.[35]
[b] Adapted with permission from the IVF-ET Registry.[4]

described in 1984 in subhuman primates.[36] Shortly thereafter, the successful tubal transfer of human zygotes with an ensuing pregnancy was reported.[37] This technique combines the advantages of the information to be gained through *in vitro* fertilization with the theoretical benefit of the ideal culture environment provided by the fallopian tube. This technique has become very popular for the treatment of male factor infertility. Excellent success rates following the transfer of preembryos at several stages including the pronuclear stage (PROST), zygote stage (ZIFT), or after embryo cleavage (TET) has been described.[38–40] Although these techniques require two procedures 24–48 hours apart, laparoscopy is performed only in those patients who have fertilized — avoiding unnecessary laparoscopies in cases of failed fertilization.

A final option may provide the patient with the benefits of a tubal transfer with the diagnostic benefits of IVF but without the need for two procedures. Patients with 8 or more oocytes can undergo GIFT with 4 oocytes at the time of retrieval, and have IVF performed on the remaining oocytes. If fertilization occurs, the embryos may be cryopreserved and transferred in a subsequent cycle. While this option has theoretical advantages, its use is restricted to those couples in whom the wife produces a large number of fertilizable oocytes.

A small number of patients are so severely oligospermic that enough sperm to meet even the minimal requirements for IVF or GIFT are unavailable. In these circumstances, technical modifications in IVF have been described that can significantly increase the concentration of sperm around the oocytes. These options include simply placing all the embryos in a single dish, performing the culture in microliter wells, culturing in 25–100 μl droplets under mineral oil, and even performing the culture in capillary tubes.[2,14,41] These techniques require very small volumes so that even a few thousand sperm can be used to attain very high local sperm concentrations around the oocytes. Although fertilizations are achieved, overall fertilization and clinical pregnancy rates are diminished in these individuals. In those individuals who either do not have enough sperm or who fail to fertilize using these microculture techniques, the final remaining option is assisted fertilization.

Assisted Fertilization

In contrast to conventional IVF that achieves its therapeutic effect by bringing the gametes together in increased concentrations, Assisted Fertilization physically alters the mechanisms of fertilization. These techniques may allow fertilization in those areas where conventional IVF has failed, or when the number of motile sperm are too low for even the microvolume culture techniques.

Physiological Impacts of Assisted Fertilization

The mechanism of fertilization in the human requires that sperm arrives at the oocyte investments with an intact acrosome. Upon contact with the ZP3 protein in the zona, the acrosome reaction is initiated and zona penetration ensues. After entering the perivitelline space, fusion between the sperm and oolemma occur. This is followed by the development of a block to polyspermy and reinitiation of the meiotic process. All of the techniques classified as Assisted Fertilization bypass one or more of these obligatory steps of fertilization.

The role of this highly ordered but complex and inefficient process in evolution is unclear. An important but unproven possibility is that gametogenesis is both imprecise and hazardous, resulting in a large number of genetically abnormal cells. The overall process of fertilization may provide the selection pressure that ensures that only normal gametes may successfully complete this process. Supportive of this concept is the fact that even the normal male ejaculate usually contains many abnormal spermatozoa.

Assisted Fertilization techniques are intrinsically more efficient than natural fertilization. The number of sperm required to sustain a high probability of fertilization decreases from the tens of millions seen in most normal fertile males to only a few. However, it must be recognized that in bypassing the normal selective pressures of natural fertilization, the likelihood of fertilization by genetically aberrant sperm may increase.

Given these concerns, the goal of Assisted Fertilization is to increase the efficiency of fertilization while still exerting, to a maximal extent, selection for the best sperm.

Finally, all forms of Assisted Fertilization have in common the physical interruption of the barrier provided by the zona pellucida. The precise role of this barrier beyond the block to polyspermy is unknown. Possible physiological roles for the zona include fostering normal blastomere association, protection from immunological attack and/or infection, and creation of a smooth surface that promotes normal tubal transport.

Development of Assisted Fertilization

The original research from which Assisted Fertilization techniques have evolved was performed by Gordon and Talansky.[42] They used the mouse model to evaluate the impact that making a small hole in the zona pellucida would have on sperm–zona interactions and fertilization rates. They used acid Tyrode's solution to "drill" a small hole in the zona. The rate of oocyte survival, fertilization, polyspermic fertilization, and development of live young were all measured against control eggs fertilized *in vitro* without drilling. Zona drilling was associated with a remarkable increase in fertilization efficiency with a 300% increase in fertilization rates at normal sperm:oocyte ratios of 1000:1. Furthermore, a decrease in the sperm:oocyte to 10:1 sustained fertilization rates equivalent to those of control eggs exposed to much higher insemination concentrations. Oocytes survived micromanipulation in >95% of cases and a normal rate of polyspermy was observed. A normal rate of live young was observed following transfer confirming that the embryos retained their ultimate reproductive potential.[42]

Although a high rate of fertilization at low sperm:oocyte ratios documented that zona drilling could compensate for oligospermia, it did not address the fact that in humans, oligospermia is frequently accompanied by asthenozoospermia and teratozoospermia. A subsequent study made use of a mutant line of mice in which the males were infertile and had grossly disordered sperm morphology. Despite the fact that the preponderance of the sperm were grossly abnormal, fertility following zona drilling was normal and offspring were produced at normal rates.[43] These highly successful animal studies inspired a number of human studies and led to the development of the area of Assisted Fertilization.

Assisted Fertilization Techniques

Assisted Fertilization techniques may be divided into two broad categories. The first involves physically altering the zona, making it easier for sperm to penetrate into the perivitelline space. These techniques still require that the sperm negotiate their way from the surrounding culture media. The second group involves bypassing the zona with direct injection of the sperm into either the perivitelline space or the ooplasm itself.

Zona Drilling and Dissection

The initial clinical trials with zona drilling followed soon after the animal trials.[44] This landmark study was restricted to patients who had previously had a 0% fertilization rate in conventional IVF. Although the fertilization rates increased to an impressive 32% of the oocytes inseminated, no clinical pregnancies ensued. Evaluation of the results of the study revealed several differences between mouse and human oocytes. Acid Tyrode's solution had a detrimental effect on oocyte quality as gauged by morphologic changes such as darkened ooplasm. Attempts at softening the zona with chymotrypsin and mechanical introduction of a microneedle followed. Here again fertilization was obtained, but the rate of polyspermy was very high and no clinical pregnancies resulted. It became apparent that the zona contributes more to the physiologic block to polyspermy in the human than in the mouse.[44,45] Although the chemical digestion of the zona pellucida had held great promise, it did not prove to be clinically effective.

Many of the initial clinical problems of altering the zona without effecting the oolemma have been resolved by using purely mechanical techniques. Partial zona dissection (PZD) is the least invasive of the techniques currently used in assisted fertilization. This technique used microinstruments to physically tear a slit in the zona, thus eliminating the potential risks of chemical treatment of the oocyte.[46]

Partial zona dissection is performed by taking a mature oocyte and removing the cumulus by incubation with hyaluronidase. The oocyte is then placed in culture media containing hypertonic sucrose, which causes the ooplasm to contract and the size of the perivitelline space to increase. This provides a larger window into which a microneedle is used to pierce the zona, travel through the perivitelline space and then exit through the zona again (Figure 28-3). Once the microneedle is placed, the holding pipet releases the oocyte and is used to rub the zona over the microneedle until the abrasive force tear the microneedle through the zona. This leaves a small slit-like opening in the zona. The dissected oocyte is then incubated with the sperm using traditional IVF incubation techniques.

Partial zona dissection has the clinical advantage of being less invasive with a lower chance for direct trauma to the oocyte.[1,6,46] However, two problems remain. First, a high incidence of polyspermy (25–35% of fertilizations) persists. Second, although the number of motile sperm required are lower than with conventional IVF, a significant number of motile sperm are still required. The largest clinical experience to date is from Cohen et al. where fertilization occurred in 79% of 47 cycles.[48] Clinical pregnancies occurred in 10 of the 47

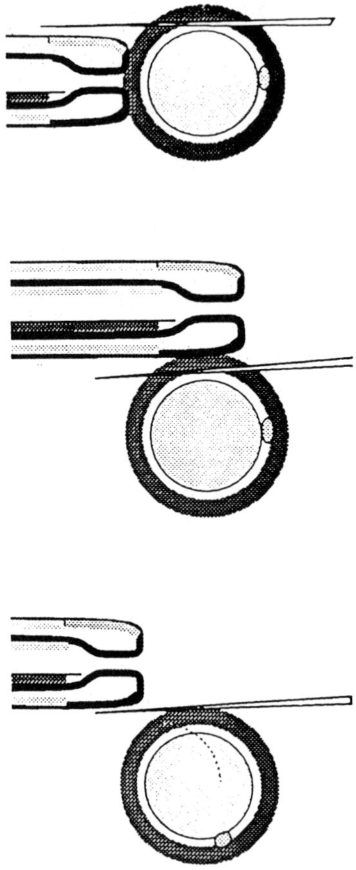

Figure 28-3 Schematic sequence of PZD: (A) the zona pellucida is pierced by the microneedle while traversing the periviteline space. The holding pipet is rubbed against the microneedle until a slit is created in the zona (B) and the oocyte detaches (C). (From Talansky,[47] with permission.)

cycles (Table 28-7). While these results are encouraging, the patient population was not limited to couples with prior IVF failures. Although fertilizations have also been reported from other centers,[49] broad applicability of this technique will await trials from multiple centers that are limited to patients with an inability to achieve fertilization with conventional IVF.

Subzonal Insertion

Subzonal insertion (SZI) is the injection of capacitated sperm directly into the perivitelline space. This technique bypasses the barriers of the cumulus and zona and requires significantly fewer sperm than PZD. The first successful fertilization of human oocytes was reported in 1987.[50] The first human pregnancy following SZI was reported soon thereafter in 1988.[51] A twin pregnancy was reported approximately one year later.[51] Since these original reports, the procedure has been performed in a number of centers and a handful of pregnancies have been reported.[52–56]

The technique of subzonal insertion has been described as being of intermediate invasiveness to oocytes.[57] Nevertheless, it is performed very similarly to PZD and induces no permanent tear into the perivitelline space. The oocyte is placed into culture media containing hypertonic sucrose, which shrinks the ooplasm and increases the size of the perivitelline space. The oocyte is then grasped with a holding pipette. Next a few sperm are aspirated into a microneedle. The zona pellucida is then pierced by the microneedle and 1 to 50 sperm are expelled into the perivitelline space. The microinjection needle is then removed and the oocyte is placed back into the culture media and returned to routine culture conditions.

Clinical fertilization and pregnancy rates following subzonal insertion remain relatively low (Table 28-8).[56–59] The high rate of polyspermy (as high as 35% of fertilized oocytes) also suggests the need for improved studies that can provide guidelines as to how many sperm should be replaced for any given patient. The

Table 28-7 Results of PZD (1988–1989) on Fertilization in the First 40 Patients (47 Cycles)[a]

	Incidence of fertilization					
	Intact control	%	PZD oocyte	%	Polyspermy (%)	Incidence of pregnancy
Oligospermic	11/24	46	19/25	76	0	3/9 (8%)
Asthenospermic	13/31	31	19/30	63	21	4/14 (28.5%)
Combined OAT	18/74	24	37/83	46	42	3/24 (12.5%)
Total	42/129	33	75/138	54	26	10/47 (21%)

[a] Adapted with permission from Cohen et al.[48]

Table 28-8 Worldwide Clinical Experience with Subzonal Sperm Insertion (SZI)

Author and reference	Cycles	Monospermic fertilization (%)	Clinical pregnancies		Deliveries	
			N	%	*N*	%
Cohen et al.[56]	47	28.0	10	21.0	8	17
Fishel et al.[58]	130	12.8	6	4.6	4	3.0
Ng et al.[59]	131	16.6	5	3.8	1	0.8
Krzyminska et al.[60]	60	21.6	14	23.3	—	—
Garrisi et al.[61]	37	23.0	6	16.2	6	16.2
Fishel et al.[66]	225	16.0	12	5.0	—	—

fact that several pregnancies have been attained in patients who would not generally be considered to be IVF candidates does establish this as a useful technique in at least some settings.

Several problems remain that limit the widespread application of SZI: Foremost is the intrinsic difficulty in selecting a genetically normal acrosome reacted sperm for insertion. Additionally, questions regarding how many sperm should be inserted for any given patient to maximize their chances for fertilization while still minimizing the risk for polyspermy must also be answered. Finally, specific patient selection criteria need to be developed to determine which patients require SZI to achieve fertilization to prevent overutilization of the technique in couples who may succeed with less invasive technologies.

Direct Ooplasmic Injection

Direct ooplasmic injection involves the injection of a single capacitated acrosome reacted sperm into the ooplasm itself. In doing so, all the physical barriers for fertilization are bypassed. The obvious clinical advantage is that only a single sperm is required. This must be weighed against the severe disadvantage that the natural mechanisms of sperm selection have been eliminated. Additionally, this may be the most invasive of the assisted fertilization techniques and operative damage to the oocyte is not uncommon.[57,62]

The technique is very similar to that used for SZI. Once the oocyte has been grasped, the microneedle is inserted through the zona and oolemma, directly into the ooplasm. A small amount of ooplasm is aspirated into the needle followed by injection back into the oocyte along with a single sperm. The microneedle is then removed. At the current time no clinical pregnancies have been reported following direct ooplasmic injection.

Summary

The role of Assisted Fertilization in the treatment of male factor infertility is evolving. Detailed, methodical, prospective, well-controlled studies will be required to determine the role of each of these techniques. Additionally, several basic questions remain to be answered. Perhaps foremost is determining the reproductive potential of abnormal sperm. If sperm that are incapable of achieving fertilization with conventional IVF are also deficient in their ability to sustain embryonic growth and development following fertilization, then the role for Assisted Fertilization will be limited. Some initial evaluations of this question have stated that once fertilization is achieved reproductive potential of the embryos is similar to embryos generated by couples with strict tubal factor infertility.[63–65] Others state that alterations in insemination conditions will allow many couples to fertilize who initially failed to fertilize with conventional IVF but that implantation rates and ongoing pregnancy rates are dramatically lower.[5]

Further evaluation and characterization of the patient populations that may benefit from these techniques are also required. Limited comparisons of clinical outcome from these techniques have been published, however, greater numbers with more stringent experimental designs will undoubtedly provide clearer guidelines in the future.

REFERENCES

1. Speroff L, Glass RH, Kase NG, eds. Male infertility. In Clinical reproductive endocrinology and infertility, 4th ed. Baltimore: Williams & Wilkins, 1989: 607.
2. Oehninger S, Hodgen GD: How to evaluate human spermatozoa for assisted reproduction. Assist Reprod Rev 1991; 1:15.
3. Patton PE, Burry KA, Thurmond A, Novy MJ, Wolf DP: Intrauterine insemination outperforms intracervical insemination in a randomized, controlled study with frozen, donor semen. Fertil Steril 1992; 57:559.
4. In vitro fertilization-embryo transfer (IVF-ET) in the United States: 1989 results from the IVF-ET registry. Fertil Steril 1991; 55:14.
5. Oehninger S, Acosta AA, Morshedi M, Veeck L, Swanson RJ, Simmons KF, Rosenwaks Z: Corrective measures and frequency outcome in IVF in patients with severe sperm morphology abnormalities. Fertil Steril 1988; 50:283.
6. World Health Organization: Laboratory manual for the examination of human semen and semen-cervical mucus interaction. Cambridge, England: Cambridge University Press, 1987.
7. Mahadevan MM, Trounson AO: The influence of seminal characteristics on the success rates of human in vitro fertilization. Fertil Steril 1984; 42:400.

8. Hirsch I, Gibbons WE, Lipshultz LI: In vitro fertilization in couples with male factor infertility. Fertil Steril 1986; 45:659.
9. Edwards RG, Fishel SB, Cohen J: Factors influencing the success of in vitro fertilization for alleviating human infertility. J IVF ET 1984; 1:3.
10. Turner SR, Yovich JM, Tuvik AI: Oligospermic infertility treated by in vitro fertilization. Aust NZ J Obstet Gynaecol 1987; 26:84.
11. Mettlar L, Bankloh V, Riedel HH: Immunological and other problems with human spermatozoa. In Edwards JG, Purdy JM, eds. Human conception in vitro. Orlando, FL: Academic Press, 1982: 181.
12. Alper MM, Lee GS, Seibel MM: The relationship of semen parameters to fertilization in patients participating in a program of in vitro fertilization. J IVF ET 1985; 2:217.
13. Meachem RB, Lipshultz LI: The impact of in vitro fertilization on male infertility. Semin Reprod Endocrinol 1990; 8:281.
14. Acosta AA, Oehninger S, Morshedi M, Swanson RJ, Scott RT, Iriani F: Assisted reproduction in the diagnosis and treatment of the male factor. Obstet Gynecol Surv 1988; 44:1.
15. Yovich JL, Stanger JD: The limitation of in vitro fertilization from males with severe oligospermia and abnormalities in sperm morphology. J IVF ET 1984; 1:172.
16. Acosta AA, Kruger T, Swanson RJ, Simmons KF, Oehninger S, Veeck LL, Hague D, Pleban P, Morshedi M, Ackerman S: The role of in vitro fertilization in male infertility. Ann NY Acad Sci 1988; 541:297.
17. Liu DY, Baker HWG: The proportion of human sperm with poor morphology but normal intact acrosomes detected with pisum sativum agglutinin correlates with fertilization in vitro. Fertil Steril 1988; 50:288.
18. Kruger TF, Menkveld R, Stander FSH, Lombard CJ, Van der Merwe M, van Zyl JA, Smith K: Sperm morphologic features as a prognostic factor in IVF. Fertil Steril 1986; 46:1118.
19. Kruger TF, Acosta AA, Simmons KF, Swanson RJ, Matta JF, Oehninger S: Predictive value of abnormal sperm morphology in in vitro fertilization. Fertil Steril 1988; 49:112.
20. Vantman D, Koukoulis G, Dennison L, Zinaman M, Sherins RJ: Computer assisted semen analysis: Evaluation of method and assessment of the influence of sperm concentration on linear velocity determination. Fertil Steril 1988; 49:510.
21. Knuth VA, Yeung CH, Jieschlag E: Computerized semen analysis: Objective measurement of semen analysis is biased by subjective parameter setting. Fertil Steril 1988; 48:118.
22. Mack SO, Wolf DO, Tash JS: Quantification of specific parameters of motility in large numbers of human sperm by digital image processing. Biol Reprod 1981; 38:270.
23. Jeulin C, Feneux D, Serres C, Jouanner P, Guillet-Rosso F, Belaisch-Allart J, Frydman J, Testart J: Sperm factors related to failure of human IVF. J Reprod Fertil 1986; 70:735.
24. Hinting A, Comhaire F, Vermeulen L, Dhont M, Vermeulen A, Vanderkerckhove D: Possibilities and limitation of techniques of assisted reproduction for the treatment of male infertility. Hum Reprod 1990; 5:544.
25. Lanzendorf SE, Toth TL, Scott RT, Veeck LL, Oehninger S: Variables that influenced the penetration of human sperm through the zona pellucida of human oocytes: Standardization of a zona penetration assay (ZPA). Submitted for presentation at the American Fertility Society, New Orleans, LA, November 1–5, 1992.
26. Yanagimachi R, Yanagimachi H, Rogers BJ: The use of zona-free animal ova as a test system for the assessment of the fertilizing capacity of human spermatozoa. Biol Reprod 1976; 15:471.
27. Swanson RJ, Mayer JE, Jones KH, Lanzendorf SE, McDowell J: Hamster ova/human sperm penetration: Correlation with count, motility, and morphology for human in vitro fertilization. Arch Androl 1984; 12:69.
28. Auzmanus M, Tureck RW, Blasco L, Kipf GS, Ribes J, Mastroianni L: The zona free hamster

egg penetration assay as a prognostic indicator in a human in vitro fertilization program. Fertil Steril 1987; 43:433.
29. Margalioth EJ, Navot D, Laufer N, Lewin A, Rabinowitz R, Schenker JG: Correlation between the zona-free hamster egg sperm-penetration assay and human in vitro fertilization. Fertil Steril 1986; 45:665.
30. Burkman LJ, Coddington CC, Franken DR, Kruger TF, Rosenwaks Z, Hodgen GD: The hemizona assay (HZA): Development of a diagnostic test for the binding of human spermatozoa to the human hemizona pellucida to predict fertilization potential. Fertil Steril 1988; 49:688.
31. Oehninger S, Coddington CC, Scott RT: Hemizona assay: Assessment of sperm dysfunction and prediction of in vitro fertilization outcome. Fertil Steril 1989; 51:665.
32. Coddington CC: The hemizona assay (HZA) and considerations for its use in assisted reproductive technology. Semin Reprod Endocrinol 1992; 10:1.
33. Smith KD, Rodriguez-Rigau LJ, Steinberger E: Relationship between indices of semen analysis and pregnancy rates in infertile couples. Fertil Steril 1977; 23:1314.
34. Collins JA, Wrixon W, Janes LB et al.: Treatment-independent pregnancy among infertile couples. N Engl J Med 1983; 309:1201.
35. In vitro fertilization-embryo transfer in the United States: 1988 results from the IVF Registry. Fertil Steril 1990; 53:13.
36. Balmaceda JP, Pool TB, Arana JB, Heitman TS, Asch RH: Successful in vitro fertilization and embryo transfer in cynomolgus monkeys. Fertil Steril 1984; 42:791.
37. Devroey P, Braeckman P, Smith J, Van Waesberghe L, Wisanto A, Van Steirteghem A, Heytens L, Camu F: Pregnancy after translaparoscopic zygote intra-fallopian transfer in a patient with sperm antibodies. Lancet 1986; 1:1329.
38. Palermo G, Devroey P, Camus M, DeGravwe E, Khan I, Staessen C, Wisanto A, Van Steirteghem AC: Zygote intrafallopian transfer as an alternative treatment for male infertility. Hum Reprod 1989; 4:412.
39. Yovich JL, Blackledge DG, Richardson PA, Matson PL, Turner SR, Draper R: Pregnancies following pronuclear stage tubal transfer. Fertil Steril 1987; 48:851.
40. Balmaceda JP, Gastaldi C, Remohi J, Borrero C, Ord T, Asch RH: Tubal embryo transfer as a treatment from infertility due to male factor. Fertil Steril 1988; 50:476.
41. van der Ven HH, Hoebbel K, Al-Hasani S, Diedrick K, Krebs D: Fertilization of human oocytes in capillary tubes with very small numbers of spermatozoa. Hum Reprod 1989; 4:72.
42. Gordon J, Talansky BE: Assisted fertilization by zona drilling: A mouse model for correction of oligospermia. J Exp Zool 1986; 239:347.
43. Gordon JW: Use of micromanipulation for increasing the efficiency of mammalian fertilization in vitro. Ann NY Acad Sci 1988; 541:601.
44. Gordon JW, Grunfeld L, Garrisi GJ, Talansky BE, Richards C, Laufer N: Fertilization of human oocytes by sperm from infertile males after zona pellucida drilling. Fertil Steril 1988; 50:68.
45. Gordon JW, Grunfeld L, Talansky BE, Garrisi GJ, Richards C, Wiczyk H, Rappaport D, Navot D, Laufer N: The human oocytes blocks polyspermy at the zone pellucida. Proc Am Fertil Soc 1988; 53a.
46. Malter HE, Cohen J: Partial zone dissection of the human oocyte: A nontraumatic method using micromanipulation to assist zona pellucida penetration. Fertil Steril 1989; 51:139.
47. Talansky BE: Microsurgical fertilization in mammals. In: Cohen J, Malter HE, Talansky BE, Grifo J, eds. Micromanipulation of human gametes and embryos. New York: Raven Press, 1992: 122.
48. Cohen J, Malter H, Wright G, Kort H, Masseh J, Mitchell D: Partial zona dissection of human oocytes when failure of zona pellucida penetration is anticipated. Hum Reprod 1989; 4:435.
49. Garrisi GJ, Talansky BE, Grunfeld L, Sapira V, Navot D, Gordon JW: Clinical evaluation of

three approaches to micromanipulation assisted fertilization. Fertil Steril 1990; 54:671.
50. Laws-King A, Trounson A, Sathananthan AH, Kola I: Fertilization of human oocytes by microinjection of a single spermatozoa under the zona pellucida. Fertil Steril 1987; 48:637.
51. Ng SC, Bongso TA, Ratnam SS, Sathananthan H, Chan CLK, Wong PC, Hagglund L, Anandakumar C, Wong YC, Goh VHH: Pregnancy after transfer of multiple sperm under the zona. Lancet 1988; 790.
52. Fishel S, Antinori S, Jackson P, Johnson J: Twin birth after subzonal insertion. Lancet 1990; 2:790.
53. Lippi J, Turner M, Jansen RPS: Pregnancies after in vitro fertilization by sperm microinjection into the perivitelline space. Abstract O-068. 46th Annual Meeting, American Fertility Society, Washington D.C., October 1990.
54. Bongso TA, Sathanathan AH, Wong C: Human fertilization by microinjection of immotile spermatozoa. Hum Reprod 1989; 4:175.
55. Reproductive Technology Update. 1991; 3:13.
56. Cohen J, Malter H, Talansky B, Tucker T, Wright G: Gamete and embryo micromanipulation for infertility treatment. Semin Reprod Endocr 1990; 8:290.
57. Buster JE, Carson SA, Minhas BS: Embryo micromanipulation in reproductive medicine. Semin Reprod Endocr 1992; 10:19.
58. Fishel S, Antinori S, Jackson P, Johnson J, Rinaldi L: Presentation of six pregnancies established by sub-zonal insemination. Human Reprod 1991; 6:124.
59. Ng SC, Bongso A, Ratnam SS: Microinjection of human oocytes: A technique for severe oligoasthenoteratozoospermia. Fertil Steril 1992; 56:1117.
60. Krzyminska UB, Leung P, O'Neill C, Pike IL: Microinsemination by sperm transfer. Lancet 1992; 339:375.
61. Garrisi GJ, Navot D, Chin A, Boyle PM, Nagler HM, Vasquez-Levin M, Gordon JW: Establishment of success in a program of micromanipulation-assisted fertilization: Analysis of variables. (Abstract) 48th Annual Meeting of the American Fertility Society, October 1992.
62. Lanzendorf SE, Maloney MK, Veeck LL, Slusser J, Hodgen GD, Rosenwaks Z: A preclinical evaluation of pronuclear formation by microinjection of human spermatozoa into human oocytes. Fertil Steril 1988; 49:835.
63. Matson PL, Turner SR, Yovich JM, Tuvik AI: Oligospermic infertility treated by in vitro fertilization. Aust NZ J Obstet Gynaecol 1984; 26:84.
64. Cohen J, Talansky BE, Malter H, Alikani M, Adler A, Reing A, Berkeley A, Graf M, Davis O, Liu H, Bedford MJ, Rosenwaks Z: Microsurgical fertilization and teratozoospermia. Human Reprod 1991; 6:123.
65. Cohen J, Alikani M, Malter HE, Adler A, Talnasky BE, Rosenwaks Z: Partial zona dissection or subzonal sperm insertion: Microsurgical fertilization alternatives based on evaluation of sperm and embryo morphology. Fertil Steril 1991; 56:696.
66. Fishel S, Timson J, Lisi F, Rinaldi L: Evaluation of 225 patients undergoing subzonal insemination for the procurement of fertilization in vitro. Fertil Steril 1992; 57:840.

ANNOTATED BIBLIOGRAPHY

Oehninger S, Hodgen GD: How to evaluate human spermatozoa for assisted reproduction. Assist Reprod Rev 1991; 1:15.

This is a comprehensive review of morphometric and functional studies available to date for the evaluation of spermatozoa for assisted reproduction. The report emphasizes the value of "strict" criteria for sperm morphology as a prognosticator for *in vitro* fertilizing capacity. The cutoff of <14% normal morphology demarcates between 88 and 49.5% fertilization. Further breakdown into "good" and "poor" patterns within the abnormal group (≤14%) yields fertilization rates of 63 and 7%, respectively. The review also summarizes the utility of the hemizona assay as a biosystem reflecting sperm capacity to bind to the oocyte and predict fertilization. They claim a 95% sensitivity and 83% specificity for the assay.

In vitro fertilization-embryo transfer (IVF-ET) in the United States: 1989 results from IVF-ET registry. Fertil Steril 1991; 55:14.

The yearly report of the Society for Assisted Reproduction on all IVF related procedures in the United States in a given year (1989). This is a very accurate reflection of the scope of male infertility and the solution provided by the novel reproductive technologies. Male infertility represented over one-third of all diagnostic categories treated by IVF. While a 15% delivery rate per transfer was attained, the rate per oocyte retrieval is a meager 6%. This discrepancy is accounted for by the high rate of complete failure of fertilization (57%).

Talansky BE: Microsurgical fertilization in mammals. In: Cohen J, Malter HE, Talansky BE, Grifo J, eds. Micromanipulation of human gametes and embryos. New York: Raven Press, 1992; 122.

This the only available comprehensive text on micromanipulation of human gametes. The book overviews the physiological processes of early embryonic development in the human, provides the reader with detailed descriptions, accompanied by elegant figures of the various techniques of micromanipulation. State of the art on mammalian micromanipulation and human gamete manipulation follows. The book also provides a practical guide for techniques and equipment needed.

29 Hormonal Abnormalities

Jonathan P. Jarow

The testis is a dual organ in both function and structure. The interstitial compartment has an endocrine function whose principal product is testosterone. The seminiferous tubule compartment has an exocrine function whose product is spermatozoa. Both of these functions are under the direct control of the hypothalamic–pituitary–gonadal (HPG) axis. In addition to adult sexual and reproductive function, the HPG axis is responsible for the phenotypic gender development during embryogenesis and sexual maturation during puberty. The HPG axis is comprised of a delicate balance between stimulation and feedback inhibition between the component parts. Abnormalities of this system may result in one of various clinical entities depending on the type of abnormality, extent of the defect, and stage of development during which it occurs. A thorough understanding of the normal function of the HPG axis is vital to the evaluation of the infertile adult male patient and the management of endocrine abnormalities.

Hypothalamic–Pituitary–Gonadal Axis

Hypothalamus

The hypothalamus serves as the integrative center for the entire HPG axis incorporating input from various sources in the control of pituitary function. Peptidergic neurons located in the preoptic area and the arcuate nucleus secrete a decapeptide hormone known as luteinizing hormone-releasing hormone (LHRH) or gonadotropin-releasing hormone (GnRH).[1] This hormone is found in other neurons and in other tissues as well.[2] However, its function outside the hypothalamus is unknown. The hypothalamus is the pulse generator for the pulsatile secretion of the gonadotropins and testosterone. Secretion of GnRH by the hypothalamus is stimulated by catecholamines[3] and dopamine.[4] Endorphins, androgens, and estrogens inhibit GnRH secretion.[5,6] GnRH is released into a portal circulation that delivers the hormone

Management of Impotence and Infertility, edited by Douglas Whitehead and Harris Nagler,

directly to the anterior pituitary gland. In addition, reverse flow through this hypophyseal–portal circulation allows for direct pituitary hormone feedback on the hypothalamus.[7]

Pituitary Gland

GnRH binds to a high-affinity cell surface receptor of the basophilic gonadotrophs located in the anterior pituitary gland. GnRH stimulates the release of gonadotropins acutely and the production of gonadotropins with chronic administration. The sensitivity of the basophilic cells for GnRH is dependent on age and the hormonal status. The primary hormones that control testicular function are luteinizing hormone (LH) and follicle-stimulating hormone (FSH). Both of these glycoprotein hormones are composed of an α and β subunit. They share the same α subunit with other pituitary hormones. The β subunit determines both the immunologic and functional characteristic of each hormone. Variation of the carbohydrate composition of these hormones may also affect the biologic and immunologic properties.

Both LH and FSH are secreted in a pulsatile fashion reflecting the pulses of GnRH secretion. The half-life of LH within the serum is much shorter than FSH. Therefore, more variation is observed in serum levels of LH than FSH.[8,9] This has clinical significance when measuring basal hormone levels in peripheral serum. Both FSH and LH act on target tissues by binding to cell surface receptors and stimulating the membrane-bound adenylate cyclase/protein kinase system.[10] The response of the target cell is determined by the products of the enzyme systems activated by the protein kinase system.

Testis

Testosterone is synthesized from cholesterol within the Leydig cell of the interstitial compartment of the testis. Although the testis produces small amounts of estradiol and dihydrotestosterone (DHT), the majority of these hormones are produced in target tissues through metabolism of circulating testosterone.[11,12] Testosterone production is stimulated by LH produced in the pituitary gland and regulated through a feedback inhibitory loop between the testis, hypothalamus, and pituitary gland. The majority of circulating testosterone is bound to plasma proteins.[13] In a normal man, approximately 2% of testosterone is unbound, 44% bound to testosterone-binding globulin (TeBG), and 54% bound to albumin. The unbound hormone was thought to be the only biologically active fraction. However, recent *in vivo* studies demonstrate that the albumin-bound fraction is also biologically active.[14]

Testosterone may be metabolized into one of two active metabolites, DHT and estradiol within the cytoplasm of the target cell.[11] The steroid hormone then binds to the steroid receptor present within the cytoplasm and the hormone–receptor complex is then transferred to the nucleus. Interaction of the hormone–receptor complex and nuclear chromatin produces the androgen action and may vary among the different target tissues.[15]

The action of FSH upon the Sertoli cell within the seminiferous tubule compartment is less well understood. However, it is clear that FSH stimulates Sertoli cell production of a variety of proteins including androgen-binding protein, transferrin, and the aromatase enzyme.[16,17] The Sertoli cell also produces a protein hormone, inhibin, which has a negative feedback on pituitary gland secretion of FSH independent of steroid hormones.[18] Both androgens and FSH are necessary for the initiation and maintenance of quantitatively normal spermatogenesis.[19] Although the process of spermatogenesis is incompletely understood, it appears that the Sertoli cell serves as the integrative center for the endocrine control of spermatogenesis since sperm cell do not have either FSH or androgen receptors. Inhibin is a heterodimer protein hormone within the transforming growth factor family. The homodimer hormone, activin, stimulates FSH secretion from pituitary cells. Activin has been shown to be produced by Leydig cells in animal studies.[20] Therefore, it appears that there is a complex paracrine and autocrine regulation present within the testis that is still not understood.

Endocrine Testing

Basal Hormones

Sampling of basal plasma hormones is frequently the only study needed to diagnose an endocrinopathy in an infertile individual. It is extremely rare to identify a clinically significant endocrinopathy in the presence of normal spermatogenesis reflected by a normal semen analysis. Therefore, endocrine studies are not felt to be necessary in men with normal semen analyses. Routine endocrine testing of the infertile man includes a plasma FSH and testosterone. The addition of routine prolactin, LH, and thyroid function studies is controversial. Since the majority of men with clinically significant elevations of prolactin have an abnormally low testosterone level,[21] some authors recommend reserving prolactin testing to only those men with low testosterone levels. Likewise, it is rare to identify abnormalities in LH or thyroid studies in the presence of normal testosterone levels. Traditionally, the hormone measurements are made on a pooled sample composed of three to four samples obtained every 15 minutes to compensate for the pulsatile release of these hormones. However, recent studies have shown that a single sample is frequently as accurate as the mean of three.[22] Therefore, pooled sampling may be reserved for those patients with borderline or questionable results on preliminary endocrine studies. Serum LH levels are helpful only in patients with abnormally low or high testosterone levels. Inhibin assays are now available, but have not yet proven to be clinically useful.

The results of basal endocrine studies may fall into one of four categories (Table 29-1). Normal basal endocrine studies are the most common results observed in the infertile population. An isolated elevation of serum FSH, reflecting an abnormality in the seminiferous tubule compartment, is the second most common endocrine finding. Total primary testicular failure is relatively rare, whereas secondary

Table 29-1 Results of Endocrine Evaluation of Basal Hormone Levels

	T	FSH	LH	PRL
Eugonadal	nl	nl	nl	nl
Primary testicular failure	↓	↑	↑	nl
Germ cell abnormality	nl	↑/nl	nl	nl
Secondary testicular failure	↓	↓	↓	nl
Hyperprolactinemia	↓	↓/nl	↓/nl	↑
Androgen insensitivity	↑	↑	↑	nl

testicular failure and androgen resistance are extremely rare findings.

The hormone measurements of FSH and LH are performed with radioimmunoassays. Unfortunately, the immunologic properties of these hormones do not always correlate with their biologic activity.[23] However, it is extremely rare for this difference to be clinically significant. Testosterone levels are also measured with a radioimmunoassay. "Free" testosterone can be measured directly from a dialysate. The biologically active fraction can be measured directly using an *in vivo* system[24] or indirectly by measuring TeBG levels. Measurement of free or bioavailable testosterone is clinically important in patients with altered binding protein levels such as liver disease or hyperthyroidism.

Dynamic Tests

Dynamic hormonal testing is used to assess the potential function of unstimulated endocrine cells, or identify subtle abnormalities in feedback inhibition. For instance, the ability of prepubertal Leydig cells to respond to gonadotropins is assessed following repeated doses of hCG.[25] A typical protocol is a daily injection of 2000 IU hCG for 5 days. A normal response documents intact Leydig cell function in the absence of endogenous gonadotropin secretion. An hCG stimulation test may also be performed in the adult to determine testicular reserve. However, this test does not frequently add much to the standard endocrine assessment of the routine infertile adult patient.

Pituitary response to LHRH is sometimes used to assess the functional integrity of the hypothalamic–pituitary–gonadal axis. There is a five-fold increase in LH with a peak level at 30 minutes following intravenous administration of 100 μg of LHRH in normal men.[26] However, the range of response is broad within normal men, making interpretation extremely difficult in patients with subtle endocrinopathies. LHRH stimulation test may be used to assess pituitary function in a patient with secondary hypogonadism or hypogonadotropic hypogonadism. However, the pituitary does not usually respond to the first test dose. This test is sometimes used to assess pituitary function, which will determine the type of therapy used for this disorder.[27] An alternative method to assess the integrity of the hypothalamic–pituitary–gonadal axis is the clomiphene citrate stimulation test. Clomiphene citrate is an antiestrogen that blocks steroidal feedback inhibition of the hypothalamus and pituitary gland. This results in a significant elevation of serum LH, FSH, and testosterone in the normal individual. However, as with the LHRH stimulation test, the response of normal men is broad. Both of these dynamic tests add very little to the diagnostic evaluation over routine basal endocrine testing.[28] Therefore, these studies are usually reserved for research protocols.

Endocrine Disorders

Hypogonadotropic Hypogonadism

Hypogonadism may be due to an intrinsic testicular abnormality (primary testicular failure) or a lack of stimulation by the hypothalamus and pituitary gland (secondary hypogonadism). In the first setting, lack of feedback inhibition on a normal pituitary gland results in elevated serum LH and FSH levels. However, hypogonadotropic hypogonadism is diagnosed by the association of low serum LH and FSH

Table 29-2 Causes of Hypogonadotropic Hypogonadism

Congenital
Kallmann's syndrome
Trauma
Tumor
Prolactinoma
Nonfunctional
Metastatic
Iatrogenic
Anabolic steroid abuse

with a low serum testosterone level. There are numerous causes of this disorder, which may be congenital or acquired (Table 29-2). The association of the familial syndrome of congenital hypogonadotropic hypogonadism with midline defects such as anosmia is known as Kallmann's syndrome.[29] The age of onset and extent of the deficit determine the presentation of this disorder. Many patients present with cryptorchidism, microphallus, or delayed puberty. However, some patients present in adulthood with primary infertility. The pattern of inheritance of this disorder is both X-linked[30] and autosomal recessive.[31] In addition, more than half of the patients lack a family history. Therefore, new mutations appear to be common.

The diagnosis is usually established by history and basal hormone studies. Concomitant deficits of other pituitary hormones are common and should be assessed. Prolactin-secreting pituitary tumors may be identified by obtaining a prolactin level. Radiologic imaging of the pituitary with either CT or MRI can rule out primary or metastatic tumors. The underlying defect is at the hypothalamic level in the congenital form, and is more frequently a pituitary disorder in the acquired form. Dynamic endocrine testing using intravenous LHRH will normalize LH and FSH in almost half of the patients with congenital disorders.[32] Repetitive treatment for at least 1 week is required in patients with a more severe deficiency.[33] Patients with pituitary abnormalities will not respond to LHRH.

There are three forms of therapy for hypogonadotropic hypogonadism. Testosterone replacement therapy is achieved using intramuscular injections of testosterone esters to virilize the individual during puberty or in adulthood. Gonadotropin and LHRH therapy are used to induce fertility. In rare patients with only partial defects in gonadotropin secretion, testosterone alone can induce spermatogenesis.[34] Patients with acquired hypogonadotropic hypogonadism frequently respond to hCG therapy alone.[35] Patients with congenital lesions usually require therapy with both hCG and hMG to induce spermatogenesis, which can then be maintained with hCG alone.[36] Alternatively, LHRH administered subcutaneously using a pulsatile pump may be employed in patients with an undamaged pituitary gland.[37] This technique is much more cumbersome and has not been documented to have a significant advantage over gonadotropin therapy.[38]

The prognosis is adversely affected by a baseline testis size less than 4 ml and history of cryptorchidism.[39] Prior testosterone therapy does not affect prognosis.[40] Spermatogenesis can be induced in greater than 80% of these patients and fertility rates are high (Table 29-3).[37,39,41–43] Interestingly, pregnancies have occurred in couples whose husbands' sperm counts would not normally be considered within the fertile range. This group of patients demonstrates that quality is more important than quantity of sperm to be able to conceive. Therefore, one can remain optimistic even when endocrine therapy does not induce normal levels of spermatogenesis.

Table 29-3 Results of Therapy for Hypogonadotropic Hypogonadism

Reference	Treatment	Sperm Production (%)	Pregnancy (%)
Burger and Baker (1985)[41]	hCG/hMG	56	44
Finkel et al. (1985)[42]	hCG/hMG	66	43
Burris et al. (1988)[39]	hCG/hMG	64	54
Morris et al. (1984)[43]	GnRH	41	18
Shargil (1987)[37]	GnRH	83	83

Hyperprolactinemia

The diagnosis of hyperprolactinemia is established with the measurement of serum prolactin levels. Hyperprolactinemia should be suspected in any patient with decreased libido, sexual dysfunction, low serum testosterone levels, or other clinical signs of hypogonadism. Many advocate screening all infertile patients for hyperprolactinemia but this is a rare cause of male factor infertility. Less than 20% of patients with clinically significant hyperprolactinemia have a normal serum testosterone level.[44,45] Therefore, it is reasonable to limit screening to those patients suspected to have the disease.

Hyperprolactinemia may be caused by a pituitary tumor, stress, medications, or medical illness (Table 29-4). Significant elevations of serum prolactin (greater than 50 ng/ml) are more frequently associated with pituitary tumors. However, microadenomas can be found in patients with only a modest elevation of serum prolactin.[46] Pituitary tumors can cause hyperprolactinemia directly through secretion or by interfering with normal inhibitory pathways. Pituitary function should be assessed in patients with hyperprolactinemia to rule out deficiencies of other pituitary hormones. Radiologic imaging of the pituitary with either CT or MRI will identify mass lesions.

Table 29-4 Causes of Hyperprolactinemia

Hypothalamic disease
Prolactinoma
Pituitary disease
Medications
Chronic renal failure
Cirrhosis
Stress
Idiopathic

Hyperprolactinemia may interfere with normal testicular function through several mechanisms. At normal levels prolactin appears to be synergistic with androgen on sex accessory gland growth.[47] However, elevated prolactin levels appear to have a direct antiandrogen effect. This has been demonstrated by the fact that testosterone therapy alone does not restore normal libido and sexual function to hyperprolactinemic men with low testosterone levels.[44] Normalization of prolactin levels is usually required. Elevated serum prolactin levels may inhibit LHRH release by the hypothalamus and produce a hypogonadotropic hypogonadism picture.[45] In addition, a mass lesion within the pituitary may destroy the normal gonadotroph cells in men with prolactin-secreting pituitary adenomas. Men frequently present late in the disease course. This

Table 29-5 Presenting Signs and Symptoms of Hyperprolactinemia

Decreased libido
Impotence
Headache
Visual impairment
Galactorrhea
Gynecomastia

may be because of the low frequency of galactorrhea and gynecomastia in men as compared to women with this disorder. The most frequent presenting sign is decreased libido or impotence (Table 29-5). However, men may also present with headaches and visual impairment due to the mass lesion.

Therapy consists of medication, surgery, and radiation. Medical therapy alone using bromocriptine is successful in the majority of patients. Radiation therapy has fallen out of favor at most centers. Surgery is indicated in patients with macroadenomas that do not respond to medical therapy. Although surgery or radiation therapy may be necessary in patients with large prolactin-secreting pituitary adenomas, these therapeutic modalities do not always result in normalization of serum prolactin levels. Bromocriptine has the highest rate of normalization of serum prolactin.[44] Unfortunately, fertility rates remain low in patients with prolactin-secreting pituitary adenomas despite normalization of serum prolactin levels.[49,50]

Androgen Resistance

Abnormalities of the androgen receptor, as documented by cultured genital skin fibroblasts, may produce varying phenotypic abnormalities in a chromosomally normal man.[51] A limited and rare form of androgen resistance results in infertility in men who have normal masculine development of the external genitalia. Some members from a family with Reifenstein's syndrome were noted to have gynecomastia and infertility with normal genitalia despite the same receptor abnormality found in more severely affected family members.[52] Androgen resistance is characterized by elevated levels of testosterone with elevated serum LH levels. Since the androgen receptor is abnormal, normal feedback inhibition does not occur. However, some feedback may occur through aromatization of testosterone to estradiol. Therefore, elevated levels of testosterone and LH are not completely reliable indicators of a receptor defect. Measurement of androgen receptor function in cultured genital skin fibroblasts is required to establish this diagnosis.

Androgen resistance is rarely diagnosed in infertility practices. However, one study of men with idiopathic azoospermia found that 40% had an androgen receptor defect.[53] Testis biopsy revealed both maturation arrest and germ cell aplasia in these patients, thus demonstrating a spectrum of abnormalities even in this small subgroup of patients with androgen resistance. Unfortunately, effective therapy for this disorder does not exist.

Congenital Adrenal Hyperplasia

An enzyme deficiency in the steroidogenic pathway results in a lack of feedback inhibition by cortisol on the pituitary gland and overstimulation of adrenal function. Precursors of cortisol will be present in excess and produce varying effects depending on the enzyme defect. The most common is a 21-hydroxylase deficiency that results in a build-up of androgenic steroidal precursors.[54] Ambiguous genitalia may be present in a female infant, whereas male children with this disorder may present with precocious puberty. In men with chronic untreated or undertreated congenital adrenal hyperplasia, gonadotropin secretion is suppressed as a result of feedback inhibition by an excess of adrenal androgens. Infertility results from a hypogonadotropic hypogonadal disorder. This diagnosis may be suspected in a patient with bilateral atrophic testes, normal testosterone levels, and low LH and FSH levels. This diagnosis is confirmed by finding markedly elevated serum levels of 17-hydroxyprogesterone and androstenedione.[54]

Not all patients with congenital adrenal hyperplasia are infertile. Some patients with documented elevated androstenedione levels have normal plasma testosterone and gonadotropin levels with normal fertility.[55] Treatment of infertile patients with congenital adrenal hyperplasia consists of adequate steroid replacement. Normalization of androstenedione levels confirms adequate suppression of endogenous adrenal function. The vast majority of these patients can become fertile with appropriate therapy, as documented by paternity and normal sperm counts in one study.[55]

Primary Hypogonadism

Primary hypogonadism may present with undervirilization, or as an isolated abnormality in spermatogenesis. In general, the Leydig cell compartment is more resistant to injury and, therefore, isolated problems with spermatogenesis are a more common cause of infertility. The presentation depends on age of onset and degree of the deficit. In a newborn, primary hypogonadism may present as ambiguous genitalia or microphallus. Delayed puberty will occur in most congenital disorders not detected at birth. Acquired hypogonadism in an already masculinized man will usually present with decreased libido or impotence. The diagnosis is established by the finding of elevated gonadotropin levels. Testosterone levels are low and both LH and FSH are elevated in complete primary hypogonadism. FSH may be elevated or normal in a patient with isolated abnormalities in spermatogenesis, while testosterone and LH levels are almost always normal. Feedback inhibition of FSH secretion is incompletely understood. Severe testicular disorders usually result in significant elevations of serum FSH. However, approximately 20% of patients with germinal-cell aplasia have a normal serum FSH level.[56]

There are numerous congenital and acquired disorders causing primary testicular failure (Table 29-6). Most of these disorders, with the exception of several acquired ones, are irreversible. The most common developmental defect of the testis is Klinefelter syndrome. This disorder is characterized by the presence of atrophic testes, gynecomastia, and elevated gonadotropin levels.[57] This is a chromosomal

Table 29-6 Causes of Primary Testicular Failure

Congenital
Chromosomal abnormalities
Anorchia
Germ cell aplasia
Cryptorchidism
Androgen resistance
Acquired
Viral orchitis
Trauma
Torsion
Radiation
Varicocele
Medication
Environmental toxins
Systemic illnesses
Idiopathic

disorder in which there is an extra X chromosome.[58] The incidence is one in 500 live male births.[59] Another congenital disorder resulting in primary testicular failure is anorchia and bilateral cryptorchidism. Trauma, torsion, and viral orchitis may also cause primary testicular failure when they occur bilaterally. Mumps orchitis is the most frequent cause of viral orchitis.[60] However, echovirus, lymphocytic choriomeningitis virus, and group B arboviruses may also cause orchitis.[61] Gonadotoxins such as chemotherapy and radiation therapy may also cause testicular failure.

Medications may cause testicular failure through direct inhibition of testosterone synthesis or blocking of androgen action. Spironolactone and cyproterone can block testos terone synthesis when administered at high dosages.[62,63] However, testerone levels do not change appreciably during the usual therapeutic regimens with spironolactone. Spironolactone, cyproterone, and cimetidine can block androgen binding to the androgen receptor.[62,64] Gynecomastia and decreased spermatogenesis may occur with the ingestion of these drugs. Ketoconazole, an antifungal agent, also blocks testosterone biosynthesis at high dosages greater than 400 mg/day.[65] In addition, ketoconazole also inhibits adrenal steroid production. Alcohol ingestion inhibits testosterone production, independent of its effects on the liver.[86] Finally, various nonprescription medications may inhibit testosterone secretion including marihuana, heroin, and methadone.

Systemic illnesses may produce testicular failure. Chronic renal failure has been associated with impairment of both testosterone synthesis and spermatogenesis.[67] Dialysis does not completely ameliorate these adverse effects. However, there is frequently complete resolution following successful renal transplantation.[68] Chronic cirrhosis of the liver results in a severe imbalance between testosterone and estradiol. Gynecomastia and testicular atrophy occur in approximately 50% of men with cirrhosis.[69] Correction of the endocrinopathy associated with cirrhosis through administration of testosterone does not reverse the testicular abnormalities. Other systemic disorders have been associated with testicular failure including sickle cell anemia,[70] amyloidosis,[71] thyrotoxicosis,[72] and myotonic dystrophy.[73]

Testicular failure with normal virilization may be congenital due to an isolated FSH deficiency or germinal cell aplasia.[74] Varicocele is the most common reversible cause of abnormal spermatogenesis. This vascular lesion is present in approximately 40% of men presenting with infertility.[75] *In vitro* studies have demonstrated a partial defect in testosterone biosynthesis in testes associated with varicoceles.[76] Correction of a varicocele results in improvement in spermatogenesis in approximately 70% of men.[77] Pregnancy rates are dependent on baseline testis size, serum FSH, and sperm counts.[78] Average pregnancy rate following varicocelectomy is approximately 40%.

Treatment of primary testicular failure consists of correction of any potentially reversible disorder, such as a varicocele, and testosterone replacement therapy for the hypogonadal patients. Testosterone replacement is important for maintaining normal libido and sexual function. In addition, androgenic steroids exert somatic effects on erythropoiesis, nitrogen balance, and prevention of osteoporosis. In the absence of androgenic or estrogenic steroids, disabling osteoporosis may develop with age. Appropriate replacement dose is 200 mg intramuscularly of a testosterone ester (enanthate or cypionate) every 2 to 3 weeks.[79] Oral androgens are poorly absorbed and may exert hepatic toxicity. Therefore, oral androgens should not be used routinely.

Summary

The hypothalamic–pituitary–gonadal axis contains complex homeostatic mechanisms of feedback inhibition to maintain a normal androgen environment. Normal levels of LH, FSH, and testosterone are critically important to normal sperm production and maturation. However, in the absence of specific deficiencies, exogenous hormone administration often results in disruption of the normal balance and potentially has a deleterious effect. Specifically, administration of testosterone in high dosages has a contraceptive effect. Likewise, high dosages of gonadotropins may lead to elevated estradiol levels, which can have a deleterious effect on the testis.

Patients with normal spermatogenesis or minor seminal abnormalities rarely have a significant endocrinopathy. Significant abnormalities of the HPG axis will usually result in either azoospermia or severe oligospermia. Measurement of serum hormone levels may be inaccurate due to pulsatile release. Therefore, abnormal results should be confirmed with a pooled sample. This is particularly true when the results do not correlate with the clinical history and physical findings. Low levels of LH and FSH in the face of either normal testosterone levels or normal semen analysis are not clinically significant. Treatment should be directed toward specific hormonal abnormalities. The results of nonspecific hormonal therapy have been extremely disappointing.

REFERENCES

1. Silverman AJ, Krey LC, Zimmerman EA: A comparative study of the luteinizing hormone releasing hormone (LHRH) neuronal networks in mammals. Biol Reprod 1979; 20:98.
2. Franchimont P: Regulation of gonadal androgen secretion. Horm Res 1983; 18:7.
3. Negro-Vilar A, Ojeda SR, McCann SM: Catecholaminergic modulation of luteinizing hormone-releasing hormone release by median eminence terminals in vitro. Endocrinology 1979; 104:1749.
4. Evans WS, Rogol AD, MacLeod RM, et al: Dopaminergic mechanisms and luteinizing hormone secretion. I. Acute administration of the dopamine agonist bromocriptine does not inhibit luteinizing hormone release in hyperprolactinemic women. J Clin Endocrinol Metab 1980; 50:103.
5. Delitala G, Giusti M, Mazzocchi G, et al: Participation of endogenous opiates in regulation of the hypothalamic–pituitary–testicular axis in normal men. J Clin Endocrinol Metab 1983; 57:1277.
6. Veldhuis JD, Rogol AD, Johnson ML, et al: Endogenous opiates modulate the pulsatile secretion of biologically active luteinizing hormone in man. J Clin Invest 1983; 72:2031.
7. Oliver C, Mical RS, Porter JC: Hypothalamic-pituitary vasculature: Evidence for retrograde blood flow in the pituitary stalk. Endocrinology 1977; 101:598.
8. Veldhuis JD, Fraioli F, Rogol AD, et al: Metabolic clearance of biologically active luteinizing hormone in man. J Clin Invest 1986; 77:1122–1128.
9. Coble YD Jr, Kohler PO, Cargille CM, et al: Production rates and metabolic clearance rates of human follicle-stimulating hormone in premenopausal and postmenopausal women. J Clin Invest 1969; 48:359–363.
10. Podesta EJ, Dufau ML, Solano AR, et al: Hormonal activation of protein kinase in isolated Leydig cells: Electrophoretic analysis of cyclic AMP receptors. J Biol Chem 1978; 253:8994–9001.
11. Wilson JD: Metabolism of testicular androgens. In: Greep RO, Astwood EB, eds. Handbook of physiology. Section 7: Endocrinology. Vol II. Female reproductive system. Part I. Washing-

ton, DC: American Physiological Society, 1976:491–508.

12. MacDonald PC, Madden JD, Brenner PF, et al: Origin of estrogen in normal men and in women with testicular feminization. J Clin Endocrinol Metab 1979; 49:905–916.
13. Dunn JF, Nisula BC, Rodbard D: Transport of steroid hormones: Binding of 21 endogenous steroids to both testosterone-binding globulin and corticosteroid-binding globulin in human plasma. J Clin Endocrinol Metab 1981; 53:58–68.
14. Pardridge WM: Serum bioavailability of sex steroid hormones. Clin Endocrinol Metab 1986; 15:259–278.
15. Williams-Ashman HG: Metabolic effects of testicular androgens. In: Greep RO, Astwood EB, eds. Handbook of physiology. Section 7: Endocrinology. Vol. V. Male reproductive system. Washington, DC: American Physiological Society, 1975:473–490.
16. Cheng CY, Musto NA, Gunsalus GL, et al: There are two forms of androgen binding protein in human testes: Comparison of their protomeric variants with serum testosterone-estradiol binding globulin. J Biol Chem 1985; 260:5631–5640.
17. Dorrington JH, Armstrong DT: Follicle-stimulating hormone stimulates estradiol-17β synthesis in cultured Sertoli cells. Proc Natl Acad Sci USA 1975; 72:2677–2681.
18. Robertson DM, McLachlan RI, Burger HG, et al: Inhibin-related proteins in the male. In: Burger H, de Kretser D, eds. The testis, 2nd ed. New York: Raven, 1989:231–254.
19. Matsumoto AM, Karpas AE, Bremner W: Chronic human chorionic gonadotropin-administration in normal men: Evidence that follicle-stimulating hormone is necessary for the maintenance of quantitatively normal spermatogenesis in man. J Clin Endocrinol Metab 1986; 62:1184–1192.
20. Lee W, Mason AJ, Schwall R, et al: Secretion of activin by interstitial cells in the testis. Science 1989; 243:396–398.
21. Micic S, Dotlic R, Ilic V, et al: Hormone profile in hyperprolactinemic in fertile men. Arch Androl 1985; 15:123–128.
22. Bain J, Langevin R, D'Costa M, et al: Serum pituitary and steroid hormone levels in the adult male: one value is as good as the mean of three. Fertil Steril 1988; 49:123–126.
23. Dahl KD, Stone MP: FSH isoforms, radioimmunoassays, bioassays, and their significance. J Androl 1992; 13:11–22.
24. Pardridge WM, Landaw EM: Testosterone transport in brain: Primary role of plasma protein-bound hormone. Am J Physiol 1985; 249:E534–542.
25. Toublanc JE, Canlorbe P, Job JC: Evaluation of Leydig-cell function in normal prepubertal and pubertal boys. J Steroid Biochem 1975; 6:95–99.
26. Wollesen F, Swerdloff RS, Odell WD: LH and FSH responses to leuteinizing-releasing hormone in normal, adult, human males. Metabolism 1976; 28:845–863.
27. Synder PJ, Rudenstein RS, Gardner DF, et al: Repetitive infusion of gonadotropin-releasing hormone distinguishes hypothalamic from pituitary hypogonadism. J Clin Endocrinol Metab 1979; 48:864–868.
28. Harman SM, Tsitouras PD, Costa PT, et al: Evaluation of pituitary gonadotropic function in men: value of luteinizing hormone-releasing hormone response versus basal luteinizing hormone level for discrimination of diagnosis. J Clin Endocrinol Metab 1982; 54:196–200.
29. Kallmann FJ, Schoenfeld WA, Barrerra SE: The genetic aspects of primary eunuchoidism. Am J Ment Defic 1944; 48:203–236.
30. Santen RJ, Paulsen CA: Hypogonadotropic eunuchoidism. I. Clinical study of the mode of inheritance. J Clin Endocrinol Metab 1973; 36:47–54.
31. Lieblich JM, Rogol AD, White BJ, et al: Syndrome of anosmia with hypogonadotropic hypogonadism (Kallmann syndrome). Clinical and laboratory studies in 23 cases. Am J Med 1982; 73:506–519.

32. Bell J, Spitz I, Slonim A, et al: Heterogeneity of gonadotropin response to LHRH in hypogonadotropic hypogonadism. J Clin Endocrinol Metab 1973; 36:791–794.
33. Dickerman Z, Prager-Lewin R, Laron Z: The effect of repeated injections of synthetic luteinizing hormone-releasing hormone on the response of plasma luteinizing hormone and follicle-stimulating hormone in young hypogonadotropic-hypogonadal patients. Fertil Steril 1976; 27:162–166.
34. Rowe RC, Schroeder M-L, Faiman C: Testosterone-induced fertility in a patient with previously untreated Kallmann's syndrome. Fertil Steril 1983; 40:400–401.
35. Santen RJ, Paulsen CA: Hypogonadotropic eunuchoidism. II. Gonadal responsiveness to exogenous gonadotropins. J Clin Endocrinol Metab 1973; 36:55–63.
36. Baranetsky NG, Carlson HE: Persistence of spermatogenesis in hypogonadotropic hypogonadism treated with testosterone. Fertil Steril 1980; 34:477–482.
37. Shargil AA: Treatment of idiopathic hypogonadotropic hypogonadism in men with luteinizing hormone-releasing hormone: a comparison of treatment with daily injections and with the pulsatile infusion pump. Fertil Steril 1987; 47:492–501.
38. Liu L, Banks SM, Barnes KM, et al: Two-year comparison of testicular responses to pulsatile gonadotropin-releasing hormone and exogenous gonadotropins from the inception of therapy in men with isolated hypogonadotropic hypogonadism. J Clin Endocrinol Metab 1988; 67:1140–1145.
39. Burris AS, Rodbard HW, Winters SJ, et al: Gonadotropin therapy in men with isolated hypogonadotropic hypogonadism: The response to human chorionic gonadotropin is predicted by initial testicular size. J Clin Endocrinol Metab 1988; 66:1144–1151.
40. Ley SB, Leonard JM: Male hypogonadotropic hypogonadism: Factors influencing response to human chorionic gonadotropin and human menopausal gonadotropin, including prior exogenous androgens. J Clin Endocrinol Metab 1985; 61:746–752.
41. Burger HG, Baker HWG: Therapeutic considerations and results of gonadotropin treatment in male hypogonadotropic hypogonadism. Ann NY Acad Sci 1984; 483:447–453.
42. Finkel DM, Phillips JL, Snyder PJ: Stimulation of spermatogenesis by gonadotropins in men with hypogonadotropic hypogonadism. N Engl J Med 1985; 313:651–655.
43. Morris DV, Adeniyi-Jones R, Wheeler M: The treatment of hypogonadotropic hypogonadism in men by the pulsatile infusion of leutinizing hormone-releasing hormone. Clin Endocrinol 1984; 21:189–200.
44. Carter JN, Tyson JE, Tolis G, et al: Prolactin-secreting tumors and hypogonadism in 22 men. N Engl J Med 1978; 299:847–852.
45. Spark RF, O'Reilly G, Bergland R, et al: Hyperprolactinemia in males with and without pituitary macroadenomas. Lancet 1982; 2:129–131.
46. Jones LA, Lipshultz LI: Hyperprolactinemia: Its role in male infertility. J Urol 1992; 147:455A.
47. Danutra V, Harper ME, Boyns AK, et al: The effect of certain stilbestrol analogues on plasma prolactin and testosterone in the rat. J Endocrinol 1973; 57:207–211.
48. David JL: Lowering prolactin level in a hyperprolacinemic man. Responses of luteinizing hormone, follicle-stimulating hormone, and testosterone. Arch Intern Med 1982; 142:146–148.
49. Segal S, Polishuk WZ, Ben-David M: Hyperprolactinemic male infertility. Fertil Steril 1976; 27:1425–1427.
50. Murray FT, Cameron DF, Ketchum C: Return of gonadal function in men with prolactin-secreting pituitary tumors. J Clin Endocrinol Metab 1984; 59:79–85.
51. Aiman J, Griffin JE, Gazak JM, Wilson JD, MacDonald PC: Androgen insensitivity as a cause of infertility in otherwise normal men. N Engl J Med 1979; 300:223–227.
52. Griffin JE, Wilson JD: The syndromes of androgen resistance. N Engl J Med 1980; 302:198–209.
53. Aiman J, Griffin JE: The frequency of androgen

receptor deficiency in infertile men. J Clin Endocrinol Metab 1982; 54:725–732.

54. Bonaccorsi AC, Adler I, Figueiredo JG: Male infertility due to congenital adrenal hyperplasia: Testicular biopsy findings, hormonal evaluation, and therapeutic results in three patients. Fertil Steril 1987; 47:664–670.
55. Urban MD, Lee PA, Migeon CJ: Adult height and fertility in men with congenital virilizing adrenal hyperplasia. N Engl J Med 1978; 299:1392–1396.
56. Rothman CM, Sims CA, Stotts CL: Sertoli cell only syndrome 1982. Fertil Steril 1982; 38:388–390.
57. Klinefelter HF Jr, Reifenstein EC Jr, Albright F: Syndrome characterized by gynecomastia, aspermatogenesis without A-Leydigism, and increased excretion of follicle-stimulating hormone. J Clin Endocrinol Metab 1942; 2:615–627.
58. Paulsen CA, Gordon DL, Carpenter KW, et al: Klinefelter's syndrome and its variants: A hormonal and chromosomal study. Recent Prog Horm Res 1968; 24:321–363.
59. Court-Brown WM: Human population cytogenetics. New York: Wiley, 1967.
60. Werner CA: Mumps orchitis and testicular atrophy. I Occurrence. Ann Intern Med 1950; 32:1066–1074.
61. Riggs S, Sanford JP: Viral orchitis. N Engl J Med 1962; 266:990–995.
62. Lorioux DL, Menard R, Taylor A, et al: Spironolactone and endocrine dysfunction. Ann Intern Med 1976; 85:630–636.
63. Neumann F, van Berswordt-Wallrabe R, Elger W, et al: Aspects of androgen-dependent events as studied by antiandrogens. Recent Prog Horm Res 1970; 26:337–410.
64. Van Thiel DH, Gavaler JS, Smith WI Jr, et al: Hypothalamic–pituitary–gonadal dysfunction in men using cimetidine. N Engl J Med 1979; 300:1012–1015.
65. Rajfer J, Sikka SC, Rivera F, et al: Mechanism of inhibition of human testicular steroidogenesis by oral ketoconazole. J Clin Endocrinol Metab 1986; 63:1193–1198.
66. Boyden TW, Silvert MA, Pamenter RW: Chronic ethanol feeding impairs human chorionic gonadotropin-stimulated testicular testosterone responses of dogs. Biol Reprod 1982; 27:652–657.
67. Holdsworth S, Atkins RC, de Kretser D: The pituitary-testicular axis in men with chronic renal failure. N Engl J Med 1977; 296: 1245–1249.
68. Chopp RT, Mendez R: Sexual function and hormonal abnormalities in uremic men on chronic dialysis and after renal transplantation. Fertil Steril 1978; 29:661–666.
69. Chopra IJ, Tulchinsky D, Greenway FL: Estrogen-androgen imbalance in hepatic cirrhosis. Studies in 13 male patients. Ann Intern Med 1973; 79:198–203.
70. Olambiwonnu NO, Penny R, Frasier SD: Sexual maturation in subjects with sickle cell anemia: Studies of serum gonadotropin concentration, height, weight, and skeletal age. J Pediatr 1975; 87:459–464.
71. Handelsman DJ, Yue DK, Turtle JR: Hypogonadism and massive testicular infiltration due to amyloidosis. J Urol 1983; 129:610–612.
72. Kidd GS, Glass AR, Vigersky RA: The hypothalamic–pituitary–testicular axis in thyrotoxicosis. J Clin Endocrinol Metab 1979; 48:798–802.
73. Takeda R, Ueda M: Pituitary-gonadal function in male patients with myotonic dystrophy-serum luteinizing hormone, follicle stimulating hormone and testosterone levels and histological damage of the testis. Acta Endocrinol 1977; 84:382–389.
74. Mozaffarian GA, Higley M, Paulsen CA: Clinical studies in an adult male patient with "isolated follicle stimulating hormone (FSH) deficiency." J Androl 1983; 4:393–398.
75. Greenberg SH, Lipshultz LI, Wein AJ: Experience with 425 subfertile male patients. J Urol 1978; 119:507–510.
76. Rodriguez-Rigau LJ, Weiss DB, Zukerman Z, Grotjan HE, Smith KD, Steinberger E: A possible mechanism for the detrimental effect of varicocele on testicular function in man. Fertil Steril 1978; 30:577–585.
77. Dubin L, Amelar RD: Varicocelectomy: 986

cases in a twelve-year study. Urology 1977; 10:446–449.
78. Marks JL, McMahon R, Lipshultz LI: Predictive parameters of successful varicocele repair. J Urol 1986; 136:609–612.
79. Snyder PJ, Lawrence DA: Treatments of male hypogonadism with testosterone enanthate. J Clin Endocrinol Metab 1980; 51:1335–1339.

ANNOTATED BIBLIOGRAPHY

Liu L, Banks SM, Barnes KM, Sherins RJ: Two-year comparison of testicular responses to pulsatile gonadotropin-releasing hormone and exogenous gonadotropins from the inception of therapy in men with isolated hypogonadotropic hypogonadism. J Clin Endocrinol Metab 1988; 67:1140.

This study compares the efficacy of pulsatile GnRH to combination hCG/hMG therapy for the treatment of isolated hypogonadotropic hypogonadism. Five men received GnRH and 11 received hCG/hMG for 2 years. GnRH-treated men had a normal but lower testosterone level and a significantly higher FSH level. Estradiol levels were slightly elevated but no different between groups. Testicular size increased more than four-fold in both groups. Sperm production began slightly earlier in the GnRH group. However, after 2 years 40% of GnRH-treated men and 80% of hCG/hMG-treated men produced sperm. The sperm concentrations were similar in both groups. The authors conclude that GnRH therapy does not provide any significant advantage over the less cumbersome management with hCG/hMG.

Murray FT, Cameron DF, Ketchum C: Return of gonadal function in men with prolactin-secreting pituitary tumors. J Clin Endocrinol Metab 1984; 59:79.

This article reviews the baseline status and response to treatment of the reproductive function of 10 men with prolactin-secreting pituitary adenomas. Baseline status revealed signs of hypogonadism including elevated LH, reduced testosterone, and reduced nocturnal penile tumescence. Semen analysis revealed diffuse abnormalities of all parameters in the 5 patients studied. Patients were treated with radiation, surgery, and/or bromocriptine. Six of eight patients followed had normalization of semen prolactin. Four of these patients had normalization of serum testosterone levels and five had normalization of nocturnal penile tumescence. Only two patients had normal semen analysis during follow-up. Their conclusion was that treatment of prolactin-secreting tumors may restore normal hormonal function but reproductive capacity does not always improve.

Snyder PJ, Lawrence DA: Treatment of male hypogonadism with testosterone enanthate. J Clin Endocrinol Metab 1980; 51:1335.

Testosterone replacement therapy is indicated for the treatment of hypogonadal men. Intramuscular administration of testosterone esters is preferred to oral administration because of greater effectiveness and lower toxicity. This article compares four different regimens of testosterone enanthate therapy for men with primary hypogonadism. (Patients received 100 mg q week, 200 mg q 2 weeks, 300 mg q 3 weeks and 400 mg q 4 weeks.) Response was measured using serum LH, FSH, and testosterone levels.

The highest average testosterone level was in the 100 mg q week group. LH was adequately suppressed in all but the 400 mg q 4 week group. The authors concluded that 200 mg q 2 weeks or 300 mg q 3 weeks were the best regimens based on testosterone levels, LH suppression, and convenience for patient.

Urban MD, Lee PA, Migeon CJ: Adult height and fertility in men with congenital virilizing adrenal hyperplasia. N Engl J Med 1978; 299:1392.

Congenital adrenal hyperplasia (CAH) may adversely affect male fertility through feedback inhibition of normal pituitary function by adrenal secretion of androgenic steroidal precursors. This review of 20 men with CAH demonstrates that fertility can be preserved or restored in these men. Two patients who had never received treatment had fathered three children. Unfortunately, semen analyses could not be obtained since both had undergone a vasectomy. Two of three patients off of therapy had documented paternity and all three had normal semen analyses. Of the 15 treated men, 10 had reproduced and 6 of 8 patients had a normal semen analysis. The authors conclude that men with CAH may be fertile without treatment and have an excellent prognosis with treatment.

30

Infections and Infertility: Significance and Treatment

Richard E. Berger
Ivan Rothman

While genital infection is an important cause of infertility in veterinary medicine[1] its role in humans is less clear. The presence of certain known lower tract pathogens has not necessarily been associated with adverse qualities in semen and sperm. Researchers have also not yet been able to consistently and accurately relate inflammation from infection in the male lower genital tract. Furthermore, evidence exists that the use of antibiotics to treat male infertility may itself have adverse effects on sperm quality.

While the role of seminal infection in male infertility is unclear, seminal inflammation or pyospermia has more clearly been associated with decreased male fertility. We will present the evidence for and against infection as inflammation. We will also discuss methods of evaluation and treatment of male lower genital tract inflammation in the context of known syndromes of symptomatic male genital infection.

Inflammation and Infertility

Genital infection with pathogenic organisms can lead to leukocytosis in the seminal fluid and expressed prostatic secretions (EPS). It is not clear whether infection is always the cause of such inflammation.[2,3] Most studies assume that white blood cells in the semen come from the prostate; however, leukocytosis could also come from the urethra, prostate, seminal vesicles, vas deferens, or epididymis. Few studies have attempted to localize the inflammation. Men with pyospermia may therefore represent a very heterogeneous group.

Quantification of leukocytes in semen can be inaccurate if care is not taken to differentiate leukocytes from the other round cells in the semen. Immature sperm can easily be confused with lymphocytes. There have been a number of methods developed to differentiate leukocytes from immature sperm.[4–7] Couture et al.[4] used a Brian–Leishman stain to differentiate

Management of Impotence and Infertility, edited by Douglas Whitehead and Harris Nagler,

white blood cells from immature sperm. Peroxidase staining has been used to identify leukocyte peroxidase and differentiate granulocytes from nonseparated spermatocytes.[5]

The most promising technique in this area has been the recent development of monoclonal antibodies to different leukocyte subsets. Wolff et al.[8] found that patients with high concentrations of monocytes and macrophages had significantly reduced ejaculate volume. He also found that patients with high numbers of T lymphocytes had decreased sperm velocity. El et al.,[9] however, found no lymphocytes in a group of infertile men. Barratt et al.[10] found both suppressor/cytotoxic and helper/inducer lymphocytes as well as B lymphocytes in many control (normal) men. Some investigators have, however, suggested that there also could be cross-reactivity of immature sperm with monoclonal antibodies supposedly specific for leukocytes.[11]

Keeping these methodological problems in mind, let us review the role of male lower genital tract inflammation and infection in male factor infertility. Berger et al.[12] did semen and 4-glass urine cultures in men with symptomatic prostatitis and idiopathic infertility, and in normal controls. Culture results among the groups did not differ significantly, although the men with idiopathic prostatitis had more leukocytes in EPS and semen. Cumming et al.[13] found that granulocyte elastase levels in semen, which correlate with inflammation, did not correlate with anaerobic or aerobic bacterial growth from the seminal plasma of infertile men. Hillier et al.[14] reported that cultures of semen samples for aerobes, anaerobes, and mycoplasmas had no correlation with any of the following results: quantitative semen analyses (SFA), numbers of white blood cells, or *in vitro* hamster penetration test (SPA) values. Some investigators have found that there is an inverse relation between the number of leukocytes and the concentration of zinc in the semen of men with bacterial prostatitis and in men with idiopathic prostatitis.[15–17] They have inferred that men with idiopathic prostatitis also have infection. However, this inference has not been proven. Guilatt-Rosso et al.[18] found a reduction and pregnancy rate per cycle in *in vitro* fertilization (IVF) with increasing amounts of any bacteria in the semen. That study, however, did not address the primary cause of infertility in the couples. On the other hand, Close et al.[19] found no relationship of inflammation to infection. They did find a positive association between the number of WBCs per 100 sperm and subjects' level of use of both cigarettes and alcohol. Cigarette smoking was also related to poor hamster sperm penetration assays. Perhaps toxic effects from substances in the genitourinary tract could manifest itself as seminal inflammation.

Under certain conditions, sperm themselves may be capable of attracting leukocytes in semen without the presence of infection. Electron microscopy by Hughes et al.[20] on semen specimens obtained from 144 infertile men demonstrated that 57 men (or 40%) had large numbers of leukocytes in their semen. White blood cells from 35 of these 57 men contained bacteria; those of the remaining 22 men contained the only phagocytized spermatozoa. Pathogenic bacteria were isolated from only two men in each group. Two authors[21,22] found normal spermatozoa interacted with serum or plasma to generate C5A, a potent chemotactic factor derived from the fifth component of the compliment. Koehler et al.[23] noted that sperm phagocytosis was common in the semen of infertile men. Pandya and Cohen[24] found spermatozoa created leukocytosis in cervical

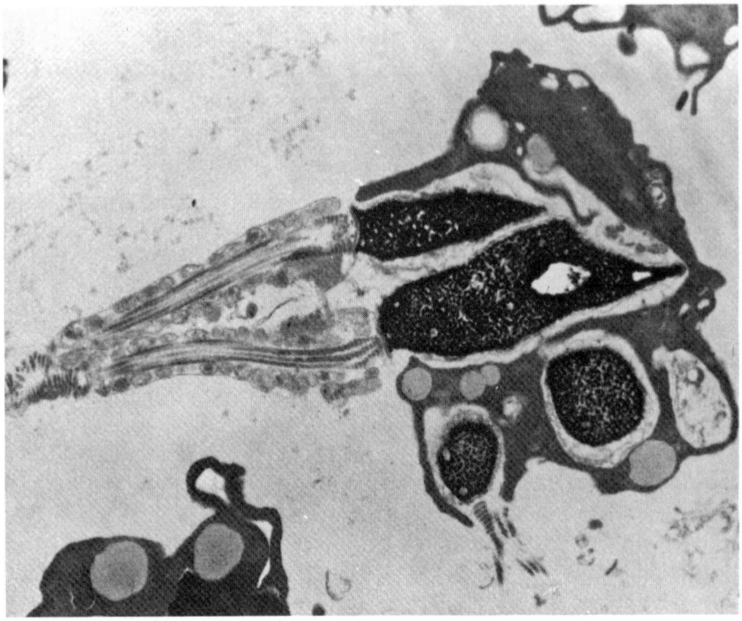

Figure 30-1 Probable polymorphonuclear leukocyte with ingested sperm heads and phagsome communicating with external milieu.

mucous after artificial insemination (Figure 30-1).

Inflammation may have an adverse effect on sperm function. Berger et al.[25] found abnormal sperm function (as measured by SPA results) to be related very highly to the number of leukocytes in semen. The risk of having an abnormal SPA was 8.7 times higher in infertile men with at least one leukocyte per 100 sperm as compared with those with less than one leukocyte per 100 sperm. They found no correlation between the number of seminal leukocytes and the results of semen cultures. Shy et al.[26] defined pyospermia as the presence of six or more white blood cells per 100 sperm. They found that 65% of the couples where the male did not have pyospermia reported pregnancies after 4 or more years (Figure 30-2). In this same time period only 17% of couples where men did have more than six white blood cells per 100 sperm had achieved pregnancies. The presence of pyospermia was associated with continued infertility as compared to those without white blood cells.

Maruyama et al.[27] found that adding white cells to the semen of fertile donors decreased sperm penetration rates (Figure 30-3). Supernatants of white blood cells also decrease SPA scores. When white cells were removed by physical means, the SPA scores were improved. Berger et al.[12] found that the number of white blood cells was inversely related to count and motility (Figure 30-4). These findings were confirmed by Wolff et al.[28] who also found that the presence of high numbers of T lymphocytes in seminal plasma was related to decreased sperm velocity. They also found higher numbers of granulocytes, monocytes, macrophages, and lymphocytes in infertile men compared to controls (Figure 30-5).

Figure 30-2 Three-year cumulative pregnancy percents according to white blood cells (WBCs) per 100 spermatozoa for men from infertile couples ($n = 74$) without female infertility factor.

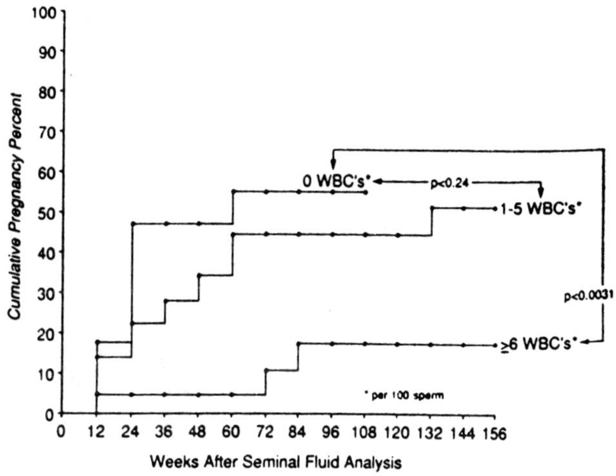

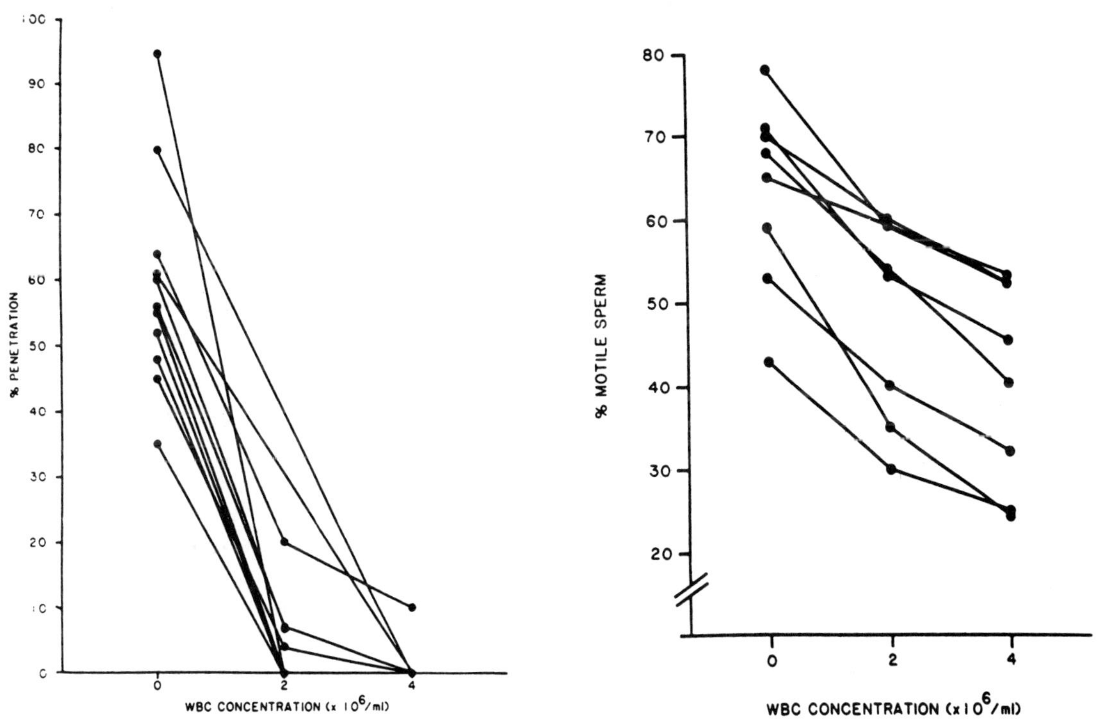

Figure 30-3 (a) The effect of white blood cell addition prior to preincubation on the percentage of eggs prepared by spermatosoa from individual serem smples. (b) The percentage of motile spermatozoa following preincubation with prepared white blood cells.

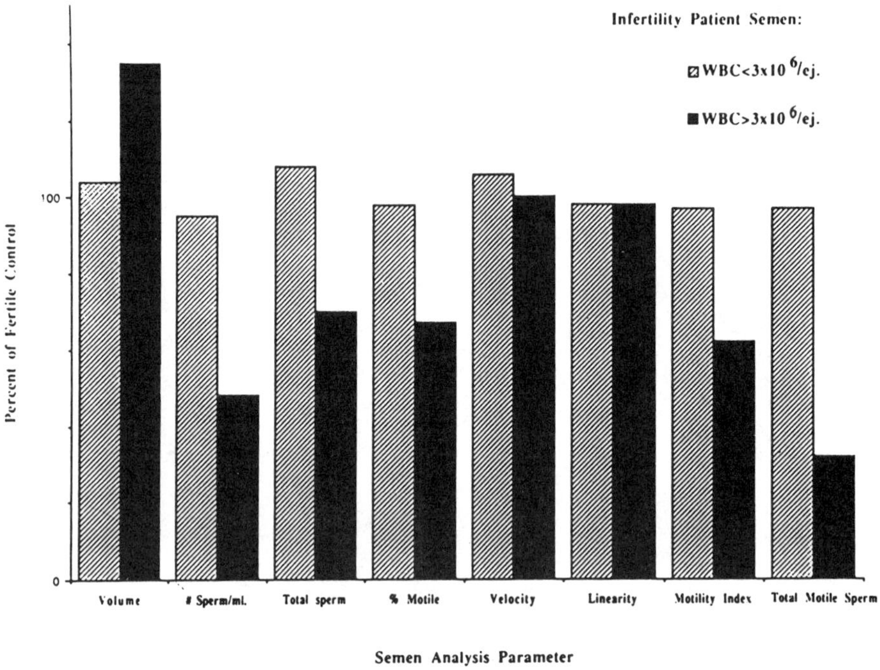

Figure 30-4 Reduction of semen parameters in infertility patients with high total WBC per ejaculate. Group medians of semen paraniters in infertility patients with high numbers (>3 × 10^4 WBC/ejaculate; $n = 44$) and low numbers (<3 × 10^6 WBC/ejaculate; $n = 135$). Of WBC are expressed as percent of the respective medians in the fertile control group ($n = 15$). WBC were identified by the MAb anti-tile-k.

Other researchers have suggested chemical and vascular causes for lower tract inflammation as well. Persson et al.[29] suggested that high concentrations of uridine and xanthine in seminal plasma could drive these components to leave solution and crystallize. They hypothesized that this could constitute the first step in the development of forms of nonbacterial prostatitis.

Gattauccio et al.[30] found a correlation between the presence of a varicocele and genital inflammation. They suggested that this inflammation could be a result of anoxic inflammation of the prostate caused by venous congestion in the pelvis.

To circumvent some of the problems in identifying leukocytes histologically, some authors have tried to use leukocyte products such as granulocyte elastase in semen to identity inflammation. Wolff et al.[28] found that high levels of granulocyte elastase correlated significantly with number of white blood cells, total sperm number, and total motile sperm number. Jochum et al.[31] also found seminal plasma elastase to be correlated with the number of bacteria on stained semen samples and on number of

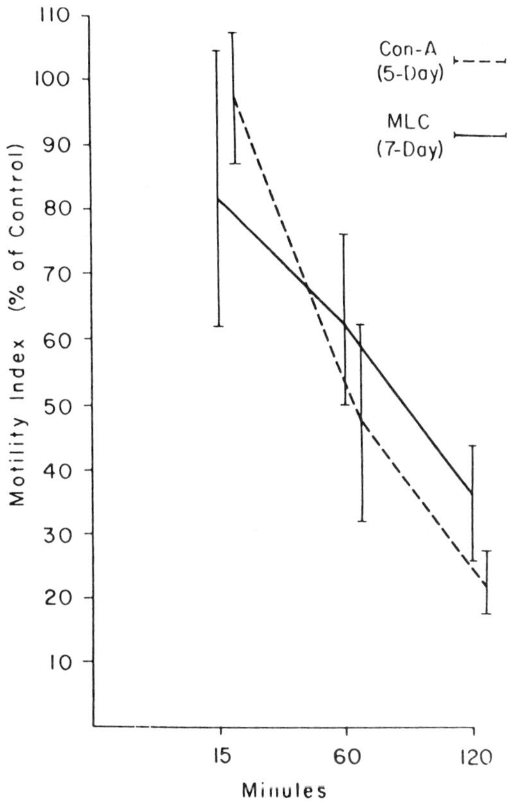

Figure 30-5 The effect of Con A and MLC-acativated lymphocyte supernatants on the index of sperm mobility.

round cells in the semen suggests a correlation of inflammation and infection.

Infertility and Asymptomatic Infection

Symptomatic infections such as orchitis and epididymitis are well defined and important causes of infertility. The role of asymptomatic infection is far less clear. Bacteria could effect semen quality by utilizing important substances, inducing phagocytosis, stimulating inflammation and causing antibodies, decreasing secretory function of the accessory sex glands, or damaging the gonads or adenexa.[32]

Unfortunately, studies have often used the presence of seminal inflammation instead of positive culture to document infection. Localization of both seminal leukocytes and bacteria to parts of the genital tract (such as are used in studies of symptomatic chronic bacterial prostatitis) are also frequently lacking. Investigators have inferred the presence of prostatic infection from biochemical abnormalities in semen or EPS such as are found in bacterial prostatitis. However, the actual relationship of such biochemical abnormalities to asymptomatic seminal colonization, inflammation, and fertility has been poorly defined.

Finally, few studies on the roles of infections and inflammation on male infertility have been well controlled. Issues of time, cost, and the difficulty of analyzing data from multiple semen specimens over time frequently force investigators to use a single semen specimen to classify men as cases or controls. Single semen specimens are probably unreliable indicators of fertility.

Several studies have tried to relate male lower genital tract asymptomatic colonization by coliform bacteria to male infertility. Harrison and Johnson[33] found gram-negative bacteria in the semen in 29 of 100 men with abnormal semen analysis but in none of the men with normal semen analysis. Toth and Lesser[34] found *Escherichia coli* in 2% of infertile men with no past history of genitourinary infection and 11% of infertile men with a history of prostatitis or urethritis. They were unable to isolate *E. coli* from any of their 30 control subjects.

Ulstein et al.[35] examined age-matched fertile and infertile men with four glass localization cultures. Gram-negative bacteria were found only in those men with abnormal SFA results. However, Berger et al.[12] found no difference in coliform colonization between infertile men and controls. Increased numbers of leukocytes have been reported in the semen of men who have coliforms present.[36,37] However, the methods that they used did not necessarily differentiate mature forms of leukocytes from immature sperm. Comhaire et al.[38] found that acid phosphatase was decreased in the semen of men with coliform bacteria. *E. coli*, when added to sperm in quantities of 10^7 or greater, can also decrease motility. A motility decreasing factor has been isolated from *E. coli* filtrates.[39,40] In summary, the role of coliform colonization as a cause of infertility is not clear.

Studies looking at gram-positive commensal organisms have not found them to be associated with male infertility.[41–44] However, one study found different gram-positive organisms in the second portions of split ejaculates than they did the first portions.[45] Findings like this suggesting that bacteria may originate from different portions of the genitourinary tract, or different antibacterial factors may be present in different parts of the split ejaculate. Morton[46] found the highest seminal white counts in men with past histories of genital infections. Bacterial counts may actually increase as semen is diluted. This is possibly due to an antimicrobial effect of the zinc on bacterial growth in antibacterial factors in semen.[47] It is even possible that increased bacterial counts may actually be due to decreased bacteriostatic effect of semen, representing accessory gland dysfunction rather than actual infection. Although there seems to be little evidence relating seminal inflammation to present infection, there is, perhaps, a relationship to infection in the past.

Infertility and Ureaplasma Urealyticum

While the role *U. urealyticum* plays in both male and female infertility has received much attention in the scientific literature, it is still poorly defined. As a result of a series of well-conceived and well-executed studies *U. urealyticum* has been strongly implicated as a cause of nongonococcal urethritis. *U. urealyticum* has been implicated as a causative factor in male infertility for reasons less rigorously attained. The support comes from three types of results obtained in studies of infection and infertility. First, some studies have been shown abnormal semen analysis to be more common among culture-positive infertile men than among culture-negative ones. Case-control studies, although poorly matched, have shown higher frequencies of isolation of *urealyticum* in infertile men than in controls. Finally, some treatment studies have shown the use of antibiotics to which *Ureaplasma* are sensitive has improved the semen analyses or fertility of cases.

It is worth noting the virtues of the body of research that has implicated *U. urealyticum* as a cause of urethritis. These include epidemiological studies with cases and controls carefully matched with respect to important confounding variables (i.e., relationship to sexual activity, past STDs), the use of quantitative cultures, the definition of a subset of urethritis not associated with pathogens such as *C. trachomatis*, experimental inoculation, and controlled therapeutic trials comparing antibiotics with and without activity against *Ureaplasma.* Most of these methods have yet to be applied to the study of the role of *Ureaplasma* in male infertility.

At present it is virtually impossible to clinically assess the role of a positive *Ureaplasma* culture in any individual case of urethritis or infertility. *Ureaplasma* is very common in the sexually active population. The presence of *Ureaplasma* in a symptomatic or asymptomatic man is directly proportional to his number of sexual partners. In patients with three to five partners, specimens in 40% of men and 70% of women will contain *Ureaplasma.*[48]

Changes in the semen analyses of men with *Ureaplasma* infection have been reported by several authors. Toth et al.[49] found fuzzy and coiled tails in 70% of men colonized with *Ureaplasma* and 19% of men not colonized. They found more men with *Ureaplasma* had a history of genital infection. They did not, however, differentiate between the role of *Ureaplasma* and the role of past infection. Using electron microscopy, Fowlkes et al.[50] found increased numbers of sperm with coiled tails in *Ureaplasma*-positive men and was able to identify *Ureaplasma* in the sperm head and midpiece. He also found decreased semen volume, decreased sperm counts, poor morphology, and decreased motility in culture positive patients. Grossgebauer and Hennig[51] demonstrated *Ureaplasma* in the heads of spermatozoa in a man with symptoms of urethritis. Swensen et al.[52] found decreased sperm motility at 3 hours in *Ureaplasma*-positive patients.

Valvo et al.[53] found the semen pH to be greater in the *Ureaplasma*-positive than in *Ureaplasma*-negative patients possibly because of the urease enzyme present in *Ureaplasma.* They also found greater numbers of white cells in *Ureaplasma*-positive men than negative. However, they found no other semen analysis difference between culture-positive and culture-negative men. With antibiotic treatment, pH levels and the number of white blood cells in semen decreased. Other investigators have found no differences in the semen analyses of culture positive and culture negative men.[54,55] Berger et al.[56] found no differences in the rate of recovery of *U. urealyticum* in men with normal or abnormal sperm function as measured by the *in vitro* hamster assay.[56] Shalhoub et al.[57] found no difference in the SFA, SPA, or bovine cervical mucous penetration in *Ureaplasma*-positive and negative men. Hargreave et al.[81] found no association with *Ureaplasma* culture and agglutinating sperm antibodies. On the other hand, Busolo and Zanchetta[58] showed that *U. urealyticum* produces a factor that hinders the penetration of zona free hamster oocytes by sperm. Guillet-Rosso[14] found that many positive semen cultures (including *Ureaplasma*) seem to have a negative effect on the results of *in vitro* fertilization.

Studies using case-control methodology have found an association between the presence of *U. urealyticum* in the male lower genital tract and infertility. Friberg and Knarpe[59] recovered *U. urealyticum* in 81% of men and 91% of women in infertile couples, and 22% of pregnant women and 20% of their male partners. Stray-Pedersen et al.[60] confirmed this finding. However, de Louvois et al.[61] found no difference in the incidence of *Ureaplasma* colonization between infertile men and controls. No studies have compared *U. urealyticum* isolation rates among fertile and infertile subjects while adjusting or controlling for sexual experience, antibiotic usage, and other potential confounders.

Cassell et al.[62] did a multivariable risk analysis among infertile couples. Male factor infertility was defined either by having two or more subfertile semen analyses, or by a history of chronic prostatitis. However, chronic prostatitis was not defined. They found ureaplasma isolation from the female to be highly correlated with a diagnosis of male factor infertility. *Ureaplasma* colonization was inversely correlated with social economic classes. A significantly higher percentage (74%) of cervical infection was found in those couples with a diagnosis of male factor infertility than in any other diagnosis. Eighty-seven percent of couples who had a male factor also had other factors related to infertility.

Some trials of antibiotics aiming to eradicate *U. urealyticum* in infertile couples have shown a positive effect on treatment of infertility, while others have not. Most, however, employed suboptimal methods. They were not placebo controlled, not randomized, or involved only a short duration of therapy. For example, Toth et al.[63] followed patients for 3 years after treatment with doxycycline. Pregnancy occurred in 60% of couples in whom *Ureaplasma* had been eradicated and in 5% of those in whom it persisted. These researchers postulated (but did not document) that the isolation of *Ureaplasma* after treatment could be attributed to doxycycline resistance. They also did not address whether other factors in the male tract possibly related to fertility and persistence after treatment could be involved in his results.

U. urealyticum is a known pathogen of the male urethra and probably does cause urethritis. More studies are needed utilizing the latest techniques in semen analysis, semen histology, and epidemiology to determine what, if any, role *Ureaplasma* plays in male infertility.

Infertility and Chlamydia Trachomatis

Chlamydia trachomatis is a sexually transmitted organism. It causes cervicitis and salpingitis in women, and urethritis, prostatitis, and epididymitis in males. Since chlamydial urethritis is quite common, it is possible that *Chlamydia* could be a common cause of male infertility. *Chlamydia* most certainly leads to many couples' infertility via salpingitis and tubal obstruction in women. There is also little doubt that *Chlamydia trachomatis* infection, by causing obstructive epididymitis, may lead to azoospermia and male infertility. However, in men presenting with infertility, it appears that acute *Chlamydia* infection is extremely rare.

Probably less than 1% of men with urethral infections get epididymal infections. Hellstrom et al.[64], Berger et al.[65], Bennett et al.,[66] and Ruijs et al.[67] all failed to find significant chlamydial infection in populations of infertile males. Soffer et al.[68] actually found *Chlamydia* to be more frequent in normal men than men with semen analysis abnormalities.

It appears that *Chlamydia trachomatis* may infect the prostate as well as the epididymis. If true, this type of infection could have long-term effects on prostate function, and possibly prostate inflammation as well. In men with the symptoms of prostatitis and urethritis, Poletti et al.[69] found that *Chlamydia* could be isolated to the prostate by transrectal aspiration in 10 of 33 men. However, Suominen et al.[70] found significantly higher seminal fluid anti-*Chlamydia* IgA levels in infertile men (51.1%) than in fertile men (23.2%). Wolff et al.[71] found granulocyte elastase to be increased in men with *Chlamydia trachomatis* antibody, but did not do cultures for *Chlamydia*. At this time, however, it appears that most men with infertility and seminal inflammation either with symptomatic or asymptomatic prostatitis do not have active *Chlamydia* infection.

Sperm Autoimmunity and Infection

Vasectomy and vasal or epididymal obstruction have been shown to lead to the generation of antisperm antibodies.[72,73] Many authors have found sperm directed autoantibodies to be related to male infertility.[74–77] These antibodies may be found in blood as IgG or IgM, or can be found in semen as locally produced secretory IgA.

Since infection of the vas and epididymis may cause obstruction, it is possible that such obstruction may be related to subsequent male infertility, even if found unilaterally. Close et al.[157] found sperm autoimmunity to be more common in men who had been exposed to *C. trachomatis* (which does cause epididymitis) (Table 30-1). Ligation of one vas deferens in the mouse may produce autoimmunity and subsequent infertility.[78] Bandhauer and Marberger[79] found that 9 of 48 men with unilateral epididymitis subsequently developed sperm antibodies. Hendry et al.[80] found that among 32 patients with unilateral epididymal obstruction, 81% had antibodies to sperm. They estimated that 37% of infertile males with antisperm antibodies have evidence of vassal or epididymal obstruction.

Soffcr ct al.[68] found increased antisperm antibody activity in men with semen culture positive to *Ureaplasma* or to any other bacteria. On the other hand, Hargreave et al.[81] found that *Ureaplasma* colonization in males was unrelated to the presence of sperm autoimmunity. Micic[82] found no significant relationship between genitourinary tract infection, inflammation, and sperm autoimmunity. Hargreave et al.[83] found no difference between fertile men and men attending an STD clinic in the prevalence of sperm antibodies. On the other hand, Witkin and Toth[84] found a higher incidence of sperm antibodies in prostatitis patients than in controls. Barratt[85] found that there was a preponderance of helper inducer T cells in the ejaculate of men with antibodies as opposed to suppressor/cytotoxic cells in men without antibodies.

There is clearly a relationship between vassal obstruction and development of antibodies in male infertility. We are unsure of how frequently this phenomenon occurs, or if it is treatable. We are also still unsure of exactly how sperm antigen–antibody complexes affect fertility. The relationship of prostatitis to sperm autoimmunity is even less clear.

Infertility and Nongonococcal Urethritis

Chlamydial infection nongonococcal urethritis (NGU) may cause infertility by spreading to cause epididymitis in the male and salpingitis in

Table 30-1 Correlations of Parameters of Male Fertility with Past Exposure to *C. trachomatis* in 270 Infertile Men[a]

	C. trachomatis— Antibody[b] Titer ≥ 16 (n = 16)	*C. trachomatis*— Antibody[b] Titer < 16 (n = 254)	p
History of NSU (%)	3/11 (27)	7/141 (5)	0.03
Median number of sex partners in lifetime	11.5 (n = 4)	3.0 (n = 74)	0.007
Number with agglutinating antibody [geometric (mean titer)] (%)	8/16 (1:21) (50%)	41/249 (1:25) (16%)	0.003

[a] From Close et al.[157]
[b] Micro-IF antibody titer ≥16 in IgM and/or IgG is considered seropositive.

the female. This syndrome therefore requires prompt diagnosis and treatment. The morbidity and complications of nongonococcal urethritis (NGU) are at least as great as that of gonococcal urethritis. Young men are prime candidates for contracting NGU, and it is probably the most common genitourinary infection in reproductive age men. The potentially most dangerous pathogen in NGU is *C. trachomatis,* which causes 25–60% of NGU.[86–88] *Chlamydia* can be isolated from the urethra in 25–60% of heterosexual men with NGU, 4–35% of men with gonorrhea, and 0–7% of men seen in STD clinics without symptoms of urethritis.[89] Asymptomatic infections occur in 50% of male contacts of women with cervical chlamydial infection.[90] Up to 80% of female sexual contacts of men with *C. trachomatis* will also have *C. trachomatis* isolated.

Between 20 and 50% of men with NGU may have infections with *Ureaplasma urealyticum.* As mentioned earlier, genital colonization with this organism in symptomatic or asymptomatic men is directly proportional to their number of previous sexual partners. Postgonococcal urethritis may develop in men who contract gonococcal urethritis and are treated with antibiotics to which only *Chlamydia* is sensitive.[91] Differential treatment studies have confirmed the role of *U. urealyticum* in these cases.[92] In another 20–30% of cases, the etiology of urethritis has not been determined.

Other factors associated with the development of NGU include the following. Smoking may be an independent risk factor for NGU.[93] Uncircumcised men are more likely to have NGU than circumcised men.[94] Finally, Hernandes et al.[95] found oral sex to be significantly associated with *Chlamydia*-negative, *Ureaplasma*-negative NGU.

The incubation period for NGU is 1 to 5 weeks, but longer incubations are possible. Symptoms usually include dysuria and discharge. The diagnosis of NGU requires demonstration of urethritis in exclusion of infection with *N. gonorrheae.* Men suspected of having urethritis should be examined after 4 hours of urinary continence. The finding on a gram stain of a urethral swab of four or more polymorphonuclear leukocytes (PMNs) per field in five fields under a 1000 power, oil immersion lens correlates with urethritis. Alternately, the presence of 15 or more PMNs in five random 400 power fields on spun first void urine sediment correlates with urethritis.[96,97] If urethral inflammation is highly suspected but initial exam is negative, the patient should be examined with a urethral swab before voiding in the morning.

Cultures for *C. trachomatis* should be employed when available. Cultures for *U. urealyticum* in the individual case are of no value except as a research tool due to the high rate of colonization in normal men who have been sexually active. Patterns of NGU epidemiology and antibiotic resistance are sure to change over time. For this reason, the reader is referred to the current Centers for Disease Control (CDC) recommendations for the treatment of NGU to find appropriate treatment options. Because of the potential for *C. trachomatis* to cause infertility in both men and women, men with pyospermia should be evaluated for urethritis and treated. Treatment of sexual partners in gonococcal and nongonococcal urethritis with the same antibiotic regimens is indicated to prevent recurrent disease and infection in the female.

Epididymitis, Orchitis, and Infertility

Epididymitis and orchitis are well documented causes of male infertility. The sexually transmitted pathogens *C. trachomatis* and *N. gonorrheae* are the most common causes of epididymitis in men of reproductive age. Although urethritis usually coexists with epididymitis in these men, men are usually unaware of any discharge.[98,99] One group isolated *Ureaplasma* from the epididymis of one 28-year-old man, suggesting that it too may also be a cause of epididymitis.[100]

Table 30-2 summarizes the relevant research into the causes of epididymitis. In older men, coliform infection also plays an important part. Epididymitis has been associated with infection bacteria such as *N. gonorrheae, C. trachomatis, U. urealyticum*, enterobacteriacae, and a number of mycobacteria.[148] Rarely members of the herpes virus groups and fungi have also been associated with epididymitis. Diagnosis of epididymitis is made by gram stain and culture of urethra to detect gonococcal and nongonococcal urethritis, and culture of mid-stream urine to detect bacteriuria. While relatively common in developed countries, epididymitis and its sequelae are even more common in developing countries. In places (such as parts of sub-Saharan Africa) where gonorrhea and *Chlamydia* infections often go untreated, epididymitis may be a leading cause of infertility.[101,102]

Epididymitis affects not only the epididymis but usually involves the testicle as well. This infection and resulting orchitis may lead to testicular atrophy. Wolin did testicular biopsies on men with epididymitis and found 20 of 28 to have decreased spermatogenesis and 9 of 28 to have testicular inflammation.[103] Nillson et al.[104] did aspiration biopsies on testicles of men with acute epididymitis and found that 16 of 20 showed inflammatory cells in the testicle. Subsequent testicular atrophy was in direct proportion to initial inflammation and occurred in two-thirds of men. Ludwig and Hasleberger[105] followed 46 patients with unilateral epididymitis from 8 days to 1 year. Two-thirds were found to have oligospermia, and 28% had long-term fertility abnormalities as reflected in semen analysis. Krishnan and Heal[106] found enlargement of the seminal vesicle on the side of epi-

Table 30-2 Etiology of Acute Epididymitis

Paper	Total No. Men	Age <35 (No./total) [%] GC (%)	Age <35 Ct (%)	Age <35 E. coli (%)	Age >35 (No./total) [%] GC (%)	Age >35 Ct (%)	Age >35 E. coli (%)
Berger et al, 1978	23	0/13 (0)	10/13 (77)	0/13 (0)	0/10 (0)	8/10 (80)	0.10 (0)
Berger et al, 1979	50	7/34 (21)	16/34 (47)	1/34 (3)	0/16 (0)	1/16 (6)	12/16 (75)
Berger et al, 1987	51	9/51 (18)	19/51 (37)	6/51 (12)[1]			
Hawkins et al, 1986	40	2/27 (19)	13/27 (48)	0/27 (0)	3/13 (23)	2/13 (15)	3/13 (23)
Scheibel et al, 1983	52	1/31 (3)	13/31 (42)	0/31 (0)	0/13 (0)	0/13 (0)	6/13 (46)
Kristensen et al, 1984	16	4/16 (25)	14/16 (88)				
Kojima et al, 1988	45	3/30 (10)	21/30 (70)	0/30 (0)	0/15 (0)	0/15 (0)	7/15 (47)
Grant et al, 1987	54	2/42 (5)	13/42 (31)	1/42 (2)	0/12 (0)	1/12 (8)	8/12 (67)
De Jong et al, 1988[2]	25	1/13 (8)	11/13 (85)	1/13 (8)	0/12 (0)	1/12 (8)	10/12 (23)
Melekos et al, 1988[3]	21		6/11 (55)	4/11 (36)		1/10 (10)	7/10 (70)

[1] Six of nine homosexual men had coliform infection: one other had infection with H. influenzae. None of 42 heterosexual men had coliform infection.
[2] Forty subjects evaluated; 25 had a single organism identified.
[3] Cut off between younger and older men was age 40.

didymis in 75% of cases, indicating seminal vesicular as well as epididymal involvement.

Osegby[107] found that after epididymitis, only 40% of men have semen samples considered adequate for conception. Nearly 27% had permanent azoospermia, and 33% had permanent oligospermia with counts less than 10 million. In a study population of 225 azoospermic men, Micic[34] found that 63% had epididymal obstruction. Campbell[108] noted that 40% of his patients with unilateral epididymitis secondary to gonorrhea were sterile. Pelouse found 11% of patients with gonococcal urethritis, 24% of men with unilateral epididymitis, and 42% of men with bilateral epididymitis were sterile.[109]

Infections that can cause destruction of testicular substance or occlusion of the tubules needed to transport spermatozoa are known to lead directly to male infertility. In mumps, testicular involvement occurs in 30% of males who are above the age of 10. Before that age, orchitis rarely accompanies mumps. After it, bilateral orchitis occurs in one-third of men with mumps. Of those with bilateral orchitis, one-third will develop azoospermia. Serum FSH are often elevated and, histologically, the testicle may be atrophic or fibrotic.[110]

Mycobacterium tuberculosis may affect both the testicle and the epididymis. Abdel and el Morsy[111] found that men with tuberculosis often had abnormalities of the epididymis. *Mycobacterium leprimodous* also frequently involves the testicle and leads to infertility.[112] Leprimodous leprosy is the only type of leprosy associated with orchitis.[113]

Damage to the epididymis or testicle on one side could affect overall fertility in several ways. Minimal or subclinical epididymitis could occur on the other side and affect epididymal function without causing obstruction. It has been shown that damage to the testicle from torsion[114,115] causes contralateral testicular abnormalities. A possible mechanism for this was described by Hendry et al.,[116] who studied 32 patients who had unilateral vasal or epididymal obstruction. Eighty-one percent of these men had antisperm antibodies. They also found that 37% of naturally infertile males with antisperm antibodies showed evidence of vasal or epididymal obstruction.

Kessler[78] also showed that unilateral vasal occlusion in mice could lead to infertility via sperm autoimmunity. Rumke et al.[117,118] have suggested that vas deferens or epididymal obstruction can be detected in 50% of men with sperm antibodies. Bandahauer and Marberger[75] found 9 of 48 with unilateral epididymitis to have sperm antibodies. Bietz[119] found toxic changes in the opposite testicle in several patients 150 to 250 days following onset of unilateral epididymitis. Animal models in rats and monkey have been developed and may be used to study the effect of epididymitis on infertility.[76,120,121]

Prostatitis and Infertility

Symptomatic prostatitis has classically been divided into four classifications: acute bacterial prostatitis, chronic bacterial prostatitis, nonbacterial or idiopathic prostatitis, and prostatodynia. Prostatic inflammation may also be asymptomatic.[121] These syndromes are often confusing, even in the absence of infertility.

Acute bacterial prostatitis usually presents with fever, signs of systemic infection, bacteriuria, difficulty urinating, and a very tender, enlarged prostate. The agents causing acute prostatitis are usually the coliform bacteria, pseudomonas, and enterococcus. Acute prostatitis can also occur from untreated gonococcal infection. The pathogen for acute prostatitis can almost always be cultured from the urine or urethra. Prostatic massage is not necessary to make the diagnosis, and may precipitate septicemia.[122,126] This syndrome is not known to be associated with infertility except acutely but, theoretically, could cause prostate damage.

Chronic bacterial prostatitis is most often characterized by the symptoms of relapsing bladder infection. Although most data concerning prostatitis concern the syndrome of chronic bacterial prostatitis, it is relatively uncommon. Less than 10% of all cases of prostatitis are of this type. Bacterial infections of this type are resistant to treatment. Even long-term treatment with antibiotics often will only suppress the infection. When treatment ceases, the organism may reemerge from the prostate to infect the bladder.[129] The diagnosis can be made by prostatic localization cultures as described by Meares and Stamey.[123] Patients must be abacteriuric but off of antibiotics to successfully perform localization cultures.

The diagnosis of prostatic infection is made by finding at least one log higher count of pathogenic bacteria in the cultures of either postprostatic massage urine or expressed prostatic secretions (EPS) as compared to the first voided (urethral) specimen.[130] Prostatic secretions obtained in chronic bacterial prostatitis usually show numerous white blood cells. The upper limit of normal is 10 white blood cells per 400 power high power field or 1000 cells per cubic millimeter on hemocytometer in EPS.

Biochemical abnormalities in the EPS of men with chronic or acute bacterial prostatitis are common.[128] Zinc concentrations are low, and have been reported to correlate with the antimicrobial properties of prostatic secretions.[124] The pH of prostatic fluid (usually acid) is alkaline, with an average pH of 8.32. Local immunity to urinary pathogens can be demonstrated in chronic bacterial prostatitis. Serum antibody titers to bacterial O specific antigens are elevated and decrease with treatment. Antigen-specific secretory immunoglobulin IgA in EPS also correlates with disease activity.[131] Chronic bacterial prostatitis is seldom a cause of male infertility. Bacterial cystitis is unusual in an infertile man.

Chronic idiopathic prostatitis (sometimes called nonbacterial prostatitis) is characterized by pain and symptoms referable to the prostate. These patients complain of dysuria, perineal pain, testicular pain, groin discomfort, urgency, nocturia, and sometimes of hematospermia and/or ejaculatory pain.[129] As its name suggests, no pathogenic bacteria can be isolated to the prostate or bladder on the four glass urine test. Findings include the presence of EPS in greater than 10 white blood cells per high power field or greater than 1000 white blood cells per cubic millimeter.

Anderson and Weller[125] found 4543 ± 650 leukocytes per cubic millimeter in EPS of patients with symptoms of idiopathic prostatitis versus 887.88 ± 11 leukocytes in controls without symptoms. Berger et al.[12] also found that more patients with symptoms than controls without symptoms had white blood cells in the prostatic secretions. Others have found a poor correlation between the EPS leukocytes concentrations and symptoms.[126] Commensal bacteria, such as *Staphylococcus epidermidis* and streptococci, are often isolated.[127] Local IgA to these commensal bacteria has been shown to be absent[128] and up to 70% of asymptomatic volunteers can have commensal bacteria isolated to the prostate by four glass urine.[12]

Sexually transmitted organisms have been implicated in the etiology of nonbacterial prostatitis. There is inconclusive evidence that the prostate may be involved as well as the urethra

Table 30-3 Review of Therapy Trials for Male Infertility

Reference	Rx	Female Criteria	Male Criteria	Faults of Study	% Pregnancies
Knudsin et al.[158]	Demeclocycline, 150 mg for 10 days	1. Unexplained infertility 2. *Ureaplasma*	1. Normal seminal fluid analysis 2. *Ureaplasma*	1. Uncontrolled 2. Patient selected on basis of *Ureaplasma* 3. Short Rx	15/36 (42%)
Quesada[159]	Antibiotics 1. 59 with antisperm antibodies 2. 50 without antisperm antibodies	Normal	Sole contributor to infertility	1. Uncontrolled 2. No definitive Rx 3. Mixed bacterial infection and nonbacterial inflammation 4. Mixed symptomatic and asymptomatic	6.8% with antibodies 24% without antibodies
Sokol et al.[140]	10 Weeks Methenamine mandelate	None	15 WBC/HPF semen	1. Rx methenamine mandelate 2. No definitive Rx 3. Uncontrolled	5/28 (18%)
Harrison and Johnson[41]	1. Doxycycline, 100 mg for 28 days 2. Placebo 3. No Rx	1. Ovulating 2. Patent tubes	No oligospermia	1. Short-duration therapy 2. Not randomized? 3. Small number studied	1. 5/30 (17%) 2. 4/28 (14%) 3. 5/30 (17%)

Matthews et al.[160]	1. Doxycycline, 100 mg for first 10 days of each cycle for 6 months 2. No Rx	1. Ovulating 2. Patent tubes	Normal seminal fluid analysis	1. Randomized? 2. No placebo	1. 13/62 (18%) 2. 10/42 (24%)
Idress[161]	1. Tetracycline, 2 g/day for 14 days 2. No Rx	1. Ovulating 2. Open tubes	Normal seminal fluid analysis	1. Not consecutive or randomized 2. Short Rx 3. No placebo	1. 10/24 (42%) 2. 23/71 (32%)
Taymor[162]	1. Tetracycline, 2 g for 10 days 2. Untreated	*Ureaplasma* present	*Ureaplasma*	1. No placebo 2. Short Rx 3. Nonrandomized	1. 10/24 (42%) 2. 17/67 (25%)
Khatanee and Decker[163]	1. Demeclocycline, 150 mg 2. Untreated	No demonstrable abnormality	No criteria	Untreated controls from gynecology clinic population and not all trying to conceive	1. 31/68 (46%) 2. 19/62 (30%)

in men with acute chlamydial urethritis. Nilsson et al.[129] found that 26 of 96 men with *Chlamydia*-positive NGU also had *Chlamydia* in the expressed prostatic secretions. These men all had greater than 20 white blood cells per high power field in EPS. However, EPS is, by necessity, contaminated with urethral secretions and any culture results must be interpreted with caution. Poletti et al.[130] was able to isolate *Chlamydia* from the prostate on transrectal aspiration in men with symptoms of urethritis and prostatitis. These cases, however, differ in that most men with symptoms of nonbacterial prostatitis do not have the symptoms of urethritis.

Based on prevalence alone, *C. trachomatis* would seem to be a likely candidate to cause nonbacterial prostatitis. However, this has never proved to be true in studies that attempt localization of infection. Berger et al. was unable to isolate chlamydia from 40 men with symptoms of chronic bacterial prostatitis.[12] Maardh et al.[131] concluded, from a study of 53 men with nonbacterial prostatitis, that *Chlamydia* was an extremely rare cause. Bruce et al.[132] studied of 70 men with chronic prostatitis and found 50% to have early morning urine specimens positive for *C. trachomatis* by immunofluorescence. However, they did not rule urethritis as the source of *Chlamydia*, and EPS specimens were not examined.

Ureaplasma urealyticum has also been investigated as a possible etiologic agent in chronic bacterial prostatitis. Weidner et al.[133] found *Ureaplasma urealyticum* to localize to the prostate in 36 of 137 men with symptomatic nonbacterial prostatitis. After treatment with tetracycline, 30 of the patients were free of *Ureaplasma* and 23 were free of symptoms. Persistence of *Ureaplasma* was related to coexistent infection in the patient's sexual partner. They concluded that *Ureaplasma* was the etiologic agent in men with the symptoms of nonbacterial prostatitis in 9% of their men.[134] It appear that asymptomatic, idiopathic, and pyospermic prostatitis is often associated with male infertility. Like symptomatic prostatitis, its cause is as yet uncertain.

Treatment of Inflammation and Infection in Male Infertility

Table 30-3 summarizes several important trials using antibiotics in the treatment of male factor infertility. The same methodological problems that hinder infertility research in general also make interpretation of these treatment studies difficult. We will attempt now to summarize these problems so that the reader will better appreciate how far we still have to go in this area of research.

Some investigators have studied only those patients with idiopathic infertility. Selection criteria for cases has generally included an abnormal SFA. Investigators have differed as to whether the absence of normal parameters for sperm, the presence of WBCs, or the presence of specific bacterial isolations from semen cultures is the main variable of interest. Microbiological evaluation has seldom been comprehensive. Criteria for success in treatment have also varied. Improved sperm counts, sperm motilities, decreased WBCs, and pregnancy have all been used by various researchers. Few studies have used the special stains needed to differentiate immature sperm from white blood cells. None has controlled for effects of past infection. Studies have not routinely assessed sperm function and semen cultures both before and after treatment. Lastly, no studies so far have controlled for effects of potential toxic exposures.

Many studies have attempted antibiotic

treatment for the eradication of *U. urealyticum.* Most of these studies have used tetracycline or tetracycline derivatives to accomplish this. When evaluating studies of this type, the reader should keep in mind that tetracyclines have effects on leukocyte migration and phagocytosis independent of their antibiotic properties[135–137] that could affect the number of leukocytes in semen on EPS samples. For example, Berger et al.[138] gave doxycycline to infertile men who had increased leukocyte concentrations and poor sperm function by the hamster penetration test. The sperm penetration tests of these men improved and they had more pregnancies than an untreated but poorly controlled group. It is therefore possible that a subset of men, based on sperm dysfunction (as identified by the hamster penetration test) and in the absence of documented infection, may benefit from tetracycline therapy.

Comhaire et al.[139] performed a double-blind, placebo-controlled doxycycline study on men with prostatic inflammation. They followed subjects for 175 months and used both pregnancy rates and SFA results as outcome measures. They found no significant differences in the pregnancy rate between cases and controls. Interestingly, both motility and morphology showed improvement in both groups and white cells disappeared in both groups. It is possible that the evaluation/treatment process including advice about toxic exposures and coital frequency may be the important factor in decreasing white cells in semen independent of drug treatment.

No consensus exists as to whether partners should or should not be treated in such studies. There is also the possibility that studies need to treat subjects longer to gain therapeutic efficacy. Sokol et al.[140] found that two-thirds of men treated for prostatic inflammation with antibiotics relapsed after therapy was terminated. Caldamone et al.[141,142] found that white cells decreased in men with asymptomatic prostatitis on antimicrobial treatment, then increased after therapy ended.

Prolonged antibiotic trials may bring their own set of problems. Several authors have found that antibiotics have an adverse effect on testicular function. D'Arcy[143] found sulfasaziline, an antibiotic commonly used to treat ulcerative colitis, decreased sperm counts in patients with that illness. Several investigators have found that tetracycline and its derivatives cause testicular atrophy in animals and may decrease sperm counts in men.[144–146] Cephalosporins, penicillins, and trimethoprim may also decrease spermatogenesis.[152] It is interesting that in the doxycycline treatment study by Berger et al.[138] all pregnancies took place in the first month after therapy. Continued therapy did not increase the pregnancy rate.

It is possible that short-term therapy is of benefit while longer term therapy causes problems with sperm production? Obviously, much more effort is needed in this area. Other areas for future development will be the use of antiinflammatory agents or laboratory manipulation to remove white blood cells and potentially increase fertility. Until the mechanisms by which inflammation and infection affect male fertility are better understood the best approach to patient care is a conservative one. Patients will be best served by those clinicians that thoroughly attempt to localize inflammation and corresponding infection if present and to treat specifically.

REFERENCES

1. Branny J, Zerabala M: Some characteristics of viruses isolated from bull semen and their possible pathogenicity. Br Vet J 1970; 127:88–92.

2. Svendsen M: Leukocytes and bacteria in human semen. J Pathol Bacteriol 1960; 60:131–135.
3. Comhaire F, Vershraegen G, Vermeulen L: Diagnosis of accessory gland infection and its possible role in male infertility. Int J Androl 1980; 3:32–45.
4. Couture M, Ulstein M, Leonhard J, Paulsen CA: Improved staining method for differentiating immature germ cells from white blood cells in human seminal fluid. Andrologia 1976; 8:61–66.
5. Endz AW: A rapid staining method for differentiating granulocytes from "germinal cells" in Papanicolaou-stained semen. Acta Cytol 1974; 18:2–7.
6. Phadke AM: Neutral red supravital staining for cellular elements in the semen. Andrologia 1978; 10:80–84.
7. Riedd HH: Techniques for the detection of leukospermia in human semen. Arch Androl 1980; 5:287–293.
8. Wolff H, Anderson DJ: Male genital tract inflammation associated with increased numbers of potential human immunodeficiency virus host cells in semen. Andrologia 1988; 20:404–410.
9. El DM, Hargreave TB, Busuttil A, James K, Chisholm GD: Identifying leukocytes and leukocyte subpopulations in semen using monoclonal antibody probes. Urology 1986; 28:492–496.
10. Barratt CL, Harrison PE, Robinson A, Cooke ID: Antisperm antibodies and lymphocyte subsets in semen—not a simple relationship. Int J Androl 1990; 13:50–58.
11. Mathur S, Goust JM, Williamson HO, Fudenberg HH: Cross-reactivity of sperm and T lymphocyte antigens. Am J Reprod Immunol 1981; 1:113–118.
12. Berger RE, Krieger JN, Kessler D, Ireton RC: Case-control study of men with suspected chronic idiopathic prostatitis. J Urol 1989; 141(2):328–331.
13. Cumming JA, Dawes J, Hargreave TB: Granulocyte elastase levels do not correlate with anaerobic and aerobic bacterial growth in seminal plasma from infertile men. Int J Androl 1990; 13:273–277.
14. Hillier SL, Rabe LK, Muller CH, et al: Relationship of bacteriologic characteristics to semen indices in men attending an infertility clinic. Obstet Gynecol 1990; 75:800–804.
15. Colleen S, Mardh P-A, Schytz A: Magnesium and zinc in seminal fluid of healthy males and patients with non-acute prostatitis with and without gonorrhoea. Scan J Urol Nephrol 1975; 9:192–197.
16. Caldamone AA, Dougherty KA, Cockett ATK: Monitoring zinc concentration in seminal plasma during treatment of prostatitis and infertility. Surg Forum 1981; 644–646.
17. Caldamone AA, Emilson LBVC, Al-Juburi A, Cockett ATK: Prostatitis: Prostatic secretory dysfunction affecting fertility. Fertil Steril 1980; 34:602–603.
18. Guillet-Rosso F, Fari A, Taylor S, et al: Systemic semen culture and its influence on IVF management. Br J Obstet Gynecol 1987; 94:543–547.
19. Close CE, Roberts PL, Berger RE: Cigarettes, alcohol and marijuana are related to pyospermia in infertile men. J Urol 1990; 144:900–903.
20. Hughes L, Ryder TA, McDenzie ML, Pryse-Davies J, Stredrouska J, Hendry WF: The use of transmission electron microscopy to study non-spermatozoal cells in semen. In: Frajese G, Hafez ESE, Conti C, Fabrini C, eds. Oligozoospermia: recent progress in andrology. New York: Raven Press, 1981:65–75.
21. Maroni MS, Symon DNK, Wilkinson PC: Chomotaxis of neutrophil leukocytes towards spermatozoa and seminal fluid. J Reprod Fertil 1972; 28:359–368.
22. Clark RA, Klebanoff SJ: Neutrophile mediated tumor cytotoxicity. Role of peroxidase system. J Exp Med 1975; 141:1442–1447.
23. Koehler JK, Berger RE, Karp LE: Spermophagy. In: Atlas of human reproduction. Berlin: MSP Press, 1983:213–218.
24. Pandya IJ, Cohen J: The leukocytic reaction of

the human uterine cervix to spermatozoa. Fertil Steril 1985; 43:417–421.
25. Berger RE, Karp LE, Williamson RA, Koeler J, Moore DE, Holmes KK: The relationship of pyospermia and seminal fluid bacteriology to sperm function as reflected in sperm penetration assay. Fertil Steril 1982; 37:557–564.
26. Shy K, Stenchever MA, Muller CH: Sperm penetration assay and subsequent pregnancy: A prospective study of 74 infertile men. Obstet Gynecol 1988; 71:685–690.
27. Maruyama DK, Hale RW, Rogers BJ: Effects of white blood cells on the in vitro penetration of zona free hamster eggs by human spermatozoa. J Androl 1985; 6:127–135.
28. Wolff H, Politch JA, Martinez A, et al: Leukocytospermia is associated with poor semen quality. Fertil Steril 1990; 53:528–536.
29. Persson BE, Sjoman M, Niklasson F, Ronquist G: Uridine, xanthine and urate concentrations in prostatic fluid and seminal plasma of patients with prostatitis. Eur Urol 1991; 19:253–256.
30. Gattuccio F, Di TD, Romano C, et al: Urogenital inflammations: Aetiology, diagnosis and their correlation with varicocele and male infertility. Acta Eur Fertil 1988; 19:201–208.
31. Jochum M, Pabst W, Schill WB: Granulocyte elastase as a sensitive diagnostic parameter of silent male genital tract inflammation. Andrologia 1986; 18:413–419.
32. Megory E, Zuckerman H, Shoham Z, Lunenfeld B: Infections and male fertility. Obstet Gynecol Surv 1987; 42:283–290.
33. Harrison KL, Johnson DK: Chronic asymptomatic genital tract infection and semen quality. Pathology 1979; 11:289–292.
34. Toth A, Lesser ML: Asymptomatic bacteriospermia in fertile and infertile men. Fertil Steril 1981; 36:88–91.
35. Ulstein M, Capell P, Holmes KK, Paulsen CA: Nonsymptomatic genital tract infection and male infertility. In: Esem G, ed. Human semen and fertility regulation in men. St. Louis: Mosby, 1976:355–362.
36. Svendsen M: Leukocytes and bacteria in human semen. J Pathol Bacteriol 1960; 60:131–135.
37. Comhaire F, Vershraegen G, Vermeulen L: Diagnosis of accessory gland infection and its possible role in male infertility. Int J Androl 1980; 3:32–45.
38. Comhaire F, Vershraegen G, Vermeulen L: Diagnosis of accessory gland infection and its possible role in male infertility. Int J Androl 1980; 3:32–45.
39. Paulson JD, Polakoski KL: A glass wool column procedure for removing extraneous material from the human ejaculate. Fertil Steril 1977; 28:178–181.
40. Linossier A, Thurmann A, Bustos-Obregon E: Sperm immobilization by dental focus microorganisms. Andrologia 1982; 14:250–255.
41. Harrison KL, Johnson DK: Chronic asymptomatic genital tract infection and semen quality. Pathology 1979; 11:289–292.
42. Ulstein M, Capell P, Holmes KK, Paulsen CA: Nonsymptomatic genital tract infection and male infertility. In Hafez ESE, ed. Human semen and fertility regulation in men. St Louis: Mosby, 1976:355–362.
43. Rehewy MSE, Hafez ESE, Thomas A, Brown WJ: Aerobic and anaerobic bacterial flora in semen from fertile and infertile groups of men. Arch Androl 1979; 2:263–268.
44. Moberg PJ, Eneroth P, Ljung A, Nord CE: Bacterial growth in samples from cervix and semen from infertile couples. Int J Fertil 1979; 24:157–165.
45. Eneroth A, Wadstrom L, Moberg PJ, Nord C-E: Studies on the bacterial flora in semen from males in infertile relations. Int J Androl 1978; 1:105–116.
46. Morton RS: White cell counts in human semen. Br J Vener Dis 1968; 44:72–74.
47. Fair WR, Cordonnier JJ: The pH of prostatic fluid: A reappraisal and therapeutic implications. J Urol 1978; 120:695–698.
48. Taylor-Robinson D, McCormack WM: The genital mycoplasmas. N Engl J Med 1980; 302:1003–1010.
49. Toth A, Swenson CE, O'Leary WM: Light

microscopy as an aid in predicting ureaplasma infection in human semen. Fertil Steril 1978; 39:586–691.
50. Fowlkes DM, Dooher GB, O'Leary WM: Evidence by scanning electron microscopy for an association between spermatozoa and T-mycoplasmas in men of infertile marriage. Fertil Steril 1975; 26:1203–1222.
51. Grossgebauer K, Hennig A: Ureaplasma-infected human sperm in infertile men. Arch Androl 1984; 12(suppl):35–41.
52. Swenson CE, Toth A, O'Leary WM: *Ureaplasma urealyticum* and human infertility: Correlation of infection with alterations in seminal parameters. Fertil Steril 1979; 31:660–665.
53. Valvo JR, Caldamone AA, Hipp S, Duncan D, Cockett A: Elevated seminal pH and *Ureaplasma urealyticum.* J Androl 1982; 3:144–148.
54. Desai S, Cohen MS, Kratamee M, Leiter E: Ureaplasma urealyticum (T-mycoplasma) infection: Does it have a role in male infertility? J Urol 1980; 124:469–471.
55. Cintron RD, Wortham JWE, Acosta A: The association of semen factors with the recovery of *Ureaplasma urealyticum.* Fertil Steril 1981; 36:648–652.
56. Berger RE, Karp LE, Williamson RA, Koeler J, Moore DE, Holmes KK: The relationship of pyospermia and seminal fluid bacteriology to sperm function as reflected in the sperm penetration assay. Fertil Steril 1982; 37:557–564.
57. Shalhoub D, Abdel LA, Fredericks CM, Mathur S, Rust PF: Physiological integrity of human sperm in the presence of Ureaplasma urealyticum. Arch Androl 1986; 16:75–80.
58. Busolo F, Zanchetta R: The effect of Ureaplasma homin and Ureaplasma urealyticum in hamster egg *in vitro* penetration by human spermatozoa. Fertil Steril 1985; 43:110.
59. Friberg J, Knarpe H: mycoplasma in semen from fertile and infertile men. Andrologia 1974; 6:45–46.
60. Stray-Pedersen B, Eng J, Mannsaker Reikvan T: Uterine T-mycoplasma colonization in reproductive failure. Am J Obstet Gynecol 1978; 130:307–311.
61. de Louvois J, Blades M, Hurley R, Stanley VC, Harrison RF: Frequency of mycoplasma in fertile and infertile couples. Lancet 1974; 1:1073–1075.
62. Cassell GH, Younger JB, Brown MB, et al: Microbiologic study of infertile women at the time of diagnostic laparoscopy. N Engl J Med 1983; 308:502–505.
63. Toth A, Lesser ML, Brooks C, Labriola D: Subsequent pregnancies among 161 couples treated for T-mycoplasma genital tract infections. N Engl J Med 1983; 308:505–507.
64. Hellstrom WJ, Schachter J, Sweet RL, McClure RD: Is there a role for Chlamydia trachomatis and genital mycoplasma in male infertility? Fertil Steril 1987; 48:337–339.
65. Berger RE, Krieger JN, Kessler D, et al: Case-control study of men with suspected chronic idiopathic prostatitis. J Urol 1989; 141: 328–331.
66. Bennett AH, Hipp SS, Alford LM: Pyosemia and carriage of chlamydia and ureaplasma in infertile men. J Urol 1982; 128:54–56.
67. Ruijs GJ, Kauer FM, Jager S, Schröder PF, Schirm J, Kremer J: Is serology of any use when searching for correlations between *Chlamydia trachomatis* infection and male infertility? Fertil Steril 1990; 53:131–136.
68. Soffer Y, Ron ER, Golan A, et al: Male genital mycoplasmas and Chlamydia trachomatis culture: Its relationship with accessory gland function, sperm quality, and autoimmunity. Fertil Steril 1990; 53:331–336.
69. Poletti F, Medici MC, Alinovi A, et al: Isolation of Chlamydia trachomatis from the prostatic cells in patients affected by nonacute abacterial prostatitis. J Urol 1985; 134:691–693.
70. Suominen J, Gronroos M, Terho P, Wichmann L: Chronic prostatitis, Chlamydia trachomatis and infertility. Int J Androl 1983; 6:405–413.
71. Wolff H, Neubert U, Zebhauser M, et al: Chlamydia trachomatis induces an inflammatory response in the male genital tract and is associated with altered semen quality. Fertil Steril 1991; 55:1017–1019.
72. Ansbacher R, Keung-Yeung K, Wurster JC: Sperm antibodies in vasectomized men. Fertil Steril 1972; 23:640–643.

73. Linnet L, Hjort T: Sperm agglutinins in seminal plasma and serum after vasectomy. Correlation between immunological and clinical findings. J Exp Immunol 1977; 30:413–420.
74. Kessler DL, Smith WD, Hamilton MS, Berger RE: Infertility in mice after unilateral vasectomy. Fertil Steril 1985; 43:308–312.
75. Bandhauer K, Marberger H: Spermagglutinins in diseases of the epididymitis. 5th World Congress on Fertility and Sterility, 1966; 781.
76. Hendry WF, Parslow JM, Stedronska J, Wallace DMA: The diagnosis of unilateral testicular obstruction in subfertile males. Br J Urol 1982; 54:774–779.
77. Mathur S, Williamson HO, Derrick FG, et al: A new microassay for spermocytotoxic antibody: Comparison with passive hemagglutination assay for antisperm antibodies in couples with unexplained infertility. J Immunol 1981; 126:905–909.
78. Kessler DL, Smith WD, Hamilton MS, Berger RE: Infertility in mice after unilateral vasectomy. Fertil Steril 1985; 43:308–312.
79. Bandhauer K, Marberger H: Spermagglutinins in diseases of the epididymitis. 5th World Congress on Fertility and Sterility 1966; 781.
80. Hendry WF, Parslow JM, Stedronska J, Wallace DMA: The diagnosis of unilateral testicular obstruction in subfertile males. Br J Urol 1982; 54:774–779.
81. Hargreave TB, Torrance M, Young H, Harris AB: Isolation of *Ureaplasma urealyticum* from seminal plasma in relation to sperm antibody levels and sperm motility. Andrologia 1982; 14:223–227.
82. Micic S: Incidence of aetiological factors in testicular obstructive azoospermia. Int J Androl 1987; 10:681–684.
83. Hargreave TB, Harvey J, Elton RA, McMillan A: Serum agglutinating and immobilising sperm antibodies in men attending a sexually transmitted diseases clinic. Andrologia 1984; 16:111–115.
84. Witkin SS, Toth A: Relationship between genital tract infections, sperm antibodies in seminal fluid, and infertility. Fertil Steril 1983; 40:805–808.
85. Barratt CL, Harrison PE, Robinson A, Cooke ID: Antisperm antibodies and lymphocyte subsets in semen—not a simple relationship. Int J Androl 1990; 13:50–58.
86. Lassus A, Paavonen J, Kousa M, et al: Erythromycin and lymecycline treatment in Chlamydia-positive and Chlamydia-negative nongonococcal urethritis: A partner-controlled study. Acta Derm Venereol 1979; 59:278.
87. Bowie WB, Wang SP, Alexander ER, et al: Etiology of nongonococcal urethritis: Evidence for *C. trachomatis* and *U. urealyticum.* J Clin Invest 1977; 59:735–742.
88. Ripa KT, Måardh P-A, Thelin I: *Chlamydia trachomatis* urethritis in men attending a venereal disease clinic: A culture and therapeutic study. Acta Derm Venereol 1978; 58:175–179.
89. Schacter J: Chlamydial infections. N Engl J Med 1978; 298:423,490,540.
90. Thelin I, Wennstrom AM, Måardh PA: Contact tracing in patients with genital chlamydial infection. Br J Vener Dis 1980; 56:259–262.
91. Stimson JB, Hale J, Bowie WR, Holmes KK: Tetracycline resistant *Ureaplasma urealyticum*: A cause of persistent urethritis. Ann Intern Med 1981; 94:192.
92. Bowie WR, Floyd JF, Miller V, et al: Differential response of chlamydial and ureaplasma-associated urethritis to sulfafurazole (sulfisoxazole) and aminocyclitols. Lancet 1976; 2:1276–1278.
93. Pessione F, Dolivo M, Casin I, et al: Sexual behavior and smoking: Risk factor for urethritis in men. Sex Transm Dis 1988; 15:119–122.
94. Smith GL, Greenup R, Takafuji ET: Circumcision as a risk factor for urethritis in racial groups. Am J Public Health 1987; 77:452–454.
95. Hernandez AI, Alvarez DC, Gili M, et al: Oral sex as a risk factor for Chlamydia-negative nongonococcal urethritis. Sex Transm Dis 1988; 15:100–102.
96. Bowie WR: Etiology and treatment of nongonococcal urethritis. Sex Transm Dis 1978; 5:27–33.
97. Swartz SL, Kraus SJ, Herrmann KL, et al: Diagnosis and etiology of nongonococcal urethritis. J Infect Dis 1978; 138:445–454.

98. Watson RA: Gonorrhea and acute epididymitis. Milit Med 1979; 144:785–786.
99. Berger RE, Alexander ER, Harnisch JP, et al: Etiology, manifestations and therapy of acute epididymitis: Prospective study of fifty cases. J Urol 1979; 121:750–754.
100. Jalil N, Doble A, Gilchrist C, Taylor RD: Infection of the epididymis by Ureaplasma urealyticum. Genitourin Med 1988; 64:367–368.
101. Arya OP, Tuder SR: Correlates of venereal disease and fertility in rural Uganda. Presented at the Medical Society for the Study of Venereal Disease. Malta, April, 1975.
102. Osegbe DN, Amaku EO: The causes of male infertility in 504 consecutive Nigerian patients. Int Urol Nephrol 1985; 17:349–358.
103. Wolin LH: On the etiology of epididymitis. J Urol 1971; 105:531–533.
104. Nilsson S, Obrant KO, Persson PS: Changes in the testis parenchyma caused by acute nonspecific epididymitis. Fertil Steril 1968; 19:748–757.
105. Ludwig VG, Haselberger J: Epididymitis and fertilat: Behandlungser-gebrisse bei akuter unspezifischer epididymitis 1977; 95:397–399.
106. Krishnan R, Heal MR: Study of the seminal vesicles in acute epididymitis. Br J Urol 1991; 67:632–637.
107. Osegbe DN: Testicular function after unilateral bacterial epididymo-orchitis. Eur Urol 1991; 19:204–208.
108. Campbell MS: Surgical pathology of epididymitis. Ann Surg 1928; 88:98–111.
109. Pelouze PS: Epididymitis in gonorrhea in the male and female. Philadelphia: Saunders, 1941:141.
110. Candel S: Epididymitis in mumps, including orchitis: Further clinical studies and comments. Ann Intern Med 1951; 34:20–36.
111. Abdel RM, el Morsy F: Genitourinary mycobacteria in infertile Egyptian men. Fertil Steril 1990; 54:713–717.
112. Ibrahiem AA, Awad HA, Metawi BA, Hamada TA: Pathologic changes in testis and epididymis of infertile leprotic males. Int J Lepr Other Mycobact Dis 1979; 47:44–49.
113. El SS, El HH, Abdel FA, El OM, Farid A: Testicular and epididymal involvement in leprosy patients, with special reference to gynecomastia. Int J Dermatol 1976; 15:52–58.
114. Chakraforty J, Jhunjhunwala J: Experimental unilateral torsion of the spermatic cord in guinea pigs. Effects on the contralateral testes. J Androl 1982; 3:117–123.
115. Krarup T: The testes after torsion. Br J Urol 1978; 30:43–46.
116. Hendry WF, Parslow JM, Stedronska J, Wallace DMA: The diagnosis of unilateral testicular obstruction in subfertile males. Br J Urol 1982; 54:774–779.
117. Rumke PH, Van Amstad N, Messer EN, Bezemer PD: Prognosis of fertility of men with sperm agglutinins in the serum. Fertil Steril 1974; 25:393–398.
118. Rumke PH, Hellinga G: Autoantibodies against spermatozoa in sterile men. Am J Clin Pathol 1959; 32:357–363.
119. Bietz O: Fertilitatsuntersuchungen bei des unspezifichen epididymitis. Hauturzt 1959; 10:134–135.
120. Kuzan FB, Patton DL, Allen SM, Kuo CC: A proposed mouse model for acute epididymitis provoked by genital serovar E, Chlamydia trachomatis. Biol Reprod 1989; 40:165–172.
121. Meares EM: Prostatitis syndromes: New perspectives about old woes. J Urol 1980; 123:141–147.
122. Meares EM, Burbalras GA: Prostatitis, bacterial, non-bacterial and prostatodynia. Semin Urol 1983; 1:146–154.
123. Meares EM, Stamey TA: Bacteriologic localization patterns in bacterial prostatitis and urethritis. Invest Urol 1968; 5:492–518.
124. Fair WR, Cordonnier JJ: The pH of prostatic fluid: A reappraisal and therapeutic implications. J Urol 1978; 120:695–698.
125. Anderson RW, Weller C: Prostatic secretion leukocyte studies in non-bacterial prostatitis (prostatosis). J Urol 1979; 121:292–294.
126. O'Shaughnessy EJ, Perrino PS, White JP: Chronic prostatitis, fact or fiction. JAMA 1956; 160:540–542.

127. Meares EM: Bacterial prostatitis vs prostatosis, a clinical and bacteriological study. JAMA 1973; 224:1372–1375.
128. Centifano VM, Drylie DM, Dearddourff SL, Kaufman HE: Herpes virus type 2 in the male genitourinary tract. Science 1972; 178:318–319.
129. Nilsson I-K, Colleen S, Mardh P-A: Relationship between psychological and laboratory findings in patients with symptoms of non-acute prostatitis. In: Davidsson D, Dublin L, Mardh P-A, eds. Genital infections and their complications. Stockholm: Almquist and Wiksell, 1975:133.
130. Poletti F, Medici MC, Alinovi A, et al: Isolation of Chlamydia trachomatis from the prostatic cells in patients affected by nonacute abacterial prostatitis. J Urol 1985; 134:691–693.
131. Maardh P-A, Ripa KT, Colleen S, Treharne JD, Darougar S: Role of *Chlamydia trachomatis* in non-acute prostatitis. Br J Vener Dis 1978; 54:330–334.
132. Bruce AW, Chadwick P, Willet WS, O'Shaughnessy M: The role of chlamydiae in genitourinary disease. J Urol 1981; 126:625–629.
133. Weidner W, Brunner H, Krause W: Quantitative culture of *Ureaplasma urealyticum* in patients with chronic prostatitis or prostatosis. J Urol 1980; 124:622–625.
134. Drummond AC: Trichomonas infection of the prostate gland. Am J Surg 1936; 31:98–103.
135. Belsheim J, Gnarpe H, Persson S: Tetracyclines and host defence mechanisms: Interference with leukocyte chemotaxis. Scand J Infect Dis 1979; 11:141–145.
136. Forsgren A, Schmeling D: Effects of antibiotics on chemotaxis of human leukocyte chemotaxis. Scand J Infect Dis 1979; 11:141–145.
137. Forsgren A, Gnarpe H: The effect of antibacterial agents on the association between bacteria and leukocytes. Scand J Infect Dis 1982; 33:115–120.
138. Berger RE, Smith D, Critchlow CW, et al: Improvement in the sperm penetration (hamster ova) assay (SPA) results after doxycycline treatment of infertile men. J Androl 1983; 4:126–130.
139. Comhaire FH, Rowe PJ, Farley TM: The effect of doxycycline in infertile couples with male accessory gland infection: A double blind prospective study. Int J Androl 1986; 9:91–98.
140. Sokol S, Kacobson CB, Derrick FC: Use of methenamine hippurate in male infertility. Urology 1975; 6:59–62.
141. Caldamone AA, Dougherty KA, Cockett ATK: Monitoring zinc concentration in seminal plasma during treatment of prostatitis and infertility. Surg Forum 1981; 644–646.
142. Caldamone AA, Emilson LBVC, Al-Juburi A, Cockett ATK: Prostatitis: Prostatic secretory dysfunction affecting fertility. Fertil Steril 1980; 34:602–603.
143. D'Arcy PF: Drug interactions and reactions update. Drug Intell Clin Pharm 1982; 16:218–221.
144. Deichmann WB, Bernal E, Anderson WAD, et al: The chronic oral toxicity of oxytetracycline HCl and tetracycline HCl in the rat, dog, and pig. Indst Med Surg 1964; 787–806.
145. Desau FI, Sullivan WJ: A two-year study of the toxicity of chloretetracycline hydrochloride in rats. Toxicol Appl Pharmacol 1961; 3:654–677.
146. Timmermans L: Influence of antibiotics on spermatogenesis. J Urol 1974; 112:348–349.
147. Berger RE, Alexander ER, Mona GD, et al: *Chlamydia trachomatis* as a cause of acute "idiopathic epididymitis." N Engl J Med 1978; 298:301–304.
148. Berger RE, Kessler D, Holmes KK: The etiology and manifestations of epididymitis in young men: Correlations with sexual orientation. J Inferect Dis 1987; 155:1341–1343.
149. Hawkins DA, Taylor-Robinson D, Thomas BJ, Harris JR: Microbiological survey of acute epididymitis. Genitourin Med 1986; 62:342–344.
150. Scheibel JH, Anderson JT, Brandenhoff P, et al: Chlamydia trachomatis in acute epididymitis. Scand J Urol Nephrol 1983; 17:47–50.
151. Kristensen JK, Scheibel JH: Etiology of acute epididymitis presenting in a venereal disease clinic. Sex Transm Dis 1984; 11:32–33.
152. Kojima H, Wang SP, Kuo CC, Grayston JT:

Local antibody in semen for rapid diagnosis of Chlamydia trachomatis epididymitis. J Urol 1988; 140:528–531.
153. Grant JB, Costello CB, Sequeira PJ, Blacklock NJ: The role of *Chlamydia trachomatis* in epididymitis. Br J Urol 1987; 60:355–359.
154. Doble A, Taylor-Robinson D, Thomas BJ, Jalil N, Harris JR, Witherow RO: Acute epididymitis: A microbiological and ultrasonographic study. Br J Urol 1989; 63:90–94.
155. De Jong Z, Pontonnier F, Plante P, et al: The frequency of Chlamydia trachomatis in acute epididymitis. Br J Urol 1988; 62:76–78.
156. Melekos MD, Asbach HW: The role of chlamydieae in epididymitis. Int Urol Nephrol 1988; 20:293–297.
157. Close CE, Wang SP, Roberts PL, Berger RE: The relationship of infection with *Chlamydia trachomatis* to parameters of male fertility and sperm autoimmunity. Fertil Steril 1987; 48(5):880–883.

ANNOTATED BIBLIOGRAPHY

Close CC, Roberts PL, Berger RE: Cigarettes, alcohol, and marijuana are related to pyospermia in infertile men. J Urol 1990; 144:900–903.

Histories, physical exams, semen analyses, and hamster ova sperm penetration assays were performed on 132 men from infertile couples attending an infertility clinic. Exposure to other substances and sexually transmitted disease history were controlled for by multiple linear regression analysis. Cigarette, marijuana, and heavy alcohol use were all associated with increased levels of seminal leukocytosis ($p < .05$). Cigarette smoking was associated with significantly lower sperm penetration assay scores as compared to nonsmokers ($p < .05$). In addition, marijuana users had higher percentages of motile sperm as compared to nonusers. The authors present possible explanations for their findings.

Hill JA, Haimovici F, Politch JA, Anderson DJ: Effects of soluble products of activated lymphocytes and macrophages (lymphokines and monokines) on human sperm motion parameters. Fertil Steril 1987; 47:460–465.

The authors conducted experimental trials to evaluate the effects of supernatants from activated leukocyte cultures and purified lymphokine and monokine preparations on sperm motion. Semen samples from fertile donors were pooled, motile sperm separated by sperm rise technique, then placed into Whitten's 2% human serum albumin and washed twice. Human peripheral blood leukocytes were isolated from heparinized blood and put into culture media stimulated with one of these four mitogens: T cell, concanavalin A, pokeweed; or mixed leukocyte culture. Cells were cultured at least 12 hours, then harvested at 1, 3, 5, and 7 days. Lymphokines and monokines of interest were obtained from commercial sources. Sperm concentration was adjusted to 100×10^6/ml, and 20 μl of suspension was mixed with an equal volume of test solution. An automated semen analyzer was used to measure percentages of motile sperm, mean swimming speed, and linearity and motility index of sperm from control (media only) and treated sperm. Differences among the groups were expressed as percentages of control values. The lymphokines human gamma interferon (culture and recombinant types) and significantly decreased sperm motility indices. Only culture-type interferon did this in a dose–response fashion. In addition, the monokine tumor necrosis factor showed a dose-dependent effect on sperm motility. B cell growth factor affected sperm linearity through agglutination, but further analysis found this effect attributable to another, unidentifiable component of the preparation. All other substances tested (interleukin-1 and -2, colony-stimulating factor) had no effects on sperm motion parameters. The authors suggest that the presence of lymphokines and monokines in the reproductive tracts of either sex could play a key role in mechanisms of unexplained infertility.

Kessler DL, Smith WD, Hamilton MS, Berger RE: Infertility in mice after unilateral vasectomy. Fertil Steril 1985; 43:308–312.

Thirty-six male DBA/1J mice, 9–10 weeks old, were randomized into three equal treatment groups: unilateral vasectomy, unilateral orchiectomy, or sham surgery. The mice were maintained under standard conditions postoperatively and during the follow-up period. Postoperative fertility was assessed monthly in a blinded fashion. Each male was placed in a cage with two females who had undergone ovulation induction 8 hours prior. The number of fertilized, unfertilized, and degenerated ova per female was determined directly. After the fourth month of follow-up, fertility was assessed by natural matings allowing term pregnancies. In addition, all mice underwent monthly serum antisperm antibody determinations and a measurement of serum testosterone at the end of the study. Mean percentages of fertilized ova were significantly decreased in unilaterally vasectomized mice at 2 and 3 months as compared to the two other groups. Antisperm antibody was also significantly increased in this group after 2 months. Serum testosterone levels were approximately equal. The authors suggest that infertility in the unilaterally vasectomized mice was immunologically mediated by antisperm antibody.

Maruyama DK, Hale RW, Rodgers BJ: Effects of white blood cells on the in-vitro penetration of zona-free hamster eggs by human spermatozoa. J Androl 1985; 6:127–135.

The authors carried out a series of experiments to measure the effects of WBCs on sperm penetration. In the first, semen samples having less than 1×10^6 WBC/ml and hamster egg sperm penetration assays of more than 25% were collected and prepared with standard methods to a dilution of 2×10^7 sperm/ml. Subjects had blood drawn at the time of semen sample collection, and WBCs were separated out using methods described in the literature. Sperm and WBC preparations were incubated for 18–22 hours prior to penetration assay performance. Ova and attached cumulus cells were recovered from superovulated golden hamsters and treated to disperse cumulus cells and remove the zona pellucidae. Then 20–30 ova were incubated for 2.5–3 hours in the prepared sperm–WBC concentrations of 0, 2.0, and 4.0×10^6 WBC/ml. In the second series, sperm were not exposed to WBC preparations until the time of *in vitro* insemination. In the third series, semen samples were exposed both during incubation and during insemination. At least 20 eggs were scored for each WBC preparation by direct examination. Penetration rates were determined at this time as well. Finally, semen samples with more than 3×10^6 WBC/ml had their WBC levels reduced to a mean of 1.25×10^6 using standard methods. Motility and penetration assays were done on these reduced WBC samples. Addition of WBCs was found to significantly decrease both sperm motility and penetration assay scores in all trials. Removal of WBCs significantly improved both these parameters of sperm function. In their discussion the authors present possible reasons for these findings.

31

Toxicants and Infertility: Identification and Prevention

Rebecca Z. Sokol

The potential hazard of toxicants to the male reproductive system is well established.[1] A toxicant, whether a chemical, physical, or biological agent, acts by interrupting biological processes either by a direct chemical action or indirectly via metabolic products by altering physiological control systems.[2] In the male reproductive system, such an interruption can occur at any level of the hypothalamic–pituitary–testicular axis, or alternatively, by altering posttesticular events such as sperm motility and/or function. Any disruption of these events by toxicants may lead to hypogonadism and/or infertility.

The most extensively studied toxicants are chemotherapeutic agents and radiation therapies used to treat malignancies.[3] Of the thousands of chemicals used in the workplace, relatively few have been examined for their effects on reproductive function.[4]

Chemotherapeutic Agents

The increasingly successful treatment of patients with malignant disease with either chemotherapy or radiation therapy has focused attention on the long-term effects of these therapies on gonadal function and fertility. Drugs used in the treatment of cancer are well known to produce a number of acute but reversible toxic effects on normal tissues. Most commonly affected are those organs containing self-renewing cell populations, such as bone marrow, skin, and the gastrointestinal tract.[5]

Cytotoxic damage to the testicular germinal epithelium by cancer treatment with chemotherapy and/or radiation is well documented.[6–10] In 1948, Spitz reported absent spermatogenesis at autopsy in 27 of 30 men treated with nitrogen mustard (mechlorethamine).[11] Since that time, a number of antineoplastic agents have been implicated as germ cell toxins.

The assessment of the adverse effects of individual cytotoxic drugs on the testes is made more difficult by the advent of combination chemotherapy. The effect of cytotoxic drugs on the testis have been studied by testicular biopsy, semen analysis, and endocrine assessment of the hypothalamic–pituitary–testicular axis.[10]

Management of Impotence and Infertility, edited by Douglas Whitehead and Harris Nagler,

Adult Male

Single Agent Chemotherapy: Cyclophosphamide or Chlorambucil

Single agent daily therapy with cyclophosphamide results in a rapidly progressive decrease in sperm count to azoospermia in approximately 90–120 days.[9] The testicular damage is dose-dependent. Limitation of the dose of cyclophosphamide from 2.5 to 4.6 mg/kg/day for 8 weeks or less minimizes this side effect. Doses greater than 3.7 mg/kg/day for greater than 3 months results in oligo or azoospermia.[12,13] Return of spermatogenesis does occur and may be related to the duration of treatment. Buchanan and co-workers reported normal spermatogenesis in 12 of 26 male patients within 15–49 months after cyclophosphamide-induced azoospermia. The return of spermatogenesis was not significantly related to the duration of therapy, total dose, or length of follow-up after stopping treatment.[14] Others do not report complete recovery of spermatogenesis.[10] Similarly, the germ cell toxicity of chlorambucil is dose-dependent with a minimal total dose of 400 mg resulting in azoospermia.[9] Thus, recovery of spermatogenesis is variable and the rapidity with which it resumes appears related to the total dose of chemotherapy administered.[5]

Combination Chemotherapy

Combination therapy has been a major therapeutic advance in the treatment of lymphoma, Hodgkin's disease, and leukemia.

In 1973, Sherins and DeVita confirmed that alkylating agents used with other agents cause sterility in most adult male lymphoma patients.[15] Testicular biopsy in 15 patients revealed complete germinal aplasia in 10, scattered spermatogonia with arrest of spermatogenesis in two, and normal spermatogenesis in three. In other studies, Chapman and co-workers reported virtually 100% azoospermia in men receiving MVPP. They documented azoospermia followed by return of active spermatogenesis in only 4 of 64 men (6%) from 15 to 51 months after treatment was stopped.[16] Sherins and DeVita observed azoospermia and testicular aplasia in patients as long as 4 years after completion of MVPP.[15]

Two prospective studies evaluating the hypothalamic–pituitary–testicular axis in men with Hodgkin's disease pre- and posttreatment with combination therapy have been published. Chapman and co-workers studied men prospectively to assess the effect of Hodgkin's disease and subsequent chemotherapy (MVPP) on gonadal function.[17] One-third (12 of 37) of the men presented with sperm counts of 50 million or more per ejaculate with greater than 40% motility before chemotherapy. Histologic abnormalities were noted in 8 of 9 pretreatment testicular biopsy specimens. After completion of 2 cycles of treatment, 14 men became persistently azoospermic. Of interest is the finding by Chapman and co-workers of decreased libido and sexual performance during chemotherapy in 74% of the men studied. Impotence occurred in 8%. These investigators noted elevated prolactin levels in 18 of 74 men treated with MVPP.[17]

In a similar study, Whitehead et al.[18] studied 19 men pre- and post-MVPP therapy for Hodgkin's disease. Fifteen of 19 men had sperm counts >20 million per ml with >40% motility. After completion of therapy, all patients were azoospermic or severely oligospermic (<1 million/ml). The median follicle-stimulating hormone (FSH) and leutinizing hormone (LH) levels and the median increments in these hormones after gonadotropin-releasing hormone (GnRH) administration were significantly elevated compared with age-matched control group. The mean testosterone level was significantly lower than controls, but not outside the lower limits of normal. No evidence of hyperprolactinemia was found.

More recently, Kreuser and co-workers evaluated the reproductive axis of 10 men with acute lymphoblastic leukemia who were in remission following aggressive combination chemotherapy with 10 chemotherapeutic agents, the majority of which were antimetabolites.[19] Elevated serum FSH levels and azoospermia were seen in all the men after completion of induction and consolidation therapy. However, serum LH, testosterone, and prolactin levels were within normal limits. These parameters were remeasured during the second year of maintenance therapy. All FSH serum levels had normalized. Sperm concentrations ranged from 20 to 108 million. In all cases motility and morphology had returned to greater than 60%. Ejaculation and erection were normal in all men. The investigators concluded that the chemotherapeutic agents used induced germ cell death with a stem cell depletion that was ultimately reversible. They suggested FSH measurement as a method to monitor germ cell depletion and recovery.

Thus, a review of the literature suggests that the severity of germ cell damage may well be related to the category of chemotherapeutic agent prescribed and to the dose and duration of therapy. Antimetabolites have been associated with less gonadal toxicity than alkylating agents.

Prepubertal and Pubertal Males

Reports concerning the effects of cytotoxic drugs on the gonadal function of children are scant and inconclusive.

Early reports suggested that the prepubertal testis was relatively insensitive to cytotoxic-induced damage. Since that time, other investigators have suggested that moderately severe damage to the tubular system of the testis unassociated with Leydig cell impairment may not be detected in the prepubertal boy using current tests of testicular function.[10]

Hsu et al. studied 24 boys and young adults who received an 8 week course of 2.5 mg/kg/day of cyclophosphamide.[12] They found no consistent relationship between the degree of gonadal dysfunction and the age of the patient when treatment was initiated. An increase in total dosage and in duration of the treatment was associated with a higher incidence of testicular dysfunction. Others have reported that pubertal germinal epithelium is susceptible to cytotoxic-induced damage, with aplasia, high FSH levels, and abnormal testicular histology.[20]

Sherins et al. reported elevated FSH and LH levels and borderline decreased T levels in pubertal boys who received MOPP treatment for Hodgkin's disease. By contrast, six prepubertal boys (3–10 years old) similarly treated showed no change in serum gonadotropins.[21] On the other hand, other investigators have noted abnormalities of testicular biopsies in prepubertal children treated with combination treatment for leukemia.[22] Recently, Levy and Sullivan reviewed studies that assessed the reproductive potential in survivors of childhood malignancy.[51] Adult reproductive potential varied according to the type of cancer diagnosed and the treatment instituted. In general, the use of alkylating agents resulted in a 50% reduction in fertility among male survivors. Radiation therapy induced the most profound damage to the testis. From their review, these investigators concluded that the prepubertal and adolescent gonad was less damaged by chemotherapy and radiation therapy than the postpubertal testis.

Gynecomastia

Gynecomastia has been described as a complication of chemotherapy. Sherins et al. reported gynecomastia and gonadal dysfunction in adolescent boys treated with MOPP.[21] The gynecomastia was associated with elevated gonadotropins, but normal prolactin and estradiol concentrations. They suggested that the gynecomastia was an accentuation of the transient breast enlargement seen normally in early puberty, enhanced by the relative decrease in serum testosterone. In contrast, Whitehead et al. noted gynecomastia in only 1 out of 12 British pubertal boys who were similarly treated with MOPP for Hodgkin's disease.[18] Similarly, Leydig cell dysfunction and gynecomastia have been reported in adult males treated with combination chemotherapy.[23–26]

Radiation Therapy

Exposure to X-rays, neutrons, and radioactive materials can cause germinal cell destruction.[20] Radiation effects on spermatogenesis depend on total dose received and the developmental stage of the germ cell at the time of exposure.[9] Rowland and Murthy studied the effects of graded doses of testicular irradiation on spermatogenesis in 67 normal men.[27] Spermatogonia were found to be the most radiosensitive cell type. The higher the dose of radiation, the lower the sperm number and the less the likelihood of recovery. Similarly, Ash noted that spermatogenesis returned to preirradiation sperm concentrations within 9–18 months for doses of <100 rads, 30 months for doses of 200 and 300 rads, and rarely after 400–600 rads.[28] Permanent sterility generally occurs after single-dose field irradiation to both testes (600–800 rads).[29] Similarly, inverted irradiation for Hodgkin's disease produces 70–100% azoospermia.[30]

Less has been published on the effects of radiation-induced gonadal damage in children. Brauner and co-workers studied 12 boys with acute lymphoblastic leukemia who had been treated with direct testicular irradiation 10 months to 8-1/2 years earlier.[31] Insufficient Leydig cell function, manifested by a low response of plasma testosterone to chorionic gonadotropin or an increased basal level of plasma LH (or both), was observed in 10 patients, 7 of whom were pubertal. Testosterone secretion was severely impaired in three pubertal boys studied more than 4 years after testicular irradiation. They concluded that testosterone deficiency is a frequent, albeit variable, complication of testicular irradiation.

Interventions to Maintain Fertility

Semen Cryopreservation

Semen cryopreservation is frequently recommended for men with Hodgkin's disease before the initiation of therapy. However, it is important to remember that some investigators have reported abnormal semen characteristics in this population before treatment.

Redman et al. reported only 3 pregnancies in 11 couples using artificial insemination of cryopreserved sperm.[32] Similar results were reported by Henry and co-workers.[33] Recently, Ragni and co-workers recommended that sperm from tumor patients are better preserved if frozen by a computerized slow-staged freezing method.[34]

Pretreatment with Synthetic GnRH Analogues

Variable results have been reported on the efficacy of pretreatment with GnRH analogues as "protector" agents against the testicular cytotoxic effects of chemotherapy.

In a mouse model, pretreatment with [D-leu6]-des-Gly-NH_2 proethylamide (a GnRH analogue) "protected" the germinal epithelium of cyclophosphamide-treated animals.[35] These investigators suggested that the interruption of the pituitary-gonadal axis may protect spermatogenesis from the effects of cytotoxic chemotherapy. In contrast, Goodpasture et al.[36] reported potentiation of the gonadotoxicity of cyclophosphamide by adjuvant treatment with a leutinizing hormone-releasing hormone (LHRH) agonist in beagle dogs.[36] The clinical use of such agents is considered experimental.

Gonadotoxins

Although numerous chemicals have been reported to alter the male reproductive axis, few have been extensively studied. However, groups of toxicants have been identified as leading to reproductive dysfunction in males. The workplace chemicals most thoroughly studied are the heavy metals, agricultural chemicals, and industrial chemicals.

Heavy Metals

The adverse reproductive effects of lead, mercury, cadmium, arsenic, lithium, antimony, boron, and manganese have been described in humans and experimental animals.[2,4] Of these, the most extensively studied is lead.

The reproductive toxicity of lead was recognized in the days of the Roman Empire.[37] Today, environmental exposure to toxic levels of lead occurs in a number of industries with potential adverse effects on the reproductive capacity of exposed men.[38–40] Clinical and animal studies indicate that abnormalities of spermatogenesis result from toxic exposure to lead.[40–43] Lancranjan et al.[38] evaluated the semen analysis, serum testosterone levels, and urinary gonadotropins of men who worked in a battery plant and were either exposed to lead on the production line or worked in the office. They found a dose-related suppression of spermatogenesis, normal or decreased serum T, and normal urinary gonadotropins. They concluded that lead was primarily a testicular toxin. Braunstein et al. reported blunted clomiphene and GnRH responses in lead poisoned men. Although the hormone data supported the concept that lead toxicity impairs hypothalamic–pituitary function, testicular biopsies revealed peritubular fibrosis, oligospermia, and vacuolation, suggesting that lead may also be a direct testicular toxin.[41] In a recent review, Cullen et al. reported on 55 patients referred for evaluation of possible lead intoxication.[39] Although a thorough and systematic analysis of reproductive function was not done, abnormalities of semen morphology were documented in five patients: two men were azoospermic and three men were oligospermic. Gonadotropin levels were normal in 12 of the 14 patients. One man had elevated LH and FSH levels whereas the other had an elevated FSH with a normal LH level. Serum testosterone levels were not reported.

In animals, lead exposure results in a dose–response suppression of serum testosterone and spermatogenesis.[42] However, investigations into the mechanisms of the toxic action of lead on the hypothalamic–pituitary–testicular axis indicate that lead exposure disrupts primarily the hypothalamic control of pituitary hormone secretion.[44] Although no human studies have investigated whether the toxic effects of lead on the reproductive system are reversible, animal studies suggest that the effects are reversible when lead exposure is removed.

Although chelation therapy using either ethylenediaminetetraacetic acid (EDTA) or 2,3-dimercaprol:British anti-lewisite (BAL) is recommended as treatments for the toxic effects of lead on the hematopoietic, renal, and neurologic systems, no data have been published on their use in the treatment of the reproductive toxicity.

Less thorough studies have been reported on the effects of the other heavy metals on male reproduction. Workers are primarily exposed to mercury during the manufacture of thermometers, mercury vapor lamps, paint, and electrical appliances and in mining. Both organic and inorganic mercury can alter spermatogenesis and decrease fertility in experimental animals.[9]

Boron is extensively used in the manufacture of many products including glass, cements, soaps, carpets, crockery, and leather. Earlier studies conducted using animal models suggested that the major adverse reproductive effect of boron is on the testes.[43] However, more recent studies conducted by Chapin and co-workers indicate that boron alters the hypothalamic–pituitary axis in a manner similar to that of lead. Clinical studies on the effects of boron have been conducted outside the United States. Oligospermia and decreased libido were reported in men working in boric acid-producing factories.[4]

Cadmium, another ubiquitous metal, is a testicular toxin. Animal studies suggest direct testicular toxicity.[9] Clinical studies associate cadmium exposure with testicular toxicity, altered libido, and infertility. As with the treatment for lead toxicity, chelation therapy has been proposed for the treatment of cadmium toxicity.

Agricultural Chemicals

Dibromochloropropane (DBCP) is a nematocide widely used in agriculture in the United States and Europe until 1977. With the documentation by Whorton and co-workers that DBCP is a testicular toxin, the American population became aware of the fact that male fertility could be adversely affected by occupation-related chemical exposures.[45]

The initial studies reported by Whorton found a direct relationship between sperm count and duration of DBCP exposure in DBCP production workers in Northern California.[15] Animal and human studies indicate that DBCP is a testicular toxin.[46] Exposed workers will usually present with hypergonadotropic hypogonadism.[45,47] Recovery of spermatogenesis and fertility is variable following removal of the exposure.[48] DBCP use is now prohibited in the United States.

Other agricultural chemicals implicated as male reproductive toxicants include epichlorhydrin, DDT, ethylene diebromide, kepone, and the dioxins.[2]

DDT, a commonly used pesticide, acts as an estrogen antagonist when absorbed, competing with estradiol for estrogen receptors. Thus DDT can alter the male reproductive system by disrupting the hypothalamic–pituitary–testicular axis.

Similarly, kepone, a chlorinated polycyclic ketone, has been demonstrated to have estrogen like actions. Low dose kepone exposure in male rats and quails adversely affects the testes. Abnormal sperm morphology and abnormal testicular biopsies have been reported in kepone production workers.

Agent orange, the most widely used of the herbicides during the Vietnam War, and 2,4,5-trichlorophenoxyacetic acid, a widely used herbicide in the United States until it was banned in 1979, have also been investigated as possible male reproductive toxicants. Data published on the toxic effects of agent orange continue to elicit controversy. In an epidemiologic study conducted by Townsend and coworkers[49] no adverse reproductive events were documented in the wives of employees exposed to chlorinated toxins. Most investigators report no differences in semen characteristics and infertility in men exposed to agent orange.[50]

Industrial Chemicals

The most thoroughly studied industrial chemical is methyl chloride, a colorless gas used primarily as a chemical intermediate in the production of organosilicate compounds and gasoline antiknock additives.[52] Acute exposure of rats to MeCl causes toxicity in both the testis and epididymis. In a series of elegant studies, investigators identified the initial testicular lesion to be delayed release of late stage spermatids from the seminiferous epithelium, followed by generalized disruption and disorganization of the seminiferous epithelium.[53] Further studies provided evidence to implicate the testicular toxicity of MeCl in the induction of the cytotoxic effects on sperm that eventually lead to failure of fertilization and concomitant increased preimplantation loss postexposure.[52]

Organic solvents have also been reported to induce deleterious changes in semen quality, testicular size, and gonadotropins.[4]

Summary

Exposure to reproductive toxicants may result in male infertility. Although a fair amount of research has been conducted in the area of the effects of chemotherapy and radiation therapy on the male reproductive system, more extensive research is warranted. Even less research has focused on the area of reproductive hazards in the workplace. Most of the data to date have been generated using animal models. Few clinical studies have been published. In one of the rare studies investigating the association between occupational group and sperm concentration in infertile men, investigators in Australia collected pertinent reproductive information from 1695 male patients. The patients were categorized into nine occupational groups: professional, administrative, clerical, sales, farmers, transport, craftsmen, service, and not employed. Mean sperm concentrations were significantly higher in the administrative and professional groups and lowest in the farming and transport groups.[54]

The clinician can and should take an active role in the identification and prevention of reproductive toxicity.[55,56] The following steps should be taken:

1. Identify the exposure and the potential health effects.
2. Characterize the extent of exposure.

3. Assess the degree of risk to the patient.
4. Initiate a plan to control or prevent the exposure.

The need to identify reproductive toxicants in the workplace is clear. More research is needed to elucidate the association between occupation and infertility in men. Without data, prediction and prevention of human reproductive hazard are impossible.

REFERENCES

1. Dixon W: Toxic responses of the reproductive system. In: Klaassen CD, Amdur MO, Doull J eds. Casarett and Doull's toxicology, ed. New York: Macmillan, 1986:453–454.
2. Mattison DR: The mechanisms of action of reproductive toxins. Am J Industr Med 1983; 4:65–79.
3. Damewood MD, Grochow LB: Prospects for fertility after chemotherapy or radiation for neoplastic disease. Fertil Steril 1986; 45:443–459.
4. Reproductive Hazards in the Workplace: Congress of the United States. Office of Technology Assessment, 1985.
5. Schilsky RL et al: Gonadal dysfunction in patients receiving chemotherapy for cancer. Ann Intern Med 1980; 83:109–114.
6. Kinsella TJ: Effects of radiation therapy and chemotherapy on testicular function. In: Burger EJ et al. (ed), Sperm measures and reproductive success. New York: Alan R. Liss, 1989:157–177.
7. Chapman R: Effects of cytotoxic therapy on sexuality in gonadal function. Semin Oncol 1982; 9:84–89.
8. Lushbaugh CC, Casarett GW: The effects of gonadal irradiation in clinical radiation therapy: A review. Cancer 1976; 37:1111–1120.
9. Barlow SM, Sullivan FM: Reproductive hazards of industrial chemicals. London: Academic Press, 1982.
10. Shalet SM: Effects of cancer chemotherapy on gonadal function of patients. Cancer Treatment Rev 1980; 7:141–152.
11. Spitz S: The histological effects of nitrogen mustards on human tumors and tissues. Cancer 1948; 1:383.
12. Hsu AC et al: Gonadal function in males treated with cyclophosphamide for nephrotic syndrome. Fertil Steril 1979; 3:173–177.
13. Etteldorf JN et al: Gonadal function, testicular histology and meiosis following cyclophosphamide therapy in patients with nephrotic syndrome. J Pediatr 1976; 88:206.
14. Buchanan JD: Return of spermatogenesis after stopping cyclophosphamide therapy. Lancet 1975; 2:156–157.
15. Sherins RJ, DeVita VT Jr: Effect of drug treatment for lymphoma on male reproductive capacity. Ann Intern Med 1973; 79:216–220.
16. Chapman RM, Sutcliffe SB, Rees LH, Edwards RW, Malpas JS: Cyclical combination chemotherapy and gonadal function. The Lancet 1979; 1:285–289.
17. Chapman RM, Sutcliffe SB, Malpas JS: Male gonadal dysfunction in Hodgkin's disease. JAMA 1981; 245:1323–1328.
18. Whitehead E, Shalet SM, Blackledge G: The effects of Hodgkin's disease and combination chemotherapy on gonadal function in the adult male. Cancer 1982; 49:418–422.
19. Kreuser ED, Hetzel WD, Heit W, Hoelzen D, Kurrle E, Xeros N, Heimpel H: Reproductive and endocrine gonadal functions in adults following multidrug chemotherapy for acute lymphoblastic or undifferentiated leukemia. J Clin Oncol 1988; 6:588–595.
20. Shalet SM: Disorders of the endocrine system due to radiation and cytotoxic chemotherapy. Clin Endocrinol 1983; 18:637–659.
21. Sherins RJ et al: Gynecomastia and gonadal dysfunction in adolescent boys treated with combination chemotherapy for Hodgkin's disease. N Engl J Med 1978; 299:12–16.
22. Blatt J, Poplack DG, Sherins RJ: Testicular function in boys after chemotherapy for acute lymphoblastic leukemia. N Engl J Med 1981; 304:1121–1124.

23. Glass AR, Berenberg J: Gynecomastia after chemotherapy for lymphoma. Arch Intern Med 1979; 139:1048–1049.
24. Friedman NM, Plymate SR: Leydig cell dysfunction and gynecomastia in adult males treated with alkylating agents. Clin Endocrinol 1980; 12:553–556.
25. Turner RA et al: Gynecomastia after cytotoxic therapy for metastatic testicular cancer. Arch Intern Med 1982; 142:896–897.
26. Trump DL et al: Gynecomastia in men following antineoplastic therapy. Arch Intern Med 1982; 142:511–513.
27. Rowland KM, Murthy A: Hodgkin's disease: Long term effects of therapy. Med Pediatr Oncol 1986; 14:88–96.
28. Ash P: The influence of radiation on fertility in man. Br J Rad 1980; 53:271–278.
29. Lushbaugh CC: The effects of gonadal irradiation in clinical radiation therapy: A review. Cancer 1976; 37:1111–1120.
30. Speiser B et al: Aspermia following lower truncal irradiation in Hodgkin's disease. Cancer 1973; 32:692–698.
31. Brauner R, Czernichow P, Cramer P, Schaison G, Rappaport R: Leydig cell function in children after direct testicular irradiation for acute lymphoblastic leukemia. N Engl J Med 1983; 309:25–28.
32. Redman JR et al: Semen cryopreservation and artificial insemination for Hodgkin's disease. J Clin Oncol 1987; 5:233–238.
33. Hendry WF et al: Semen analysis and testicular cancer in Hodgkin's disease: Pre- and post-treatment findings and implications for cryopreservation. Br U Urol 1983; 55:769–773.
34. Ragni G et al: Computerized slow-staged freezing of semen from men with testicular tumors of Hodgkin's disease preserves sperm better than standard vapor freezing. Fertil Steril 1990; 53:6:1072–1075.
35. Glode LM, Rolinson J, Gould SF: Protection from cyclophosphamide-induced testicular damage with an analogue of gonadotropin-releasing hormone. Lancet 1981; 1:1132–1134.
36. Goodpasture JC et al: Potentiation of gonadal toxicity of cyclophosphamide in the dog by adjuvant treatment with an LRH agonist. J Androl 1987; 8:30–35.
37. Gilfillan SC: Lead poisoning and the fall of Rome. J Occup Med 1965; 7:53–60.
38. Lancranjan I, Popescu HI, Gavanescu O et al: Reproductive ability of workmen occupationally exposed to lead. Arch Environ Health 1975; 30(8):396–399.
39. Cullen MR, Robins JM, Esbencizi B: Adult inorganic lead intoxication: Presentation of 31 new cases and a review of recent advances in the literature. Medicine 62:221–247.
40. Winder C: Reproductive and chromosomal effects of occupational exposure to lead in males. Reprod Toxicol 1989; 3:221–233.
41. Braunstein GD, Dahlgren J, Loriaux DO: Hypogonadism in chronically lead poisoned men. Infertility 1978; 1:33–35.
42. Sokol RZ, Madding CE, Swerdloff RS: Lead toxicity and the hypothalamic–pituitary–testicular axis. Biol Reprod 1985; 33:722–728.
43. Weir RJ, Fisher RS: Toxicologic studies on borox and boric acid. Toxicol Appl Pharmacol 1972; 23:251–364.
44. Sokol RZ: Hormonal effects of lead acetate in the male rat: Mechanism of action. Biol Reprod 1987; 37:1135–1138.
45. Whorton MD, Krauss RM, Marshall S: Infertility in male pesticide workers. Lancet 1977; 2:1259–1261.
46. Whorton D, Foliart D: DBCP: Eleven years later. Reprod Toxicol 1988; 3:155–161.
47. Lipschultz LT, Ross EC, Whorton MD et al: DBCP and its effects on testicular function in man. J Urol 1980; 124:464–468.
48. Lantz GO, Cunningham GR, Huckins C et al: Recovery from severe oligospermia after exposure to dibromochloropropane. Fertil Steril 1981; 35:46–54.
49. Townsend JC, Bodner KM, Van Peenen PFD et al: Survey of reproductive events of wives of employees exposed to chlorinated dioxins. Am J Epidemiol 1982; 115:695–713.
50. Suskind RR, Hertzung VS: Human health effects of 2,4,5-T and its toxic contaminants. JAMA 1984; 251(18):2372–2380.
51. Levy MJ, Stillman RJ: Reproductive potential in

survivors of childhood malignancy. Pediatrician 1991; 18:61–70.
52. Chellman GJ, Hurtt ME, Bus JS, Working PK: Role of testicular versus epididymal toxicity in the induction of cytotoxic damage in Fischer-344 rat sperm by methyl chloride. Reprod Toxicol 1987; 1:25–36.
53. Chapin RE, White RD, Morgan KT, Bus JG: Studies of lesions induced in the testes and epididymis of F-344 rats by inhaled methyl chloride. Toxicol Appl Pharmacol 1984; 76:328–343.
54. Henderson J, Rennie GC, Baker HWG. Association between occupational group and sperm concentration in infertile men. Clin Reprod Fertil 1986; 4:275–281.
55. Paul M, Himmelstein J: Reproductive hazards in the workplace: What the practitioner needs to know about chemical exposures. Obstet Gynecol 1988; 71:921–938.
56. Clegg ED, Sakai CS, Voytek PE: Assessment of reproductive risks. Biol Reprod 1986; 34:5–16.

ANNOTATED BIBLIOGRAPHY

Damewood MD, Grochow LB: Prospects for fertility after chemotherapy or radiation for neoplastic disease. Fertil Steril 1986; 45:443.

This is a review article that comprehensively covers the effects of radiation therapy and chemotherapy on the male and female reproductive axis. Included are discussions of animal studies as well as clinical studies dealing with these topics. Information is included regarding the effects of radiation on testicular function based on the testicular dose of radiation. Theoretical interventions to maintain fertility prior to therapy are discussed. A comprehensive bibliography can be found at the end of the article.

Whorton D, Foliart D: DBCP: 11 years later. Reprod Toxicol 1988; 3:155.

In this article, the authors review the identification of DBCP as a reproductive toxicant. The article summarizes the animal and human investigations of the reproductive effects of DBCP. Included are tables describing DBCP thresholds for reproductive effects on rats, mice, and rabbits, as well as a summary of the human DBCP studies from 1977 to 1978. The discussion includes an analysis of the role of route exposure, duration of exposure, and dose exposure on subsequent fertility, pregnancy outcome, and chromosomal analysis of children conceived during or after parental exposure to DBCP.

Included is an extensive reference list of 55 articles, all dealing with the effects of DBCP on the reproductive system.

Winder C: Reproductive and chromosomal effects of occupational exposure to lead in males. Repro Toxicol 1989; 3:221.

In this article, Dr. Winder reviews extensively the reproductive and chromosomal effects of occupational exposure to lead in males. Included are animal as well as clinical studies. Discussions regarding the pathophysiology and mechanisms by which lead exerts its toxicity on the male reproductive axis are discussed.

32 Immunologic Infertility: Significance and Treatment Options

Richard Bronson

Both spermatozoa and mature oocytes are short lived cells that only transiently make their appearance, in a periodic manner, within the female reproductive tract. Their interaction, if successful, may lead to the development of a zygote, initiating a potential chain of events resulting in successful reproduction. However, the evanescent nature of gametes makes them especially susceptible to damage. Spermatozoa must also have an unusual relationship with the immune systems of both men, of whom they are a part, yet can be immunologically rejected due to new developmental antigens to which the immune system is not tolerant, and of women, whose bodies they periodically invade as foreigners.

Spermatogenesis begins during puberty, long after the immune system has learned to distinguish between itself, the antigenic expression of its own tissues, and extra corporeal antigens. Despite this circumstance, an autoimmune response against spermatozoa is uncommon, occurring only in approximately 7–8% of unselected men from infertile couples.

Following their intravaginal deposition, spermatozoa pass through various immunocompetent compartments of the female reproductive tract yet fail to elicit an immune response, even with frequent coital activity. Clues to the lack of immunologic responsiveness in both males and females reside within the immune system itself. Populations of lymphocytes with putative T suppressor signatures have been detected both with semen and the submucosal regions of the epididymis. Activated macrophages (Ia^+), which are capable of acting as antigen-processing cells, have access to spermatogonia that express unique antigens and exist in the basal compartment of the seminiferous tubule outside of the protective sequestration of the blood–testis barrier. Furthermore, macrophages and Ia^+ epithelial cells have been found in contact with sperm in the rete testis and regions of the epididymis. These findings suggest that active immunosuppression may normally protect sperm from immunologic rejection in the male. Conversely, both the male and female reproductive tracts have

Management of Impotence and Infertility, edited by Douglas Whitehead and Harris Nagler,

been shown to be capable of a local immune response and to participate, at a more general level, in mucosal immunity.

This immune response may not be geographically restricted, and the concept recently has developed of a common mucosal immunity, that encompasses several mucosal surfaces of various organs. The trafficking of lymphocytes between distant mucosal sites has been demonstrated. The local mucosal immune response may, in addition, influence and suppress the systemic humoral response. In addition, the immunoglobulins produced at the mucosal level are of different classes (primarily secretary IgA). That an isolated mucosal immunity to sperm can exist in the male, in the absence of systemic circulating antibodies directed against spermatozoa, has also been suggested by the presence of antisperm antibodies in semen, while absent in serum.

Regulation of Immunoglobulin Secretion

Secretory IgA is the major immunoglobulin present in tears, saliva, colostrum, as well as respiratory, gastrointestinal, and genital urinary tract secretions.[1] It is the product of two distinct cell types. Secretory IgA is synthesized by plasma cells, and epithelial cell produce secretory component (SC), which acts as a regulatory transport protein for IgA. A membrane SC–IgA complex forms, due to the presence of an SC binding site on polymeric IgA, which is then internalized and transported to the apical region of the epithelial cell. The SC–IgA complex is then released into the external secretions.

In humans, passive transudation rather than active transport of plasma-derived immunoglobulin is primarily responsible for the presence of monomeric IgA and IgG in external secretions. However, the vast majority of polymeric IgA found in external secretions is derived from local synthesis by plasma cells, rather than selective transport from blood. Radiolabeled polymeric IgA administered intravenously appears in very small quantities in nasal and intestinal secretions.

Locally secreted IgA released by subepithelial plasma cells interacts with SC on the surfaces of epithelial cells via noncovalent binding. This complex is internalized and stabilized by the formation of disulfide bridges. The internalized SC–IgA complex is transported in the form of a vesicle through the epithelial cell (a process that takes approximately 30 minutes). Intracytoplasmic IgA-containing vesicles move toward the apical surface of epithelial cells and fuse with the apical membrane, releasing the SC–IgA complex.

That the male reproductive tract can participate in a local immune response to infections has been suggested by the finding that total IgA concentration is greater in the prostatic secretions than IgG or IgM. Total IgA in the presence of prostatitis has been found to be greater than total IgA in men with urinary tract infection. Greater than 50% of the total prostatic fluid IgA contains secretory component, suggesting either its local production or active transport from serum by prostatic epithelium. In prostatitis caused by *Escherichia coli*, 90% of total IgA and IgG is anti-*E. coli* specific. *E. coli*-specific IgA concentration is 40 times higher in prostatic fluid, when compared with serum, providing further circumstantial evidence that active IgA transport occurs in the prostate. Measurement of the IgA antibody response in men following vasectomy also supports the fact that the epididymis is capable of local IgA secretion.

Characterization of Specific Antisperm Antibodies in the Male Reproductive Tract Secretion

The ejaculates of men with autoimmunity to sperm commonly contain a mixture of IgA and IgG antisperm antibodies. Antisperm IgG is derived primarily as a transudate from serum, and its presence in the ejaculate would be expected to correlate with the titer of circulating antisperm antibodies. The local production of antisperm IgA in the male genital tract has been suggested both by its detection in semen while absent from sera, and the presence of antisperm antibodies with unique regional binding specificities on the sperm surface, different from those present in serum. In a study of approximately 850 matched serum and semen samples, immunoglobulins were detected solely on the sperm surface in 15% of cases. Hellstrom and associates have also demonstrated the presence of IgA on sperm despite its absence in serum, as detected by immunobead binding.[2]

Using a new application of the immunobead binding technique, in which monoclonal antibodies (MAbs) directed against IgA subclasses were first used to probe the sperm surface, and then secondarily, antimurine immunoglobulin immunobeads used to detect MAbs, Bronson and Cooper demonstrated a preponderance of the IgA_1 subclass of antisperm antibodies in the ejaculates of men with autoimmunity sperm. A wide variation was noted, however, in the ratio of antisperm IgA_1 relative to IgA_2 between different men. In some individuals, this ratio approached one. They suggested that the varying proportion of antisperm IgA subclasses in different men could be a reflection of varying etiologies or different routes of immunization.

Lymphocytes that produce IgA_1 and IgA_2 subclasses display a varying distribution in lymphoid organs. While IgA_1 cells predominate in varying degrees in most glandular and secretory tissues, IgA_2-containing cells are more frequent within the large intestine. The intrarectal inoculation of rabbits with spermatozoa and gastric inoculation in rats have both been shown to lead to antisperm autoantibody production, the latter associated with decreased fertility.

Several studies have documented a higher incidence of antisperm antibodies (ASA) in homosexual men than in heterosexual men from infertile couples. The ratio of ASA isotypes is also different; a higher incidence of antisperm IgM relative to IgG and IgA immunoglobulins classes has also been noted in sera of homosexual men. It has been postulated that the etiology of autoimmunity to sperm, or the route of immunization might account for these observations. Could intrarectal deposition of semen in these men then lead to the development of IgA_2-secreting lymphocytes that subsequently home to the male genital tract, where they contribute to the local production of antisperm antibody?

Effect of Antisperm Autoantibodies on Sperm Function

Proof that autoimmunity to sperm plays a significant role in male infertility requires documentation of the presence of immunoglobulins on the sperm surface, as well as evidence of alteration in the ability of such antibody-labeled sperm to either enter the female reproductive tract or to fertilize eggs. It is now clear that 5–10% of men from unselected infertile couples will manifest autoimmunity to sperm.[3] Approximately 85% of these men with circulating humeral antisperm antibodies (ASA) will also have ASAs in their ejaculates. While these antibody-labeled sperm move well within seminal fluid, their ability to penetrate and survive within human cervical mucus is impaired. Hence, the more sperm that are coated with immunoglobulins, the fewer will enter cervical mucus and populate the female reproductive tract (Table 32-1).[4] This impairment appears to be mediated through the Fc portion of the

Table 32-1 Correlation between Extent of Autoimmunity and Number of Motile Spermatozoa in Cervical Mucus at Postcoital Testing[a]

Antibody-Bound Sperm in Ejaculate Detected by Immunobead Binding (%)	Total Number of Motile Sperm in Ejaculate $\times 10^6$	Number of Motile Sperm/hpf in Postcoital Cervical Mucus
100	42	0–3[b]
	45	0–3[b]
	69	0–1
	80	0–4
	82	0–4
	127	0
	157	0–8
	176	0–1
	345	0
	472	0
	638	7
>50 but <100	15	15
	35	3
	45	2–7
	49	3
	49	0–1
	63	6–15
	67	4
	715	8
<50	94	7
	118	15–40
	150	12
	153	15–26
	158	15–30

[a] Cervical mucus was examined within 48 hours preceding the thermal shift, 8 to 12 hours after coitus.

[b] Spermatozoa in cervical mucus are listed as the average observed or as a range in each high power field (c 400).

immunoglobulin molecule. Hence, spermatozoa exposed to Fab preparations of antisperm IgG are able to swim through cervical mucus, while those labeled with intact antibody do not. Similarly, we demonstrated that immunoglobulins of the IgA class bound to the sperm surface could be degraded by an IgA_1 protease derived from *Neisseria gonorrhea.*[5] This enzyme is limited in its substrate specificity to IgA_1, cleaving the heavy chain at amino acid bond 235–236 of the hinge region. The Fc portion of IgA is liberated from the sperm surface. However, utilizing Fab-directed monoclonal antibody probes, we demonstrated that such sperm remain coated by IgA Fab. These protease-treated spermatozoa showed an improved ability to penetrate into and sustain motility within human cervical mucus. On this basis, we postulated that a solid phase moiety of human cervical mucus possesses an as yet identified receptor for a ligand on the Fc portion of the immunoglobulin molecule. That this effect is not species specific was demonstrated in a study of the effects of a number of antisperm monoclonal antibodies, provided by the WHO Task Force on vaccines for fertility regulation, on the ability of human sperm to penetrate bovine cervical mucus *in vitro.* Those MAbs directed against epitopes present on the living sperm surface (as detected by immunobead binding) impaired sperm penetration through a column of bovine cervical mucus, while monoclonal antibodies directed against subsurface epitopes (detected by indirect immunofluorescence with permeabilized sperm) did not. Antisperm antibodies may also impair sperm function through the mediation of a premature acrosome reaction (AR). Capacitated mammalian sperm must undergo an acrosome reaction prior to penetration of the zona pellucida. The timing of this process varies between species. In the hamster, the acrosome reaction appears to occur as spermatozoa pass through the cumulus oophorus, and these sperm subsequently adhere to the zona pellucida. In mice, and possibly in humans, acrosome-intact sperm initially bind the zona pellucida where they subsequently undergo an acrosome reaction that is stimulated by the zona glycoprotein ZP3. Should acrosome-reacted sperm in humans prove to be unable to bind to the zona pellucida, antisperm antibodies that cause the premature loss of the plasma membrane and acrosomal contents could impair the ability of such sperm to bind to and fertilize eggs.

We have provided preliminary evidence that certain sperm head-directed antibodies in the presence of complement may promote an acrosome reaction ultrastructurally similar to that seen following incubation of spermatozoa in media containing human serum albumen at concentrations that lead to capacitation. The mechanism of plasma membrane shedding and release of acrosomal contents in these experiments is different from that noted in the "classical" acrosome reaction of other mammals, in that fusion of plasma membranes (PM) and outer acrosome membranes (OAM) did not occur. Rather, vesiculation of the outer acrosomal membrane (rather than formation of a hybrid vesicle of PM and OAM) occurs concomitantly with ballooning of the plasma membrane and release of acrosomal matrix. That these ultrastructural alterations are physiologically relevant is suggested by the increased ability of such antisperm antibody-complement-treated sperm to penetrate zona-free hamster eggs. Recent evidence has been presented that certain antisperm antibodies can also promote an acrosome reaction in the absence of complement. In addition, sera containing sperm head-directed ASAs may promote or inhibit the penetration of zona-free eggs by mechanisms that do not involve an alteration of the proportion in acrosome-reacted sperm.

Sperm Oocyte Penetration: Role of Fc and Complement Receptors

During experiments to determine the effects of ASAs on human sperm-fertilizing ability, we noted a paradoxical promotion by antibody labeling of the penetration of human spermatozoa into zona-free hamster eggs. This result was surprising, in light of prior circumstantial clinical evidence that antisperm antibodies were associated with infertility, and other preliminary laboratory studies that appeared to indicate that antisperm antibodies inhibited fertilization. Although we assumed that the results between different laboratories could have been on the basis of antibody specificities to different epitopes in the different sera studied, this explanation did not explain why promotion of egg penetration could occur in some cases. Given that the weight of evidence, at that time, was against the presence of specific oolemmal sperm receptors playing a role in fertilization (in contrast to the zona pellucida, where species-specific sperm receptors had been identified), we turned toward the spermatozoan for an explanation. Initially, we speculated that epitopes against which antisperm antibodies were directed possessed lateral mobility within the sperm plasma membrane. Antibody binding could lead to clustering of antigen, similar to the patching and capping formation of glycoprotein-free zones within the plasma membrane, that might promote the acrosome reaction.

Subsequently, Aitken et al. demonstrated that IgG purified from different human sera containing antisperm antibodies could either inhibit or promote the penetration of zona-free hamster eggs by ASA-labeled human spermatozoa.[6] Lansford et al. also provided evidence that an increased proportion of acrosome-reacted sperm was seen in ejaculates of men with autoimmunity to sperm and that their sera promoted the release of acrosomal contents in the absence of complement. Unfortunately, this study was performed in the absence of a control (a supervital dye) to document alterations in sperm permeability related to pathologic sperm damage due to autoimmunity to sperm. Nor was evidence presented of an enhancement of the egg-penetrating ability of these sperm.

When we studied the ultrastructural appearance of a highly motile population of sperm from a fertile donor, following antibody labeling with each of several sperm head-directed ASAs, and after incubation in capacitating medium *in vitro*, no difference was observed in the proportion of spermatozoa acrosome reacted between treatment groups, despite a varying degree of enhancement of inhibition in the ability of antibody-labeled human sperm to penetrate zona-free hamster eggs.

Given these concerns, we postulated that some other mechanism independent of the acrosome reaction promoted fertilization by antibody-labeled sperm. The majority of human spermatozoa that adhere to the oolemma of zona-free hamster eggs are acrosome-reacted. Hence, if the proportion of acrosome-reacted sperm were not increased following antibody labeling, then ASA was either promoting the binding of antibody-labeled sperm to the egg surface, or the ability of such oolemmal bound sperm to penetrate the egg.

When zona-free hamster eggs were coincubated with a highly motile population of sperm obtained by swim-up from the same ejaculate, either antibody-labeled or antibody-free, an increased number of the former sperm became adherent to the oolemma vs. those antibody-free. This confirmed that antisperm antibodies were promoting sperm adherence to the egg surface. To determine whether the increased penetration of eggs was associated solely with increased binding, or was related to an alteration in the mechanism of incorporation, increasing the likelihood of penetration, experiments were performed in which eggs were exposed for short periods of time to populations of antibody-labeled or antibody-free sperm. Immediately after sperm adherence to the egg surface, eggs were washed out of sperm suspension and further observed in sperm-free medium. In this manner, a limited population of sperm on the egg surface could be studied. The ratio of penetrating to the total number of adherent sperm (penetrated plus oolemmal bound) was compared in both treatment groups and found to be similar. The mechanism of sperm incorporation by the egg, as determine by scanning electron microscopy, was no different from that of antibody-free sperm.

As promotion of acrosome reaction may be expected to increase the number of oolemmal adherent sperm following antibody labeling and overnight incubation under capacitating conditions, *Pisum savitum* agglutinin (PSA) staining was utilized to document that equal numbers of acrosome-reacted sperm were present in the ASA-labeled and ASA-free groups, for each serum tested, at the time of insemination. The percent acrosome reacted sperm ranged from 6 to 12% and there was no difference between treatment groups.

At least two separate mechanisms could account for this phenomenon of increased sperm oolemmal adherence following antibody labeling. A common epitope could be present on sperm and egg surfaces, which would allow antibody bridging between gametes. Alternatively, the oolemma may possess Fc receptors. Evidence for both mechanisms exists. Immunization of laboratory animals with sperm has been found to lead to the production of antibodies that react with unfertilized or fertilized eggs, or preimplantation embryos as well as sperm. Oncofetal antigens have also been shown to be present on both sperm and egg surfaces.

Recently, we have shown that zona-free hamster and human eggs bind monomeric IgG Fc fragments as well as hear aggregated IgG. The finding of an Fc receptor on a nonimmune cell is not unique, in that Fc receptors have been documented on syncytiotrophoblast and gastrointestinal epithelium. Whether these receptors play a functional role in sperm interaction is currently unknown.

The antibody-mediated promotion of sperm penetration of zona-free hamster eggs has important clinical implications. Previous studies have suggested that antisperm antibodies may cause reproductive dysfunction by impairing sperm-fertilizing ability at the level of either the zona pellucida or oolemma, depending on the epitopes against which they are directed. Our present results suggest that antisperm antibodies, through their enhancement of sperm adherence to the egg surface, may increase the risk of polyspermy, leading to reproductive failure through this mechanism. Triploid human eggs have been shown to have both diminished developmental competence during their preimplantion growth as well as a higher likelihood of postimplantation loss, increasing the possibility of occult or clinically manifest spontaneous abortion.

Fertilization Failure Associated with Immunities to Sperm

Several investigators have utilized zona-free hamster eggs as a model to determine whether antisperm antibodies from infertile couples may alter the fertilizing ability of human sperm. Alexander et al. exposed spermatozoa to whole serum containing antisperm antibodies or to an IgG fraction of the serum. Penetration rates in the presence of such sperm antibodies were 15% compared with 59% for control sera. Six sera completely blocked penetration of zona-free hamster eggs. Haas et al. studied the effect of plasma containing antisperm IgG on spermatozoa when added at the time of insemination of zona-free hamster eggs. Four of six samples significantly reduced sperm penetration. As noted previously, Aitkin and associates investigated the effects of immunoglobulins obtained from a large group of sera containing antisperm antibodies on sperm egg penetrating ability.[6] Approximately 25% of these samples promoted penetration of zone-free hamster eggs by human sperm, 25% were neutral, and the remainder inhibited penetration. Whether these effects were in part mediated by alterations in the effective concentration of motile sperm, due to agglutination, or direct effects at the level of the gamete membranes was unclear. These results do emphasize, however, that as the immunologic response to spermatozoa is polyclonal, individuals can make antibodies directed against different epitopes that may have varying effects on sperm function. This is well illustrated by the investigation of the effects of monoclonal antibodies raised against spermatozoa of several species on sperm function. These various antibodies can affect the ability of the spermatozoa to bind to and penetrate the zona pellucida or the oolemma itself. The specificity of such immunoglobulin-mediated interactions has been demonstrated recently by the characterization of two monoclonal antibodies, each reactive with the same plasma membrane glycoprotein of living, motile guinea pig sperm, but different antigenic epitopes, one functionally significant and the other not.

The realization that sera contain antibodies directed against not one but several different sperm surface antigens has emphasized the need to identify and characterize these antigens. Several preliminary studies have already been performed, in which solubilized surface moieties have been characterized by polyacrylamide gel electrophoresis and high-pressure liquid chromatography. These include PH20, isolated from guinea pig spermatozoa, RSA-1 isolated from rabbit sperm, and FA-1 isolated from human and mouse sperm, as well as mouse testis.

An alternative approach has been to utilize clinically derived sera from men and women likely to be infertile on an immunologic basis due to the presence of antisperm antibodies, to identify sperm surface antigens that play a role in human fertilization. Following labeling the sperm surface proteins of living human sperm with ^{125}I, Primakoff et al. used sera from 27 infertile males, 18 infertile females, and 4 vasectomized males (each possessing antisperm antibodies detected by immunobead binding) for immunoprecipitation of solubilized sperm surface glycoproteins.[7] The sera were remarkably similar in their surface antigen recognition, and specifically immunoprecipitated the same small group of ^{125}I-labeled surface proteins, which included polypeptides in the region of 90, 40–45, and 26 kDa. Treatment with *N*-glycanase showed that the proteins were glycoproteins with N-linked carbohydrates. When separated on two-dimensional gels, the 90-kDa polypeptide was shown to be a major sperm surface component, whereas the other peptides are minor components. Two-dimensional gel comparison also indicated that the 90-, 40 to 45-, and 26-kDa glycoproteins are a small subset of the total ensemble of sperm surface proteins.

To determine whether antisperm antibodies alter the ability of human sperm to penetrate the zona pellucida, we exposed populations of motile sperm obtained from fertile men to sera containing antisperm antibodies reactive with the sperm head. Other spermatozoa from the same ejaculate were exposed to the same panel of sera, following their absorption with spermatozoa, to lower sperm antibody levels. Nonviable human eggs were previously retrieved from surgical specimens of human ovaries, which had been minced and filtered serially through nylon mesh gauze, and salt stored until further use. These zonae were then first exposed to a population of spermatozoa completely antibody labeled over their heads as determined by immunobead binding. Numbers of ASA-labeled sperm adherent to the zona pellucida were determined. They were subsequently exposed to a second population of sperm from the same ejaculate, but exposed to absorbed sera, in which the majority of sperm were now antibody-free. The number of sperm bound to the zona pellucida was again observed following serial washing. When all sperm were antibody-labeled, it was rare to find more than 5–10 spermatozoa attached to the zona pellucida. That sperm zona receptors were intact in the salt-stored eggs was documented by the second sperm challenge, following which usually more than 100 sperm could be seen attached to the zona surface. This was true for each of the six sera studied. In two cases, although IgA antibodies were completely absorbed, IgG remained detectable on all sperm, yet sperm zona binding increased markedly. These observations suggested that either the isotype of antisperm antibody bound to the head or the total immunoglobulin bound to the sperm surface was important in determining the degree of impairment of sperm zona binding. Whether these antibodies were directed against epitopes of the zona receptor on the sperm surface, or to a neighboring epitope, inhibiting sperm zone binding through steric hindrance, could not be determined.

Further evidence that circulating antisperm antibodies present in sera of infertile men and women may impair the binding of human spermatozoa to the human zona pellucida, when directed against the sperm head, has recently been observed by Mahoney et al.[8] A hemi-zona assay was used in which bisected, salt-stored human zona pellucida was used to assess the effects of labeling sperm from known fertile men with antisperm antibodies (ASA). The power of this approach is that the variation in sperm binding between men is eliminated. Immunobead binding was used to confirm that at the semen dilution chosen that minimized sperm agglutination, nearly all sperm were labeled with immunoglobulin over their heads. Hemizonas from the same egg were inseminated with antibody-free or antibody-labeled sperm from the same donor. Of note, a wide range in effect was observed, several sera markedly lowering the number of tightly bound sperm observed after seral zona washing, while other sera were completely without effect. These results further emphasize that the functional effects of ASAs in different individuals may vary, despite their same regional localization of binding on the spermatozoan surface. These observations emphasize the need for the utilization of more specific tests that allow one to determine the antigenic moieties against which ASAs are directed.

Also of note, in no case was sperm zona binding completely inhibited, suggesting that clinical *in vitro* fertilization as a treatment of immunologically mediated infertility due to immunity to spermatozoa might succeed, even in the face of high levels of circulating antisperm antibodies (see below).

Evidence That Antisperm Antibodies Impair Sperm Penetration of Living Human Eggs

While previous investigations using zona-free hamster eggs or salt-stored zona pellucidae have indicated that ASAs may impair the ability of human sperm to attach to the zona, several reports have now documented that fertilization of viable human oocytes is also impaired.

In two independent studies, Clarke et al.[9] and DeAlmeida et al.[10] studied the relationship between antisperm antibodies in the ejaculate and *in vitro* fertilization (IVF) rates. Their results suggested that IVF was adversely affected if antisperm antibodies were present on more than 70–80% of spermatozoa.

Given the small number of couples with antisperm antibodies available for study in an individual IVF program, nonimmunologic factors may interfere with the interpretation of results. Oocytes may not fertilize due to an inherent defect in the spermatozoan, the egg, or the culture medium rather than the ASAs. To eliminate these variables, Clarke et al.[9] utilized "spare" oocytes in which excess unfertilized eggs in couples undergoing intrafallopian transfer were studied rather than cryopreserved. One oocyte was inseminated with donor sperm, preincubated in normal serum that did not contain antisperm antibodies, and another oocyte was inseminated with the same sperm donor, but labeled with ASAs. A group of six positive sera from women was tested, in 17 experiments. The overall rate of fertilization *in vitro* for ASA-labeled sperm was 41 versus 84% for ASA-free sperm.

Mechanisms That Prevent Immunities to Spermatozoa

The first line of defense against the development of a sperm-specific autoimmune response in men is the blood–testis barrier between Sertoli cells (Table 32-2). The tight

Table 32-2 Factors Limiting an Antisperm Autoimmune Response in Men

Sequestration of antigens within the seminiferous tubules by tight junctions between Sertoli cells
T suppressor preponderance of cells within the male genital tract
Immunoregulatory effect of seminal plasma
Inhibition of T and B lymphocyte proliferation by mitogens and target antigens
Block of antibody-dependent cell-mediated cytotoxicity
Inhibition of NK and T cytotoxic lymphocyte recognition of tumors and PMNs
Inhibition of macrophages and PMN phagocytosis
Inhibition of the action of complement
Blockade of the Fc portion of IgG

junctions between Sertoli cells divide the seminiferous tubules into adlumental and basal compartments, excluding the passage of lymphocytes and high-molecular-weight proteins such as immunoglobulins and complement. In addition, they form an immunologic barrier by actively phagocytosing and degrading sperm and residual products of spermatogenesis that would be a major source of antigenic stimulation if absorbed. Only approximately one-fifth of sperm produced leave the testis, the remaining four-fifth being resorbed. Additionally, Sertoli cells probably produce immunoregulatory factors, in that they secrete transferrin, which has been shown to inhibit lymphocyte blastogenesis and complement-mediated cell lysis. The barrier between the reproductive system and the immune system is less effective in the rete testis and the ductus efferentes, so that these sites are more accessible to cellular immune components, as demonstrated in mice by the ability of sperm-sensitized activated T lymphocytes, transferred to recipient males, to react with autoantigens in this region, as well as the vas deferens. Conversely, dilution of sperm antigens in the rete testis, and its poor vascularization, may limit the interchange between intraluminal and intravascular compartments.

In addition to the barrier mechanisms that limit the contact of sperm antigens with both male and female immune systems, an active semen-related immunosuppression appears to exist. Several line of evidence have been presented for the existence of immunosuppressive factors within the seminal fluid.[11] Seminal plasma inhibits the ability of T and B lymphocytes to proliferate in response to mitogen or antigen challenge, impairs antibody-dependent cell-mediated cytotoxicity, and blocks the recognition of tumor cells or virally infected cells by NK and cytotoxic T lymphocytes. In addition, it inhibits phagocytosis by macrophages and PMNs and the action of complement. Soluble receptors for IgG (Fc RIII) have detected within human seminal plasma, raising the possibility of their role in blocking antibody-mediated sperm damage through their binding to the Fc portion of the immunoglobulin molecule. Spermatozoa have also been demonstrated to be immunosuppressive, as judged by their ability to induce tolerance *in vitro* in an autologous system. Since they are able to induce the activation of complement by the alternative pathway, it is possible that spermatozoa modulate the immune response via C3a, which suppresses antibody production by B lymphocytes *in vitro.*

Evidence also exists for active cellular immunosuppressive activity within the male reproductive system and in semen. T suppressor lymphocytes have been detected in the interstitium of the testis and in the submucosal region of epididymis,[12] and the ratio between T suppressor and T helper lymphocytes in semen indicates the prevalence of suppressing activity.[13]

Vasectomy: Immunologic Consequences

Approximately 75% of men who have undergone vasectomy will develop autoimmunity to spermatozoa (Table 32-3). That return of fertility is high after vasovasostomy has been adequately documented. Cos et al. surveyed the results of 943 vasovasostomies performed by 19 urologists. The average patency rate was 82% and an overall pregnancy rate of 53% was achieved. Silber documented a pregnancy rate of 71% at 15 years following sterilization reversal. He found only a weak correlation between

Table 32-3 Conditions Associated with the Production of Antisperm Antibodies in Men

Disruptions of the blood–testis barrier
Vasectomy
Testicular trauma
Tumors
Testis biopsy
Testicular torsion
Genital tract infections
Obstruction
Cystic fibrosis
Failure of the mechanisms of immunosuppression
Decrease of T suppressor lymphocyte activity
Lack of immunosuppressive factors in the seminal plasma?
Abnormal expression of antigens on the sperm surface?
Gastrointestinal exposure to spermatozoa

the sperm concentration present in the ejaculate following vasovasostomy and the likelihood of fathering a child. Neither was there a relationship between the presence of circulating antisperm antibodies and pregnancy rates following sterilization reversal.

However, the impact of autoimmunity to sperm on male fertility subsequent to vasovasostomy remains controversial. Sullivan and Hane noted that while approximately 50% of men with serum antisperm antibodies were fertile following vasovasostomy, there was a strong association of autoimmunity to sperm and persistent infertility. Rolye et al. also observed a correlation between the time of circulating antisperm antibodies (ASA) as determined by tray agglutination test, and the chance of fathering a child.

The key question is whether men who manifest autoimmunity to sperm following sterilization reversal exhibit these antisperm antibodies in their ejaculates. Linnet et al. documented, in 1981, a pregnancy rate of 85% among vasovasostomies men with no ASA in seminal plasma versus 14% for ASA-positive men. Parslow et al. confirmed this work, in part, but also documented that higher titers of ASA needed to be present in seminal plasma to affect fertility. They also showed that men from infertile couples with spontaneous autoimmunity to sperm, in contrast to vasectomized men, had higher levels of IgA and more SC on their sperm than men following vasectomy reversal. They postulate that secretory IgA, in these men, was more likely to compromise sperm function then those antibodies detected in vasectomized men.

More recently, Menertz et al. studied 26 men following sterilization reversal using a mixed agglutination reaction.[14] They found that in a subgroup of men with a pure IgG response, the conception rate was 85%, while only 43% of men who also had IgA on their sperm fathered children. The conception rate was reduced even further when 100% of sperm were coated with IgA (21.7%). The combination of IgA on all sperm and a high serum titer (greater than 1:250), as detected by agglutination tests, was associated with a zero conception rate. The median time since vasectomy was 58 months and the median time since sterilization reversal was 44 months.

As IgA-coated spermatozoa exhibit a significant impairment in their ability to penetrate cervical mucus, the ability of such spermatozoa to populate the female reproductive tract will be impaired. This finding, as documented either by *in vitro* cervical mucus penetration testing or *in situ* at postcoital testing, should alert one to the need for the utilization of assisted reproductive techniques, such as IUI, IVF, or GIFT.

There has been debate as to whether the preoperative documentation of antisperm antibodies is of any prognostic value as regards the fertility potential of a vasectomized individual, following sterilization reversal. As the majority of vasectomized men will have ASA in their serum, this test offers no useful information. In addition, those antibodies will often not be detected in the seminal fluid, while present in serum. There is strong evidence for a major source of antisperm antibodies within the ejaculate in the epididymis. High levels of ASAs have been detected in the proximal vas deferens (the epididymal efficient), at the time of vas reanastomosis. Witkin[13] has previously documented, in rabbits, that the epididymis can be a source of IgA immunoglobulins. Unfortunately, the contribution of the epididymis to the semen in vasectomized men can become apparent only following vasovasostomy. While prostatic secretions contain IgA and IgG immunoglobulins, and secretory IgA has been detected in the secretions in men with prostatitis, there has been no evidence presented that antisperm antibodies are locally transported from serum by the prostatic epithelium. Hence, preoperative analysis of semen for antisperm antibodies, in vasectomized men, is often of limited value. Given the association of antibody coating of spermatozoa and impaired fertility in men following sterilization reversal, tests of the ejaculate for antisperm antibodies should be performed postoperatively, if pregnancy does not occur in a reasonable period of time.

Methods of Detecting Antisperm Antibodies

Until the late 1970s most laboratories attempted to diagnose immunities to spermatozoa by using one of three major forms of serologic tests: sperm agglutination, either macroscopic or microscopic, complement-dependent sperm immobilization, or indirect immunofluorescence. Although several studies documented a clear difference in the prevalence of antisperm antibodies in infertile couples as compared with fertile men and women, other studies could not make this distinction between these groups. Hence, for agglutination assays, the range of positive results varied from 2% to more than 30%, with a large overlap between fertile and infertile groups. Although complement-dependent immobilization assays had more discriminating power, in that the incidence of positive results was far lower in sera of fertile men and women, this test suffered from an inability to detect non-complement-fixing immunoglobulins, such as IgA. It is now apparent that these serologic tests are subject to a number of pitfalls, so that it was not unexpected to find a lack of discriminating power in their results.

One important recent realization has been that naturally occurring antisperm antibodies exist in the sera of many species, including man. As detected by indirect immunofluorescence, the sera of approximately 60% of men and women possess immunoglobulins that react with sperm. The naturally occurring antibodies are readily absorbed by sperm and testicular extracts, but not by other human tissues. Of importance, they do not stain the surface of viable sperm in suspension, but rather are directed against intracellular antigens. Sera possessing antiacrosomal antibodies, when absorbed with bacteria of several species, no longer react with sperm. In one study, these naturally occurring antisperm antibodies were shown to be present only at low titer (only 3 of 80 sera were positive at 1:16 or greater). Conversely, in women with unexplained infertility, 15 of 29 sera tested possessed at least one antisperm antibody at a titer of 1:16 or greater. The antibodies detected the indirect immunofluorescence with methanol fixed, permeabilized sperm are directed against antigens that are internal rather than present on the sperm surface. In contrast to their high incidence in the general population, antibodies directed against the sperm surface, as detected by agglutination tests, MAR tests, and immunobead binding, are uncommon and present in less than 10% of infertile men and women.

Several methods are now clinically available to determine whether spermatozoa themselves are coated with antibodies. These include a direct antiglobulin assay using ^{125}I-radiolabeled heterologous antibodies, mixed agglutination reaction (MAR), and immunobead binding. Although each of these tests allows one to determine, in a semiquantitative way, the extent of autoimmunity to sperm, immunobead binding in particular provides a measure of the proportion of spermatozoa in the ejaculate antibody bound by each of the three major immunoglobulin classes (IgG, IgA, IgM). The precise amount of immunoglobulin associated with an individual spermatozoan surface, however, still cannot be determined by current methods.

Detection of Humoral Antibodies

Antibodies that mediate sperm immobilization through their interaction with complement were initially described by Fjalbrant in 1965 and in Isojima in 1968. In these assays, sperm are washed and incubated with serially diluted heat-inactivated test serum or secretions. A source of complement, usually guinea pig serum, is added. A time end point for immobilization of 90% sperm or a percentage of motile sperm at a standard time is compared microscopically with sperm incubated and control sera and complement alone. Complement-dependent immobilization, while highly specific in that false positive reactions are in common, will not detect the presence of non-complement-fixing immunoglobulins, such as IgA. The amount of antibody present on the sperm surface also appears to play a role in the extent of complement-dependent immobilization. Hence, results obtained from immobilization tests have a definite relationship to immunologic infertility and are highly specific; however, not all antisperm antibodies are detected. In addition, as seminal plasma contains complement inhibitors, complement-dependent cytotoxicity tests can not be applied to detection of autoantibodies to sperm in semen.

Agglutination tests are a relatively insensitive means of detecting sperm antibodies, as a relatively large number of immunoglobulins must be present on the sperm surface to lead to the crosslinking of highly motile sperm. The two main procedures for sperm agglutination are the gelatin agglutination test of Kibrick and the microagglutination test. Failure to give careful attention to controls can often lead to misleading results, and nonspecific agglutination can occur in undiluted or only minimally diluted serum.

While a number of enzyme-linked immunosorbent assays have been developed to detect the presence of antisperm antibodies in serum, there has recently been increasing dissatisfaction with this approach. The high incidence of naturally occurring sperm-reactive antibodies in the sera of fertile men and women of all ages has posed a major problem of "immunologic background noise" for the ELISA. The method of fixing sperm is critical in determining which antigens are "presented" to the test serum sample. A marked variation in the ability of ELISA to detect sperm-reactive antibodies has been documented when sperm were fixed in different manners.[15] Although this assay lends itself technically to the rapid analysis of larger numbers of serum, and hence has been a favorite in commercial laboratories, results have not been shown to correlate well with the clinical status, in several studies.

Treatment of Immunities to Spermatozoa

Effective treatment of immunities to sperm rests on the accuracy of diagnosis. Of the newer assays that have become available in clinical laboratories in the past decade, to test for the presence of antisperm antibodies, immunobead binding has gained popularity due to its ability to probe the surface of living spermatozoa for the presence of immunoglobulins.[16] This assay uses micron-size plastic microspheres to which antibodies produced against human antibodies are chemically coupled. The antihuman antibodies on the immunobead surface bind to the human antibodies present on the sperm surface. Hence, they act as antibody detector particles, which can be visualized with an ordinary microscope. This test can be utilized to analyze sperm recovered from semen specimens, or can be used indirectly to study serum for the presence of antisperm antibodies. In the latter case, spermatozoa must be first documented free of antibodies on their surface, by a direct immunobead assay. They are then incubated in serum at various dilutions and subsequently washed free and retested, to see if they have acquired antibodies on their surface during this time. Immunobead binding allows one to determine the proportion of sperm that is coated with antibodies, the region of the sperm surface to which antibodies bind (head versus tail), and the type of antibody present (IgG, IgA, IgM).

Three approaches have been used to treat couples with antisperm antibodies: corticosteroids, intrauterine insemination, and *in vitro* fertilization or GIFT. The weight of present evidence is that the risk-to-benefit ratio of the use of corticosteroids is still not well known for either men or women. Preliminary evidence suggests that this approach is relatively ineffectual. While intrauterine insemination (IUI), when carefully timed to follicular maturation in superovulated and hormonally and sonographically monitored cycles, results in an increased chance of pregnancy, this is at best no greater than 35–40% within six treatment cycles. Currently, if IUI fails, *in vitro* fertilization, although technically intense and expensive, offers the greatest likelihood of achieving fertilization, both in the presence of autoantibodies on the sperm, in men, or circulating antisperm antibodies in women. Early evidence indicates that GIFT may also be effective in treating couples in whom the husband has developed antisperm antibodies. These results with the newer assisted reproductive techniques suggest that immunities to sperm impair the ability of spermatozoa to reach the site of fertilization within the fallopian tubes to a far greater extent than their ability to penetrate eggs, should the gametes meet in the presence of these antibodies.

The first report of the successful treatment of a man with autoimmunity to sperm with corticosteroids in the United States was published in 1976. Although subsequently, varying success has been described, most of these earlier reports suffer from their inability to document a change in antibody binding on the spermatozoa themselves. Hence, a basic premise in medical investigation was violated, that is, success of treatment was often not judged on an observed quantitative change in the status of autoimmunity, but rather on the rate of pregnancy during treatment. Given the now well-documented spontaneous pregnancy rates (15–50% over a 2-year period of observation) depending on the extent of antisperm autoantibodies, the use of pregnancy as a validation of treatment is misleading, without adequate placebo controls (Table 32-4).[17]

Studies have recently documented a variable suppression of antisperm antibodies within seminal plasma in some men treated with corticosteroids. A single study has also reported changes in the amount of antibody bound to sperm. Whether the degree of suppression of autoimmunity in these case would be sufficient to increase the number of antibody-free sperm in a semen specimen to a clinically significant level is yet unproven. Given the side effects of corticosteroids, such as mood changes, leg muscle cramps, hypertension, reactivation of ulcers, alteration of glucose tolerance, and rare but severe aseptic hip joint necrosis, one must currently remain conservative about their use, pending further well-controlled studies.

The rationale for intrauterine insemination is the placement of a large population of living sperm within the uterine cavity, which had been excluded following coitus, due to the presence of antisperm antibodies either on the surface or within cervical mucus. In theory, this should increase the likelihood that sperm enter the fallopian tube and reach the egg. Utilizing careful sonographic and hormonal monitoring of follicular maturation, insemination can be timed to within a few hours of the expected ovulation (approximately 36 hours following administration of hCG). The accuracy of timing is theoretically important in that antibody-bound spermatozoa have a shortened survival time within the female reproductive tract. Cumulative pregnancy rates have varied in different clinical series over the range of 20–40%, but occur rapidly within 4–6 cycles. They appear to be higher in gonadotropin-stimulated cycles. Thereafter, the likelihood of con-

Table 32-4 Pregnancy Outcome in 198 Couples Where Husbands Manifested Autoimmunity to Spermatozoa

	Proportion of Couples Pregnant		
Clinical Category	More than 50% Sperm Antibody Bound[a]	Less than 50% Sperm Antibody Bound[a]	Level of Significance[b]
Normal men and women	4/26	06/09	0.005
Normal men and abnormal women	6/16	13/31	NS[c]
Abnormal men and normal women	0/06	3/04	0.01
Abnormal men and women	2/07	1/09	NS
All groups	12/55	23/53	0.05

[a] As determined by immunobead binding of sperm washed free of seminal fluid.
[b] Chi-square analysis.
[c] NS, not significant.

ception following IUI falls considerably. This clinical experience suggests that either antibody-coated sperm may not always reach the fallopian tubes following IUI, despite their placement high within the uterus, or that they are unable to fertilize despite successfully meeting the egg.

If IUI fails, *in vitro* fertilization currently appears to offer the best chance of conception in couples with documented immunities to sperm. In men with autoimmunity to sperm, the diminished number of antibody-coated sperm within cervical mucus after coitus markedly lowers the chances that the gametes will meet. IVF circumvents these problems of sperm transport, ensuring the meeting of spermatozoa and egg. However, in contrast to women with antisperm antibodies, which although present within follicular fluid may be washed from the egg, in men, immunoglobulins remain bound to the sperm surface following their recovery from semen. While antibodies present on the sperm tail do not play a significant role in preventing fertilization *in vitro*, sperm head-directed antibodies have the potential to alter the spermatozoan's egg penetrating ability. Fortunately, these effects become important only when more than 75% of a sperm population used in IVF are coated with immunoglobulins. If more than one-quarter of sperm recovered in semen for IVF are free of antisperm antibodies, the likelihood that fertilization rates will not be impaired is high. Results will also depend on the sperm antigens against which the antibodies are directed. In other words, should the antibodies be directed against antigens that play no role in fertilization, the process of egg penetration by the spermatozoan may not be impaired. Unfortunately, there are no clinical tests currently available to predict this prior to an actual attempt at *in vitro* fertilization. Again, as a technique to minimize the amount of antibody binding on the sperm after ejaculation, it is good practice to produce the semen specimens directly on hospital premises, rather than transporting it from home, during which time immunoglobulins may continue to accumulate on the sperm from the seminal fluid. The technique of producing semen directly into washing buffer appears to be beneficial, both in terms of maximizing sperm recovery and minimizing the proportion of antibody-coated sperm. Finally, the number of sperm placed in culture with eggs for IVF can also be increased, in an attempt to increased the likelihood of fertilization.[18] As the percent of eggs fertilized by antibody-coated sperm may be diminished, the use of hormonal stimulus protocols leading to the formation of a greater number of mature follicles yielding fertilizable eggs would increase the likelihood that some of these eggs would be fertilized. In those instances where spermatozoa failed to attach to and penetrate the zona-pellucida, preliminary studies suggest that fertilization may be successful by partial "zona-dissection" or subzonal microinjection of sperm into the perivitelline space surrounding the egg.[19] However, the effectiveness and safety of these procedures need to be clearly documented.

Future Treatment Directions

The recent reassessment of the use of corticosteroids in the treatment of autoimmunity to sperm, in which immunoglobulin levels on the sperm surface are currently being determined, will allow one to judge the clinical usefulness of the approach. If a significant proportion of men do show a decrease in the percent of spermatozoa coated with immunoglobulins, the next step will be to establish criteria as to who might benefit from this approach. It is at present unclear whether a therapeutic response will depend on the isotype of antisperm antibodies (IgA or IgA) or the source of immunoglobulins within the male reproductive tract (epididymis versus accessory gland secretions), or perhaps the etiologic mechanisms that might account for antisperm antibody production in the first place.

As IVF remains expensive and inefficient, there is a continuing need to develop newer treatment options for the majority of men who do not respond to corticosteroid regimens. The use of more sophisticated techniques of sperm processing, in association with intrauterine insemination, are likely to become more prevalent in the near future. Direct ejaculation into wash buffers and immediate Percoll gradient centrifugation appears, in preliminary reports, to minimize the amount of antibody on spermatozoa during their recovery. Several investigators have attempted to degrade immunoglobulins on the spermatozoan surface enzymatically with preliminary success, although concern exists that concurrent damage to sperm receptors or ligands that play a role in fertilization must be avoided. Unfortunately, this very direct approach to the problem has not yielded a clinically useful treatment to date.

REFERENCES

1. McGhee JR, Mestecky J: In the defense of mucosal surfaces. Infect Dis Clin North Am 1990; 4:315–341.
2. Hellstrom WJG, Overstreet JW, Samuels SJ, Lewis EI: The relationship of circulating antisperm antibodies to sperm surface in infertile men. J Urol 1988; 140:1039–1044.
3. Clarke GW, Elliott PJ, Smaila C: Detection of sperm antibodies in semen using the immunobead test. Am J Reprod Immunol 1985; 7:118.
4. Bronson RA, Cooper GW, Rosenfeld DL: Autoimmunity to spermatozoa: effect on sperm penetration of cervical mucus as reflected by postcoital testing. Fertil Steril 1984; 41:609–614.
5. Bronson RA, Cooper GW, Rosenfeld DL, Gilbert JV, Plaut AV: The effect of an IgA_1 protease on immunoglobulins bound to the sperm surface and sperm cervical mucus penetrating ability. Fertil Steril 1987; 47:985–991.
6. Aitken RJ, Parslow JM, Hargreave JB, Hendey WF: Influence of antisperm antibodies on human sperm function. Br J Urol 1988; 62:367–373.
7. Primakoff P, Lathrop W, Bronson RA: Identification of human sperm surface glycoproteins recognized by autoantisera from immune infertile men, women and vasectomized men. Biol Reprod 1990; 42:929–xxx.
8. Mahoney MC, Blackmore PF, Bronson RA, Alexander NJ: Inhibition of human sperm-zona pellucida tight binding in the presence of antisperm antibody positive polyclonal patent sera. J Reprod Immunol 1991; 19:287–301.
9. Clarke GN, Lopata A, McBain JC, Baker HWG, Johnston WIH: Effect of sperm antibodies in males in human in vitro fertilization (IVF). Am J Reprod Immunol 1985; 8:62–66.
10. DeAlmeida M, Gazagne I, Jeulin C, Herry M, Balaisch-Allart J, Frydman R, Jouannet P, Testart J: In vitro processing of sperm with autoantibodies and in vitro fertilization results. Human Reprod 1989; 4:49–53.
11. James K, Hargreave TB: Immunosuppression by seminal plasma and its possible clinical significance. Immunol Today 1984; 5:357–xxx.
12. El-Demry M, James K: Lymphocyte subjects and macrophages in the male genital tract in health and disease. Eur J Urol 1988; 14:226–245.
13. Witkin SS: Selective activation of functional suppressor cells by human seminal fluid. Clin Exp Immunol 1988; 64:364.
14. Meinertz H, Linnet L, Fogh-Anderson P, Hjort

T: Antisperm antibodies and fertility after vasovasostomy. Fertil Steril 1990; 54:315–321.
15. Bronson RA, Cooper GW, Hjort T et al: Antisperm antibodies detected by agglutination, immobilization, microcytotoxicity and immunobead binding assays. J Reprod Immunol 1985; 8:279.
16. Bronson RA, Cooper GW, Rosenfeld DL: Sperm antibodies: Their role in infertility. Fertil Steril 1984; 42:171–183.
17. Ayvaliotis B, Bronson RA, Cooper GW, Rosenfeld DL: Conception rates in couples where auto-immunity to sperm is detected. Fertil Steril 1985; 43:739.
18. Bronson RA: Immunity in sperm and in vitro fertilization. J In Vitro Fertil Embryo Trans 1987; 4:195.
19. Cohen J, Malter H, Wright G, Kort H, Massey J, Mitchell D: Partial zona dissection of human oocytes when failure of zona-pellucida penetration is anticipated. Human Reprod 1989; 4:432.

ANNOTATED BIBLIOGRAPHY

Bronson RA: Immunology of infertility. In: Seibel MM, ed. Infertility, a comprehensive text. Norwalk, CT: Appleton and Lange, 1991:217–234.

This chapter reviews basic concepts in immunology as applied to clinical human reproduction. It discusses the structure of immunoglobulin molecules, the regulation of their secretion within the reproductive tract, the role of the complement system in mediating cell damage, and the detection of antisperm antibodies, and summarizes evidence that antibodies directed against spermatozoa alter their ability to fertilize. It possesses an extensive bibliography of 122 references.

Bronson RA: Laboratory diagnosis of male fertility. In: Soules MR, ed. Controversies in reproductive endocrinology. New York: Elsevier Science Publishers, 1989:165–182.

This chapter reviews the physiology of normal gamete interactions leading to fertilization. Laboratory methods of judging male reproductive potential are discussed, including immunologic techniques.

Landers DV, Bronson RA, Pavia CS, Stites DP: Reproductive immunology. In: Stites DP, Terr AI, eds. Basic clinical immunology, 7th ed. Norwalk, CT: Appleton and Lange, 1991:200–216.

This chapter reviews the relationship of the immune system to human reproduction in men and women. It focuses on natural immunities to spermatozoa, the etiology of autoimmunity spermatozoa, a comparison of clinical diagnostic tests, and their pitfalls and the immunologic consequences to health of vasectomy.

Index

ISBN 0-397-51153-1
90000
9 780397 511532